Inte

Contemporary Pain Medicine

Integrative Pain Medicine: The Science and Practice of Complementary and Alternative Medicine in Pain Management

Series Editor

Steven Richeimer, MD

Director, USC Pain Center, University of Southern California, Los Angeles, California, USA

Integrative Pain Medicine

The Science and Practice of Complementary and Alternative Medicine in Pain Management

Edited by

Joseph F. Audette, MA, MD

Department of Physical Medicine and Rehabilitation, Spaulding Rehabilitation Hospital, Spaulding, Massachusetts, Harvard Medical School, Boston, Massachusetts

Allison Bailey, MD

Department of Physical Medicine and Rehabilitation, Spaulding Rehabilitation Hospital, Massachusetts General Hospital, Harvard Medical School, Boston, Massachusetts

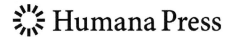

Editors
Joseph F. Audette
Harvard Medical School
Boston, MA, USA

Allison Bailey
Harvard Medical School
Boston, MA, USA

Series Editor
Steven Richeimer
USC Pain Center
University of Southern California
Los Angeles, CA, USA

ISBN: 978-1-61737-778-5   e-ISBN: 978-1-59745-344-8

Cover Illustration: The cover image is called a Sri Yantra or "great object" and belongs to a class of meditation
devices used mainly by those belonging to the Hindu tantric tradition. The central diagram consists of nine interwoven
isosceles triangles, with four pointing upwards to represent Sakti, the primordial female essence of dynamic energy,
and five pointing downwards to representing Siva, the primordial male essence of static wisdom. The image represents
the continuous process of Creative Generation, with indwelling Mahavidya Devatas in all the triangles and stupa and
lingam motifs combining Buddhist and Hindu symbolism (Nepal, c. 1700). The pattern is also a symbolic manifestation
of the Fibonacci series or phi, the golden ratio, which is a mathematical representation of repeating patterns found
throughout nature. In this way, the Sri Yantra can be viewed as a graphic representation of the integration of ancient
knowledge (CAM) and Modern Science, which is the aspiration of this book and Integrative Medicine.

Printed on acid-free paper

9 8 7 6 5 4 3 2 1

springer.com

This book is dedicated in loving memory of Grace Peterson Audette and Mary Frances McConathy.

PREFACE

The field of Pain Medicine has evolved over the last 20 years to include an increasing array of sophisticated and technologically complex diagnostic and therapeutic procedures. Concurrent to this advancement has been the development of a battery of pharmacological options to treat pain, from extended-release formulations of analgesics to antidepressants and anticonvulsants designed to treat specific types of pain syndromes. Despite (and perhaps because of) this phenomenal growth, it is not uncommon for patients with persistent pain to find themselves having gone through a number of procedures and taking a growing list of medications without ever experiencing true resolution of the condition or a return to a normal lifestyle and function. Inherent in this approach is the viewpoint that the clinician's role is to *do* something to the patient that will reduce symptoms rather than to work in concert *with* the patient to either resolve the root causes or ameliorate the functional consequences of their pain condition. Although motivated by the desire to help, this model of pain management neglects individual choice and personal responsibility.

This approach is of even greater concern in special populations such as the elderly. By the year 2030, people older than 65 years will comprise 20% of the total population in the United States. The most common explanation for disability reported by older persons is musculoskeletal pain. Whether due to arthritic or non-arthritic causes, pain is a major factor in disability in this age group even when other impairments and symptoms are taken into account. Although pain, in and of itself, is a primary concern of the elderly, it is the associated impairments that have the most devastating impact on quality of life, morbidity, and mortality. The elderly are also more likely to be on multiple medications for other chronic conditions. The addition of pain medications and invasive procedures to this growing list may have dangerous and possibly fatal outcomes.

This problem in Pain Medicine has two sides, however. Many patients who come to pain management clinics are seeking quick fixes. They may lack the motivation or interest to devote time and effort toward lifestyle changes that could have a more profound impact on the root causes of their pain. Patients may feel that they do not have the time to care for themselves or to work with the clinician in a collaborative model of care. They may want to be at the end of treatment before it has started and without having to experience a process of healing. They may want the physician to prescribe a medication or perform a procedure that will reduce or eliminate pain quickly, even when there may be little chance of success. Unfortunately, physicians are all too often ready to make such heroic attempts, sometimes at the expense of patient wellness.

As new treatments are attempted to relieve painful symptoms without improvement, patients may become increasingly passive and can develop a sense of hopelessness and despair. This is the current culture of technological medicine in which we live. Our society believes that everything can be fixed and that patients have a right to never experience pain. Advanced imaging, invasive procedures, and surgery are viewed as superior forms of diagnosis and treatment, while emphasis on self-care and optimization of the body's natural healing process is minimized. However, when technologically advanced treatments fail, clinicians may become dismissive, blaming the patient for lack of success. Given this kind of feedback, patients may find themselves without the ability to cope with the uncertainty of a journey through life with pain. Without the help of a guide, they may be unable to negotiate this difficult path that demands personal growth, lifestyle change, and acceptance. When this occurs, patients may begin to disregard the painful body part, seeing it as separate from themselves. The painful part may never be integrated back into the whole of consciousness and being, but is left to atrophy.

In this pain management quagmire, *Integrative Pain Medicine: The Science and Practice of Complementary and Alternative Medicine in Pain Management* offers an alternative that can provide a perfect counterbalance to the paternalistic, technological medicine predominant today. Jon Kabat Zin speaks to this concept in his book, *Full Catastrophe Living*, when discussing the concept of rehabilitation. The word comes from the Latin root *habilitare*, which means "to enable," but is also related to the French verb *habiter*, which means "to live in, to inhabit, to dwell." Thus to rehabilitate someone means not only to re-enable them, but also to teach them how to re-inhabit, to live or dwell in, their body again. The goal is to help patients to accept their limitations and become an integrated whole again. The ideals of integrative medicine help reintroduce a model of care that is more process oriented and whole body in nature.

This should not be taken to mean that science does not play an important role in developing novel treatments for pain. However, a scientific approach to pain management need not be based entirely on reductionism. The current trend of the science–medicine interface trains clinicians to analyze something into simpler elements or organized systems. Neck pain can be best assessed and evaluated by looking at the patient's X-ray or MRI image, while factors such as the candy bars and coffee consumed all day long, the computer work station, the stress of work and home, or the grief over the loss of a family member are just noise to be filtered out of the assessment. Instead, an enhanced scientific view can be adopted. This view recognizes that there remains much that we have yet to learn about the complexity of the human experience of pain and its treatment. For example, structures such as fascia and muscle tissue appear capable of generating pain that can be at times severe and may become chronic. Yet, within conventional medicine, the muscle and fascia are essentially invisible to standard methods of imaging. Therefore, little emphasis has been placed on understanding how this type of pain arises and ways in which to treat it. Many integrative treatments discussed in this book have mechanisms of action that appear to work at the level of the muscle or the fascial tissue.

Another important concept in this enhanced scientific view is that the body is an integrated whole. Pain in one part of the body must be the result of a complex series of whole body structural and psycho-biological changes that leads to the surfacing of this symptom in one region. To the pure reductionist this may appear unscientific. In our enhanced scientific model, however, a more thorough understanding of the interconnectedness of the various structures and regulatory systems and the ways that they may affect pain syndromes is integrated into our comprehension. Through basic science research and an appreciation of the complexity of pain and the inter-relationships between structure and function, we can develop a model of pain management that is both scientific and integrative in its approach.

This is the model presented in *Integrative Pain Medicine: The Science and Practice of Complementary and Alternative Medicine in Pain Management*. We begin with several chapters that discuss pain and its management from a mechanistic standpoint. These chapters present a scientific basis for potential mechanisms of action that can be applied to an array of integrative therapies. In the following section, specific therapeutic approaches are discussed in terms of their application to pain management. Whenever possible, authors have attempted to propose hypotheses regarding mechanisms of action for these therapies, incorporating information from the introductory basic science chapters. Finally, two integrative models of care are put forward as examples of how these principles may be applied in a pain management clinic setting. Ultimately, our hope is that this book will fulfill both scientific and philosophic purposes in the ongoing development of the field of Pain Medicine and serve as a guide to help both clinicians and patients reconnect with a model of care that takes as primary the concept of rehabilitation.

Joseph F. Audette, MA, MD
Allison Bailey, MD

CONTENTS

Contributors

JOSEPH F. AUDETTE • Department of Physical Medicine and Rehabilitation, Spaulding Rehabilitation Hospital, Spaulding, MA; and Harvard Medical School, Boston, MA

ALLISON BAILEY • Department of Physical Medicine and Rehabilitation, Harvard Medical School, Spaulding Rehabilitation Hospital, Massachusetts General Hospital, Boston, MA

BRUCE E. BECKER • Department of Rehabilitation Medicine, University of Washington School of Medicine, Seattle, WA; College of Veterinary and Comparative Anatomy, Pharmacology and Physiology, Washington State University, Pullman, WA

ALEXIOS G. CARAYANNOPOULOS • Department of Neurosurgery, Lahey Clinic, Burlington, MA

MICHAEL H. COHEN • Principal, Law Offices of Michael H. Cohen, Cambridge, MA; Assistant Professor, Department of Health policy and Management, Harvard School of Public Health, Boston, MA

RUPALI P. DHOND • Martinos Center for Biomedical Imaging, Massachusetts General Hospital, Boston, MA

TIERAONA LOW DOG • Director of Education, Program in Integrative Medicine, Department of Medicine, University of Arizona College of Medicine, Tucson, AZ

DAVID EULER • Harvard Medical School Continuing Medical Education Course, Structural Acupuncture for Physicians, Kiiko Matsumoto International, Newton, MA

SALOMAO FAINTUCH • Staff Interventional Radiologist, Harvard Medical School, Beth Israel Deaconess Medical Center, Boston, MA

LOREN FISHMAN • Department of Physical Medicine and Rehabilitation, Columbia College of Physicians and Surgeons, New York, NY

JAMES H. GRONEMEYER • Spaulding Rehabilitation Hospital, Arlington, MA

AMBER C. ISENHART • Absolute Health and Nutrition, LLC, Sierra Madre, CA

CHARISE L. IVY • Physical Medicine and Rehabilitation, Proactive Care Partners, LLC, Sierra Madre, CA

JANET R. KAHN • Integrated Healthcare Policy Consortium, Burlington, VT

NORMAN W. KETTNER • Department of Radiology, Logan College of Chiropractic, Chesterfield, MO

DOUGLAS W. KINNAIRD • Mittleman Jewish Community Center, International Council for Aquatic Therapy and Rehabilitation Industry Certifications, Portland, OR

ELVIRA V. LANG • Chief, Interventional Radiology, Harvard Medical School, Beth Israel Deaconess Medical Center, Boston, MA

HELENE M. LANGEVIN • Department of Neurology, University of Vermont, Burlington, VT

ERIC LESKOWITZ • Integrative Medicine Project, Spaulding Rehabilitation Hospital, Department of Psychiatry, Harvard Medical School, Boston, MA

ARTHUR MADORE • Muscular Therapy of Boston, Osher Clinical Center for Complementary and Integrative Medical Therapies, Boston, MA

GLORIA MARIA MARTINEZ SALAZAR • Department of Radiology, Beth Israel Deaconess Medical Center, Harvard Medical School, Boston, MA

JOSEPH MOSQUERA • University of Arizona School of Medicine; St. Michaels Medical Center, University of Medicine and Dentistry of New Jersey, Newark, NJ

VITALY NAPADOW • Martinos Center for Biomedical Imaging, Massachusetts General Hospital, Boston, MA

STEVE PARCELL • NatureMed, LLC, Boulder, CO

ELLEN SALTONSTALL • Anusara Yoga Foundation, New York, NY

JAY P. SHAH • Rehabilitation Medicine Department, National Institutes of Health, Bethesda, MD

MERYL STEIN • Director of South Jersey Sports and Spine Medicine, Voorhees, NJ; and Clinical Assistant Professor, Department of Physical Medicine and Rehabilitation, University of Pennsylvania, Philadelphia, PA

MARIA SULINDRO-MA • Anti-Aging Specialist, Physical Medicine and Rehabilitation, Sierra Madre, CA

TIM TAKKEN • Department of Pediatric Physical Therapy and Exercise Physiology, Wilhelmina Children's Hospital, University Medical Center, Utrecht, The Netherlands

DAVID WANG • Department of Physical Medicine and Rehabilitation, Harvard Medical School, Boston, MA

FRANK WILLARD • Department of Anatomy, College of Osteopathic Medicine, University of New England, Biddeford, ME

HARRIËT WITTINK • University of Applied Sciences Utrecht, The Netherlands

JOSHUA WOOTTON, • Department of Psychiatry, Harvard Medical School, Arnold Pain Management Center, Beth Israel Deaconess Medical Center, Boston, MA

I Introduction

1

Legal and Ethical Issues in Integrative Pain Management

Michael H. Cohen

CONTENTS

INTRODUCTION
LEGAL RULES
MALPRACTICE DETAIL
MANAGING LIABILITY RISKS
FEDERATION OF STATE MEDICAL BOARD GUIDELINES
ETHICAL ANALYSIS
CONCLUSION

Summary

Use of complementary and alternative medical (CAM) therapies (such as acupuncture and traditional oriental medicine, chiropractic, herbal medicine, massage therapy, and mind-body therapies such as hypnotherapy and guided imagery) may be more common in pain management as compared with other clinical specialties, because of medical recognition that pain has psychological (and perhaps even spiritual) and physical dimensions. Nonetheless, the integration of CAM therapies into pain management raises legal issues for clinicians who may be initiating delivery of CAM therapies, referring patients to CAM providers, or simply responding to patient requests concerning specific CAM modalities. This review addresses some of the key legal issues and liability risk management strategies that may be helpful in integrative pain management.

Key Words: liability, legal issues, pain management.

1. INTRODUCTION

Clinical integration of CAM therapies into pain management also raises legal issues for institutions, which must negotiate between the competing demands of their various constituencies to satisfy administrative, legal, and patient care concerns *(1–3)*. For both individual clinicians and institutions, neither the "ostrich approach" (pretending that the problem does not exist) nor unbridled advocacy can be considered viable ways to meet growing interest in applying CAM therapies to pain management. This review addresses some of the key legal issues and liability risk management strategies that may be helpful in integrative pain management.

From: *Contemporary Pain Medicine: Integrative Pain Medicine: The Science and Practice of Complementary and Alternative Medicine in Pain Management*
Edited by: J. F. Audette and A. Bailey © Humana Press, Totowa, NJ

2. LEGAL RULES

Basic principles of health law apply whether a therapy is labeled "conventional" or CAM *(4)*. The critical arenas of legal analysis are 1) licensure; 2) scope of practice; 3) malpractice liability; 4) professional discipline; 5) access to treatments; 6) third-party reimbursement; and 7) healthcare fraud. These areas are broadly described with case examples elsewhere *(4)*, although it is worth briefly summarizing some of the major legal rules that would apply whether discussing integrative pediatrics, oncology, cardiology, or any other specialty, and identifying how these rules might specifically apply to pain management.

2.1. Licensure and Credentialing

Licensure refers to the requirement in most states that health care providers maintain a current state license to practice their professional healing art. Historically, medical licensing statutes made the unlicensed practice of medicine a crime and defined the practice of medicine broadly in terms of the diagnosis and treatment of any human disease or condition *(4)*. This put non-licensed practitioners of the healing arts at risk of prosecution for unlawful medical practice. Over time, chiropractors, massage therapists, naturopathic physicians, acupuncturists, and other CAM providers attempted to gain licensure on a state-by-state basis.

Today, while a few states have enacted statutes authorizing non-licensed CAM providers to practice with certain restrictions *(5)*, in most states, licensure serves as the first hurdle to professional practice. The existence of licensure for the various CAM providers varies by state; chiropractors, for example, are licensed in every state, whereas massage therapists and acupuncturists are licensed in well over half the states, and naturopathic physicians in at least a dozen states *(6)*.

Credentialing refers to the verification of practitioner credentials to ensure competence, whether the practitioner is considered a conventional healthcare provider delivering a CAM therapy (such as a physician-acupuncturist needling a patient) or a CAM provider (such as a licensed massage therapist) *(6)*. The first step in credentialing often involves verifying that the practitioner maintains a valid, current license in the state in which he or she wishes to practice *(6)*. Licensure itself is not a guarantee of competence, although licensure suggests that the practitioner has passed examinations necessary to demonstrate the level of skill and training required by the state in order to practice the healthcare profession *(4,6)*. For example, non-physician acupuncturists seeking state licensure are required to undergo extensive training and to pass a comprehensive examination, which in many states includes a hands-on practicum component *(6)*.

As discussed below under referral liability, it is important to understand the licensure requirements for various CAM professions when a licensed practitioner refers the patient to, or co-manages the patient with, a licensed CAM provider. The referring pain management specialist should know, for example, whether the non-physician acupuncturist receiving a referral is licensed within the state, as well as what level of training and skill is required as a prerequisite to such licensure.

Additional legal complications may be present if the practitioner receiving the referral is not licensed and is practicing within a state that lacks legislation authorizing non-licensed practice of the healing arts. Just as the unlicensed practice of medicine is a crime in all states, similarly "aiding and abetting" unlicensed medical practice can also be considered criminal *(4)*. For example, aiding and abetting unlicensed medical practice could be a concern if a court found that a physician had referred the patient to a non-licensed practitioner who the state deemed was diagnosing and treating disease. These terms are broadly defined and interpreted, and their boundaries are unclear *(4)*. This is not to say that such referrals are inherently and always illegal, but rather that practitioners should flag this practice as potentially raising a legal issue and consider consulting an attorney. There may in fact be situations, for instance, where it is in the patient's best interest to have a referral to someone such as a tai chi or yoga instructor. Assuming the instructor has solid professional boundaries, exercises good judgment and common sense, watches for contraindications and adverse reactions, and refrains from making medical recommendations, or interfering with the physician's medical orders, liability concerns should not unduly deter a sensible referral.

2.2. Scope of Practice

Scope of practice refers to the legally authorized boundaries of care within the given profession *(4)*. State licensing statutes usually define a CAM provider's scope of practice; regulations promulgated by the relevant state licensing board (such as the state board of chiropractic) often supplement or interpret the relevant licensing statute; and courts interpret both statutes and administrative regulations *(4)*. For example, chiropractors can give nutritional advice in some states but not others, and typically, massage therapists are prohibited from mental health counseling *(4)*.

Scope-of-practice limitations can create liability issues in pain management, as scope of practice places limits on the modalities a practitioner can legally offer. For instance, some states authorize acupuncturists to offer herbal medicine, whereas other states prohibit such practices. Exceeding one's scope of practice can lead to charges of practicing other healing arts (for example, medicine) without a license *(4)*.

Some institutions will further limit the practice boundaries of affiliated CAM providers beyond the existing limitations of the practitioner's legally authorized scope of practice *(1,3)*. For example, the state licensing statute may authorize acupuncturists to practice herbal medicine, but the hospital hiring the acupuncturist into the pain management department may, as a matter of institutional policy, contractually prohibit the acupuncturist from employing herbal medicine. Although the relevant liability concerns are canvassed below, such decisions vary across institutions and are matters of institutional judgment, based on a combination of liability concerns (or sometimes fears), administrative issues, and local politics within the care organization *(1,3)*.

Scope-of-practice issues can frequently arise when devising schemes for credentialing practitioners within the organization. For example, consider the physical therapist, working for a pain management practice, who takes a weekend course in the Upledger method for craniosacral therapy and wishes to provide that service to in-hospital patients. The physical therapist would probably maintain that state licensure entitles the physical therapist to deliver craniosacral therapy within the institution and that the weekend course provides the requisite level of skill and training needed to offer this therapy.

The first part of the argument (that licensure authorizes the physical therapist to provide craniosacral therapy) depends on how state law defines the practice of physical therapy. As noted, definitions vary by state. For example, Oregon defines physical therapy as "the evaluation, treatment and instruction of a human being to assess, prevent, correct, alleviate and limit the signs and symptoms of physical disability, bodily malfunction and pain," and clarifies that "physical therapy does not include chiropractic" as defined in the statute *(7)*. Furthermore, the statute provides that "physical therapy" includes "(a) The performance of tests and measurements as an aid to evaluation of function and the administration, evaluation, and modification of treatment and instruction, including the use of physical measures, activities, and devices, for preventive and therapeutic purposes; and (b) The provision of consultative, educational, and other advisory services for the purpose of reducing the incidence and severity of physical disability, bodily malfunction, and pain." *(7)*

The physical therapist in this case might be able to argue that craniosacral therapy is not the practice of chiropractic (or medicine); is similar to other modalities regularly taught in the educational curriculum for physical therapists and tested on the state exam; and involves "treatment … of a human being to assess, prevent, correct, alleviate and limit … pain," which is what the Oregon licensing statute authorizes physical therapists to do. This is the kind of argument that might ultimately be tested in court, if the physical therapist becomes subject to prosecution based on a complaint to a state regulatory board for one health profession or another that the physical therapist has exceeded allowable scope-of-practice boundaries *(4)*.

But, even if the argument has merit and is likely to succeed, the institution must evaluate whether it wishes to allow practitioners with the physical therapist's licensure to provide such a service to patients based on the limited instruction in the craniosacral modality given at the weekend workshop. Again, the institution would probably take into account not only the level of medical evidence, if any, supporting or cautioning against the designated modality but also the possibility for patient injury (including undue reliance on a treatment lacking in efficacy), liability concerns related to the foregoing, and other factors including the effect on the institution's marketing and credibility *(1,3)*.

Similar issues and controversies would arise in deciding whether and how to credential physician acupuncturists who may have different or perhaps more limited training (e.g., again a weekend workshop) than the training required for state licensure of non-physician practitioners of acupuncture and traditional oriental medicine. Some institutions may address such issues by either limiting scope of practice beyond what the licensing statute requires, as suggested above, or by adding training standards as prerequisites to practitioners offering designated therapies within the institution (e.g., requiring that the physician-acupuncturist has to have completed 300 h of a continuing medical education course on clinical acupuncture theory and practice). Such requirements can also serve as liability management tools *(1,3)*.

2.3. Malpractice

Malpractice refers to negligence, which is defined as failure to use due care (or follow the standard of care) in treating a patient, and thereby injuring the patient. While medical standards of care specific to a specialty are applied in medicine, each CAM profession is judged by its own standard of care; for example, claims of chiropractic malpractice will be judged against standards of care applicable to chiropractic *(4)*. In cases where the provider's clinical care overlaps with medical care—for example, the chiropractor who takes and reads a patient's X-ray—then the medical standard may be applied *(4)*.

2.4. Professional Discipline, Third-Party Reimbursement, and Healthcare Fraud

Professional discipline refers to the power of the relevant professional board to sanction a clinician, most seriously by revoking the clinician's license. The concern over inappropriate discipline, based on medical board antipathy to inclusion of CAM therapies, has led consumer groups in many states to lobby for "health freedom" statutes, laws providing that physicians may not be disciplined solely on the basis of incorporating CAM modalities *(4)*. More recently, the Federation of State Medical Boards has issued Model Guidelines for Physician Use of Complementary and Alternative Therapies, reaffirming this same principle and urging physicians to develop a sound treatment plan justifying any inclusion of CAM therapies (see discussion below) *(8)*.

Third-party reimbursement typically involves a number of insurance policy provisions, and corresponding legal rules, designed to ensure that reimbursement is limited to "medically necessary" treatment; does not, in general, cover "experimental" treatments; and is not subject to fraud and abuse *(4)*. In general, insurers have been slow to offer CAM therapies as core benefits—largely because of insufficient evidence of safety, efficacy, and cost-effectiveness—although a number of insurers have offered policyholders discounted access to a network of CAM providers.

Healthcare fraud refers to the legal concern for preventing intentional deception of patients. Overbroad claims sometimes can lead to charges of fraud, and its related legal theory, misrepresentation *(4)*. If the clinician or institution submits a reimbursement claim for care that the clinician knew or should have known was medically unnecessary, this also might be grounds for a finding of fraud and abuse under federal law *(4)*.

3. MALPRACTICE DETAIL

Malpractice appears to cause enormous concern among clinicians and institutions considering the integration of CAM therapies into conventional medical settings *(1,3)* and is therefore worth reviewing in more detail. Few judicial opinions address malpractice and CAM therapies; the legal landscape is subject to rapid change as CAM therapies increasingly penetrate mainstream healthcare *(9)*. Yet, general principles from malpractice in conventional care still should apply *(10)*. As noted, malpractice (or negligence) generally consists of two elements: 1) providing clinical care below generally accepted professional standards and 2) thereby causing the patient injury. The plaintiff (who is suing) usually hires a medical expert to testify that the defendant physician practiced below generally accepted standards of care. There are multiple possible claims of health care malpractice, including misdiagnosis; failure to treat; failure of informed consent; fraud and misrepresentation; abandonment; vicarious liability; and breach of privacy and confidentiality *(11)*. Of these, misdiagnosis, failure to treat, failure of informed consent, and referral liability are often dominant concerns.

3.1. Misdiagnosis in Pain Management

Misdiagnosis refers to failure to diagnose a condition accurately, or at all, and constitutes malpractice when the failure occurred by virtue of providing care below generally accepted professional standards, and the patient was thereby injured *(11)*. A conventional provider who fails to employ conventional diagnostic methods where such methods could have averted unnecessary patient injury, or who substitutes CAM diagnostic methods for conventional ones and thereby causes patient injury, risks a malpractice verdict *(11)*.

Adding complementary diagnostic systems (such as those of chiropractic or acupuncture, either by referral or by using modalities within the scope of one's clinical licensure) is not itself problematic, so long as the conventional bases are not neglected *(10)*. In particular, a physician should take a conventional history and physical in their assessment of a patient to ensure patient safety and optimal treatment, including reviewing or ordering relevant diagnostic tests and consultations, as one would in the normal execution of their practice, before making a pain diagnosis and embarking on a series of CAM treatments. Similarly, it is not malpractice for a CAM provider to use modalities within his or her legally authorized scope of practice, so long as the provider refers to medical care where necessary and appropriate *(4)*. For example, it would be perilous to treat headaches as subluxations or displaced *chi* if the patient turns out to have a brain tumor. Continuing to monitor conventionally (or for the CAM provider, referring for conventional care) may be useful in reducing this liability risk *(4,10)*.

3.2. Failure to Treat in Pain Management

The law does not currently distinguish between medical malpractice in conventional care and medical malpractice in "integrative" care. Although some have questioned whether a "mixed" standard of care should apply in the latter case (i.e., taking into account that the clinician "mixed" conventional and CAM therapies) *(9)*, courts are likely to apply the same legal rule as applied to conventional care: malpractice means providing substandard care and thereby injuring the patient *(4,12)*. Thus, it is not the use of CAM therapies that is problematic in itself but, rather, inducing the patient to rely on such therapies to the exclusion of necessary medical care where such conventional care might have prevented further harm.

In general, the following framework may help the clinician (or institution) classify any given therapy (conventional or CAM) used for pain management into one of four regions *(10)* (see Figure 1):

A. The medical evidence supports both safety and efficacy.
B. The medical evidence supports safety, but evidence regarding efficacy is inconclusive.
C. The medical evidence supports efficacy, but evidence regarding safety is inconclusive.
D. The medical evidence indicates either serious risk or inefficacy.

In A, clinicians can recommend the CAM therapy, as a therapy deemed both safe and effective could be recommended regardless of whether it is classified as conventional or CAM. In A, liability is unlikely, because inclusion of the therapy is unlikely to fall below prevailing standards of care (as it is effective), and unlikely to injure the patient (as it is safe). Conversely, in D, a therapy that is either seriously risky or ineffective should be avoided and discouraged, whether the therapy is medically accepted or considered part of CAM.

Many CAM therapies will fall within either B or C, where liability is conceivable but probably unlikely, particularly in B, where the therapy presumably is safe. If, however, the patient's condition deteriorates in either case B or C, then the physician should consider implementing a conventional intervention or risk potential liability if the patient becomes injured through reliance on the CAM therapy. The best strategy

EFFICACY

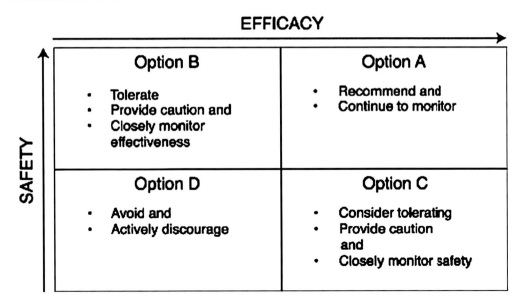

Option B • Tolerate • Provide caution and • Closely monitor effectiveness	**Option A** • Recommend and • Continue to monitor
Option D • Avoid and • Actively discourage	**Option C** • Consider tolerating • Provide caution and • Closely monitor safety

SAFETY

Fig. 1. Decision tool for balancing the safety versus efficacy of a complementary and alternative medical (CAM) treatment.

in B and C is to caution the patient and while accepting the patient's choice to try the CAM therapy, continue to monitor efficacy and safety, respectively *(10)*.

In pain management, some CAM therapies, such as mind-body techniques, have been shown safe and/or effective for conditions such as chronic pain and insomnia, and thus can be recommended *(13)*. Overall, the evidence of efficacy for many standard therapies in pain management may be poor (i.e., region C), but if such therapies are generally medically accepted as the best available, and not known to be inherently unsafe or ineffective, then liability is probably unlikely. On the contrary, inclusion of some CAM therapies can raise the specter of direct harm from the therapy or from adverse interactions with conventional care, or of indirect harm from diverting the patient from necessary conventional care. For example, some herbal products may contain "undisclosed drugs or heavy metals, interaction with the pharmacokinetic profile of concomitantly administered drugs, or association with a misidentified herbal species" *(14)*. Thus, the clinician must remain alert to the medical evidence regarding CAM therapies, and particularly herbal therapies that may contain previously unclassified hazards; the categorization of therapies over time into any given region of the framework may change according to new medical evidence *(10)*.

Again, the above framework should be applied across the board no matter whether the therapy is labeled conventional or CAM. This is consistent with the key recommendation of the 2005 Report by the IOM) at the National Academy of Sciences entitled *Complementary and Alternative Medicine*: "The committee recommends that the same principles and standards of evidence of treatment effectiveness apply to all treatments, whether currently labeled as conventional medicine or CAM" *(15)*. At the same time, recommendations involving herbal products remain problematic, because under the Dietary Supplement Health Education Act of 1994, dietary supplements—containing vitamins, minerals, amino acids, and herbs—generally are regulated as foods, not drugs. In addition to issues of contamination and adulteration, and lack of batch-to-batch consistency, clinicians have to consider the possibility of adverse herb–herb as well as herb–drug interactions. The literature on efficacy is sparse compared with comparable pharmaceutical medications, and concerns have been raised about patient use of dietary supplements during care for serious conditions.

Sales of dietary supplements as ancillary to treatment also are especially troublesome (16). So too are any arrangements whereby clinicians receive any percentage or profit from sales of supplements recommended to patients (16). Such sales can trigger legal anti-kickback considerations. Sales of dietary supplements also can suggest that the clinician has been not only negligent, but potentially reckless, a higher state of culpability, triggering the possibility of punitive as well as compensatory damages (17). In addition to legal culpability are ethical questions pertaining to conflict of interest (16). The American Medical Association has opined that physician sale of dietary supplements for profit may present an impermissible conflict of interest between good patient care and profit, and thus be ethically objectionable. Several states have enacted laws limiting or prohibiting physician sales of dietary supplements (16). Yet, another concern is potential discipline by the relevant state regulatory boards, such as the state medical board for physicians, as many of the relevant statues contain generic provisions that allow physician discipline, for example, for such acts as: "failure to maintain minimal standards applicable to the selection or administration of drugs, or failure to employ acceptable scientific methods in the selection of drugs or other modalities for treatment of disease" (18).

3.3. Informed Consent in Pain Management

The legal obligation of informed consent is to provide the patient with all the information material to a treatment decision—in other words, which would make a difference in the patient's choice to undergo or forgo a given therapeutic protocol. This obligation applies across the board, whether CAM or conventional therapies are involved (19). Materiality refers to information about risks and benefits that is reasonably significant to a patient's decision to undergo or forgo a particular therapy; about half the states judge materiality by the "reasonable patient's" notion of what is significant, whereas the other half judge materiality by the "reasonable physician." Presumably, materiality in the latter half means evidence-informed judgments concerning what therapies may be potentially useful (19).

The principle of shared decision-making takes informed consent a step further, by ensuring that there are not only disclosures by physicians to patients, but also full and fair conversations in which patients feel empowered and participatory. The Institute of Medicine (IOM) Report on Complementary and Alternative Medicine encouraged shared decision-making as a means of patient empowerment (15). Updating the patient about changes in medical evidence also is an important part of the informed consent obligation. If the discussion involves an herbal product, the physician should try to deconstruct the notion that "natural" necessarily means "safe" (19–21).

An interesting question is how the law might treat clinicians who fail to make recommendations for patients regarding nutrition, mind-body, and other readily accepted CAM therapies as adjuncts to conventional care. As medical evidence begins to show safety and efficacy for such therapies, and these therapies become more generally accepted within the medical community, there may be liability for clinicians who fail to make helpful, adjunctive recommendations involving CAM therapies (4). The case would likely depend on the court's view of whether the medical profession generally accepted the CAM therapy as safe and effective for the patient's condition, and possibly, as a safer and more effective therapeutic option than the conventional drug or treatment route otherwise prescribed *(4)*. For example, given the recent evidence from large randomized trials in the USA and Germany showing the efficacy of acupuncture for pain related to knee osteoarthritis (OA), it is interesting to consider what the legal implications would be if a pain physician offered an elderly patient with intractable knee pain from OA an oral pain medication such as morphine, rather than acupuncture, and the patient subsequently developed cognitive impairment, fell, and fractured his hip.

In short, engaging the patient in a conversation about options, and suggesting or agreeing to a trial run with a CAM therapy that may have some evidence of safety and/or efficacy in the medical literature, while continuing to monitor conventionally, is a strategy that makes sense. The IOM Report suggested:

The goal should be the provision of comprehensive medical care that is based on the best scientific evidence available regarding benefits and harm, that encourages patients to share in decision making about therapeutic options, and that promotes choices in care that can include CAM therapies, when appropriate (15).

3.4. Referral Liability in Pain Management

A major concern involves the potential liability exposure for referral to a CAM provider. While there are few judicial opinions setting precedent regarding referrals to CAM therapists, the general rule in conventional care is that there is no liability merely for referring to a specialist. It makes sense to apply this rule across the board whether referral is to a practitioner labeled conventional or CAM *(9)*.

The major exceptions to this no-liability rule involve a negligent referral (one that delays necessary care and thereby causes harm to the patient—in this case referral to a CAM provider that delays necessary conventional care); a referral to a practitioner that the referring provider knew or should have known was incompetent; and a referral involving joint treatment, in which the referring clinician and the practitioner receiving the referral actively collaborate to develop a treatment plan and to monitor and treat the patient *(9)*. For example, a pain management specialist or a neurologist who referred a patient complaining of persistent headaches to a chiropractor, but then failed to follow the patient conventionally, might be held liable for a negligent referral delaying necessary medical care, if it turned out the patient's headaches were the result of a brain tumor that should have been diagnosed conventionally. Similarly, referral to a practitioner who makes exaggerated claims and lacks even minimum standards of training and skill might be considered negligent referral to a "known incompetent." And finally, integrative pain management suggests a sufficiently high degree of coordination between the referring provider and the one receiving the referral that a court could find the joint treatment necessary for shared liability *(9,17)*. In this regard, ensuring that referred-to providers have competence and a good track record in their area of expertise may help reduce potential liability risk *(17)*.

4. MANAGING LIABILITY RISKS

As suggested, a principal strategy to help reduce liability risk involves paying attention to the therapeutic relationship, as injury to the patient and a poor physician–patient relationship can lead to litigation. Safe practice also includes monitoring for potential adverse reactions between conventional and CAM therapies, for example, monitoring for adverse herb–drug interactions. The few judicial opinions on-point suggest the importance of conventional diagnosis and monitoring when CAM therapies are recommended or allowed, as a means of ensuring that patients do not receive substandard care *(4,10)*. Continuing to monitor conventionally, and intervening conventionally when medically necessary, means that the standard of care likely will be met, and the possibility of patient injury minimized.

Thus, the physician and patient may wish to try a CAM pain management therapy for a pre-defined period of time instead of conventional care (e.g., acupuncture and hypnotherapy) and return to conventional care (e.g., pain medication) when it becomes necessary. From a liability perspective, the more acute and severe the condition, the more important it would be to monitor and treat conventionally. Another risk reduction measure is the practice of obtaining consultation and documenting this in the patient's record to help establish the standard of care in the community *(23)* and keeping clear medical records that show how treatment options were discussed and decisions made with patients. Physicians also should familiarize themselves with documentation standards suggested by the Federation of State Medical Board Guidelines, and whether these are applicable in their state or home institution.

Finally, there is a legal doctrine known as "assumption of risk" that can, in some states, provide a defense to medical malpractice where the patient has chosen a therapeutic course despite the physician's efforts to dissuade and discourage *(17)*. Assumption of risk has been allowed as a defense in at least one case involving patient election of a CAM therapy instead of conventional care (i.e., of a nutritional protocol in lieu of conventional oncology care) *(24)*. In this case (*Schneider v. Revici*), the court allowed the patient's signing of an appropriate consent form to serve as an express assumption of risk and therefore a complete defense to the claim of medical malpractice. In another case (*Charell v. Gonzales*), a New York court found that the patient had "impliedly" assumed the risk because she was aware of and voluntarily chose a CAM protocol for cancer care, even without signing the requisite form *(25)*.

Based on these cases, some attorneys might advise physicians to have the patient sign a waiver, expressly stating that the patient knowingly, voluntarily, and intelligently chose the CAM therapy or regimen—for example, energy healing and a nutritional protocol—instead of the recommended conventional treatment. Courts, however, tend to disfavor waivers of liability in medical malpractice cases, taking the perspective that medical negligence cannot be waived away, and that the physician remains responsible for the patient's treatment *(23)*. Physicians should, nonetheless, engage in clear conversations with patients concerning options involving CAM therapies, because such an approach is likely to satisfy informed consent concerns, respect an ideal of shared decision-making, and encourage positive relationships that can help mitigate the prospect of litigation.

5. FEDERATION OF STATE MEDICAL BOARD GUIDELINES

As noted, the Federation has passed model guidelines for "1) physicians who use CAM in their practices and/or 2) those who co-manage patients with licensed or otherwise state-regulated CAM providers" *(26)*. These guidelines are not binding but rather offer a framework for individual state medical boards to regulate physicians integrating CAM therapies. They should be read in conjunction with existing medical board guidelines in the state in which the physician practices, as the guidelines may provide ways for medical boards to think about integrative practices.

The guidelines "allow a wide degree of latitude in physicians' exercise of their professional judgment and do not preclude the use of any methods that are reasonably likely to benefit patients without undue risk" *(26)*. The guidelines also recognize that "patients have a right to seek any kind of care for their health problems," and that "a full and frank discussion of the risks and benefits of all medical practices is in the patient's best interest" *(26)*. In trying to assess whether an integrative care practice is violative and should trigger physician discipline, the guidelines ask whether the therapy selected is:

- Effective and safe? (having adequate scientific evidence of efficacy and/or safety or greater safety than other established treatment models for the same condition);
- Effective, but with some real or potential danger? (having evidence of efficacy, but also of adverse side effects);
- Inadequately studied, but safe? (having insufficient evidence of clinical efficacy, but reasonable evidence to suggest relative safety);
- Ineffective and dangerous? (proven to be ineffective or unsafe through controlled trials or documented evidence or as measured by a risk/benefit assessment).

The guidelines further provide other requirements, such as that medical documentation include a record as what medical options have been discussed, offered, or tried, and if so, to what effect, or a statement as to whether certain options have been refused by the patient or guardian; that proper referral has been offered for appropriate treatment; and that the risks and benefits of the use of the recommended treatment to the extent known have been appropriately discussed with the patient or guardian; that the physician has determined the extent to which the treatment could interfere with any other recommended or ongoing treatment *(26)*. The guidelines also provide that the CAM treatment should

- Have a favorable risk/benefit ratio compared with other treatments for the same condition;
- Be based on a reasonable expectation that it will result in a favorable patient outcome, including preventive practices;
- Be based on the expectation that a greater benefit will be achieved than that which can be expected with no treatment.

Again, the guidelines are suggestive but not binding in any given state, unless adopted by that state's medical board.

6. ETHICAL ANALYSIS

In general, integrative care suggests a balancing of three major ethical values: beneficence (the obligation to help the patient), non-maleficence (the obligation to "do no harm"), and autonomy (the obligation to honor a patient's freely made medical choices) *(4)*. Sometimes, CAM therapies force physicians to confront a medical paternalism that insists on doing no harm to the detriment of patient autonomy interests *(4)*. Thus, if a CAM therapeutic intervention actually succeeds in helping a patient in pain, such an intervention may satisfy the three ethical values above, even if the literature regarding the therapy's efficacy may be sparse.

As suggested earlier, the legal requirement of informed consent obligates the clinician to disclose to the patient all material treatment possibilities, including CAM therapies that have some evidentiary support, and to discuss, in a process of shared decision-making, potential risks, benefits, and unknowns. The ethical choices are more complicated than labeling the provision of certain CAM therapies unethical simply because the evidence base is not as satisfactory as may exist for some standard therapies. Moreover, the borderline between conventional and CAM therapies may be difficult to detect *(5)*. For example, allied health providers such as physical and occupational therapists may offer the patient non-opioid alternatives to pain management that are still considered to fall within the framework of a standard pain practices; they may also offer services such as Therapeutic Touch, Reiki, and other modalities generally denoted as "energy healing" *(12)*, looking for subtle cues to patient improvement even if the medical literature does not definitively conclude whether such techniques have efficacy. It can be difficult, but not impossible, for institutions to credential such practitioners and allow these therapies, and still ensure that the boundaries of professional practice are respected—e.g., limiting practitioner claims and patient expectations, honoring whatever contraindications may exist, and referring back for conventional pain management (or other monitoring and care) when necessary *(1–3,12)*.

More generally, the literature offers one way to break the ethical/unethical dichotomy by instead asking the clinician to review seven factors in assessing the ethics of whether to offer the patient CAM therapies *(22)*:

- Severity and acuteness of illness
- Curability with conventional treatment
- Invasiveness, toxicities, and side effects of conventional treatment
- Quality of evidence of safety and efficacy of the CAM treatment
- Degree of understanding of the risks and benefits of conventional and CAM treatments
- Knowing and voluntary acceptance of those risks by the patient
- Persistence of patient's intention to utilize CAM treatment

The above factors dovetail with the liability approach described earlier. Thus, if the illness is not severe or acute, and not easily curable with conventional treatment, and/or the conventional treatment is invasive and carries toxicities or side effects that are unacceptable to the patient, then, assuming the CAM therapy is not proven unsafe or ineffective, it may be ethically compelling to try the CAM approach for a limited period of time, while monitoring conventionally *(22)*. The ethical posture is even further improved if the patient understands the risks and benefits, is willing to assume the risk of trying such an approach, and insists on this route. In this case, a monitored, wait-and-see approach respects the patient's autonomy interest, while satisfying the clinician's obligation to do no harm *(22)*.

For example, the use of hypnotism in an effort to reduce the need for painkillers and anesthesia, and to reduce anxiety would, if safe and effective, be ethically compelling, assuming the clinician held a full and fair conversation with the patient about the potential benefits and risks of such an approach. In similar fashion, conversations about the possibility of acupuncture to relieve chronic pain may be warranted.

The IOM report cited this framework with approval and highlighted five ethical values to be held in balance in public policy conversations about integration of CAM therapies: a social commitment to public welfare; a commitment to protect patients and the public from hazardous health practices; a respect for patient autonomy; recognition of medical pluralism (acknowledgment of multiple valid modes of healing); and public accountability *(15)*.

7. CONCLUSION

Historically, many medical practitioners characterized CAM therapies as a whole as unproven and the matter ended there. But the medical evidence regarding safety and efficacy is in flux, and both medical research and legislative developments reflect a shifting environment for integrative pain management.

One stated ideal is to respond to patient interest in CAM therapies in a way that is "clinically responsible, ethically appropriate, and legally defensible" *(27)*. This can be done by assessing the literature and then determining whether to recommend, approve, or avoid and discourage a given CAM therapy; by asking patients, as part of the medical history, what dietary supplements and other CAM therapies they are currently using; by evaluating the extent to which such concurrent regimens may either accelerate or interfere with conventional care; by discussing risks, benefits, and unknowns; and by then advising the patient accordingly within a framework of shared decision-making.

ACKNOWLEDGMENTS

This paper was supported by grants from the Helen M. and Annetta E. Himmelfarb Foundation and the Frederick S. Upton Foundation to the Institute for Integrative and Energy Medicine. The author acknowledges the fellowship and support of Harvard colleagues Joseph F. Audette, M.D.; Roger Fisher, J.D.; Eric D. Leskowitz, M.D.; Ted J. Kaptchuk, O.M.D.; Mary Ruggie, Ph.D.; Daniel L. Shapiro, Ph.D.; and the late John E. Mack, M.D.; and dedicates this paper to them.

REFERENCES

1. Cohen MH, Ruggie M. Overcoming legal and social barriers to integrative medicine. Med Law Int 2004:6:339–393.
2. Cohen MH. Negotiating integrative medicine: a framework for provider-patient conversations. Negotiation J 2004;30:3;409–433.
3. Cohen MH, Ruggie M. Integrating complementary and alternative medical therapies in conventional medical settings: legal quandaries and potential policy models. Cinn L Rev 2004; 72(2):671–729.
4. Cohen MH. Complementary and alternative medicine: legal boundaries and regulatory perspectives. Baltimore: Johns Hopkins University Press; 1998.
5. Cohen MH. Healing at the borderland of medicine and religion: regulating potential abuse of authority by spiritual healers. J Law Relig 2004;18(2):373–426.
6. Eisenberg DM, Cohen MH, Hrbek A, Grayzel J, van Rompay MI, Cooper RA. Credentialing complementary and alternative medical providers. Ann Intern Med 2002;137:965–973.
7. Oregon Revised Statutes s. 688.010(4).
8. Federation of State Medical Boards, Model Guidelines for Physician Use of Complementary and Alternative Therapies in Medical Practice (available at www.fsmb.org, accessed 02 May 2004).
9. Studdert, DM et al. Medical malpractice implications of alternative medicine. J Am Med Assoc 1998;280(18):1620–1625.
10. Cohen MH, Eisenberg DM. Potential physician malpractice liability associated with complementary/integrative medical therapies. Ann Intern Med 2002;136:596–603.
11. Schouten, R, Cohen MH. Legal issues in integration of complementary therapies into cardiology. In: Frishman WH, Weintraub MI, Micozzi MS, editors. Complementary and Integrative Therapies for Cardiovascular Disease (Elsevier, 2004); pp. 20–55.
12. Cohen MH. Future medicine: ethical dilemmas, regulatory challenges, and therapeutic pathways to health and healing in human transformation. Ann Arbor: University of Michigan Press; 2003.
13. NIH Technology Assessment Statement. Integration of Behavioral and Relaxation Approaches into the Treatment of Chronic Pain and Insomnia. 1995. Bethesda, National Institutes of Health. NIH Pub #PB96113964.

14. Isnard Bagnis C, Deray G, Baumelou A, Le Quintrec M, Vanherweghem JL. Herbs and the kidney. Am J Kidney Dis. 2004;44(1):1–11.

15. Institute of Medicine (Board on Health Promotion and Disease Prevention), Complementary and Alternative Medicine in the United States (National Academies Press, 2005).

16. Dumoff A. Medical Board Prohibitions Against Physician Supplements Sales, Alternative/Complementary Therapies 2000;6(4):226–236.

17. Cohen MH. Beyond complementary medicine: legal and ethical perspectives on health care and human evolution. Ann Arbor: University of Michigan Press; 2000:47–58.

18. Ohio Rev. Code Ann. § 4731.22 (18).

19. Ernst EE, Cohen MH. Informed consent in complementary and alternative medicine. Arch Intern Med 2001;161:19:2288–2292.

20. Ernst E. Second thoughts about safety of St John"s wort. Lancet 1999;354:2014–2016; Fugh-Berman A. Herb-drug interactions. Lancet 2000;355:134–138.

21. Piscitelli SC, Burstein AH, Chaitt D, Alfaro RM, Falloon J. Indinavir concentrations and St John's wort. Lancet 2000;355:547–548.

22. Adams KE, Cohen MH, Jonsen AR, Eisenberg DM. Ethical considerations of complementary and alternative medical therapies in conventional medical settings. Ann Intern Med 2002;137:660–664.

23. Tunkl v. Regents of the Univ. of Calif., 383 Pacific Reporter 2d 441 (Cal. 1963).

24. Schneider v. Revici 817 Federal Reporter 2d 987 (2d Cir. 1987).

25. Charell v. Gonzales, 660 New York Supplement 2d 665, 668 (S.Ct., N.Y. County, 1997), affirmed and modified to vacate punitive damages award, 673 New York Supplement 2d 685 (App Div., 1st Dept., 1998), reargument denied, appeal denied, 1998 New York Appellate Division LEXIS 10711 (App. Div., 1st Dept., 1998), appeal denied, 706 Northeastern Reporter 2d 1211 (1998).

26. Federation of State Medical Boards, Model Guidelines for Physician Use of Complementary and Alternative Therapies in Medical Practice (available at www.fsmb.org).

27. Cohen MH. Legal issues in integrative medicine: a guide for clinicians, hospitals, and patients. National Acupuncture Foundation; 2005.
    Future legal and regulatory updates and related resources may be found on the Complementary and Alternative Medicine Law Blog (available at www.camlawblog.com).

II   FUTURE TRENDS IN CAM RESEARCH

2   Basic Mechanisms of Pain

Frank Willard

Contents

Summary

Pain itself occurs in the central nervous system (CNS), while the peripheral nervous system reports on tissue damage via a mechanical event, termed nociception, characterized by the discharge of high-threshold primary afferent fibers. Neuronal responses in these peripheral fibers drive spinal cord activity and result in signals ascending to the brainstem and thalamus through spinal cord tracts. It is from the patterned activity of these ascending signals, distributed throughout a cerebral neuromatrix, that the brain assembles a feeling of pain. This may or may not be directly associated with nociceptive events occurring in peripheral tissue. Nociception can occur in peripheral tissue and not be detected as pain by the central nervous system; this typically is due to the activation of powerful inhibitory systems in the spinal cord and brainstem. Conversely, pain can be perceived in the brain in the absence of any peripheral nociception; a situation that can be fostered by a powerful facilitating system in the brainstem. The mechanisms by which these processes occur are outlined in this chapter.

Key Words: chronic pain, central sensitization, peripheral sensitization, hormones, spinal cord

1. INTRODUCTION

1.1. Acute Pain Is a Common Occurrence in Daily Activity

Pain is characteristically thought of as something unpleasant and to be avoided whenever possible. Yet despite its disagreeable nature, there are aspects of pain that are extremely useful to us as well as necessary for our survival. Rather than think of

From: *Contemporary Pain Medicine: Integrative Pain Medicine: The Science and Practice of Complementary and Alternative Medicine in Pain Management*
Edited by: J. F. Audette and A. Bailey © Humana Press, Totowa, NJ

pain as a single system functioning to give unpleasant warnings, perhaps a better way to perceive pain is as one product of a complex, interoceptive system, recording events as they occur in the tissue of the body and informing the brainstem and cerebrum, particularly the limbic system, of conditions within our body. In fact, pain could simply be one extreme representation of an interoceptive system that is reporting regularly on the current state of our tissue *(1)*, with the central nervous system providing feedback by adjusting the output of the endocrine and autonomic nervous systems. In many ways, pain is a necessary event for the healthy survival of our tissues and ourselves. The value of pain can be seen by examining the situation where pain is not present due to a congenital absence of the small-caliber primary afferent nociceptors. Patients with this disorder are self-mutilating to an extent that leads to premature death *(2)*.

1.2. Distinction Between Pain and Nociception

Pain itself is a central nervous system (CNS) event; pain does not happen in the peripheral tissue. Instead, the peripheral nervous system reports on tissue damage via a mechanical event, termed nociception, characterized by the discharge of high-threshold primary afferent fibers. Neuronal responses in these peripheral fibers drive spinal cord activity and result in signals ascending to the brainstem and thalamus through spinal cord tracts. It is from the patterned activity of these ascending signals, distributed throughout a cerebral neuromatrix, that the brain assembles a feeling of pain. Thus all pain exists solely as a construct of the brain *(3)* and may or may not be directly associated with nociceptive events occurring in peripheral tissue. Although the activity in the interoceptive system at the spinal cord and brainstem level is often referred to as "pain" or the "pain pathways," it is technically nociception until it reaches the thalamocortical level, at which point we begin perceiving it as pain. Because nociception and pain are actually two separate events, they can be disassociated. Nociception can occur in peripheral tissue and not be detected as pain by the central nervous system; this typically is due to the activation of powerful inhibitory systems in the spinal cord and brainstem. Conversely, pain can be perceived in the brain in the absence of any peripheral nociception—a situation that can be fostered by powerful facilitating system in the brainstem. Perception of pain in the absence of peripheral generators lies at the root of numerous chronic pain states.

1.3. Two Categories of Pain

Fundamentally, pain can be divided into two major categories: that which is good for you (protective) and that which is not (maladaptive). Good pain is commonly designated as acute pain; it has also been termed *eudynia*. It is protective in nature and lessens in intensity as the tissue returns to normal. Chronically recurring or unremitting pain is not a normal experience and is an indicator that something has gone seriously wrong with the interoceptive or pain-processing system. Either tissue is very abnormal in its composition (chronic inflammation) and thus a constant nociceptive signal is being generated, or the neural pathways of the interoceptive system, which lie between the tissue and the cerebral cortex, have suffered a significant change in organization and are malfunctioning. A combination of both peripheral tissue and central system malfunction is also possible. Ultimately, this abnormal activity can result in the system over-responding to noxious or even non-noxious stimuli or, in some cases, simply generating spontaneous activity that the brain then interprets as pain. This form of pain, often called chronic pain (not necessarily the best choice of words), represents a pathological state. Chronic pain states often arise due to structural or functional changes in the nervous system, which in some cases can be permanent. This type of pain has also been termed *maldynia* or bad pain. Simply put, acute pain is an expected symptom of a problem that typically will resolve with time; chronic pain represents an unexpected disease that is a pathologic entity in and of itself and often is not being driven by a triggering stimulus any longer *(4)*. This chapter will review the normal anatomy and physiology of the interoceptive system. The focus throughout the chapter will be to elucidate the mechanisms whereby a normally functioning system can become altered pathologically such that the patient enters into a state of maldynia or chronic pain.

2. THE PERIPHERAL NERVOUS SYSTEM

2.1. Components of the Peripheral Nervous System

In this chapter, the term *peripheral nervous system* will refer to those peripheral sensory neurons that have their cell bodies in the either the dorsal root ganglia or a cranial ganglion. Specifically, it will not cover the auditory or vestibular ganglia nor will it address the sensory neurons involved in taste. In this section, the peripheral sensory system will be considered to have two major components: somatic fibers that innervate somatic tissue and visceral fibers that innervate the organs of the body. Both types of primary sensory neurons have their cell bodies located in the dorsal root ganglia. A third category includes the vascular afferent fibers that innervate the blood vessels of both the somatic tissue and the visceral organs; their cell bodies are also located in the dorsal root ganglia.

2.2. Primary Afferent Neurons Innervate Peripheral Tissue

The sensory cells of the peripheral nervous system are termed primary afferent neurons. Their cell bodies are located in a dorsal root ganglion. The central processes of these cells terminate in the spinal cord or brainstem (Figure 1). In general, these primary afferent neurons are divided into four fundamental types of fibers based on the size of their axon and the type of peripheral ending. (Table 1). The four fiber types of the peripheral nervous system can be grouped into roughly two general categories: large-caliber myelinated fibers with encapsulated endings and small-caliber unmyelinated or lightly myelinated fibers with naked nerve endings. Although this division is not perfect, it is supported by evidence that suggests the cell bodies of the two types differ in size, the development of the two groups occurs on differing timetables, and their immuno-histochemistry is differentiated *(5,6)*.

2.3. The large fiber system is mainly involved in discrimination and proprioception

The large fiber sensory system is composed of A-alpha and A-beta fibers. Of these, the A-alpha fibers are the largest and feature muscle spindle and Golgi tendon organs at their distal endings, while the A-beta fibers are slightly smaller in diameter and are typically attached to cutaneous touch corpuscles or related endings located in deeper tissues. Table 1 compares the properties of these two rapidly conducting fiber systems. Typically, members of the largest fibers are easily activated, being sensitive

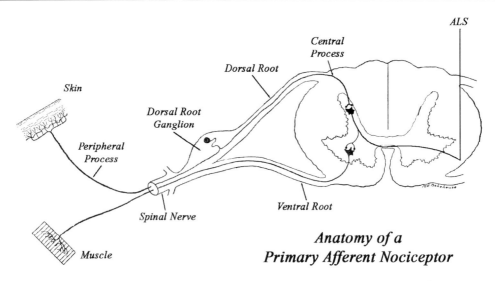

Fig. 1. Peripheral afferent fiber with its cell body located in the dorsal root ganglion (from: Ranson SW and Clark SL. 1959. The Anatomy of the Nervous System: Its Development and Function. Philadephia: W.B. Saunders Co.)

to low levels of mechanical energy, and have the fastest conduction velocities. The ascending projections of the large fiber system are mapped through the dorsal column–medial lemniscus system and spinocerebellar systems to the thalamus and somatic sensory cortex (Figure 2). This mapping is fairly precise and supports the homunculus representation on the postcentral gyrus of the cerebral cortex *(7)*. Collectively, the large-fiber system gives us the sensory modalities of vibratory sense, discriminative touch, and proprioception. Individual fibers of this system are said to be line-labeled in so much as they represent a specific modality, varying the intensity of the stimulus for this fibers does not significantly alter the modality that they represent. Thus an A-beta fiber associated with a Pacinian corpuscle, when activated, gives the individual a sense of vibration regardless of the intensity of the activation. This consistency in sensory perception contributes to the accuracy and precision of the system. An additional property, prominent in the large fiber system, is the adaptability of many of its endings to undergo adaptation to repetitive stimuli. In such fibers, repetitive stimuli initially

Table 1
Small-Caliber Fiber Types and Their Response Properties

Name	Description	Properties
CMH	C-fiber	Sensitive to mechanical and heat stimuli
C-MIA	C-fiber	Mechano-insensitive (chemoreceptors)
A-MIA	Aδ-fibers	Mechano-insensitive (chemoreceptors)
MSA	Aδ- and C-fibers	Mechanosensitive
AMH	Type I Aδ-fibers	High threshold mechanosensitive, slow response
AMH	Type II Aδ-fibers	High threshold mechanosensitive, rapid response
	Aδ-fibers	Gentle cooling
	Aδ- and C-fibers	Cold responders

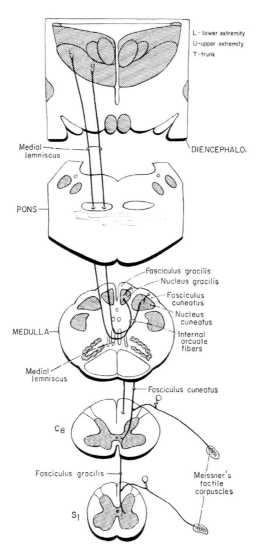

L – lower extremity
U – upper extremity
T – trunk

Medial lemniscus

DIENCEPHALO₁

PONS

Fasciculus gracilis
Nucleus gracilis
Fasciculus cuneatus
Nucleus cuneatus
Internal arcuate fibers

MEDULLA

Medial lemniscus

Fasciculus cuneatus

C₈

Fasciculus gracilis

Meissner's tactile corpuscles

S₁

Fig. 2. Dorsal column–medial lemniscal system (from Crosby EC, Humphrey T, Lauer EW. 1962. Correlative Anatomy of the Nervous System. New York: The Macmillan Company.)

activate the fiber ending, which then adapts to the stimulus by altering its shape in such a way that it becomes non-responsive to that particular stimulus. Adaptation of these fibers facilitates the detection of novel stimuli in the environment.

2.4. The Large Fiber System Is Active in Pain Control

Although the major target of A-beta fibers is the dorsal column nuclei of the brainstem, many of these fibers, as they enter the spinal cord, give collateral branches that invade the dorsal horn as well. Through an inhibitory mechanism, these collateral branches can block the transmission of information in the small fiber system and thereby prevent nociceptive information from entering the spinal cord. This mechanism has been termed the gate-control theory of pain modulation and appears to play a significant role in control of the small fiber system *(8)*. Conversely, under situations of intense peripheral stimuli involving inflammation, some members of the large fiber system have been observed to undergo a phenotypic change such that they can now activate dorsal horn neurons and produce a neuropeptide termed substance-P, a marker for the small fiber system *(9)*. This alteration in fiber function would have profound effects on the amplification of signal in the dorsal horn and the patient's perception of pain.

2.5. The Small Fiber System Is Mainly Involved in Warning Information

The small fiber sensory system is composed of A-delta and C-fibers; collectively these fibers have been referred to as primary afferent nociceptors (PANs). The A-delta fibers have a thin myelin sheath; whereas the C-fibers only have a thin wrapping derived from the Schwann cell but no myelin. A common feature of these fiber types is their termination in a naked nerve ending, also termed free nerve ending, embedded in the extracellular matrix of the surrounding tissue. In general, many of these small-caliber fibers have high thresholds of activation, requiring tissue-damaging or potentially tissue- damaging levels of energy before generating action potentials. However, there are some A-delta fibers with thresholds of activation in the same range as the large fiber systems previously described *(10)*. These low-threshold fibers will not be considered further.

2.6. The Small Fiber System Targets the Dorsal Horn

The central process of the small-caliber fibers terminates in the ipsilateral dorsal horn of the spinal cord (Figure 1) or if the fiber is in the trigeminal territory of the head, it terminates in spinal trigeminal nucleus of the medullary brainstem. Specifically these small-diameter afferent fibers reach laminae I, II, and V of the dorsal horn as well as the central portion of the gray matter around lamina X. Ascending projections from the dorsal horn cross the midline in the anterior white commissure of the spinal cord and course upward in the anterolateral tract or system to reach the brainstem and thalamus (Figure 3). Low-level activation of the small fiber systems (most likely A-delta fibers) gives us the perception of touch without much localizing capability; however, increasing the activity of this system transforms the perception from that of touch to the sensation of pain. Thus instead of being line labeled such as the large fiber system, some members of the small fiber system appear to change their specificity with the intensity of activation.

2.7. The Output of the Small-Fiber System Is Protective in Nature

In addition to the warning signals (pain sensation), the small-caliber system activates a complex response from the brainstem, termed by Hans Selye the general adaptive response *(11)*. This response involves alterations in the autonomic nervous system and the hypothalmic–pituitary–adrenal axis, which will be discussed toward the end of the chapter. An additional distinctive property of the small-caliber system is its ability to sensitize to repetitive stimuli. Unlike the large-fiber system, which tends to adapt to a stimulus, many of the components in the small-fiber system—either at the level of the peripheral neuron, spinal cord neurons, or even higher in the CNS—will increase their sensitivity to the stimulus. This enhanced activity has significant implications for the small fiber system in the pathology of chronic pain.

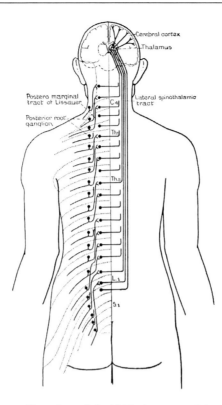

Fig. 3. The anterolateral system (from Larsell O. 1942. Anatomy of the Nervous System. New York: Appleton-Century Crofts, Inc.)

2.8. Summary

Both small- and large-fiber systems can play a role in the human perception of pain. However, typically, the small-caliber system has by far the greatest impact. In normal tissue only small fibers transmit nociceptive information and only their activity is perceived as pain. In addition, normally the large-fiber system helps to gate the activity of the small-fiber system and control the amount of nociceptive information gaining access to the spinal cord neurons. However, in injured tissue the situation changes dramatically. The large-fiber system can now become a key player involved in generating the perception of pain. Much of the remainder of this review will be focused on the anatomical organization and functional properties of the small fibers and their interaction with the large-fiber system in pathologic situations.

3. SMALL-FIBER LOCATION

PANs terminate with naked nerve endings in numerous tissues throughout the body. Specific locations of importance in pain medicine will be presented.

3.1. Skin and Fascia

PANs are present in the dermis and underlying fascia throughout the body *(12)*. Upon entering the dermis much branching of these fibers occurs before their termination. A variety of molecular receptor types are present on cutaneous afferent fibers *(13)*. The

PANs in the deep fascia are mostly associated with blood vessels, while a few in the dermis can have small terminal branches that actually penetrate the epidermis to end embedded between cells of the squamous epithelium; these are termed intraepithelial endings. PANs also reach the specializations of the integument such as the nail beds, tympanic membrane, and cornea.

3.2. Muscle

Muscle nerves can be as much as 50% small fibers in composition *(14)*. Within the muscle, PANs are seen to course in the connective tissue surrounding the vasculature. While PANs do not directly innervate myocytes, they do remain in the surrounding connective tissue termed the perimycium and are thought to play a major role in regulating the vascular dynamics of the muscle. Many of these small fibers contain neuropeptides such as substance-P and calcitonin gene-related peptide consistent with their role as sensory fibers and neurosecretory fibers. Thresholds for activation muscle PANs are usually somewhat lower than that necessary actually to damage the surrounding muscle tissue. Distribution of the PANs is complex; many of these fibers have more than one receptive field in the peripheral tissue, and often the two fields are not contiguous. Muscle PANs appear to be sensitive to inflammatory substances and to the breakdown products resulting from intense muscle activity. Finally, muscle PANs are well noted for their ability to increase activity in the spinal cord, leading to sensitization of the dorsal horn neurons *(15)*.

3.3. Tendon

The PANs found in tendons are not very well characterized at this time. Mense describes small fibers in the peritendineum and in the enthesis but not in the body of the tendon *(14)*. Alpantaki described nerve networks extending the length of the human bicep tendon and especially dense at the enthesis, but not in the tendon–muscle junction *(16)*. The small fibers in these neural networks contained several neuropeptides typically associated with sensory fibers such as PANs. Concentration of these fibers at the enthesis could be related to the notably painful presentation of enthesiitis.

3.4. Blood Vessels

Somatic and visceral blood vessels receive small-caliber sensory fibers as well as a sympathetic innervation. PANs follow the sympathetic nervous system coursing in the tunica adventitia of these blood vessels. PANs release vasodilatory neuropeptides and can act as a counter-regulatory force to the vasoconstrictive nature of the sympathetic system. This is especially interesting in light of the fact that the somatic peripheral vasculature does not receive a parasympathetic innervation; thus the PANs could be providing some, if not most, of the dilatory signals to the vasculature *(17)*.

3.5. Nerves

The connective tissue sheath surrounding nerves contains a PAN innervation *(18)*. Where studied, these fibers contain and release proinflammatory neuropeptides and have high thresholds of activation similar to nociceptors. It is possible that some of the pain arising from chronic injury of a nerve could be arising from the PANs in the connective sheath surrounding the nerve rather than from the discharge of axons contained within the nerve itself.

3.6. Joints

Joints typically receive multiple articular nerves. These nerves have been demonstrated to contain as much as 80% small-caliber (C-fiber range) axons; of these, there is approximately an even split between those of the sympathetic nervous system and PANs *(19)*. Fibers of all calibers innervate the joint capsule, ligaments, menisci, and surrounding periosteum; however, only small-caliber, peptide-containing fibers are typically seen in the synovial membranes. Increased density of innervation is a feature in abnormal, osteoarthritic joints and suggests that the PAN system is plastic and dynamic and can respond to injury by proliferating into the damaged tissue along with the blood supply *(20)*.

3.7. Viscera

The axons entering viscera are typically small in size, being in the Aδ- and C-fiber range *(21)*. Afferent fibers enter the thoracoabdomenopelvic cavity either with the vagus nerve or the splanchnic nerves. These fibers are distributed via suspensory ligaments (mesenteries and mesocolons) to the hollow viscera. Sensory innervation can be found in the suspensory ligament as well as in the muscular wall and mucosa of the organ. Solid organs, such as the liver, are primarily innervated in the region of the fibrous capsule with very little projecting into the organ parenchyma. Many fibers are mechano-*insensitive*, responding only to inflammatory compounds in the tissue. As such, they have been termed silent nociceptors to denote the lack of initial response to mechanical deformation *(22)*, for example, during surgery. Although the total number of visceral afferent fibers is marginal compared to the somatic afferent system, the visceral system makes up for this by heavy branching and ramification of the central terminals in the spinal cord and brainstem *(23)*.

3.8. Meninges

Small-caliber fibers innervate the dura and extracerebral blood vessels surrounding the brain. These small fibers are components of the trigeminovascular system. Their cell bodies are located in the trigeminal ganglion and their peripheral processes follow the cerebrovascular system until it penetrates the brain. Inflammatory irritation of these fibers plays a crucial role in migraine and other vascular head pains *(24)*.

3.9. Annulus Fibrosis

PANs penetrate approximately one-third of the way into the disc, reaching most of the annulus fibrosis but do not extend into the nucleus pulposis *(25,26)*. These fibers are derived from the sinu vertebral nerve (recurrent meningeal) posteriorly and from the prevertebral plexus (somatosympathetic nerves) anteriorly *(27)*. Many of these fibers contain neuropeptides typical of small caliber primary afferent fibers and are involved in discogenic pain. In addition, PANs are found in the anterior and posterior longitudinal ligaments and in the facet joint capsules as well as in other ligaments of the vertebral column. This network of small caliber fibers surrounding the vertebral column is involved in the axial pain syndromes *(28)*.

3.10. Summary

From the above presentation it is apparent that PANs have an almost universal distribution in the body. Only a few areas have been demonstrated to been free of

PANs; these include such regions an central nervous system, articular cartilage, the parenchyma of the liver, and lung and the nucleus pulposis. The density of small-fiber distribution is not uniform throughout the tissue of the body, being greatest in the dermis and more scattered in distribution through the visceral organs. The widespread and plentiful nature of these fibers is a testament to their importance in our health.

4. SMALL-FIBER ACTIVATION

4.1. Small Fibers Respond to Mechanical, Heat, and Chemical Irritation

PANs have several different forms of membrane bound receptor mechanisms and a variety of events can activate these fibers (Table 2). However, not all PANs have the same constellation of receptors. Mechanical distortion of tissue can open ion channels of some PANs and initiate depolarization of the fiber. Thermal stimuli also open ion channels on some PAN fiber membranes. These heat-sensitive channels have been identified and are known as vanilloid receptors (V1) or, as more recently termed, transient receptor potential channels (TRPV1). Perhaps more important for the types of chronic pain seen in the musculoskeletal system are the chemoreceptive fibers. Substances released in the environment of the chemoreceptive PANs during tissue injury or inflammation activate receptors located on the exposed membrane (Figure 4). Many different substances (called alodynogens) can activate or sensitize PANs, either directly through their receptors or indirectly by stimulating the production of other compounds that in turn can activate their receptors; thus chemoreceptive PANs are responsive to a wide range of modifications in the chemical milieu of the surrounding tissue *(29)*. Receptors are of three general types: ion-channels, G-protein-coupled receptors, and cytokine-type receptors (Table 2). This section will focus on the growing list of alodynogens that have been demonstrated to interact with PAN receptors (Table 3).

4.2. Bradykinin

Bradykinin is a plasma protein produced in the liver. It circulates in a blocked state termed kininogen. Unblocking kininogen by the action of the enzyme kallikrein produces bradykinin. Kallikrein exits normally in a blocked state called prekallikrein, which is converted to kallilrein by the Hagman factor (clotting factor XII) in association

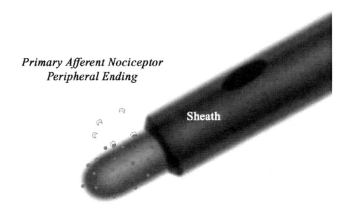

Fig. 4. Primary afferent nociceptor ending.

Table 2
PAN Receptors and Their Activating Substances

Pan receptor classes	Activating substances	Examples	Function
Ion-channels	Heat, mechanical force	Transient receptor potential channels (vanilloid receptors); Proton-gated channels; Sodium channels; Potassium channels; Calcium channels; Serotonin (5-HT3) channel	$Na+$, $Ca++$ influx
G-proteins	Bradykinin, prostaglandin, endocannabinoids	BK-1, BK-2, DP, EP, FP, IP, TP,	Second messenger cascades
Cytokine receptors	Growth factors, cytokines	TrkA, Trk-B, Trk-C, NT-4/5, NT-3, IL-1RI, sIL-6R, TNFR1	Modify surrounding ion channel activity

with tissue injury. Paradoxically, kininogen itself acts as a cofactor or activator for Hagman factor, creating a feedforward system. Finally, kallikrein is also a potent activator of Hagman factor further, contributing to the feedforward nature of this cascade. Once produced, bradykinin can be inactivated by circulating kininases and by angiotensin converting enzyme in the lung. PANs have bradykinin receptors on their exposed membrane and bradykinin is a potent stimulant for these fibers. The bradykinin receptor is a G-protein system and can modify the activity of surrounding ion channels. Two types of bradykinin receptors have been documented, BK1 and BK2. The later is constitutively expressed on PANs, while the BK1 receptor is only seen on PANs following inflammatory tissue injury. The BK1 receptor is thought to play a major role in the exacerbation of the inflammatory response *(30)*.

4.3. Histamine

Mast cells are found through out connective tissue (fascia). These cells produce histamine and contain histamine-loaded granules. Histamine is released when the mast cell is stressed or when release is triggered immunologically. In addition, neuropeptides

Table 3
List of Alodynogens and their Receptors

Alodynogen	Receptor	Origin
Bradykinin	BK1 and BK2	Plasma protein from liver
Histamine	H1	Mast cells
Serotonin		Platelets
Prostaglandins	DP, EP, FP, IP and TP	Vascular endothelial cells
ATP	Purine	Local cell rupture
H+	Vanilloid receptor (VR1)	Local cell rupture and stasis

released from PAN terminals can degranulate mast cells resulting in histamine release. Histamine receptors on PANs have also been termed pruriceptors and as such are responsible for the sensation of itch *(31,32)*.

4.4. Tryptase and Trypsin

Along with histamine, mast cells also release tryptases and trypsin from their secretory granules. PANs have receptors for proteases termed protease-activated receptors (PARs). Activation of PAR-3 triggers a G-protein system of intracellular messengers. Ultimately, this mechanism can increase sensitization of the PAN contributing to hyperalgesia *(33)*.

4.5. Prostaglandins

Any form of cellular injury leads to the release of arachidonic acid (AA) from the plasma membranes by the enzyme phospholipase A2. Decomposition of AA by cyclooxygenase (COX) enzymes yields members of the prostaglandin family and the lipoxygenase family. Receptors for prostaglandins typically do not open ion channels to depolarize the afferent terminal; instead, they interact with G-protein systems to sensitize the fiber and make it more responsive to other alodynagins *(34)*. Lipoxygenase end-products have structural similarities to capsaicin, a hydrophobic molecule that is a potent stimulant of PANs. Capsaicin works through the vanilloid receptors, members of a large group of ion channels termed the transient receptor potential family (TRPV1). Like capsaicin, lipoxygenase end products of AA metabolism also activate the vanilloid receptors but only weakly *(13)*.

4.6. Serotonin

Injury to tissue is usually accompanied by vasodilatation and platelet extravasation. Platelets, as well as mast cells, produce and release serotonin; thus levels of this neuromodulatory agent can be elevated at an injury site. Since various types of serotonin receptors are found on the terminal portions of PANs, serotonin can have multiple and differing effects depending on where in the body it is released. In the extracerebral vasculature, $5\text{-HT}_{1B/D}$ receptors act to stabilize trigeminovascular PANs and block the release of neuropeptides thus aborting neurogenic inflammatory events. However, somatic PANs express 5-HT_{1A}, 5-HT_3, and 5-HT_{2A} receptors; these receptors are known to be involved in the production of peripheral mechanical and thermal hyperalgesia, respectively *(35,36)*. Most 5-HT receptors on somatic PANs appear to act through G-protein-coupled mechanisms, causing sensitization of the fiber terminal; however, the 5-HT_3 receptor is known to increase neuronal activity by act directly through an ion channel *(37)*.

4.7. Adenosine Triphosphate and Adenosine

When cells are injured, ATP is released into the extracellular fluids and acts on purine receptors to influence PANs. Most PANs respond to the presence of ATP in the surrounding extracellular fluid *(38)*. Two types of purine receptors have been described on PAN membranes: ion channel (P2X) and G-protein-coupled (P2Y). Activation of the P2X ion channel receptors is directly excitatory, while the P2Y G-protein-coupled receptors appear to modulate PAN sensitivity. In this way, the purine receptors would represent an excellent method for detecting injury serious enough to evoke cell destruction.

4.8. Protons

Injury, inflammation, and swelling can create areas of stasis in tissue. Indeed, in some ischemic conditions, tissue pH can drop to 5.0. Under these circumstances, the extracellular environment becomes acidic: that is, its proton concentration $[H^+]$ increases. Excess proton concentration in the areas of stasis can activate and sensitize TRPV1 channels as well as activate special acid sensing ion channels (ASIC). The ASICs are proton-gated ion channels that allow cations, such as Ca^{+2} and Na^+, to flux into the cell. Proinflammatory compounds, such as nerve growth factor, serotonin, or bradykinin, can increase the sensitivity of PANs to protons by increasing the number of ASIC channels expressed on the PAN membrane *(38)*. NSAIDs act on ASIC channels to inhibit their activity and diminish the sensation of pain during inflammation.

4.9. Norepinephrine

The interaction of norepinephrine with the interoceptive sensory system of PANs is exceedingly complex. In non-injured tissue, norepinephrine is not effective in activating or sensitizing PANs; nor are catecholamines effective in activating PANs in acutely inflamed tissue. However, in conditions of chronic inflammation or nerve injury, PANs increase the expression of alpha$_2$ receptors *(10,39–43)*. In an area of an ongoing inflammation, the PAN response to norepinephine application is enhanced by the presence of bradykinin, suggesting that PAN sensitization could be made worse by the interaction of inflammatory agents *(44)*. In nerve injury, PANs increased the expression of alpha-2-adrenergic receptors, thus increasing their sensitivity to circulating norepinephrine *(45)* as well as norepinephrine released from postganglionic sympathetic efferent fibers *(46)*. Sensitization could also occur through indirect action of norepinephrine on the production of prostaglandins from postganglionic sympathetic neurons. Sensitization of PANs to norepinephrine could explain at least some of the patients with complex regional pain syndrome *(47)*. Finally, it has been noted that activation of alpha 2B-adrenergic receptors can produce hyperalgesia in a PAN, while activation of the alpha 2C-adrenergic receptor has anti-nociceptive properties *(48)*. Thus norepinephrine has a complex interaction with PANs that could lead to either increased on decreased pain, depending on the adrenergic receptor type expressed on the fiber ending and the clinical setting.

4.10. Excitatory Amino Acids

Excitatory amino acids, such as glutamate, are found in the peripheral tissues. These amino acids are secreted by macrophages and epithelial, dendritic, and Schwann cells *(10)*. It has also been suggested that neuronal endings in joints could potentially release glutamate *(49)*. Receptors for glutamate have been detected on PAN peripheral membranes and are found to be manufactured in the dorsal root ganglion cell bodies of PANs and then transported to the periphery *(50)*. Centrally, presynaptic *N*-methyl-D-aspartate (NMDA)-linked glutamate receptors have been reported to be present on the PAN central terminals and activation of these receptors increases the secretion of neuropeptide (substance-P) from the terminal *(51)*. Glutamate (non-NMDA) channels have also been detected on the peripheral terminals of PANs. The presence of glutamate receptors on the peripheral terminal of the PANs could allow these fibers to detect glutamate spilled from damaged or dying cells in areas of tissue injury *(37)*.

4.11. Proinflammatory Cytokines

During tissue injury, proinflammatory cytokines are released by a variety of cell types, including macrophages, fibroblasts, and synoviocytes amongst others. Members of the cytokine receptor family are present on PAN membranes *(52)*. Typically cytokine receptors are not ion channels themselves, but their activation modifies the excitability of surrounding ion channels such as the TRPV1 channel. Indirectly, proinflammatory cytokines can also modify PAN excitability by imitating the action of prostaglandins. Through these routes, proinflammatory cytokines can influence the sensitization of PANs and increase the hyperalgesia experienced by the patient.

4.12. Growth Factors

Nerve growth factor (NGF) is necessary for the development and differentiation of classes of small-caliber primary afferent neurons, especially those that contain the neuropeptides substance-P (SP) and calcitonin gene-related peptide (CGRP) *(53)*. NGF not only plays a significant role in the development of the peripheral nervous system, it also has a function in the mature fibers, especially in the induction of hyperalgesia in inflamed tissue *(54)*. When injected in sufficient dosage into human skin, NGF is an algogen, producing mild to moderate myalgias akin to post-exercise soreness in axial muscles *(55)*; it can also regulate the chemosensitivity of the PAN by increasing the expression of receptors on their membrane, causing sensitization of PANs with prolonged exposure. Since NGF can induce mast cells to degranulate, the increased PAN sensitivity could, in part, be orchestrated though activation of surrounding cells such as mast cells or neutrophils. NGF is increased in areas of inflammation by the presence of cytokines and free radicals. Thus NGF acts through a variety of mechanisms—both direct and indirect—to activate and sensitize PANs. Blocking the activity of NGF can prevent the induction of inflammation and significantly reduce ongoing inflammation in experimental situations *(56)*. Thus it is clear that growth factors such as NGF play a significant role in the sensitization of PANs.

4.13. Neuropeptides

Since the early part of the 20th century it has been thought that PANs might secrete a proinflammatory substance. It is now known that numerous neuropeptides are produced by dorsal root ganglion neurons and secreted by a vesicle-release process from the peripheral terminal of the cell following repeated depolarization *(57–59)*. The two best-understood of these neuropeptides are substance-P (SP), calcitonin gene-related peptide (CGRP), and somatostatin. SP is a member of the tachykinin family and is present in some PANs found in dermis but is far more plentiful in PANs of the skeletal muscle and viscera. SP has a proinflammatory effect when it is released into surrounding tissue. Specific actions of SP are many and varied *(29)*, including such things as degranulating mast cells, vasodilation, and fluid extravasation from blood vessels. SP can stimulate the proliferation of synoviocytes in joints along with the release of prostaglandin E2 and collagenases from these cells and from endothelial cells in blood vessel walls. Also, SP is chemoattractant to immune cells and stimulates their secretion of proinflammatory cytokines. If SP release occurs in the setting of an ongoing inflammation, it will exacerbate the situation; however, if it is released into non-inflamed tissue, it will generate an inflammation de novo, this later condition is termed *neurogenic inflammation* and could be the pathophysiological basis for some forms of mirror pain, for example, that seen in rheumatoid arthrtitis, as well as complex regional pain syndrome.

5. SUMMARY

5.1. PANs Are Activated by the Chemical Soup That Is Released Upon Tissue Injury

Inflammation releases a cascade of chemicals, many of them capable of helping cleanse the tissue and stimulating wound repair in short-term exposure. PANs have receptors for many of these chemicals and can record their release into the tissue by depolarization and action potential formation. Peripheral release of neuropeptide alodynogens from PANs can initiate or exacerbate an inflammatory response (Figure 5). Some of these same substances are also used as neurotransmitters or neuromodulators, released from the central process of the PAN in the dorsal horn (Figure 5). PAN activation serves as a warning and initiates spinal cord and brainstem level reflexes to protect the injured area. In addition, exposure to some of these compounds activates G-protein-signaling cascades capable of sensitizing the PAN.

5.2. PANs Contribute to a Feed-Forward Allostatic Process Involved in Tissue Repair

When activated, PANS secrete potent, proinflammatory neuropeptides that enhance the release of histamine, prostaglandins, and cytokines. A feed-forward loop is established, with the PANS releasing substances that ultimately provoke additional activity from the fiber. Importantly, this feedback loop has no established end-point or set-point.

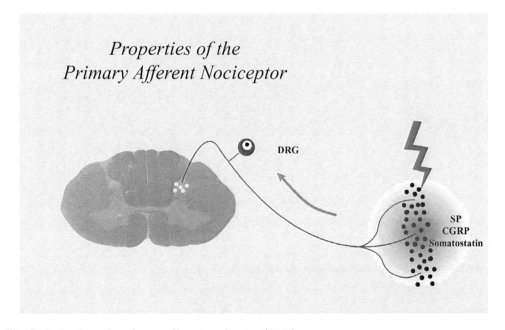

Fig. 5. Activation of a primary afferent nociceptor (PAN).

These types of reactions, rapidly fulminating with no established end-point, epitomize a process characterized by the term *allostasis (60)*. In allostatic processes, rapid change in the tissue chemistry is protective and contributes to the long-term survival of the individual. This is contrary to homeostasis, in which inhibitory feedback control establishes boundary parameters that oscillate around a defined set-point. Allostatic processes lack immediate boundaries or set-points; thus this inflammatory process can potentially get out of control and become a chronic issue. Eventually the increasing systemic levels of norepinephrine and glucocorticoids, due to long-loop inhibitory feedback systems, will aid in controlling the inflammatory response. Acute exposure to allostatic process such as this one can be very protective, creating an area of increased sensitivity to pain and hyperalgesia, and initiating protective reflexes.

6. CLINICAL CONSIDERATIONS

6.1. Sensitization of PANs

With repeated or tonic activation, PANs can lower their threshold and become easily excited, a processes termed peripheral sensitization. The process of sensitization has been demonstrated to involve a number of mechanisms: (1) the addition of new and different receptors on the cell membrane, (2) the overexpression of existing receptors, or (3) the modification of existing receptors on the PAN membrane. Sensitization of PANs accounts in part for the development of primary hyperalgesia at the site of injury. Desensitization of PANs is a natural process as well and normally will occur as the surrounding inflammatory condition subsides.

6.2. Peripheral Nerve Injury

Acute damage to a peripheral nerve fiber is usually relatively painless and when done experimentally, rarely produces more than a few seconds of rapid firing. Acute damage to the dorsal root ganglion can produce long periods of excitation and rapid firing lasting 5 to 25 minutes. Acute compression of a chronically injured, inflamed nerve represents a different situation and will produce several minutes of repetitive firing; it has been suggested that this long-duration rapid firing is the basis for radicular pain *(61)*. Injury to a nerve can facilitate sprouting from the peripheral terminal of fibers within the nerve; this can be accompanied by the invasion of sympathetic axons into the dorsal root ganglion with inappropriate synapse formation and abnormal sprouting of axon terminals in the dorsal horn *(62–64)*. All of these scenarios can contribute to the development of an intense chronic pain condition, termed *neuropathic pain*.

7. THE SPINAL CORD AND PAIN

When PANs become active, they transmit a signal to the dorsal horn of the spinal cord via their central process (Figure 5). Various cells, including both neurons and glia in the dorsal horn, are influenced by this sensory information. Interestingly, the response of the dorsal horn cells can outlast the activity of the PAN. The sustainability of this activity pattern in the dorsal horn represents central sensitization and is believed to be a major component of numerous pain syndromes. The interaction in the spinal cord of the central process of PANs from various regions in the body can create altered pain patterns and a state of chronic pain.

7.1. Central Process of the PANs

7.1.1. PANs Terminate in the Dorsal Horn of the Spinal Cord

The central process of the PANs enters the spinal cord by coursing in the lateral aspect of the dorsal root entry zone, entering the dorsal most aspect of the dorsal horn and extending inward to terminate generally in laminae I, II, and V of the dorsal horn. Conversely low-threshold, mechanoreceptive fibers tend to terminate deep in laminae III through VI. The organization of the PANs in the dorsal horn is orderly, forming a somatotopic body map extending roughly from medial to lateral across the dorsal horn *(65)*.

It is worth noting that not all PANs are the same in terms of anatomy and neurochemistry. Beyond the size difference seen between Aδ-fibers and C-fibers, the C-fibers divide into two groups: those that contain neuropeptides such as calcitonin gene-related peptide or substance-P and those that do not contain neuropeptides *(66,67)*. The neuropeptide-containing fibers seem to terminate principally in laminae I, while the non-peptide containing fibers terminate in laminae II. This dichotomy of fiber types and distributions suggests that differing aspects of nociception could be carried by specialized PANs; specifically, the peptidergic PANs terminating in lamina I are thought to be involved in localization, and the non-peptidergic fibers in lamina II are more associated with the affective nature of the pain *(68)*.

7.1.2. Dorsal Horn Neurons Receive the PAN Central Synapses

The three anatomical types of dorsal horn neurons are projection cells, interneurons, and propriospinal cells. Projection cells, the best studied of the three types, send their axons upstream in the ascending tracts to reach brainstem and thalamus. Local circuit interneurons confine their projections to the segment that their cell body is located within, while propriospinal cells represent a combination of the first two types; their axons ramify in the spinal cord, interconnecting the various segments, but do not extend out of the spinal cord. Several different forms of projection cells exist in the spinal cord *(69)*; each form of these cells receives synaptic endings from the PANs. Projection cells in the superficial layer of the dorsal horn are relatively specific to PAN input and have been termed *nociceptors-specific* cells. Projection cells located deep in the dorsal horn typically respond to a wide range of inputs, including Aβ–, Aδ–, and C-fibers, and have therefore been termed *wide-dynamic-range* (WDR) neurons *(70)*. Gentle mechanical stimulation can activate a WDR neuron; however, maximal response from these cells can only be obtained from noxious stimuli *(71)*. Although still a controversial area, evidence does support the concept that our affective perception of pain is related to the activity of the WDR neuron, while our perception of the pain location is due to the activity of the nociceptor-specific cells *(72)*.

7.2. Examination of a PAN Central Synapse

7.2.1. Central PAN Synaptic Terminals Contain at Least Two Types of Neurotransmitters

The central process of the neuropeptide-containing PANs forms terminals on dorsal horn neuronal processes. A closer look at the neurochemistry of these PAN synapses will help in understanding the central sensitization of dorsal horn neurons. Neuropeptide-containing PAN synaptic terminals produce excitatory amino acids, such as glutamate or aspartate, and neuropeptide neurotransmitters, such as substance-P or calcitonin gene-related peptide *(73)*. These transmitters are co-released from the terminal; however, while the amino acid is released during any sufficient depolarization of the ending, neuropeptide release requires more prolonged summation of depolarization such as would occur during tonic discharges *(74)*.

7.2.2. EXCITATORY AMINO ACID

The most common excitatory amino acid (EAA) in the PAN central terminal is glutamate. Release of glutamate activates the alpha-amino-3-hydroxy-5-methyl-4-isoxazolepropionic acid (AMPA) receptors on the postsynaptic surface. AMPA receptors are ion channels that allow sodium to enter the cell when open, as such these channels can cause a rapid depolarization of the postsynaptic process when activated. This type of transmission is relatively quick, involving milliseconds at most, and has thus been termed fast transmission. Most neurons in the dorsal horn express AMPA receptors on their membranes.

7.2.3. NEUROPEPTIDE

A specific population of PAN central terminals also contain neuropeptides. Upon release, these peptides diffuse onto receptors located on the postsynaptic membrane, but not necessarily in the synaptic cleft. Tonic or repeated activation of the PAN is required to cause enough peptide release to activate the peptide receptors. Thus the time required to obtain adequate volume of peptide release and the longer diffusion route to a more distant receptor complex combine to increase the time required for a response *(74)*. When activated by attachment to the peptide, the peptide-receptor complex internalizes into the postsynaptic neuron through a process of endocytosis *(75)*. Thus the peptide is acting on the postsynaptic neuron in a way that is similar to some hormones in that it physically enters the postsynaptic cell to effect changes at the cytosolic and nuclear levels. Once across the cell membrane, the peptide-receptor complex can act as an enzyme and initiate second-messenger cascades leading to the phosphorylation of the AMPA receptor as well as surrounding NMDA receptors. Phosphorylation of EAA receptors facilitates the activity of the dorsal horn neuron. This type of transmission requires seconds to minutes and has thus been termed slow transmission. The result of this cascade of events is a potentiation of the responsiveness of dorsal horn cells that contributes to *central sensitization* that is the response properties of these dorsal horn neurons undergo a leftward shift on the stimulus-response curve. Interestingly, excessive activation of the PANs can lead to the spread of neurons expressing receptors for SP in the dorsal horn *(76)*; this change would also facilitate the response of the dorsal horn neurons to afferent stimuli.

7.3. Behavior of Nociceptive Neurons in the Dorsal Horn

7.3.1. TRANSIENT CHANGE IN DORSAL HORN CIRCUITRY—ACTIVITY-DEPENDENT PLASTICITY

An outstanding feature of the spinal cord dorsal horn is its ability to demonstrate a plasticity that is directly related to the activity to which it is exposed *(76)*. Afferent activity involving PANs can result in sensitization of the dorsal horn circuitry. These rapid changes in sensitivity represent a form of allostasis, similar to that already described in the periphery, and can be very protective in the short term. Numerous cellular mechanisms contribute to the plasticity of the dorsal horn system *(77)*. Initially, dorsal horn cells show a progressive increase in activity to a train of constant stimuli, an event termed *wind-up*, which will cease when the stimulus ceases. Prolonged exposure to the stimulus leads to the development of a classic form of *central sensitization*, where the heightened central neural response outlasts the end of the peripheral stimulus by tens of minutes. High-frequency PAN stimulation of dorsal horn neurons can result in a much longer lasting response termed *long-term potentiation*; in fact the duration of the response exceeds that of most experimental studies. Other events contributing to the sensitization of the dorsal horn neuron include the activation of protein kinase enzymes. Within the postsynaptic neurons, protein kinase activation with subsequent phosphorylation events can lead to the induction of numerous genes; this form of sensitization is referred to as transcription-dependent and can be very long lasting in nature. While the large projection neurons are undergoing an excitatory form of sensitization, their surrounding inhibitory neurons can also be changing their activity. Long-term depression can occur in inhibitory interneurons located in the dorsal horn, resulting in reduced inhibition on the projection neurons and thus, more information traveling upstream to the brainstem, thalamus, and cerebral cortex. Finally, two additional events can lead to a permanent form of sensitization: inhibitory cell loss *(78)* and rearrangement of synaptic connections *(76,79)*.

7.3.2. CENTRAL SENSITIZATION AND SECONDARY HYPERALGESIA

Sensitization of dorsal horn neurons can alter their response properties, typically shifting the response versus stimulus intensity curve to the left. An additional prominent feature of sensitization is the expansion of the neuron's receptive field. Expansion of the cell's receptive field outside of the area of immediate injury will contribute to the formation of secondary hyperalgesia *(80–84)*. That is, non-injured tissue contiguous with the primary site of injury will develop increased sensitivity to stimuli. In addition to field expansion, some dorsal horn neurons, particularly those driven by skeletal muscle afferent fibers, can develop new and, in some cases, non-contiguous receptive fields. Irritation of the non-contiguous receptor fields results in the sensation of pain in the area of primary and secondary hyperalgesia *(14,85)*. While the expansion of the receptive field contributes to the phenomena of secondary hyperalgesia, the development of new, non-contiguous receptive fields could contribute to the expression of either tender points or trigger points.

7.3.3. CENTRAL SENSITIZATION AND GLIAL CELL ACTIVATION

The classic notion is that a neuronal synaptic chain extends from periphery to cerebral cortex representing the pathways for processing nociception and generating the sensation of pain. However, recent evidence has forced a revisal of this concept to include other cells, such as glia, that can modify the information processing in the neuronal chain *(86)*. Glial cells form a matrix surrounding all dorsal horn neurons. Multiple types of glia are present but the ones most associated with immune responses are the astrocytes and microglia. In the dorsal horn (and to date only in this region), these two glial cell types express receptors for substance-P *(87)*. Interaction with SP can activate these two forms of glia. Activated glial cells release proinflammatory cytokines such as tumor necrosis factor-α and interleukins 1 and 6. Although it is not clear at this time how proinflammatory cytokines work in the dorsal horn, it is certain that they contribute to increasing spinal facilitation and hyperalgesia. Activated glia also increase the production of NO and PGE_2 in the dorsal horn; both substances are known to increase spinal facilitation and the resulting hyperalgesia; interesting, these glial cells also increase the release of SP from the central terminals of the PANs, thus creating another feed-forward loop in the interoceptive system pathways. Neurons in the dorsal horn have been demonstrated to express receptors for proinflammatory cytokines and IL-1 is known to increase the influx of calcium ions through the NMDA receptor, also increasing spinal facilitation. Thus multiple factors occurring within the dorsal horn are combining to create plastic changes in the dorsal horn neurons.

Finally, glial cell–neuron interaction can explain the formation of mirror-image pain, that is, pain that occurs contralateral to injured tissue *(88)*. Spinal cord glial cells are interconnected with each other by gap junctions, thereby constructing a large and complex syncytical matrix that extends across the midline in the spinal cord. Blocking the spread of information through these glial gap junctions prevents the development of mirror-image pain in experimental models. From all of this it is clear that glia cell activity in the dorsal horn can modify the processing of nociceptive information and increase the sensation of pain. While protective in the short-term, this response has the potential to fulminate and become part of a chronic problem.

7.3.4. Permanent Change in the Dorsal Horn Circuitry

All of the changes in dorsal horn circuitry discussed so far appear to be reversible; however, excessive PAN stimulation or peripheral nerve injury can also result in a permanent alteration in the dorsal horn. The smallest neurons in the dorsal horn, typically GABAergic neurons, appear to undergo an apoptotic cell death following excessive activation *(78)*. Loss of these neurons would create an easily excited circuitry, possibly one that displays spontaneous activity. A second method of permanent change in the dorsal horn involves the sprouting of Aβ-afferent fibers following peripheral nerve injury *(89)*. The normal distribution of the Aβ-afferent fibers is focused on the deeper layers of the dorsal horn. In animal models, following nerve injury, the terminals of the Aβ-afferent fibers can be seen in the superficial layers replacing sites occupied typically by PANs. Both of the above alterations in the dorsal horn circuitry would create permanent change and could contribute to chronic pain scenarios.

7.4. Dorsal Horn Involvement in Modified Pain Presentation Patterns

7.4.1. Dorsal Horn Alteration in Chronic Pain States

Normal plasticity in the dorsal horn circuitry is necessary to insure adequate warning information and protective reflexes during the healing process. To be protective, these changes have to occur rapidly; they typically involve numerous feed-forward events without an immediate set-point, thus fitting the definition of an allostatic process as put forward by Schulkin *(60)*. However, excessive activation of the dorsal horn or inadequate control mechanisms (to be discussed below) can turn the normal plasticity into a pathologic response that leads to the development of chronic pain. Adaptive changes that can become pathologic include the spread of neurons expressing receptors for SP *(76)*, expansion of dorsal horn neuron receptive fields, the loss of GABAergic inhibitory interneurons, and the sprouting of Aβ-fibers into the superficial layer of the dorsal horn. Thus the chronic pain state can be considered as a failure of normal allostatic mechanisms leading to a pathological condition similar to other chronic stress-related diseases such as depression *(90,91)*, type 2 diabetes mellitus *(92)*, and cardiovascular disease *(93)*.

7.4.2. Clinical Expression of Sensitization

Following the onset of central sensitization, the activity pattern of neurons in the dorsal horn is altered. Expanding receptive fields of dorsal horn neurons create a zone of increased sensitivity that surrounds the initial injury termed secondary hyperalgesia. Many dorsal horn neurons have projections or at least collateral axons that terminate in the ventral horn. Sensitization of dorsal horn neurons then alters the activity patterns of the large ventral horn alpha motoneurons *(94,95)*. The ventral horn output can produce muscle spasms and, when prolonged, increased muscle tone and hyperreflexia akin to that seen in spasticity.

7.4.3. Convergence of Visceral and Deep Somatic Input in the Dorsal Horn

Visceral afferent fibers from thoracoabdominal and pelvic organs enter the spinal cord through the dorsal root and terminate in the lateral aspect of the deep dorsal horn (Figure 6). Visceral PAN input overlaps with much of the somatic PAN input and many cells in the dorsal horn can be driven by both visceral and somatic input *(96,97)*. Somatic input can sensitize dorsal horn neurons eliciting specific reflexes. Subsequent visceral input can activate the previously facilitated circuit, eliciting a similar pain pattern and some of the same reflexes. The reverse situation is also often seen clinically, as pointed out by Sir Henry Head many years ago *(98)*: that is, visceral input first sensitizes the dorsal horn circuitry and subsequent somatic injury elicits the previous visceral pain pattern and associated reflexes *(99)*.

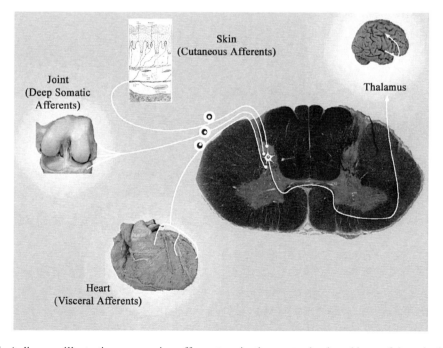

Fig. 6. A diagram illustrating converging afferernt projections onto the dorsal horn of the spinal cord.

7.4.4. INFLUENCE OF PRIMARY AFFERENT FIBERS ALONG THE SPINAL CORD

As PANs enter the spinal cord through the dorsal root entry zone, they undergo a trifurcation (Figure 7). One branch enters the dorsal horn at that segment, one branch ascends, and one descends along the dorsal margin of the dorsal horn in a bundle of fibers termed Lissauer's tract *(100)*. Older diagrams of PAN termination clearly indicated this branching pattern *(101)*, although it has been removed from most modern text for simplification. The division of the PAN is important since it can result in the spreading of information up and down the spinal cord to reach distant segmental levels. How far this information can spread is not clear, cutaneous PANs spread out at least two to three segments, while visceral PANs have reported distributions involving greater than five segments *(102)*; however, even greater distances are possible *(103)*.

The three-dimensional distribution of PAN information in the spinal cord allows for the interpretation of otherwise confusing pain patterns. Patients can have existing areas of spinal facilitation from old injuries or diseases processes such as spinal facilitation in the midthoracic region consequent to a history of gall bladder pain. A recent revival of this old pain pattern, despite the prior removal of the gall bladder, could be due to the new onset of another disease process such as myocardial ischemia or gastric ulcer. The visceral PANs from the myocardium or the stomach enter the spinal cord in the upper thoracic region; early in the disease processes their input may be present in lower thoracic segments due to segmental spread of afferent input, but below the threshold of detection by the patient. However, spread of low-grade neural activity in the caudal direction could easily activate the portion of the spinal cord originally sensitized by the remote history of gall bladder disease. The patient perceives the

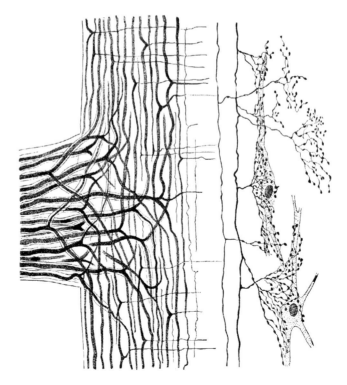

Fig. 7. Trifurcations of primary afferent fibers.

gall-bladder-associated pain pattern, but this time it is arising in the myocardium and not the gall bladder. In essence, the recent and otherwise unexplained revival of an old pain pattern should be considered the harbinger of new disease until proven otherwise.

7.4.5. The Dorsal Horn and Dorsal Root Reflexes

Normally one thinks of the dorsal root as a strictly afferent system carrying action potentials from the peripheral tissue into the spinal cord only; however, it is now known that under appropriate conditions, the dorsal root can act as an efferent pathway from the spinal cord; when this type of antidromic activity occurs in an intact sensory nerve it has been termed a dorsal root reflex *(104)*. Centrifugally conducted activity on dorsal rootlets has been known since the late nineteenth century but was not really in detail examined until the middle of the 20th century *(105)*. Dorsal root reflexes can are present in both large myelinated as well as in small myelinated and unmyelinated fibers (see *(105)* for a discussion of the difficulties in recording DRRs from the smallest fibers); in this review we will focus on those reflexes present in the small fibers such as PANs. To trigger these reflexes in PANs, the initial input stimulus to the spinal cord has to be in the range required to activate the PANs (C-fiber range). When such an afferent barrage reaches the dorsal horn, a wave of depolarization, termed *primary afferent depolarization* (PAD), occurs and is spread outward for several segments up and down the spinal cord. Interestingly, dorsal horn depolarization is facilitated by central sensitization of dorsal horn neurons, thus past experience can influence the magnitude of this depolarization event. When an area of the dorsal horn depolarizes, the central terminals of other primary afferent fibers contained within this area also depolarize. This mechanism is most likely a spin-off event of presynaptic inhibition and is known to involve GABAa receptors and GABA released by local interneurons as well as being influenced by serotonin receptors *(106)*. Significant depolarization of the central terminals of primary afferent fibers can result in the generation of an action potentials within these fibers that move antidromically (outward) to invade the peripheral terminals of this PAN. The resulting antidromic output from the dorsal horn can be recorded as a compound action potential, termed *dorsal root potential* (DRP) on adjacent dorsal rootlets that have been truncated. In the peripheral terminals of these PANs, the antidromic action potentials act similar to those involved in an classic

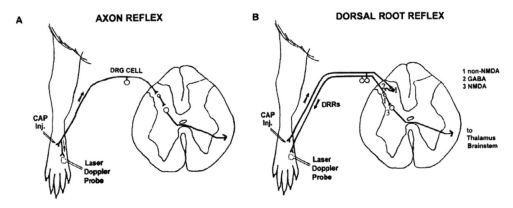

Fig. 8. Dorsal root reflex compared to an axon reflex (taken from Willis WD. Dorsal root potentials and dorsal root reflexes: a double-edged sword. Exp Brain Res 1999;124:395–421).

axon reflex, that is they trigger the release of neuropeptide into the peripheral tissue (Figure 8) thus either initiating or exacerbating an inflammatory reaction. Antidromic activity over dorsal roots can occur both ipsilateral and contralateral to the input root *(107)*. DRR have been demonstrated to play a significant role in the spread of peripheral inflammation *(108)*. Finally, recent studies have revealed that DRRs can be enhanced by stimulation of the periaqueductal gray region of the midbrain *(106)*; this finding has significant implications with respect to the generation of diffuse pain patterns and will be reconsidered in the section on descending pain control mechanisms.

8. ASCENDING PATHWAYS FOR PAIN

8.1. The Anterolateral System in the Spinal Cord and Brainstem

A population of projection neurons arising mainly in laminae I, IV-V, and VII-VIII in the dorsal horn send their axons contralaterally to reach the anterior and lateral quadrant of the spinal cord *(109)*. Most of these neurons represent either nociceptive-specific cells located in lamina I or wide-dynamic-range cells located in the deeper laminae of the dorsal horn. Axons from these neurons ascend diagonally across the spinal cord, crossing the midline in the anterior white commissure. The tract formed by these axons has been termed the anterolateral tract (ALS); within the ALS axons are arranged such that the cervical fibers are positioned most medially and the sacral fibers are most lateral. Also anterior-lateral segregation of axons occurs within the tract such that the anterior portion of the ALS contain fibers activated by light touch and

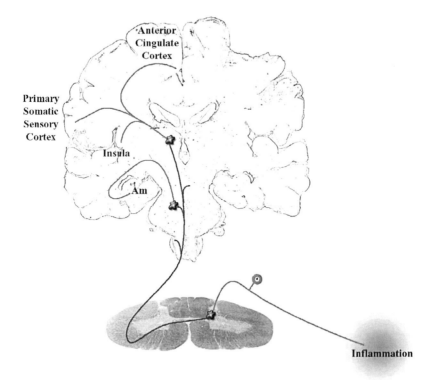

Fig. 9. Ascending pain pathways.

the lateral portions of the ALS contain more of the pain and temperature responsive fibers. Finally, based on target site, two components of the anterolateral tract can be identified: the spinoreticular and spinothalmic tracts.

8.1.1. SPINORETICULAR TRACTS

The spinoreticular fibers terminate in specific nuclei of the medulla, pons, and midbrain. Specific sites targeted by the spinoreticular fibers include the catecholamine cell groups (A1–A7), subnucleus reticularis dorsalis, the ventrolateral medulla, the parabrachial nucleus, periaqueductal gray, and the anterior pretectal area *(109,110)*. Since these areas are thought to regulate much of the descending brainstem-spinal cord projections, they therefore could play a significant role in the modulation of pain. Of these two tracts, the spinoreticular appears to be the most important in regulating the arousal system of the brainstem.

8.1.2. SPINOTHALAMIC TRACT

Dorsal horn neurons that project to the thalamus form the spinothalamic tract, their axons are also embedded in the ALS system along with those projecting to the brainstem. In fact many of the brainstem terminals can be collateral branches of the spinothalamic fibers. Spinothalmic axons located in the lateral most portion of the ALS tend to be most responsive to pain and thermal stimuli. At the rostral end of the spinothalmic tract a division occurs; the larger fibers in the tract remain laterally positioned to enter the thalamus, while the finer fibers in the tract segregate and enter the medial thalamus, thus medial and lateral pain systems exist in the thalamus. Finally, many of the ascending fibers entering the medial thalamus appear to be of brainstem origin rather than spinal cord.

8.2. Thalamic Representation of Pain

The thalamus is a major relay of ascending information from the spinal cord and brainstem to the cerebral cortex. Two pain systems can be identified in the thalamus, separated from each other anatomically and having differing functions *(111)*.

8.2.1. LATERAL PAIN SYSTEM

The spinothalamic tract (often termed the *neospinothalamic tract)* innervates some of the laterally and ventrally positioned nuclei of the thalamus including the ventroposterior lateral nucleus, ventromedial nucleus and portions of the posterior nuclear group, and portions of the ventrolateral nucleus forming lateral pain system (Figure 10). These structures rapidly relay information to somatic sensory and insular cortex and play a role in the localizing qualities and intensity of the pain perception. In one published case of a patient with a lesion involving the postcentral gyrus of the cerebral cortex (a significant target of the lateral pain system of the thalamus, the individual lost the ability to accurately localize painful stimuli but retained the ability to experience the affective nature of the pain *(112).*

8.2.2. MEDIAL PAIN SYSTEM

The medial fibers of the spinothalamic tract (often termed the paleospinothalmic fibers) pass medially in the thalamus (Figure 10) to innervate the centromedian nucleus, centrolateral nucleus, dorsomedial nucleus, nucleus submedius, and the intralaminar

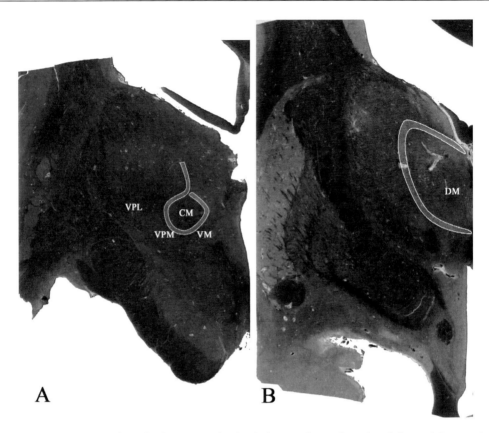

Fig. 10. The representation of pain systems in the thalamus. Coronal section **A** is caudal to section **B**. The shaded region represents the internal meduallary lamina of the thalamus. Abbreviations: DM, dorsomedial thalamic nucleus; VM, ventromedial thalamic nucleus; VPM, ventroposterior medial; VPL, ventroposterior lateral thalamic nucleus.

nuclei *(111)*. In the hypothalamus this system innervates the parventricular nucleus. Included in this ascending system would be projections from lower brainstem areas that have themselves been innervated by the spinoreticular axons. These connections form the medial pain system and are primarily relayed to the prefrontal cortex and anterior cingulate cortex. The medial pain system is slower than its lateral counterpart and is more closely related to the affective and emotional nature of pain *(113)*.

9. CEREBRAL REPRESENTATION OF PAIN

Pain is a complex perception arising from a widely distributed cortical network termed the pain neuromatix *(114)*. Areas involved with the pain neuromatrix include the somatic sensory cortex, insula, anterior cingular cortex, prefrontal cortex, and amygdala. No one portion of the cortex can entirely account for the perception of pain. The perception is most likely a construct that emerges from simultaneous activity in numerous cortical areas of this matrix *(3)*. Most information on human cortical pain representation comes from recent imaging studies and will be described in another chapter of this text. Only a basic anatomical description of the pain neuromatrix will be presented in this review.

9.1. Somatic Sensory Cortex

The somatic sensory portion of cerebral cortex is divided in to two major regions—SI and SII (Figure 11). SI is located on the postcentral gyrus, while SII is positioned at the base of the postcentral gyrus wrapping over the operculum and reaching into the insula lobe. Projections to the somatic sensory cortex arise in the ventroposterior lateral thalamic nucleus. Representation of pain is found in the contralateral SI, but can be bilateral in SII *(74,115)*. Lesions of the SI can leave a person capable of feeling pain but incapable of localizing that pain very accurately *(112)*, emphasizing role of SI in localizing painful stimuli. The SII cortex could be acting as a bridge, receiving information from the spinothalamic tract and transmitting this information to the insular cortex.

9.2. Insular Cortex

Located in the depths of the lateral sulcus, between the frontoparietal cortex above and the temporal cortex below (Figure 12), the insula is a major area in the pain cortical neuromatrix *(116)*. The insula receives thalamic projections from the ventromedial nucleus and posterior nuclei *(117)*, areas that are innervated by the spinothalamic tract *(118)*. The insula also receives cortical projections from adjacent somatic sensory areas. In primates, SI and SII project to the rostral and caudal portions of the insula *(117)*. The same regions of insular cortex that receive pain-related projections feed this information into the limbic forebrain, including such structures as the hypothalamus,

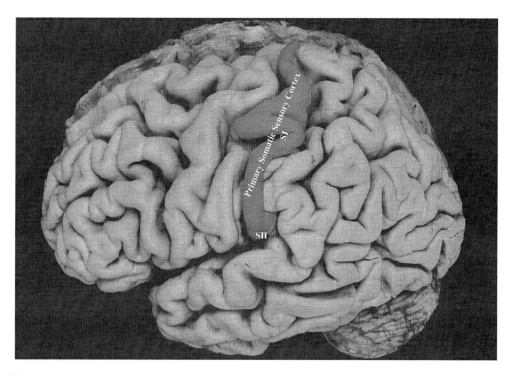

Fig. 11. Primary somatic sensory cortex. The postcentral gyrus is shaded in blue. SI occupies the convexity of the postcentral gyrus while SII extends into the posterior regions of the insula.

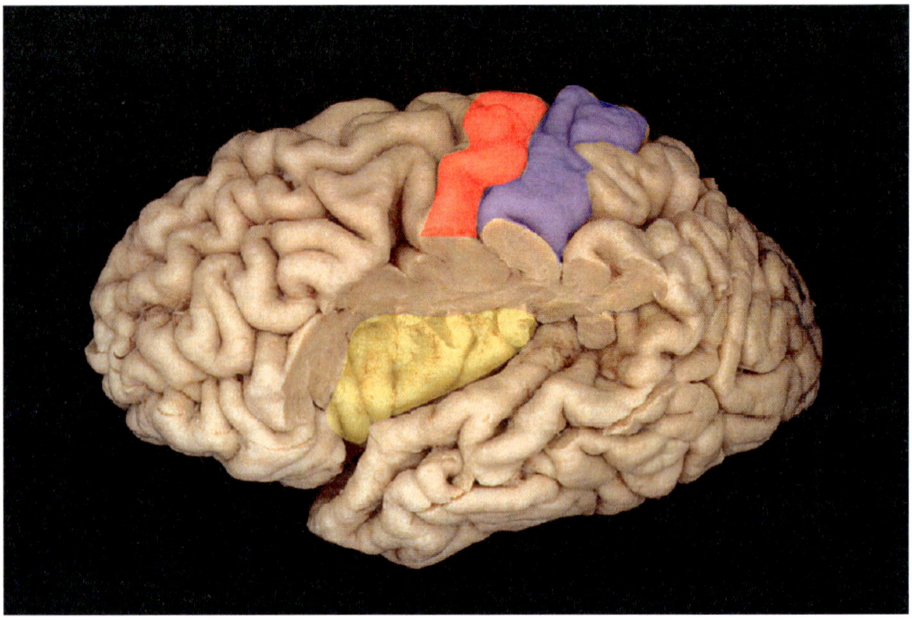

Fig. 12. Insular cortex. The insula cortex is shaded in yellow. To obtain this view, the superior operculum of the lateral sulcus had to be removed. Precentral gyrus is seen in red and postcentral gyrus in blue.

amygdala, anterior cingulate cortex, and medial prefrontal cortex *(119,120)*. Finally, the insula also has descending projections to the brainstem through which it exerts control over the autonomic nervous system *(120)* as well as apparently regulating the descending pain control systems. Recent studies have documented the presence of opioids such as dynorphin and enkephalin in the insular cortex and suggested a role for these opioid systems in the generation of cortically-mediated analgesia *(121)*. One possible interpretation of this arrangement is that the insula helps to orchestrate the bodies physiological response to pain, including pain control or enhancement depending n the situation *(118)*.

Interestingly, disruption of the deep white matter at the caudal border of the insula can produce an intense central pain, similar in quality to thalamic pain. It has been termed pseudothalamic syndrome. *(122)*. Conversely, a tumor compressing the posterior aspect of the insula altered tactile perception and the perception of mechanical and thermal pain by raising pain thresholds *(123)*. Finally, damage to the insula or disconnection of the somatic sensory areas of parietal cortex from the insula has been proposed as the mechanism for the presentation of asymbolia for pain *(124*, pp. 269–270). In asymbolia patients can localize the painful stimulus but do not experience the normal emotional or affective nature of the pain. In this state, it is proposed that the link between the somatic sensory system and the limbic system has been interrupted.

Besides interoceptive (somatic and visceral) input, the insula also is the target of olfactory, gustatory, and vestibular information *(125)*. Thus the insula could be pooling a wide range of information and passing it on to the limbic system as well as regulating autonomic response patterns.

9.3. Anterior Cingulate Cortex

The anterior cingulate cortex is located on the medial aspect of the cerebral hemisphere, wrapped around the genu of the corpus callosum (Figure 13). A major contribution to the anterior cingulate cortex arises in the dorsomedial nucleus of the thalamus and constitutes a significant portion of the medial pain system. Other contributions arise in the intralaminar nuclei of the thalamus and involve the medial thalamic pain system. The anterior cingulate cortex is associated with the anticipatory and emotional or affective aspects of pain *(113,126)*. Lesions of the ACC do not destroy our ability to perceive acute pain, but they do blunt the affective nature of the pain *(127)*.

9.4. Prefrontal Cortex

In humans, the rostral pole of the cerebrum is very prominent and forms the prefrontal cortex. This cortex receives projections from the medial pain system of the thalamus, specifically the dorsomedial nucleus. The prefrontal cortex is said to be involved with executive functions and appears to play a significant role in the attentive and cognitive aspect of pain *(128)*.

9.5. Amygdala

The amygdala is located on the medial aspect of the temporal lobe, forming a prominent enlargement termed the uncus which is visible externally (Figure 13). The amygdala receives numerous projections from most associative portions of the cerebral cortex as well as a set of subcortical projections from the parabrachial

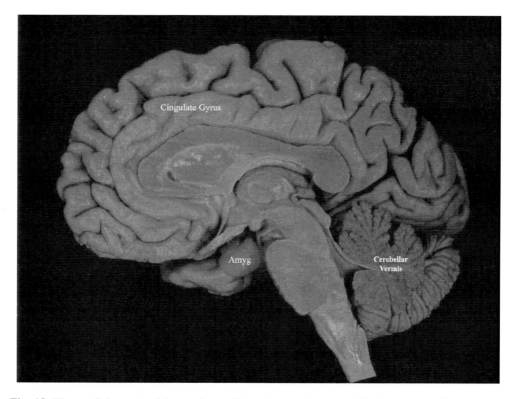

Fig. 13. The medial aspect of the cerebrum illustrating major areas of pain representation.

region of the pontomesencephalic border of the brainstem termed the spinoparabra-chioamygdalaoid pathway *(120)*. Intensely painful stimuli, acting through the spino-parabrachioamygdaloid pathway, exert a strong drive on portions of the amygdala *(129)*. This aspect of the medial temporal lobe is known for its ability to facilitate (a form of central sensitization) and it is also known to form memories of fear-provoking stimuli *(130)*. Efferent fibers from the amygdala provide a strong drive on hypotha-lamic and brainstem areas involved in control of the sympathoadrenal system. In this manner, the amygdala is capable of initiating a strong arousal response to a painful stimuli or even to the threat of a painful stimulus *(131)*.

Some of the input to the amygdala is subcortical in nature—that is, it passes from the posterior thalamus to the amygdala without cortical processing. This mechanism provides an explanation for patients who, having been exposed to a traumatic event at some point in their life, now experience strong emotional arousal over seemingly inconsequential stimuli. The initial traumatic event or events facilitated areas in the medial temporal lobe. Subsequently, innocuous stimuli that might only tangentially be related to the initial event can now evoke a major protective response from the amygdala.

The amygdala has strong connections to the prefrontal and cingulate cortex *(132)*. This medial temporal lobe structure is known to play a significant role in anxiety and depressive disorders *(133)*. Given its plasticity, it is possible that the amygdala is a junction point between chronic pain states and those of depression and anxiety along with the concomitant physiological responses *(134)*.

9.6. Cerebellum

The cerebellum arises from the ponitine portion of the brainstem (Figure 13). While not typically considered part of the cortical pain neuromatrix, the cerebellum is often seen to contain neural activity in pain imaging studies of pain states *(135)*. Nociceptive events have also been demonstrated to alter neuronal activity in the cerebellar vermis and portions of the hemispheres. Descending pathways from the deep cerebellar nuclei reach several brainstem locations that contribute to the control of nociceptive activity. Nociceptive-related cerebellar activity could relate to the coordination of motor programs necessary to control the individual's pain-related movements. However, the cerebellum is very clearly involved in learning and memory related to the motor system, and recent studies have suggested that the cerebellum can control of large areas of the cerebral cortex, extending much beyond pure motor function *(136,137)*. Supporting this contention is the observation that patients suffering cerebellar damage can present with cognitive and behavioral deficits as well as with ataxic movements *(138,139)* Thus, it is possible that the cerebellar activity evoked by pain is involved in cognitive learning processes controlling pain. Much more data on the cerebellum is necessary before a really clear picture emerges *(135)*.

9.7. Central Post-Stroke Syndromes

Strokes anywhere in the spinothalamic tract and its cortical connections can cause intense central or neuropathic pain syndromes, as a collective entity these have been termed central post-stroke pain syndromes *(140,141)*. Particularly, isolated lesions in the medial thalamus have been known to cause an intense pain typically refractive to medications, initially termed the Dejerine-Roussy syndrome *(140)*. Damage involving the anterolateral tract in the spinal cord has also been known occasionally to result in intense neuropathic or funicular pain syndromes. In addition, strokes in the peri-insular region, between the insular and the opercular portion of the parietal cortex, can result in intense central pain. Central pain most likely has varying pharmacology *(142)* and is therefore particularly difficult to treat since much of it is typically poorly responsive to conventional analgesics and opioids *(141)*.

10. THE BRAINSTEM AND DESCENDING PAIN MODULATION SYSTEMS

10.1. Endogenous Pain Control Systems

The ascending pain pathways reach areas in the medulla, rostral pons, and midbrain that can initiate an elaborate descending pain control system capable of significantly suppressing the ascending pain signals. Conversely, as has been recently demonstrated, this same system is also capable of enhancing our sensitivity to pain, an event that can also be protective in some situations *(143)*. Controlling components of the descending system are found in the limbic forebrain, hypothalamus, midbrain, and medullary regions.

10.1.1. MEDULLARY–SPINAL PROJECTIONS

The rostroventral medial medulla (RVM) is a source of descending projections to the dorsal horn of the spinal cord *(143)*. These axons descend within the dorsolateral funniculus of the cord and terminate in both the dorsal and ventral horn. The initial impression of this system was that the RVM was capable of gating activity in the dorsal horn and diminishing the ascending activity in the spinothalamic and spinoreticular tracts. However, more recent studies have found that RVM has both *Off-cells*, which are active during suppression of ALS activity and *On-cells* that are active during facilitation of dorsal horn activity *(144)*. Thus the RVM can either enhance or suppress pain control in the spinal cord. Beyond pain, the neurons in the RVM most likely have a more complex job of coordinating homeostatic reflexes, of which pain and the response to it are just one part *(145)*.

10.1.2. CONTROL OF RVM

Control of RVM emanates from the periaqueductal (central) gray of the midbrain *(143)* as well as associated areas of the tegmentum at the pontomesencephalic boundary *(146)*. This region of the midbrain has been related to analgesia and pain control, as well as fear and anxiety modulation, vocalization, lordosis, and cardiovascular control *(147)*. PAG has a rich population of opioid-producing neurons that are involved in regulating the descending pain control systems. Stimulation of PAG can strongly enhance pain suppression while blocking the opioid system will prevent pain modulation *(148)*. Stimulation of PAG can also influence the formation of dorsal root reflexes *(149)*.

10.1.3. FOREBRAIN CONTROL

The PAG is strongly influenced by projections from the hypothalamus as well as from the prefrontal cortex, cingulate cortex, and amygdala, all major sites in the limbic forebrain *(150,151)*. This limbic forebrain-midbrain system appears to represent a mechanism through which hormones, emotions, and past negative experiences can adversely influence the way in which we perceive pain (Figure 14).

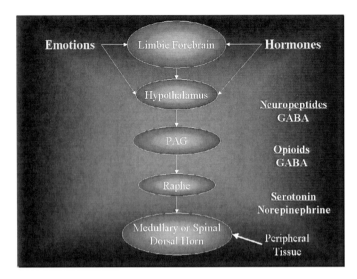

Fig. 14. Descending pain control system.

10.2. Hormones Involved in Pain Modulation

10.2.1. HORMONES INFLUENCE PAIN PERCEPTION AT MULTIPLE LEVELS

Hormonal influence on pain can occur at two distinct levels: initially hormones could alter the activity of the primary afferent nociceptor or its terminal connections in the dorsal horn; or conversely, hormones could also influence the precept of pain by altering the state of emotions in the limbic forebrain. Evidence exists supporting both methods of involvement. Although many hormonal systems have been reported to influence the processing of nociceptive information, the data is very sketchy and often conflicting in nature *(152)*. However, two major hormonal systems have the strongest data relating them to altered pain sensation: the sex steroids and the hypothalamic–pituitary–adrenal (HPA) axis (see the section on allostatic mechanisms).

10.2.2. SEX STEROIDS AND PAIN PERCEPTION

It is a common observation that many chronic pain patterns, such as migraine headache, rheumatoid arthritis, fibromyalgia, and temporomandibular joint disorder, have a strong sexual preference and that these pain patterns can alter significantly either with the onset of menses in young women, with the changes in sex steroid levels during the cycle *(153–155)*, or with the cessation of the cycling pattern in menopause *(156)*. Furthermore, hormone replacement therapy is a risk factor for developing low back pain syndromes *(157)* as well as for temporomandibular joint pain syndromes *(158)*. Finally, drug therapy also has a strong sexual dimorphism, as presented in an extensive review by Craft *(159)*. Just how these sexual dimorphisms in pain and pain management occur is not so clear.

10.2.3. ESTROGEN AND THE MODULATION OF PAIN PERCEPTION

Sex steroids appears to influence the processing of nociceptive information at multiple levels in the neuraxis. Estrogen receptors are expressed in neurons of the trigeminal ganglion *(160)* as well in the dorsal root ganglia of the lumbosacral spinal cord *(161)*. In the trigeminal ganglion, the estrogen receptors are capable of modulating the expression of pain-related peptides such as neuropeptide-Y and galinin *(160)*. Estrogen and testosterone can also modulate the sensitivity of the opioid system to increase analgesia in peripheral neurons; however, this modulation is very dependent on the type of opioid receptor system present and the results for estrogen can be somewhat inconsistent *(162)*. In the central nervous system, estrogen receptors are located on neurons in laminae I and II of the trigeminal dorsal horn in the medulla *(163)*, where they appear to modulate delta-opioid receptor activity *(164)*. Estrogen receptor α is present in the DRG and in the dorsal and lateral horn of the lumbosacral spinal cord. Expression of these receptors is regulated with the levels of estrogen in the mensus cycle as well as during pregnancy *(165)*. Interaction of estrogen and progesterone with kappa and delta opioid receptors in the spinal cord is recruited to mediate the pregnancy-associated increase in pain threshold *(166)*. Estrogen has a duel activity on neurons: first it can initiate slow, gene-regulated, nuclear transcriptional activity, and second it can trigger immediate, non-nuclear, mitogen-activated membrane effects that result in increased neuronal excitability *(167)*. Exposure to estrogen activated extracellular-signaling protein kinase (ERK-1) in cultured trigeminal ganglionic neurons *(167)*; it is also known that activation of ERK-1 in dorsal horn neurons facilitates activity and contributes to the development of central sensitization in these neurons *(77)*. These observations taken together suggest that estrogen could have two very different actions; high estrogen levels could predispose neurons in the dorsal horn to sensitization even while simultaneously enhancing opioid systems to suppress activity of primary afferent nociceptors in the spinal cord. Rapidly falling levels of estrogen could release the opioid block on PAN activity, allowing them to discharge while leaving the dorsal horn neurons vulnerable to sensitization. This would create a marked decrease in pain threshold and a increased sensitivity to noxious (hyperalgesia) and possibly innocuous (allodynia) stimuli as well.

10.2.4. THE SEX STEROIDS ALSO APPEAR TO INFLUENCE THE PROCESSING OF NOCICEPTIVE INFORMATION AT LEVELS HIGHER THAN THE SPINAL CORD

The rostral ventrolateral medulla contains neuronal systems that control, through descending projections, the activity of neurons in the dorsal horn of the spinal cord. Estrogen can modulate the activity of ON/OFF cells located in the rostral ventromedial medulla *(168)*. Estrogen also modulates opioid control systems that regulate the RVM and can cause states of increased hyperalgesia *(169)*. These changes were observed at the level of the thalamus, nucleus accumbens, and amygdala using PET scanning techniques in healthy young women and men. Thus not only is there sufficient evidence to conclude that the sex steroids modulate activity in the nociceptive pathways of the peripheral nerves, spinal cord, and brainstem, but it also appears that these same steroids can influence processing in the pain perception systems of the forebrain.

10.3. Endogenous Pain Control Systems and Diffuse Pain

The formation of diffuse pain patterns are difficult to understand given our current knowledge of the neuromusculoskeletal system. The mechanism of diffuse pain in fibromyalgia has been attributed to a defect in the central nervous system that leads to increased central sensitivity *(170)*. However, barring sensitization of dorsal horn neurons to the point of spontaneous activity, simple sensitization of these neurons would still not be expected to cause diffuse pain unless there was some type of accompanying increased activity in peripheral pain generators. This is especially true

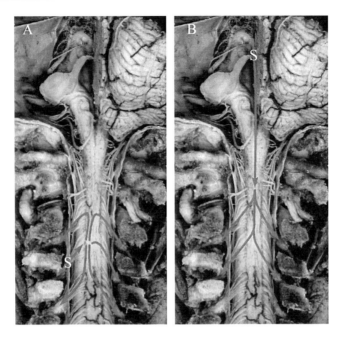

Fig. 15. Dorsal Root Reflexes: Section **A** demonstrates a intense input on a cervical nerve triggering DRRs on surrounding cervical nerves. Section **B** demonstrates a intense input from the dorsal midbrain region triggering DRRs on cervical nerves.

since fibromyalgic patients typically do not feel continuous or spontaneous pain in the diagnostic tender points, such as they would if central neurons where spontaneously active; instead, the pain is easily provoked by the examiner suggesting that thresholds have been lowered but have not reached threshold for spontaneous activity. Recent studies of the periaqueductal gray (PAG) and its descending systems provide some insight into this conundrum *(149)*. Stimulation of the PAG can lead to enhanced output of DRRs from the spinal cord (Figure 15). When these DRRs reached the peripheral terminal field of the fiber in which it is traveling, it would initiate the release of neuropeptide such as SP and CGRP. Mild tissue perfusion of these peptides would be expected to create areas of low-grade inflammation and establish a sensitizing environment surrounding the peripheral fibers. This is becoming an attractive model for fibromyalgic pain, especially given the strong emotional and hormonal input in the this system via the prefrontal cortex and medial aspect of the temporal lobe *(152,171)*.

11. PAIN AS AN ALLOSTATIC MECHANISM

There is an interesting analogy between the pain-response axis and the stress-response system as described in *(60)*. Both are feed-forward systems that are adaptive in nature. When activated, neither the stress-response axis or the pain-response system has an established set-point around which it operates; thus both are open-ended responses that meet the definition for an allostatic event. Both are protective in the short-term or acute response. Acute pain and acute stress are symptoms of a problem that has occurred and that typically will resolve. Both can become pathologic (disease) when prolonged. Chronic pain and chronic expression of the stress responses represent diseases that no longer are responding to a triggering stimulus. In essence the system is stuck in the "on" position. Both responses can result in depression when in the chronic state. There is strong crossover between each system, patients with chronic pain chronically activate the stress response system, often resulting in the onset of depression, while those caught in a chronic stress response often develop chronic pain as well *(172)*. These relationships lead to insights for treatment. The remainder of this chapter will outline the pathways linking the ascending interoceptive system with the output pathways of the arousal and stress-response system.

11.1. Ascending Pain Pathway Projections to the Midbrain and Hypothalamus

The spinoreticular fibers in the ALS terminate in portions of the medulla, pons, and midbrain and play a major role in activating the brainstem arousal system. Those terminating in the medulla are part of a system that eventually ascends through a multisynaptic route to reach the midbrain and specifically to activate the catecholaminergic neurons in the locus coeruleus, a small cluster of neurons located dorsolaterally at the pontomesencephalic junction. This noradrenergic structure is a significant component of the brainstem arousal system and the resultant stress response.

11.2. Midbrain Production of Catecholamines

The locus coeruleus supplies noradrenergic axons to much of the central nervous system above the pons, including the hypothalamus. Activation of the LC results in enhanced activity of the sympathetic nervous system and the concomitant release of norepinepherine systemically. The locus coeruleus–norepinephrine axis (LCNE) is part of a defensive, protective response; it is also part of a long-loop feedback control system that functions to modulate the inflammation cascade occurring in the peripheral tissue *(173,174)*.

11.3. Hypothalamic Production of Corticotropin-Releasing Hormone

Spinohypothalamic fibers carrying nociceptive information can stimulate the paraventricular nucleus in the hypothalamus, resulting in the production and release of corticotropin-releasing hormone (CRH) and activation of the hypothalamic–pituitary–adrenal axis (HPA). CRH acts on the anterior pituitary to stimulate the production and release of adrenocorticotropin (ACTH) that ultimately drives the adrenal cortex to secrete glucocorticoids and, to a lesser extent, mineralocorticoids. In addition, the release of CRH from the paraventricular neurons is enhanced by the presence of NE released from the LC. Finally CRH acts as a stimulant to the LC to enhance NE release (HPA-LCNE axis); thus the two structures are engaged in a powerful feed-forward system *(174)*. As such this HPA-LCNE axis is capable of mounting a rapid, powerful response to challenge—again very protective in acute situations but destructive to tissue in a chronic condition.

11.4. Amygdaloid Influence on the Hypothalamus and Locus Coeruleus

As previously described, the amygdala responds strongly to painful stimuli. Interestingly, portions of the amygdala produce CRH as a neurotransmitter *(90)*. The amygdala projects CRH-containing fibers to both the paraventricular nucleus of the hypothalamus and locus coeruleus of the midbrain. CRH release in the paraventricular nucleus fosters the production of more CRH; and in the locus coeruleus, it enhances the production of NE. Thus the amygdala, which is responsive to fear and involved in creating fear memories can, through this network of descending CRH-containing projections, facilitate the feed-forward or allostatic nature of the stress response *(90)*.

11.5. Influence of NE and Cortisol on Body Functions—Allostasis

The rapid release of adrenal cortical steroids and catecholamines represents two major effector arms of the brainstem arousal system; these arms are often termed the stress-response system *(175)*. Critical to this response is the redistribution of energy in the body, providing muscles with readily available energy metabolites. This hyperglycemia is accomplished in part by increasing the resistance of the insulin receptor to circulating insulin. In addition, the stress-response system contributes to elevating blood pressure and pulse rate, enhancing breathing, suppressing the gastrointestinal system, facilitating wound healing, and optimizing the function of the immune system in the short term. The stress response, driven by arousal, is a rapid, feed-forward event lacking boundaries and has therefore been termed allostasis to distinguish it from the traditional feedback control of homeostasis *(60)*. Allostatic responses are characterized by their quick nature, rapid rise in intensity due to feed-forward mechanisms, and lack of limitations or boundary conditions. Allostatic responses can be very protective when used in the short term. However, long-term exposure or repeated exposure to allostatic chemical milieu is pathologic and fosters disease in multiple organ systems in the body *(93,176)*.

11.6. Summary

Pain—and the responses it creates in the body—is, in essence, an allostatic mechanism. This allostatic response can be seen at all levels of the interceptive system. At the level of PANs, peripheral sensitization can occur, in a feed-forward process, enhancing the activity of the fiber. In the spinal cord, central sensitization occurs, again in a feed-forward process, creating regions of segmental facilitation. Similar facilitation also occurs, again using feed-forward mechanisms, in the forebrain areas such as the amygdala. At this level, emotional experiences surrounding the painful event can facilitate amygdaloid activity, resulting in enhanced fear memories and increased drive on the NE and CRH systems of the hypothalamus and midbrain. Finally the NE and CRH systems are interrelated in a feed-forward mechanism that results in an enhanced protective response to arousal-provoking stimuli such as pain. Thus painful stimuli trigger an allostatic response in the body that is, in itself, very protective in the short term. Long-term exposure to allostactic mechanisms is known to be pathologic to the body, facilitating cardiovascular disease, the metabolic syndrome, renal disease, and such psychiatric disorders as depression and anxiety. Viewed in this light, chronic pain becomes the end product or disease that occurs in the interoceptive system when a normal allostatic response such as acute pain goes out of control and becomes fixed in a pathologic state.

REFERENCES

1. Craig AD. Pain mechanisms: labeled lines versus convergence in central processing. Annu Rev Neurosci 2003;26:1–30.
2. Nagasako EM, Oaklander AL, Dworkin RH. Congenital insensitivity to pain: an update. Pain 2003;101:213–219.

3. Chapman CR. 2005. Psychological aspects of pain: a consciousness studies perspective. In The Neurological Basis of Pain. Pappagallo M, Ed. New York: McGraw-Hill. pp. 157–167.
4. Loeser JD. Pain as a disease. Hdbk Clin Neurol 2006;81:11–20.
5. Prechtl JC, Powley TL. B-afferents: a fundamental division of the nervous system mediating homeostasis? Behav Brain Sci 1990;13:289–331.
6. Fitzgerald M. The development of nociceptive circuits. Nat Rev Neurosci 2005;6:507–520.
7. Kandel ER, Schwartz JH, Jessell TM. 2000. Principles of Neural Sciences. New York: Elsevier.
8. Melzack R, Wall PD. Pain mechanisms: a new theory. Science 1965;150:971–979.
9. Neumann S, Doubell TP, Leslie T, Woolf CJ. Inflammatory pain hypersensitivity mediated by phenotypic switch in myelinated primary sensory neurons. Nature 1996;384:360–364.
10. Meyer RA, Ringkamp M, Campbell JN, Raja SN. 2006. Peripheral mechanisms of cutaneous nociception. In Wall and Melzack's Textbook of Pain. McMahon SB, Koltzenburg M, Eds. Elsevier Churchill Livingston, pp. 3–34.
11. Selye H. The general adaptive syndrome and the diseases of adaptation. J Clin Endocrinol 1946;6:117–173.
12. Munger BL, Ide C. The structure and function of cutaneous sensory receptors. Arch Histol Cytol 1988;51:1–34.
13. Julius D, Basbaum AI. Molecular mechanisms of nociception. Nature 2001;413:203–210.
14. Mense S, Simons DG. 2001. Muscle pain: understanding its nature, diagnosis, and treatment. Philadelphia: Lippincott, Williams and Wilkins.
15. Wall PD, Woolf CJ. Muscle but not cutaneous C-afferent input produces prolonged increases in the excitability of the flexion reflex in the rat. J Physiol (Lond.) 1984;356:453–458.
16. Alpantaki K, McLaughlin D, Karagogeos D, Hadjipavlou A, Kontakis G. Sympathetic and sensory neural elements in the tendon of the long head of the biceps. J Bone Joint Surg Am 2005;87:1580–1583.
17. Premkumar LS, Raisinghani M. Nociceptors in cardiovascular functions: complex interplay as a result of cyclooxygenase inhibition. Mol Pain 2006;2:26.
18. Bove GM, Light AR. Calcitonin gene-related peptide and peripherin immunoreactivity in nerve sheaths. Somatosens Mot Res 1995;12:49–57.
19. Schaible HG, Grubb BD. Afferent and spinal mechanisms of joint pain. Pain 1993;55:5–54.
20. Fortier LA, Nixon AJ. Distributional changes in substance P nociceptive fiber patterns in naturally osteoarthritic articulations. J Rheumatol 1997;24:524–530.
21. Bielefeldt K, Gebhart GF. 2006. Visceral pain: basic mechanisms. In Wall and Melzack's Textbook of Pain. McMahon SB, Koltzenburg M, Eds. Elsevier Churchill Livingston, pp. 721–736.
22. Cervero F, Jänig W. Visceral nociceptors: a new world order? Trends Neurosci 1992;15:374–378.
23. Cervero F. Mechanisms of acute visceral pain. Br Med Bull 1991;47:549–560.
24. Sanchez del Rio M, Moskowitz MA. 2000. The trigeminal system. In The Headaches. Olesen J, Tfelt-Hansen P, Welch KMA, Eds. Baltimore: Lippincott, Williams and Wilkins, pp. 141–150.
25. Stilwell DL. The nerve supply of the vertebral column and its associated structures in the monkey. Anat Rec 1956;125:139–169.
26. Groen GJ, Baljet B, Drukker J. Nerves and nerve plexuses of the human vertebral column. Am J Anat 1990;188:282–296.
27. Jinkins JR, Whittermore AR, Bradley WG. The anatomic basis of vertebrogenic pain and the autonomic syndrome associated with lumbar disk extrusion. Am J Roentgenol 1989;152:1277–1289.
28. Willard FH. 1997. The muscular, ligamentous and neural structure of the low back and its relation to back pain. In Vleeming A, Mooney V, Snijder CJ, Dorman T, Stoeckart R, Eds. Movement, Stability and Low Back Pain. Edinburgh: Churchill Livingstone, pp. 3–35.
29. Levine JD, Fields HL, Basbaum AI. Peptides and the primary afferent nociceptor. J Neurosci 1993;13:2273–2286.
30. Couture R, Harrisson M, Vianna RM, Cloutier F. Kinin receptors in pain and inflammation. Eur J Pharmacol 2001;429:161–176.
31. Schmelz M, Schmidt R, Bickel A, et al. Specific C-receptors for itch in human skin. J Neurosci 1997;17:8003–8008.
32. Paus R, Schmelz M, Biro T, Steinhoff M. Frontiers in pruritus research: scratching the brain for more effective itch therapy. J Clin Invest 2006;116:1174–1186.
33. Vergnolle N, Bunnett NW, Sharkey KA, Brussee V, Compton SJ, Grady EF, Cirino G, Gerard N, Basbaum AI, Andrade-Gordon P, Hollenberg MD, Wallace JL. Proteinase-activated receptor-2 and hyperalgesia: a novel pain pathway. Nat Med 2001;7:821–826.

34. Samad TA, Sapirstein A, Woolf CJ. Prostanoids and pain: unraveling mechanisms and revealing therapeutic targets. Trends Mol Med 2002;8:390–396.

35. Tokunaga A, Saika M, Senba E. 5-HT receptor subtype is involved in the terminal hyperalgesic mechanism of serotonin in the periphery. Pain 1998;76:349–355.

36. Sommer C. Serotonin in pain and analgesia: actions in the periphery. Mol Neurobiol 2004;30: 117–125.

37. Wood JN, Docherty R. Chemical activators of sensory neurons. Ann Rev Physiol 1997;59:457–482.

38. Voilley N. Acid-sensing ion channels (ASICs): new targets for the analgesic effects of non-steroid anti-inflammatory drugs (NSAIDs). Curr Drug Targets Inflamm Allergy 2004;3:71–79.

39. Sato J, Perl E. Adrenergic excitation of cutaneous pain receptors induced by peripheral nerve injury. Science 1991;251:1608–1610.

40. Jänig W. 1992. Pain and the sympathetic nervous system: pathophysiological mechanisms. In Autonomic Failure. Bannister R, Mathias CJ, Eds. Oxford: Oxford Medical Publications, pp. 231–251.

41. Petersen M, Zhang J, Zhang JM, LaMotte RH. Abnormal spontaneous activity and responses to norepinephrine in dissociated dorsal root ganglion cells after chronic nerve constriction. Pain 1996;67:391–397.

42. Perl ER. Causalgia, pathological pain, and adrenergic receptors. Proc Natl Acad Sci USA 1999;96:7664–7667.

43. Banik RK, Sato J, Giron R, Yajima H, Mizumura K. Interactions of bradykinin and norepinephrine on rat cutaneous nociceptors in both normal and inflamed conditions in vitro. Neurosci Res 2004b;49:421–425.

44. Banik RK, Sato J, Giron R, Yajima H, Mizumura K. Interactions of bradykinin and norepinephrine on rat cutaneous nociceptors in both normal and inflamed conditions in vitro. Neurosci Res 2004a;49:421–425.

45. Abdulla FA, Smith PA. Ectopic α_2-adrenoceptors couple to N-type Ca^{2+} channels in axotomized rat sensory neurons. J Neurosci 1997;17:1633–1641.

46. Tracey DJ, Cunningham JE, Romm MA. Peripheral hyperalgesia in experimental neuropathy: mediation by α2-adrenoreceptors on post-ganglionic sympathetic terminals. Pain 1995;60:317–327.

47. Koltzenburg M. The changing sensitivity in the life of the nociceptor. Pain Suppl 1999;6:S93–S102.

48. Khasar SG, Green PG, Chou B, Levine JD. Peripheral nociceptive effects of α_2-adrenergic receptor agonists in the rat. Neuroscience 1995;66:427–432.

49. Lawand NB, McNearney T, Westlund KN. Amino acid release into the knee joint: key role in nociception and inflammation. Pain 2000;86:69–74.

50. Davidson EM, Coggeshall RE, Carlton SM. Peripheral NMDA and non-NMDA glutamate receptors contribute to nociceptive behaviors in the rat formalin test. Neuroreport 1997;8:941–946.

51. Liu HT, Mantyh PW, Basbaum AI. NMDA-receptor regulation of substance P release from primary afferent nociceptors. Nature 1997;386:721–724.

52. Knotkova H, Pappagallo M. 2005. Periheral Mechanism. In The Neurological Basis of Pain. Pappagallo M, Ed. New York: McGraw-Hill, pp. 53–60.

53. Crowley C, Spencer SD, Nishimura MC, Chen KS, Pitts-Meek S, Armanini MP, Ling LH, McMahon SB, Shelton DL, Levinson AD. Mice lacking nerve growth factor display perinatal loss of sensory and sympathetic neurons yet develop basal forebrain cholinergic neurons. Cell 1994;76:1001–1011.

54. McMahon SB, Bennett DLH, Bevan S. 2006. Inflammatory mediators and modulators of pain. In Wall and Melzack's Textbook of Pain. McMahon SB, Koltzenburg M, Eds. Elsevier Churchill Livingston, pp. 49–72.

55. Petty BG, Cornblath DR, Adornato BT, Chaudhry V, Flexner C, Wachsman M, Sinicropi D, Burton LE, Peroutka SJ. The effect of systemically administered recombinant human nerve growth factor in healthy human subjects. Ann Neurol 1994;36:244–246.

56. McMahon SB, Cafferty WB, Marchand F. Immune and glial cell factors as pain mediators and modulators. Exp Neurol 2005;192:444–462.

57. Pernow B. Substance P. Pharmacol Rev 1983;35:85–141.

58. Holzer P. Local effector functions of capsaicin-sensitive sensory nerve endings: involvement of tachykinins, calcitonin gene-related polypeptide and other neuropeptides. Neuroscience 1988;24:739–768.

59. Maggi CA. Tachykinins and calcitonin gene-related peptide (CGRP) as co-transmitters released from peripheral endings of sensory nerves. Prog Neurobiol 1995;45:1–98.

60. Schulkin J. 2003. Rethinking Homeostasis. Cambridge: The MIT Press.
61. Howe JF, Loeser JD, Calvin WH. Mechanosensitivity of dorsal root ganglia and chronically injured axons: a physiological basis for the radicular pain of nerve root compression. Pain 1977;3:25–41.
62. Amir R and Devor M. Chemically mediated cross-excitation in rat dorsal root ganglia. J Neurosci 1996;16:4733–4741.
63. McLachlan EM, Jänig W, Devor M, Michaelis M. Peripheral nerve injury triggers noradrenergic sprouting within dorsal root ganglia. Nature 1993;363:543–546.
64. Ramer MS, Bisby MA. Rapid sprouting of sympathetic axons in dorsal root ganglia of rats with a chronic constriction injury. Pain 1997;70:237–244.
65. Wilson P, Kitchener PD. Plasticity of cutaneous primary afferent projections to the spinal dorsal horn. Prog Neurobiol 1996;48:105–113.
66. Hunt SP, Rossi J. Peptide- and non-peptide-containing unmyelinated primary afferents: the parallel processing of nociceptive information. Philos Trans R Soc Lond B Biol Sci 1985;308:283–289.
67. Todd AJ. Anatomy and neurochemistry of the dorsal horn. Handbook of Clinical Neurology 81 (3rd Series), 2006, pp. 61–76.
68. Braz JM, Nassar MA, Wood JN, Basbaum AI. Parallel "pain" pathways arise from subpopulations of primary afferent nociceptor. Neuron 2005;47:787–793.
69. Cervero F. Pain and the spinal cord. Hdbk Clin Neurol 2006;81(3rd Series):77–92.
70. Mendell LM. Physiological properties of unmyelinated fiber projection to the spinal cord. Exp Neurol 1966;16:316–332.
71. Willis WD. 1979. Physiology of dorsal horn and spinal cord pathways related to pain. In Mechanisms of Pain and Analgesic Compounds. Beers RF, Bassett EG, Eds. New York: Raaven Press, pp. 143–156.
72. Mayer DJ, Price DD, Becker DP. Neurophysiological characterization of the anterolateral spinal cord neurons contributing to pain perception in man. Pain 1975;1:51–58.
73. Basbaum AI. Spinal mechanisms of acute and persistent pain. Reg Anesth Pain Med 1999;24:59–67.
74. Millan MJ. The induction of pain: an integrative review. Prog Neurobiol 1999;57:1–164.
75. Mantyh PW, DeMaster E, Malhotra A, Ghilardi JR, Rogers SD, Mantyh CR, Liu H, Basbaum AI, Vigna SR, Maggio JE, et al. Receptor endocytosis and dendrite reshaping in spinal neurons after somatosensory stimulation. Science 1995;268:1629–1632.
76. Abbadie C, Trafton J, Liu HT, Mantyh PW, Basbaum AI. Inflammation increases the distribution of dorsal horn neurons that internalize the neurokinin-1 receptor in response to noxious and non-noxious stimulation. J Neurosci 1997;17:8049–8060.
77. Ji RR, Kohno T, Moore KA, Woolf CJ. Central sensitization and LTP: do pain and memory share similar mechanisms? Trends Neurosci 2003;26:696–705.
78. Scholz J, Broom DC, Youn DH, Mills CD, Kohno T, Suter MR, Moore KA, Decosterd I, Coggeshall RE, Woolf CJ. Blocking caspase activity prevents transsynaptic neuronal apoptosis and the loss of inhibition in lamina II of the dorsal horn after peripheral nerve injury. J Neurosci 2005;25: 7317–7323.
79. Doubell TP, Mannion RJ, Woolf CJ. Intact sciatic myelinated primary afferent terminals collaterally sprout in the adult rat dorsal horn following section of a neighbouring peripheral nerve. J Comp Neurol 1997;380:95–104.
80. Cook AJ, Woolf CJ, Wall PD, McMahon SB. Dynamic receptive field plasticity in rat spinal cord dorsal horn following C-primary afferent input. Nature 1987;325:151–153.
81. Laird JM, Cervero F. A comparative study of the changes in receptive-field properties of multi-receptive and nocireceptive rat dorsal horn neurons following noxious mechanical stimulation. J Neurophysiol 1989;62:854–863.
82. Hylden JLK, Nahin RL, Traub RJ, Dubner R. Expansion of receptive fields of spinal lamina I projection neurons in rats with unilateral adjuvant-induced inflammation: the contribution of dorsal horn mechanisms. Pain 1989;37:229–243.
83. Grubb BD, Stiller RU, Schaible HG. Dynamic changes in the receptive field properties of spinal cord neurons with ankle input in rats with chronic unilateral inflammation in the ankle region. Exp Brain Res 1993;92:441–452.
84. Koerber HR, Mirnics K. Plasticity of dorsal horn cell receptive fields after peripheral nerve regeneration. J Neurophysiol 1996;75:2255–2267.
85. Hoheisel U, Mense S, Simons DG, Yu XM. Appearance of new receptive fields in rat dorsal horn neurons following noxious stimulation of skeletal muscle: a model for referral of muscle pain? Neurosci Lett 1993;153:9–12.

86. Watkins LR, Wieseler-Frank J, Hutchinson MR, Ledeboer A, Spataro L, Milligan ED, Sloane EM, Maier SF. 2007. Neuroimmune interactions and pain: the role of immune and glial cells. In Psychoneuroimmunology. Vol. 1. Ader R, Ed. Amsterdam: Elsevier Academic Press, pp. 393–414.

87. Marriott DR, Wilkin GP, Wood JN. Substance P-induced release of prostaglandins from astrocytes: regional specialisation and correlation with phosphoinositol metabolism. J Neurochem 1991;56: 259–265.

88. Wieseler-Frank J, Maier SF, Watkins LR. Immune-to-brain communication dynamically modulates pain: physiological and pathological consequences. Brain Behav Immun 2005;19:104–111.

89. Neumann S, Woolf CJ. Regeneration of dorsal column fibers into and beyond the lesion site following adult spinal cord injury. Neuron 1999;23:83–91.

90. Schulkin J, McEwen BS, Gold PW. Allostasis, amygdala, and anticipatory angst. Neurosci Biobehav Rev 1994;18:385–396.

91. McEwen BS. Mood disorders and allostatic load. Biol Psychiatry 2003;54:200–207.

92. Stumvoll M, Tataranni PA, Stefan N, Vozarova B, Bogardus C. Glucose allostasis. Diabetes 2003;52:903.

93. McEwen BS. Protective and damaging effects of stress mediators. N Engl J Med 1998;338:171–179.

94. Grigg P, Schaible HG, Schmidt RF. Mechanical sensitivity of group III and IV afferents from posterior articular nerve in normal and inflamed cat knee. J Neurophysiol 1986;55:635–643.

95. He X, Proske U, Schaible HG, Schmidt RF. Acute inflammation of the knee joint in the cat alters responses of flexor motoneurons to leg movements. J Neurophysiol 1988;59:326–340.

96. Sato A, Sato Y, Schmidt RF, Torigata Y. Somato-vesical reflexes in chronic spinal cats. J Auton Nerv Syst 1983;7:351–362.

97. Sato A. Somatovisceral reflexes. J Manipulative Physiol Ther 1995;18:597–602.

98. Head H. 1920. Studies In Neurology (Vol. II). London: Henry Frowde and Hodder & Stoughton, Ltd.

99. Henry JA, Montuschi E. Cardiac pain referred to site of previously experienced somatic pain. Br Med J 1978;2:1605–1606.

100. Carpenter MB, Sutin J. 1983. Human Neuroanatomy. Baltimore: Williams and Wilkins.

101. Ramon y Cajal S. 1909. Histologie du Systeme Nerveux de l'Homme et des Vertebres, (L. Azoulay, trans). Madid, (1952–1955): Instituto Ramon y Cajal del C.S.I.C.

102. Sugiura Y, Terui N, Hosoya Y. Difference in distribution of central terminals between visceral and somatic unmyelinated (C) primary afferent fibers. J Neurophysiol 1989;62:834–840.

103. Wall PD, Bennett DL. Postsynaptic effects of long-range afferents in distant segments caudal to their entry point in rat spinal cord under the influence of picrotoxin or strychnine. J Neurophysiol 1994;72:2703–2713.

104. Rees H, Sluka KA, Westlund KN, Willis WD. Do dorsal root reflexes augment peripheral inflammation? Neuroreport 1994;5:821–824.

105. Willis WD. Dorsal root potentials and dorsal root reflexes: a double-edged sword. Exp Brain Res 1999;124:395–421.

106. Peng YB, Wu J, Willis WD, Kenshalo DR. GABA(A) and 5-HT(3) receptors are involved in dorsal root reflexes: possible role in periaqueductal gray descending inhibition. J Neurophysiol 2001;86:49–58.

107. Rees H, Sluka KA, Lu Y, Westlund KN, Willis WD. Dorsal root reflexes in articular afferents occur bilaterally in a chronic model of arthritis in rats. J Neurophysiol 1996;76:4190–4193.

108. Lin Q, Wu J, Willis WD. Dorsal root reflexes and cutaneous neurogenic inflammation after intradermal injection of capsaicin in rats. J Neurophysiol 1999;82:2602–2611.

109. Dostrovsky JO, Craig AD. 2006. Ascending projection systems. In Wall and Melzack's Textbook of Pain. McMahon SB, Koltzenburg M, Eds. Elsevier Churchill Livingston, pp. 187–203.

110. Westlund KN. 2005. Neurophysiology of pain. In The Neurological Basis of Pain. Pappagallo M, Ed. New York: McGraw-Hill, pp. 3–19.

111. Dostrovsky JO. Brainstem and thalamic relays. Hdbk Clin Neurol 2006;81:127–139.

112. Ploner M, Freund HJ, Schnitzler A. Pain affect without pain sensation in a patient with a postcentral lesion. Pain 1999;81:211–214.

113. Sewards TV, Sewards MA. The medial pain system: neural representations of the motivational aspect of pain. Brain Res Bull 2002;59:163–180.

114. Melzack R. From the gate to the neuromatrix. Pain Suppl 1999;6:S121–S126.

115. Casey KL, Tran TD. 2006. Cortical mechanisms mediating acute and chronic pain in humans. Handbook of Clinical Neurology 81(Chapter 12), pp. 159–177.

116. Hofbauer RK, Rainville P, Duncan GH, and Bushnell MC. Cortical representation of the sensory dimension of pain. J Neurophysiol 2001;86:402–411.
117. Friedman DP, Murray EA. Thalamic connectivity of the second somatosensory area and neighboring somatosensory fields of the lateral sulcus of the macaque. J Comp Neurol 1986;252: 348–373.
118. Craig AD. How do you feel? Introception: the sense of the physiological condition of the body. Nat Rev Neurosci 2002;3:655–666.
119. Augustine JR. Circuitry and functional aspects of the insular lobe in primates including humans. Brain Res Rev 1996;22:229–244.
120. Jasmin L, Burkey AR, Granato A, Ohara PT. Rostral agranular insular cortex and pain areas of the central nervous system: a tract-tracing study in the rat. J Comp Neurol 2004;468:425–440.
121. Evans JM, Bey V, Burkey AR, Commons KG. Organization of endogenous opioids in the rostral agranular insular cortex of the rat. J Comp Neurol 2006;500:530–541.
122. Schmahmann JD, Leifer D. Parietal pseudothalamic pain syndrome. Clinical features and anatomic correlates. Arch Neurol 1992;49:1032–1037.
123. Greenspan JD, Winfield JA. Reversible pain and tactile deficits associated with a cerebral tumor compressing the posterior insula and parietal operculum. Pain 1992;50:29–39.
124. Geschwind N. Disconnection syndrome in animals and man. Part I. Brain 1965;88:237–294.
125. Shipley MT, Geinisman Y. Anatomical evidence for convergence of olfactory, gustatory, and visceral afferent pathways in mouse cerebral cortex. Brain Res Bull 1984;12:221–226.
126. Wager TD, Rilling JK, Smith EE, Sokolik A, Casey KL, Davidson RJ, Kosslyn SM, Rose RM, Cohen JD. Placebo-induced changes in FMRI in the anticipation and experience of pain. Science 2004;303:1162–1167.
127. Johansen JP, Fields HL, Manning BH. The affective component of pain in rodents: direct evidence for a contribution of the anterior cingulate cortex. Proc Natl Acad Sci USA 2001;98:8077–8082.
128. Lorenz J, Minoshima S, Casey KL. Keeping pain out of mind: the role of the dorsolateral prefrontal cortex in pain modulation. Brain 2003;126:1079–1091.
129. Neugebauer V, Li W. Processing of nociceptive mechanical and thermal information in central amygdala neurons with knee-joint input. J Neurophysiol 2002;87:103–112.
130. Schafe GE, LeDoux JE. 2004. The neural basis of fear. In The Cognitive Neurosciences. Gazzaniga MS, Ed. Cambridge, MA: A Bradford Book, MIT Press, pp. 987–1003.
131. Gauriau C, Bernard JF. Pain pathways and parabrachial circuits in the rat. Exp Physiol 2002;87: 251–258.
132. Cavada C, Company T, Tejedor J, Cruz-Rizzolo RJ, Reinoso-Suarez F. The anatomical connections of the macaque monkey orbitofrontal cortex. A review. Cereb Cortex 2000;10:220–242.
133. McEwen BS. Glucocorticoids, depression, and mood disorders: structural remodeling in the brain. Metabolism 2005;54:20–23.
134. Neugebauer V, Li W, Bird GC, Han JS. The amygdala and persistent pain. Neuroscientist 2004;10:221–234.
135. Saab CY, Willis WD. The cerebellum: organization, functions and its role in nociception. Brain Res Brain Res Rev 2003;42:85–95.
136. Fiez JA. Cerebellar contributions to cognition. Neuron 1996;16:13–15.
137. Barinaga M. The cerebellum: Movement coordinator or much more? Science 1996;272:482–483.
138. Schmahmann JD, Sherman JC. The cerebellar cognitive affective syndrome. Brain 1998;121 (Pt 4):561–579.
139. Schmahmann JD. Disorders of the cerebellum: ataxia, dysmetria of thought, and the cerebellar cognitive affective syndrome. J Neuropsychiatry Clin Neurosci 2004;16:367–378.
140. Schott GD. From thalamic syndrome to central poststroke pain. J Neurol Neurosurg Psychiatry 1996;61:560–564.
141. Frese A, Husstedt IW, Ringelstein EB, Evers S. Pharmacologic treatment of central post-stroke pain. Clin J Pain 2006;22:252–260.
142. Yamamoto T, Katayama Y, Hirayama T, Tsubokawa T. Pharmacological classification of central post-stroke pain: comparison with the results of chronic motor cortex stimulation therapy. Pain 1997;72:5–12.
143. Fields HL, Basbaum AI, Heinricher MM. 2006. Central nervous system mechanisms of pain modulation. In Wall and Melzack's Textbook of Pain. McMahon SB, Koltzenburg M, Eds. Elsevier Churchill Livingston, pp. 125–142.

144. Heinricher MM, Morgan MM, Tortorici V, Fields HL. Disinhibition of off-cells and antinociception produced by an opioid action within the rostral ventromedial medulla. Neuroscience 1994;63:279–288.
145. Mason P. Ventromedial medulla: pain modulation and beyond. J Comp Neurol 2005;493:2–8.
146. Carlson JD, Selden NR, Heinricher MM. Nocifensive reflex-related on- and off-cells in the pedunculopontine tegmental nucleus, cuneiform nucleus, and lateral dorsal tegmental nucleus. Brain Res 2005;1063:187—-194.
147. Behbehani MM. Functional characteristics of the midbrain periaqueductal gray. Prog Neurobiol 1995;46:575–605.
148. Basbaum AI, Fields HL. Endogenous pain control mechanisms: review and hypothesis. Ann Neurol 1978;4:451–462.
149. Peng YB, Kenshalo DR, Gracely RH. Periaqueductal gray-evoked dorsal root reflex is frequency dependent. Brain Res 2003;976:217–226.
150. Amaral DG, Price JL, Pitkänen A, Carmichael ST. 1992. Anatomical organization of the primate amygdaloid complex. In The Amygdala: Neurobiological Aspects of Emotion, Memory, and Mental Dysfunction. Aggleton JP, Ed. New York: Wiley-Liss Publications, pp. 1–66.
151. Devinsky O, Morrell MJ, Vogt BA. Contributions of anterior cingulate cortex to behaviour. Brain 1995;118:279–306.
152. Blackburn-Munro G, Blackburn-Munro R. Pain in the brain: are hormones to blame? Trends Endocrinol Metab 2003;14:20–27.
153. Unruh AM. Gender variations in clinical pain experience. Pain 1996;65:123–167.
154. Hapidou EG, Rollman GB. Menstrual cycle modulation of tender points. Pain 1998;77:151–161.
155. Riley JL, Robinson ME, Wise EA, Price DD. A meta-analytic review of pain perception across the menstrual cycle. Pain 1999;81:225–235.
156. Mogil JS. Sex, gender and pain. Hdbk Clin Neurol 2006;81:325–342.
157. Brynhildsen JO, Björs E, Skarsgård C, Hammar ML. Is hormone replacement therapy a risk factor for low back pain among postmenopausal women? Spine 1998;23:809–813.
158. LeResche L, Saunders K, Von Korff MR, Barlow W, Dworkin SF. Use of exogenous hormones and risk of temporomandibular disorder pain. Pain 1997;69:153–160.
159. Craft RM. Sex differences in drug- and non-drug-induced analgesia. Life Sci 2003;72:2675–2688.
160. Puri V, Cui L, Liverman CS, Roby KF, Klein RM, Welch KM, Berman NE. Ovarian steroids regulate neuropeptides in the trigeminal ganglion. Neuropeptides 2005;39:409–417.
161. Papka RE, Storey-Workley M. Estrogen receptor-alpha and -beta coexist in a subpopulation of sensory neurons of female rat dorsal root ganglia. Neurosci Lett 2002;319:71–74.
162. Stoffel EC, Ulibarri CM, Folk JE, Rice KC, Craft RM. Gonadal hormone modulation of mu, kappa, and delta opioid antinociception in male and female rats. J Pain 2005;6:261–274.
163. Amandusson Å, Hermanson O, Blomqvist A. Estrogen receptor-like immunoreactivity in the medullary and spinal dorsal horn of the female rat. Neurosci Lett 1995;196:25–28.
164. Dawson-Basoa M Gintzler AR. Involvement of spinal cord δ opiate receptors in the antinociception of gestation and its hormonal simulation. Brain Res 1997;757:37–42.
165. Papka RE, Hafemeister J, Puder BA, Usip S, Storey-Workley M. Estrogen receptor-alpha and neural circuits to the spinal cord during pregnancy. J Neurosci Res 2002;70:808–816.
166. Horvath G, Kekesi G. Interaction of endogenous ligands mediating antinociception. Brain Res Brain Res Rev 2006;52:69–92.
167. Welch KM, Brandes JL, Berman NE. Mismatch in how oestrogen modulates molecular and neuronal function may explain menstrual migraine. Neurol Sci 2006;27(Suppl 2):S190–S192.
168. Craft RM, Morgan MM, Lane DA. Oestradiol dampens reflex-related activity of on- and off-cells in the rostral ventromedial medulla of female rats. Neuroscience 2004;125:1061–1068.
169. Smith YR, Stohler CS, Nichols TE, Bueller JA, Koeppe RA, Zubieta JK. Pronociceptive and antinociceptive effects of estradiol through endogenous opioid neurotransmission in women. J Neurosci 2006;26:5777–5785.
170. Vierck CJ, Jr. Mechanisms underlying development of spatially distributed chronic pain (fibromyalgia). Pain 2006;124:242–263.
171. Neugebauer V, Li W. Differential sensitization of amygdala neurons to afferent inputs in a model of arthritic pain. J Neurophysiol 2003;89:716–727.
172. Magni G, Moreschi C, Rigatti-Luchini S, Merskey H. Prospective study on the relationship between depressive symptoms and chronic musculoskeletal pain. Pain 1994;56:289–297.

173. Elenkov IJ, Chrousos GP. Stress hormones, Th1/Th2 patterns, pro/anti-inflammatory cytokines and susceptibility to disease. Trends Endocrinol Metab 1999;10:359–368.
174. Charmandari E, Tsigos C, Chrousos GP. Endocrinology of the stress response. Ann Rev Physiol 2005;67:259–284.
175. Tsigos C, Chrousos GP. Hypothalamic-pituitary-adrenal axis, neuroendocrine factors and stress. J Psychosom Res 2002;53:865–871.
176. Seeman TE, Singer BH, Rowe JW, Horwitz RI, McEwen BS. Price of adaptation—allostatic load and its health consequences. MacArthur studies of successful aging. Arch Intern Med 1997;157: 2259–2268.
177. Woolf CJ, Salter MW. 2006. Plasticity and pain: role of the dorsal horn. In Wall and Melzack's Textbook of Pain. McMahon SB, Koltzenburg M, Eds. Elsevier Churchill Livingston, pp. 91–105.

3

The Functional Neuroanatomy of Pain Perception

Norman W. Kettner

Summary

Pain is usually a source of warning and protection; this is not the case for chronic pain. The experience of pain is a form of consciousness consisting of integrated physical and psychological neural inputs. It typically originates with the spinal transmission of noxious sensory stimuli arising from damaged tissues; this level of processing is termed nociception. Signals are conveyed from the spinal cord to supraspinal networks that include the brainstem, subcortical, and cortical regions. This processing network is termed the pain neuromatrix. It is the supraspinal network that transforms the sensation of nociception into the complex and uniquely individual experience that is pain. Pain modulation (inhibitory or facilitatory) is emerging as an important clinical target for pharmacologic and non-pharmacologic interventions. This chapter outlines the neuroanatomical and physiological mechanisms underlying the experience of acute (physiological) and chronic (pathological) pain. It also highlights the theoretical role of CAM techniques in pain modulation. Finally, in order to provide an integrative view of pain perception, the dimensions of the pain experience are presented and contrasted, including the discriminative, cognitive, and affective elements.

Key Words: acute pain, chronic pain, nociception, pain modulation, neuroplasticity, anti-nociception, pain neuromatrix, pain dimensions, CAM

1. INTRODUCTION

Pain is a conscious multidimensional experience that typically arises from threat or actual damage to tissue *(1)*. The language of pain can be confusing, as a variety of terms

From: *Contemporary Pain Medicine: Integrative Pain Medicine: The Science and Practice of Complementary and Alternative Medicine in Pain Management*
Edited by: J. F. Audette and A. Bailey © Humana Press, Totowa, NJ

may be employed in its description (Table 1). Acute pain, however, may be readily contrasted with chronic pain. Acute pain usually occurs with tissue injury or disease. The value of acute pain perception arising from tissue damage in muscles, ligaments, or nerves is obvious; it is a warning of imminent danger. Chronic pain, however, typically

Table 1

Pain Classification

Pain	An unpleasant sensory and emotional experience that is associated with actual or potential tissue damage, or described in terms of such damage (IASP). Pain may be modulated by affect and cognitive factors such as attention.
Acute pain (nociceptive pain)	Acute pain is a symptom with a recognizable cause, which will continue until tissue damage is repaired, usually within a time period of several months. An ankle sprain would be an example of a disorder producing acute pain. This is physiological pain and serves an important adaptive function.
Chronic pain	This is pain that persists beyond the expected time course of tissue healing. Chronic pain may also be recurrent, as with rheumatoid arthritis. It often occurs in the absence of identifiable tissue damage and may be termed non-nociceptive pain. In this case, there is no biological value; the pain is pathological.
Neuropathic pain (central pain)	This is a pain arising in association with damage or dysfunction within the peripheral or central nervous system. Unfortunately this type of pain is often difficult to treat and may become a source of chronic pain. Diabetic neuropathy is an example of neuropathic pain.
Deafferentation pain	The reduction or loss of afferent input into the central nervous system will trigger pain. This pain condition may arise in association with peripheral or central nervous system pathology.
Somatic pain	The presence of injury or disease in skin or musculature causes somatic pain. The sensation from deep musculature is felt as aching or throbbing and more burning or stinging if superficial. A torn quadriceps muscle would trigger somatic pain.
Visceral pain	This pain is diffuse, poorly localized, and felt as cramping or pressure. It is produced by nociceptive responses within internal organs, which are diseased or injured. Visceral pain could be the result of malignant infiltration of the liver.

has no survival value; it is itself a disorder of the anatomy and function of the central nervous system. There are then two major categories of pain: acute pain, which is physiologic and nociceptive, and chronic pain that is the result of persistent nociceptive input or neuropathic pain (lesions or dysfunction of the peripheral or central nervous system). Persistent or chronic pain may also arise from a continuous nociceptive tissue injury and inflammation, such as inflammatory arthritis or malignant disease. Central pain is a form of chronic neuropathic pain arising from a lesion anywhere within the central nervous system, but usually involving the spinothalamic tract in the spinal cord or brain. It is among the most difficult pain syndromes to treat. Multiple causes of tissue injury can lead to the state of chronic pain, wherein pain and dysfunction characteristically persist beyond the expected healing period of injured tissue.

Pain perception emerges as a unified mental state consisting of several interactive biological influences, including genetic, molecular, synaptic, anatomic, physiologic, and psychosocial inputs, which usually arise in association with nociceptive generators. Pain perception is not just a sensation, but an integrated state composed of mental activity that evokes emotion, memory, attention, expectation, motor activity, autonomic responses, and an awareness of the extent of physically injured or diseased anatomy. It is this multilevel neural integration, involving nociception, input modulation, and neuroplasticity, that gives rise to the uniquely individual perception associated with the pain experience. Pain states in general are compelling personal experiences that are imposed onto both the somatic and psychosocial domains of our being with a potentially devastating impact.

The potential benefit of pain research lies in reducing the enormity of humanity's burden of pain. Chronic pain in particular appears to represent a model for the study of mind–body interactions and because of the dearth of effective treatments within traditional medical models, opens the door for the research of complementary and alternative medicine (CAM) strategies. Some important pain related research questions might include—*(1)* How do we maintain balance and homeostasis in nervous system function while encountering the myriad of mental and physical stressors arising from our external and internal environment during states of pain? *(2)* Which clinical interventions promote change in the injured brain or spinal cord by using sensory or motor conditioning inputs that trigger beneficial neuroplasticity? *(3)* How much of a role will CAM or integrative techniques such as acupuncture or manual therapy play in pain management, either acute or chronic?

The study of pain neurobiology also promises to elevate our understanding of how the body and mind interact in health and disease. The study of pain consciousness promises to provide important insights into the mind–body problem. Increasing evidence demonstrates that psychosocial factors (stress, anticipation, coping, beliefs) are better predictors of prognosis for recovery, especially in chronic pain, than the patient's specific disease and the extent of pathophysiology *(2)*.

It is the conscious awareness of tissue injury that typically results in the perception of pain. The presence of threat or actual damage to tissue initiates a signaling cascade of coded neural activity in the periphery that is transmitted to spinal and supraspinal sites. This evoked neural activity, which arises in association with inflammatory, thermal or mechanical tissue damage, is known as nociception, and evokes the accompanying pain perception. The magnitude of pain perception is not necessarily proportional to the extent of tissue injury or damage. Nociceptive processing (tissue damage) may occur independently of the perception of pain and the inverse is also true; pain may be perceived in the absence of peripheral or central damage-induced nociception. This latter circumstance, known as non-nociceptive pain, is common in chronic pain states such as psychogenic pain.

How can nociception arising from inflammatory or mechanical tissue injury occur without triggering pain perception? The pain system (like other neural systems) is arranged in a hierarchy of cortical, subcortical, and spinal neural networks that process nociceptive input to generate pain perception. Higher-order cognitive and affective pain modulatory neural networks may fire with sufficient intensity and duration in a variety of settings, i.e., sports competition, religious ritual, and combat environments, to produce significant antinociceptive or analgesic effects. This descending inhibitory influence is possible, as pain perception is the interaction of multiple excitatory and inhibitory spinal and supra-spinal processing nodes throughout the central nervous system (CNS). An extensive CNS network thus modulates the nociceptive input at the spinal cord and medullary dorsal horn (trigeminal) with both facilitatory and descending inhibitory (antinociceptive) pathways. The net output of these opposing networks and the influence of other pain-processing factors will determine the intensity and color of the pain perception. What about pain perception in the absence of tissue injury and nociception? Since the pain system is bi-valent, it may serve to amplify and even generate pain perception so under some circumstances pain perception can become independent of the presence of tissue damage.

As a result, the cortex plays a critical role in both the amplification and suppression of pain. These effects appear to be mediated by the endogenous opioid system. The role of the cortex in pain processing is a familiar experience to the marathon athlete who is able to suppress pain perception by triggering inhibitory cognitive and affective neural pathways activated by rigorous exercise. However, the role of the cortex in pain processing was not a historically accepted view in neuroscience. Only since the latter years of the 20th century has this view become established (3). The role of the cerebral cortex in pain perception evaded scientific recognition until the early 1990s. It was the introduction of powerful anatomical and functional neuroimaging techniques such as PET and fMRI that identified cortical activity in pain studies. Prior to this period, the 20th-century view by Head and later Penfield was dominant (4,5). In their view, the cerebral cortex played a limited role in the production of pain; the thalamus was believed to be the primary site of pain activation. Their view was supported by evidence that during neurosurgical ablation in the somatosensory cortex, patients failed to demonstrate any change in pain perception. In addition, they also observed little change in pain intensity in patients who had sustained trauma to the somatosensory cortex. Today, we know from functional neuroimaging studies that supraspinal pain processing occurs in a widespread, hierarchically distributed network of cortical, sub-cortical, and brainstem processing nodes. This network has been termed the pain neuromatrix (6). The pain experience then is not encoded in a discretely localized area of the brain, such as the thalamus, as posited by Head, Penfield and others (see Chapter 4).

The neural hierarchy of spinal and supraspinal neuroanatomy is an important prerequisite for understanding nociception and pain perception. The functioning of spinal and supraspinal anatomic networks gives rise to the perception of pain regardless of whether it is acute or chronic. Neuroanatomy of the spinal pathway includes the nociceptor or primary afferent nerve, dorsal root ganglion (DRG), dorsal horn of the spinal cord, and ascending and descending tracts. The ascending and descending spinal pathways connect nociceptive traffic between the spinal cord and brain and also play a critical role in the function of nociceptive modulation, which is convergent upon the dorsal horn (see Chapter 2).

Supraspinal neuroanatomy and its functions are related to higher-order nociceptive processing, the generation of pain perception and its bivalent modulation. The complexity of supraspinal pain processing is daunting and many questions remain unanswered in this complex and challenging frontier of pain research. What is the role of placebo or nocebo in healing encounters? How does the frontal cortex enhance the chronicity of pain? Can placebo induction become a therapeutic intervention? Do CAM practices somehow enhance or optimize the placebo response to pain? How can a patient's belief translate into pathophysiological or healing states? Although still under investigation, the supraspinal neuroanatomical components of the pain neuromatrix appear to include an extensive array with elements arising in the brainstem, cerebellum, thalamus, basal ganglia, subcortical and cortical regions. This chapter will focus on the spinal and supraspinal anatomy and function related to pain and its perception.

2. NOCICEPTOR

The perception of acute pain originates in the context of threatened or actual damage to visceral or peripheral tissue, including nerve fibers. Following tissue damage, peripheral and spinal neural pathways are synaptically activated and signals are then supraspinally transmitted throughout the pain system.

The most peripheral aspect of the pain system consists of nerves with specialized receptors known as nociceptors; they are associated with mostly small unmyelinated or thinly myelinated afferent nerve fibers. Their cell bodies are located in the dorsal root ganglion. Nociceptors are the gatekeepers of noxious afferent information, translating tissue damage and inflammation into nerve impulses. These impulses are transmitted through the spinal nerves and their trigeminal equivalent into the spinal and medullary dorsal horn respectively. Peripheral tissue damage arising from trauma or inflammation, including nerve injury, normally triggers the release of numerous nociceptive provoking or algesic agents. This inflammatory "soup" sensitizes local nociceptors, an event known as peripheral sensitization, which enhances peripheral neural input. There is an expanding array of algesics, including biochemical, neurotrophic, and cytokine agents (Table 2) *(7)*. Peripherally, sensitized nociceptors may alter their function and begin to demonstrate spontaneous firing, lowered thresholds of depolarization, and increased responses to noxious stimuli. Clinically, the change in sensitization of the peripheral nociceptor can lead to heightened responses to painful sensation known as hyperalgesia. This enhanced state of afferent barrage may then trigger abnormal functional and structural changes in the spinal and supraspinal pathways, a state known as central sensitization. This state can initiate allodynia, the experience of pain linked to normally non-painful sensation. Both peripheral and central sensitization phenomena are important as they contribute (along with neuroplastic mechanisms) to the transformation of acute pain to persistent and chronic pain.

Peripheral nociceptive signaling has additional routes. As mentioned above, another important afferent pathway mediating nociception is the trigeminal sensory nucleus (nucleus caudalis). It receives nociceptive peripheral afferents from the head and is analogous in function to the dorsal root ganglion. The trigeminal nociceptive pathway is activated with episodes of facial pain and during headache syndromes. There is also

Table 2

Inflammatory Pain Mediators

Bradykinin
Prostaglandin
H+
Adenosine
Serotonin
Nitric oxide
Noradrenaline
Growth factors
Chemokines
Cytokines
Bradykinin
Prostaglandin

evidence of nociceptive functioning in the afferents of cranial nerve X, i.e., the vagus nerve *(8)*. Autonomic responses such as elevated blood pressure and tachycardia occur during the perception of pain. In addition, both excitatory and inhibitory effects on spinal nociceptive processing, depending on the intensity of the stimulus, have been reported with vagal afferents *(9)*. These effects are probably mediated through bulbo-spinal pathways. Electrical stimulation of the vagus has been reported to reduce pain *(10)*. Vagal stimulation is also proposed as a mechanism of action for several CAM techniques such as acupuncture, and manual therapy *(11,12)*.

3. PERIPHERAL NERVE

Nerve cell fibers have long processes known as peripheral nerves. The constituents of the peripheral nerve include sensory, motor, and autonomic fibers. Nociceptive neural activity arising from tissue damage and inflammation in the periphery is initially transmitted to the dorsal horn of the spinal cord along variable-sized primary afferent nerve (PAN) fibers. These cell bodies are located in the dorsal root ganglion or the trigeminal ganglion. A central axon projection of the PAN synapses in the spinal or medullary dorsal horn. Fiber types of PAN mediating nociception include the A-delta and unmyelinated C-fibers. A-delta fibers conduct cold and localized nociceptive stimuli while C-fibers conduct poorly localized mechanical and heat stimuli. The size of the afferent fiber is clinically relevant because small fibers conduct an excitatory effect resulting in nociception, while the large diameter fibers (A-alpha, A-beta) arising from proprioceptors and muscle spindles have an inhibitory or gating effect on spinal cord nociceptive transmission, reducing nociceptive barrage *(13)*.

Following tissue injury, primary afferent nerve fibers convey coded noxious peripheral and visceral stimuli to the spinal cord dorsal horn, and then, in parallel pathways, to distributed supraspinal sites including the brainstem, cerebellum and multiple sites in the cortical and subcortical pain neuromatrix. As a result of the processing in this neuromatrix, a sensory stimulus arising in the primary afferent nerve undergoes transformation into a conscious state of pain perception.

4. SPINAL CORD

Nociception at the level of the spinal cord is important because of its critical role in states of pathological pain. A powerful pain modulatory mechanism originates in a network of supraspinal centers thought to be located in the cortex and brainstem. Through descending pathways, excitatory or inhibitory control is exerted on the afferent neural transmission within the dorsal horn neurons of the spinal cord.

Neurons of the spinal cord are organized into ten (I–X) gray matter layers, or laminae, first described by Rexed *(14)*. The substantia gelatinosa (lamina II) is an important node in the network of pain modulation since it is capable of blocking input from nociceptors segmentally (gating) and also through the supraspinal influence of the descending inhibitory pathways arising in the cortex and brainstem. Lamina II maintains a high concentration of opiate receptors responsible for analgesic effects. Inputs to the dorsal horn include several cell types including low threshold mechanoreceptors, low threshold thermoceptors, and nociceptive specific neurons. Wide dynamic range (WDR) neurons are second-order neurons that encode a wide range of stimuli from innocuous to noxious (low and high threshold) and have been implicated in the development of chronic pain. Neurochemicals modulating dorsal horn nociception include excitatory and inhibitory agents released by the terminals of the primary afferents, interneurons, and descending axons originating from a number of supraspinal sites *(15)*. Neurotransmitters such as glutamate and substance P mediate the synaptic transmission between nociceptors and dorsal horn neurons. Gamma-amino butyric acid (GABA) is released by interneurons and can modulate locally the response of the second-order neuron to the primary afferent barrage. Long-lasting nociceptive input from peripheral nerve injury or other damaged tissues may elicit windup and central sensitization in the dorsal horn (see Chapter 2). Peripheral sensitization of the nociceptors may be one factor that can lead to a sustained activation of the WDR and contribute to the heightened responsiveness of the second-order neuron called wind-up. This response is mediated by activation of N-methyl-D-aspartate (NMDA) receptors *(7)*. If sustained for a long enough period of time, a resultant increase in neuronal excitability throughout the spinal and supraspinal networks can occur known as central sensitization. A model for the maintenance of central sensitization is a form of increase in synaptic activity known as long-term potentiation (LTP). Its counterpart is reduced synaptic activity and known as long term depression (LTD). These mechanisms are thought to underlie the activities of learning and memory in the hippocampus and might also explain the transformation of acute to chronic pain *(16,17)*. This prolonged state of excitation may induce activity-dependent neuroplastic changes that impair the supraspinal modulation of pain. Excessive excitation may then increase the signal gain throughout the pain system elevating the risk for chronic pain (Fig. 1) *(15)*. When nociception is persistent, in addition to central sensitization, another mechanism promoting chronic pain has been recently identified based on a pathologic neuroimmune response. The response includes glial activation, pro-inflammatory cytokine release and increased release of pain mediators *(7,15)*. These factors also enhance neural sensitivity and increase the likelihood of chronic pain. In another recent study, chronic pain processing was reported to promote astrogliosis in the cingulate cortex associated with dysfunction of the cortical delta-opioid receptors *(18)*.

The gate control theory was a breakthrough concept in pain research *(13)*. It suggested that the pain experience was not a passive, static mechanism, but a dynamic

Chronic Pain Evolution

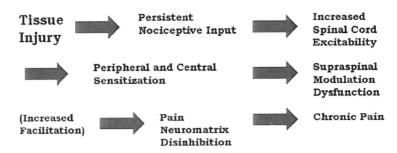

Fig. 1. Chronic pain evolution.

one, wherein afferent nociceptive signaling could be modified and influenced by neurons in the CNS acting as inhibitory or excitatory gates with both a segmental (spinal) and a central influence. Their theory described dorsal horn transmission cells as the convergence site of signals from a variety of peripheral afferent fibers (Fig. 2). Transmission cells project nociceptive signals into the supraspinal centers. The gate was a reference to either inhibition or facilitation of nociceptive signals by large and small fibers, respectively, within the substantia gelatinosa of the dorsal horn. Large diameter fibers act segmentally, and along with the supraspinal descending pathways, block nociceptive signaling in small diameter fibers. This gating mechanism serves as a potential model for the peripheral and central action of several CAM techniques. These techniques include therapies that trigger rhythmic afferent neural discharges in large-diameter mechanoreceptor fibers such as acupuncture, manual therapy, massage, exercise and transcutaneous electrical nerve stimulation (TENS).

Gate Theory

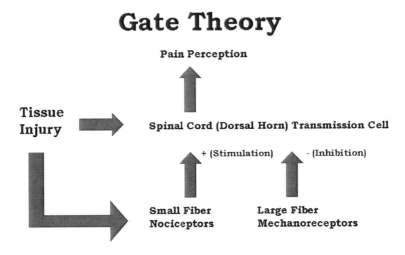

Fig. 2. Gate theory.

5. ASCENDING PATHWAYS

The anterolateral column of the spinal cord plays an important role in the ascending transmission and processing of nociceptive signaling (Figure 3). The spinothalamic tract (STT) is regarded as the most important ascending pathway for nociceptive transmission in humans. Lesions that block the anterolateral quadrant of the spinal cord result in the contralateral loss of pain and temperature and may result in ipsilateral loss of discriminative touch below the segmental level of the lesion. Such a lesion also blocks the spinoreticular, spinomesencephalic, and spinohypothalamic tracts that provide connections to the medulla, brainstem, and hypothalamus. STT cells originate in laminae I, III, IV, V, and to a lesser extent IX and X. Most cross within one or two segments and pass through the central white commissure to the opposite ventrolateral funiculus and ascend rostrally as the lateral STT. Deeper dorsal horn neurons give rise to the ascending anterior STT *(15)*.

There is an analogous pathway for the nociceptors originating in the face arising from the three divisions of the trigeminal nerve. The trigeminothalamic tract (TTT) originates from cells in the subnucleus caudalis. Second-order neurons of the STT and TTT arise from the dorsal horn of the spinal cord, (or brainstem), and ascend supraspinally to synapse in several ventral thalamic nuclei. In addition to the STT and TTT tracts, additional ascending nociceptive pathways arise in the dorsal horn that project to a variety of targets including the brainstem reticular formation, mesencephalic periaqueductal gray, thalamus, hypothalamus, amygdala, and indirectly to the frontal cortex. Third order neurons originating from the thalamus project in a wide distribution to cortical and subcortical targets as nociceptive signals are integrated throughout the supraspinal pain system *(15)*.

Inhibition of the STT in the dorsal horn can be triggered by the activation of noxious stimuli delivered to areas that are remote from the site of tissue damage. This inhibitory mechanism is known as the diffuse noxious inhibitory control system (DNIC) and is associated with activity in nociceptive neurons that recruits supraspinal inhibitory pathways *(19)*. This type of nociceptive inhibition may also be considered a tenable

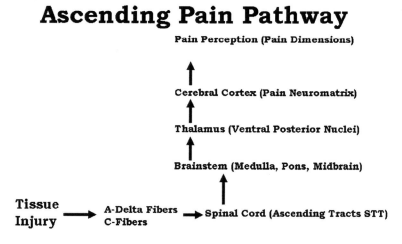

Fig. 3. Ascending pain pathway.

mechanism explaining the analgesic effects underlying counterirritant CAM techniques including TENS, acupuncture, and manual therapy.

Another major afferent spinal system, which extends to the brainstem, is the dorsal spinal (posterior) columns. Neurons in this pathway synapse in the dorsal column nuclei of the medulla oblongata. The dorsal column carries fibers activated by innocuous touch, proprioception and visceral nociception. As already mentioned, this system may also play an important role in pain modulation by activating inhibitory interneurons in the dorsal horn (15,20).

6. DESCENDING PATHWAYS

Multiple neuroanatomic levels are known to be associated with the descending pain inhibitory system (Figure 4). They include the cortex, diencephalon, limbic system, mesencephalic periaqueductal gray (PAG), rostroventral medulla (RVM), and nucleus raphe magnus (NRM), and dorsal horn. The arrival of ascending spinal nociceptive synapses in the mesencephalon triggers inhibitory substrates in the PAG. These signals are then relayed to the nucleus raphe magnus (NRM) and then send descending fibers to the dorsal horn where modulation of nociception occurs. This descending influence on nociception can be either inhibitory or facilitatory. The dorsal horn receives NRM terminals in laminae I, II, and V with the capability of inhibiting nociceptive neurons of the STT, spinoreticular and spinomesencephalic tracts. Inhibition in lamina II (substantia gelatinosa) occurs following the release of 5-HT (serotonin) and norepinephrine from the descending inhibitory fibers. The inhibition of substance P is blocked by either inhibitory interneurons and/or opioid release (7,15).

Cells in the NRM and RVM change their firing rates in response to modulatory inputs from higher cortical centers. Some cells are described as "off ," leading to descending inhibition (anti-nociceptive), while others are "on," causing descending facilitation (pro-nociception), with neutral cells also present (21). Thus, the descending pain modulatory system maintains opposing influences, anti-nociception or pain

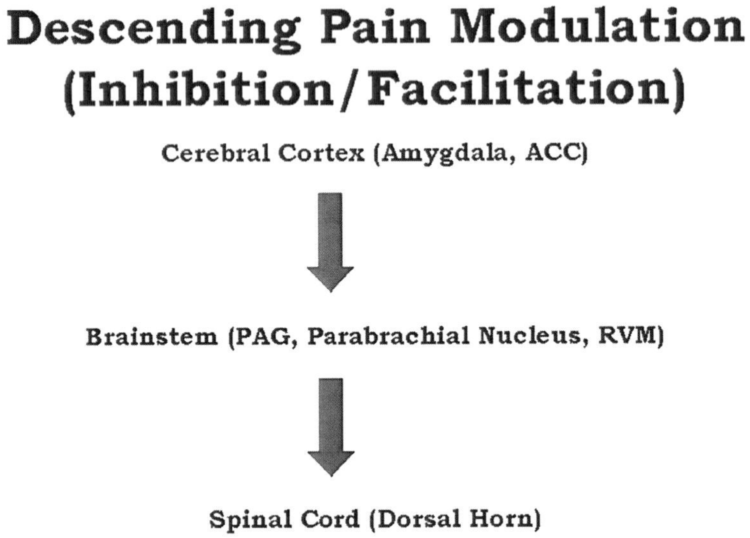

Descending Pain Modulation (Inhibition/Facilitation)

Cerebral Cortex (Amygdala, ACC)

Brainstem (PAG, Parabrachial Nucleus, RVM)

Spinal Cord (Dorsal Horn)

Fig. 4. Descending pain modulation (inhibition/facilitation).

inhibitory, and a pro-nociceptive or a pain facilitatory system. The neural architecture provides for both an ascending nociceptive and descending inhibitory or facilitatory pathway; a balance is normally maintained that provides an appropriate response level to nociceptive input. However, dysfunction arising from an increased duration of nociceptive input, failure of descending inhibition or an enhanced facilitatory tone, or all of these factors may be important in the evolution of chronic pain disorders *(22–24)*. The final balance of these pathways significantly influences the amplitude and character of the individual pain experience.

Descending modulatory pain processing is found at multiple levels of the neuraxis *(25)*. Recently, it was reported that the frontal cortex and brainstem interact to play important roles in descending pain modulation *(26)*. One mechanism for the placebo response is thought to involve the descending inhibitory pathways originating from the prefrontal and anterior cingulate cortices *(27)*. Using a thermal pain model, functional neuroimaging revealed that cortical sites can modulate afferent nociceptive input likely through the activation of the endogenous opioid network located in the brainstem. Activation of the descending inhibitory pathway appears to be operational in CAM techniques such as acupuncture and possibly in manual therapy *(28,29)*. While there are preliminary reports on spinal functional neuroimaging, until these techniques mature, the imaging evaluation of spinal cord pain processing and the study of the descending modulatory system will require more limited and invasive techniques *(30)*. Functional neuroimaging data is minimal in the descending inhibitory pathways. Some functional neuroimaging work in the brainstem, however, is underway *(31–34)*.

It is probable that a variety of mechanisms modulate nociceptive transmission at almost every synaptic relay site in the neuraxis. Modulation is accomplished by dynamic interaction between numerous neurotransmitters, their receptors and the neural inputs from the periphery, spinal interneurons and the brainstem's descending inhibitory and facilitatory control systems. This endogenous system of analgesia has been termed the anti-nociceptive system *(35)*. To summarize, three principles of endogenous anti-nociception have been identified: *(1)* supraspinal descending inhibition, where depressed discharge rates of nociceptive spinal dorsal horn neurons are detected during stimulation in the mesencephalic periaqueductal gray (PAG) or medullary nucleus raphe magnus. Higher-order descending supraspinal interactions are likely involved with this type of anti-nociception, which under certain circumstances can actually lead to pro-nociception or descending facilitation. *(2)* Propriospinal, heterosegmental inhibition resulting from the heterosegmental interneurons that are activated by a noxious conditioning stimulation. This is the DNIC mechanism *(19)*. Only A-delta or C fibers can trigger the DNIC. Convergent, but not nociceptive, neurons are impacted in the dorsal horn by DNIC. Higher-order descending input may also have an influence. In particular, stress may be a natural trigger for the activation of the endogenous pain inhibitory systems. Stress-induced analgesia (SIA) occurs following threat, restraint, rotation, and forced swim in animals. In humans, athletic competition, sexual stimulation, and combat exposure have been shown to elicit the SIA response. What role the endogenous opioids play in SIA, however, is still unclear, since the response to naloxone (an opioid antagonist) blockade is frequently quite variable. Some forms of SIA, elicited by continuous afferent input, probably act to diminish nociceptive transmission. The CAM techniques of acupuncture, manual therapy, and even rigorous aerobic exercise may utilize these mechanisms to provide pain relief. Given this analgesic effect, these techniques could decrease nociceptive sensitization in the dorsal horn and thus diminish the risk of chronic pain *(36)*. *(3)* Long-term depression (LTD) of synaptic transmission in spinal cord dorsal horn nociceptors can be induced by low-frequency stimulation of primary afferent A-delta-fibers. The role of inputs from the higher descending pathways if any is still unclear in this segmental type of gating.

7. SUPRASPINAL NEUROANATOMY

It is now clear that no single cortical or subcortical area exclusively processes nociceptive input. Instead, human functional neuroimaging studies show that multiple supraspinal targets are activated in a distributed sensory, motor, affective, and cognitive pain network. This integrated network also provides the basis for evoked states, including anxiety, expectancy, and fear that may accompany pain processing. The supraspinal component of the pain system is where the physiology of nociception is transformed into the psychology of pain.

Although some neuroimaging evidence distinguishes acute from chronic pain, there is much overlap. Chronic pain, however, is typically characterized by neuroplastic mechanisms that sustain activation of brain regions associated with emotional and cognitive evaluation *(37,38)*. Unfortunately, there is minimal functional neuroimaging evidence identifying impaired neural circuitry underlying states such as pathological pain. This is certainly an important objective for future research. Attempts have been made to classify the extensive array of neuroanatomical substrates in the supraspinal pain system in order to provide models for experimental study. Melzack coined the widely utilized term *pain neuromatrix* to describe the cortical and subcortical neural network involved in the multidimensional pain experienced by phantom limb patients (Table 3) *(6)*. He also coined the term *neurosignature* to express the influence of neuroplastic modulation in the pain neuromatrix, recognizing the dynamics of synaptic connections that become altered as the pain experience varies over time.

Treede has proposed a supraspinal neuroanatomical classification consisting of two functional subsystems within the pain neuromatrix, the lateral and medial (Figure 5) *(39)*. The lateral pain system consists of inputs from the spinal Rexed lamina I (additional inputs from lamina V) projection fibers, lateral thalamic nuclei and the

Table 3

Pain Neuromatrix

Somatosensory cortex (S-1, S-2)
Supplementary motor cortex
Insula
Anterior Cingulate Cortex
Prefrontal cortex
Posterior parietal
Striatum
Thalamus
Cerebellum
Periaqueductal gray
Hypothalamus
Amygdala

Medial and Lateral Pain Pathways

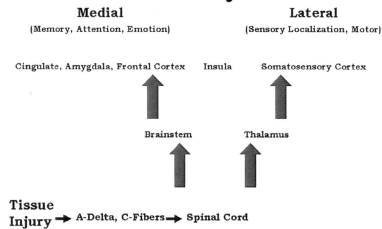

Fig. 5. Medial lateral pain pathways.

primary and secondary somatosensory cortices. The lateral subsystem subserves the sensory-discriminative function of pain. The medial pain system consists of both Rexed laminae I and V projection fibers, the medial thalamic nuclei, and the ACC. The medial pain system is involved with the emotional and motivational aspects of pain. Although the insula is clearly involved in pain processing, it is not associated with either the medial or lateral subsystems of pain processing, but is identified as an intermediate region *(3)*.

It has been reported that the medial pain system is more susceptible to exogenous and endogenous opioid neuromodulation than the so-called lateral pain system *(40)*. This finding has direct clinical relevance. A reduction in opioid receptor-binding capacity has been demonstrated in neurons within central neuropathic pain patients *(41)*. The areas of the pain matrix involved included the dorsolateral prefrontal cortex, anterior cingulate, and insula, along with the thalamus. The reduction in opioid receptor-binding capacity may have resulted in a state of disinhibited nociceptor activity within some of the structures associated with the medial nociceptive system. Persistence of such an abnormal state could contribute to the development of neuropathic pain.

The definition of supraspinal (cortical and subcortical) targets and their under-lying neurotransmitter systems triggered by CAM techniques is still a topic of intense ongoing functional neuroimaging and clinical investigation. The antinociceptive effects of acupuncture appear to be related to effects arising from the endogenous opioid network. The analgesic quality of opioids has been recognized throughout history. The discovery in modern times of the opioid receptor *(42)* and the endogenous opioid ligand, enkephalin, served as a major catalyst in the understanding of pain and its modulation *(43)*. A few years later, the endogenous opioid neuromodulatory system was identified as the mechanism underlying the nonspecific effects of placebo analgesia *(44)*. However, the relative contribution, of the specific and nonspecific effects arising from the opioid network in CAM techniques awaits additional investigation. Other neurotransmitters, such as serotonin, norepinephrine, and dopamine, are also likely to play an antinociceptive role. Disorders of the endogenous opioid network are becoming more recognized. There is recent evidence indicating that sustained pain can be the result of altered endogenous opioid regulation or abnormal opioid receptor regulation or both *(45)*.

8. BRAINSTEM

The role of the brainstem in selective pain modulation became recognized following the technique of stimulation-produced analgesia. This technique utilized intracranial electrical stimulation of the mesencephalic periaqueductal gray (PAG) *(46)*. Pain modulation induced in the dorsal horn by the brainstem was an important advance in the understanding of pain modulation by the endogenous opioid system. Today, the regions of the PAG and RVM are recognized as a circuit known to provide bi-directional influence (inhibitory and facilitatory) for the regulation of the endogenous descending pain modulatory system. Nociceptive activation in brainstem centers also triggers concomitant physiological processes involving spinal sensory modulation, autonomic and motor circuits in an effort to maintain homeostasis *(47)*.

9. THALAMUS

The thalamus is located in the diencephalon. Until the advent of functional neuroimaging, it was considered to be the highest level of pain processing, since the cortex was felt to play a limited, if any, role in nociceptive processing. Nociceptive projection pathways in the spinothalamic and trigeminothalamic tracts ascend from the spinal cord to the thalamus. Synapses are eventually formed with many supraspinal targets, including the brainstem reticular formation, hypothalamus, basal ganglia, amygdala, limbic system, and the thalamic nuclei. The thalamus transmits afferent input to the cortex and is divided into several distinct nuclei that are linked to the cortex through bidirectional tracts. The thalamus can be divided into medial and lateral components. The medial thalamus includes the medial and intralaminar nuclei, which receive input from the spinal cord and reticular system. With selected areas of the cortex, they make up the medial pain subsystem. The lateral or ventrobasal thalamus receives somatotopically organized receptive fields and projects to the primary somatosensory (S-1) and secondary somatosensory (S-2) cortex to provide discrimination of the spatial and temporal characteristics of painful stimuli. Thalamic nuclei have widespread cortical efferents projecting to frontal, parietal and limbic regions throughout the cortical and subcortical pain system *(36)*.

Until recently, deep brain thalamic stimulation was a technique utilized in neuropathic pain patients who were refractory to conservative treatment *(48,49)*. Thalamic stimulation of the sensory nuclei was shown to produce analgesia and reduce some, but not all, types of neuropathic pain. Today, deep brain stimulation for chronic central neuropathic pain has largely been replaced by motor cortex stimulation (MCS). Motor cortex stimulation is effective because it increases regional cerebral blood flow in the ipsilateral ventrolateral thalamus. It is in this area that corticothalamic connections from the motor and premotor areas are concentrated *(49)*. Pain relief following MCS also correlated with an increase of blood flow in the cingulate gyrus suggesting that MCS stimulation reduced the affective component experienced in chronic neuropathic pain.

10. CEREBRAL CORTEX

The primary somatosensory cortex consists of Brodmann subdivisions 1, 2, 3a, and 3b. Neurons in S-1 are somatotopically organized with each area of the body distinctly, but dynamically, represented by a homunculus. The map size on the cortical surface correlates with the peripheral density of somatosensory receptors in the various body regions. S-1 plays a role in the detection and discrimination of noxious stimuli. It is, however, variably activated by noxious input during functional neuroimaging studies *(3)*. The secondary somatosensory cortex (S-2) displays another complete somatotopic map in the parietal lobe. It is located on the superior bank of the Sylvian fissure. Both S-1 and S-2 receive thalamic sensory input and participate in the integration of innocuous and noxious mechanical, thermal, and electrical stimuli. The somatosensory cortices are responsible for encoding the sensory discriminative aspects of pain that include temporal, spatial and the intensity characteristics *(36)*.

The CNS is known to adapt to peripheral and central injury during development as well as throughout adult life *(50)*. Alteration in sensory inputs following stroke, nerve injury (deafferentation), phantom pain, or other highly relevant sensory input, such as chronic pain, appear to modify the functional and structural organization of cortical somatosensory somatotopic maps *(51–53)*. These altered representations, or states of cortical and subcortical neuroplastic reorganization, are capable of promoting adaptive, as well as maladaptive, clinical outcomes. The latter may result in lowered pain thresholds, lowered pain tolerance and the development of phantom pain. The underlying dynamic mechanisms involve both short and long-term neuroplastic changes. Preliminary work indicates that interventions that alter peripheral input by utilizing a correlated conditioning afferent stimulus may trigger beneficial sensorimotor reorganization and improve clinical outcomes in chronic pain *(54,55)*.

The anterior cingulate cortex (ACC) a component of the limbic system is related to many pain processing functions including anticipation, anxiety, attention and the distress of pain *(56)*. The ACC has extensive connections with the autonomic system and is also widely connected to relevant regions of the descending pain modulation system. In a study of affective modulation, Rainville used PET to measure the modulation of the ACC under hypnotic suggestion *(57)*. The level of pain unpleasantness, an affective function, was positively correlated with pain-evoked activity in the ACC. More recently, Petrovic described the shared relationship between the opioid analgesia and placebo neural networks. This study also revealed a positive ACC covariation with the pons *(27)*. The ACC as a higher cognitive center is implicated in the placebo analgesic response, and may serve as the trigger for descending modulation of pain.

The insula is located in the parietal lobe within the Sylvian fissure and consists of an anterior and posterior component; it is commonly involved in supraspinal pain processing. The anterior portion has been identified by fMRI to be related to pain attention, while the posterior is associated with sensory discrimination *(39,58)*. The insula receives thalamocortical projections and has extensive reciprocal corticocortical connections. The insula occupies an intermediate position between the lateral and medial subsystems in the supraspinal pain system *(39,59)*. The insula receives lateral system nociceptive input ascending from the spinal cord Rexed lamina I. It also receives medial thalamic input. The insula projects fibers to the amygdala, the lateral hypothalamus and important sites in the brainstem such as the nucleus tractus solitarius, parabrachial nucleus and ventral lateral medulla. The connectivity of this network supports the view that the insula plays a role in the affective processing of pain. In addition to processing nociceptive input, the insula also processes visceral sensory and motor activity *(59)*. The insula is frequently activated by noxious stimuli during functional neuroimaging studies *(3)*.

The medial orbitofrontal cortex (mOFC) maintains reciprocal connections with the thalamic nuclei involved in nociceptive processing and reciprocally connected with the somatosensory cortex (S–1). The mOFC is activated by noxious stimulation from mechanical, visceral or thermal (cold) stimuli. Along with other sites in the cortex, there is evidence that the orbitofrontal cortex is involved with pain modulation *(36,60)*.

Other sites, thought to be important in supraspinal pain processing, include the cerebellum, hypothalamus, and basal ganglia. A brief discussion of their influence in pain processing follows. Recent animal and human neuroimaging studies have shown that the cerebellum has a role in pain related processing *(61)*. Cerebellar activation in pain studies is apparently related to awareness and escape behaviors but may also play a pain modulatory role. The hypothalamus integrates and regulates the autonomic nervous system and neuroendocrine responses to painful stimuli. Dysfunctional regulation in the hypothalamus is a source of stress. It also organizes visceral and somatic reaction patterns triggered by tissue damage and pain. The hypothalamus is connected to limbic forebrain structures (cingulate, hippocampus, amygdala and septal region). It receives ascending input through the dorsal longitudinal fasciculus formed by fibers from the PAG, segmental nucleus (midbrain) and visceral, motor and autonomic centers in the caudal medulla, nucleus tractus solitarius (NTS), and vagus. A reticulohypothalamic connection allows for the brainstem influence on the hypothalamus and the limbic forebrain *(36)*.

The basal ganglia are interconnected nuclei, including the caudate, putamen, globus pallidus, and substantia nigra. The subthalamic nucleus, nucleus accumbens, claustrum, and amygdala are associated nuclei. Nociceptive information reaches the basal ganglia and associated nuclei from the cerebral cortex, posterior thalamus, amygdala, parabrachial nucleus, and dorsal raphe nucleus. Basal ganglia and associated nuclei appear to play a role in the cognitive, affective-motivational, and evaluative-discriminative dimensions of pain. They also participate in evoked motor responses, and there is evidence for pain modulation in the basal ganglia *(36)*. Abundant opiate receptors are present in the amygdala, suggesting an important role in pain processing related to states of negative emotion and affect. The central nucleus of the amygdala receives afferent input from the hypothalamus and thalamus and has been termed the nociceptive amygdala because of its participation in pain modulation *(62)*. Environmental and affective contexts allow the amygdala to play a role in either facilitatory or inhibitory pain behavior.

Characterizing pathological neural activity in multiple cortical, subcortical, and spinal pathways across distributed neural networks defines a major research objective in pain research. The complexity of pain processing is daunting and most research has been historically based on clinical, behavioral, electrophysiological, and animal models. Modern functional neuroimaging techniques have made dramatic contributions in the identification of the main components of the cortical and subcortical pain neuro-matrix in human experimental and clinical pain trials. Eventually, the brainstem and spinal cord pain circuitry will also be displayed using imaging techniques. An imaging perspective of the entire pain system would provide the first integrative view of pain pathophysiology. As the integrated anatomy and function of the spinal and supraspinal pain circuitry is revealed, new treatment models will evolve which promise to more precisely target the underlying pathophysiology of acute and chronic pain.

11. DIMENSIONS OF PAIN PERCEPTION

Pain perception is a complex conscious phenomena resulting from the integration of neural activity arising in multiple peripheral and CNS networks which process nociceptive activity. An integrative model of the pain experience must incorporate the multidimensional anatomic and physiological levels of organization arising from genetic, biochemical, histological, neurophysiological, autonomic, psychological, and behavioral inputs (Figure 6). These multidimensional anatomic and physiological levels of pain physiology constitute the various targets of CAM interventions in previous and ongoing research.

At least three definable neural states or dimensions contribute to the perceptual components of pain: discrimination, affect and cognition (Table 4). "Discrimination" refers to the anatomic localization of the nociceptive activity, that is, "Where is the pain and what tissue is involved?" In order to answer this question, the brain is required to refer interoceptively to its somatosensory somatotopic surface maps, to access an awareness of the site of injury. Unfortunately, it appears that the primary somatosensory somatotopy undergo maladaptive neuroplastic changes that may promote chronic pain states, as seen in phantom pain. The other question addressed by pain discrimination is "How much pain is present?" The intensity of pain often signals its biological significance. "Is it trivial or a threat to survival?" The discriminative dimension may often dominate the clinical encounter because the patient may be entirely focused on the personal interpretation of pain and its intensity.

Another dimension of pain perception is described as the "affective"; it may lie in parallel with the sensory or discriminative dimension *(63)*. Affective refers to the experience of emotional distress, unpleasantness and the evoked accompanying motivational responses to cope with the pain stimulus. Autonomic responses are a frequent concomitant of affective pain experience because the limbic system processes

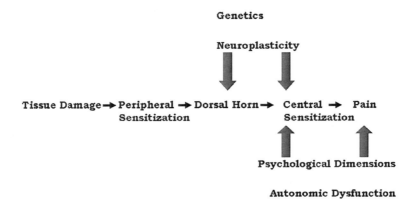

Fig. 6. Integrative pain model.

Table 4

Dimensions of Pain

Sensory-discriminative
Affective-motivational
Cognitive-evaluative
Motor
Autonomic

both affective and autonomic functions *(64)*. Patients in pain are often fearful that their pain will persist and even incapacitate them. The experience of pain then, is a perceived threat accompanied by a negative emotion. Suffering refers to the negative meaning and perceived threat directed at the integrity of one's self *(65)*. In the face of such a threat, there is typically an accompanying sense of helplessness and often exhaustion of the biological and psychosocial resources necessary for coping.

As chronic pain is a chronic stress, chronic pain patients often have disturbances of the hypothalamic–pituitary–adrenal (HPA) axis, with abnormal cortisol levels. In addition, chronic pain patients display an increased incidence of depression and anxiety. These stress-related disorders are frequently accompanied by disturbances in the limbic system including the regions of the hippocampus, amygdala and HPA axis *(66)*.

The "cognitive dimension" of pain perception includes the allocation of attentional resources to pain experience. Turning attention towards or away from a painful stimulus is known to modulate its perceived intensity. Pain can frequently captivate and dominate our attention to the extent that its persistence becomes anticipated or expected. This heightened degree of attentional allocation is termed *catastrophizing*. It may fuel persistent or chronic pain states, because attention amplifies some supraspinal pain circuitry and influences pain perception as described in a recent study *(67)*. The results suggested that catastrophizing influenced pain perception by increasing attention to and anticipation of pain, as well as heightening emotional responses to pain. The antithesis of attention is distraction, which is known to have analgesic effects. The processing capacity of the CNS is finite, so that the analgesic effects of distraction may occur when attentional resources for "distracting" stimuli are prioritized over those associated with nociceptive processing. Cognitive processing also includes the important role of previous pain experiences, as these episodic memories may color pain perception. Clinicians who learn to interact with chronic pain patients across all of the pain dimensions are more likely to increase the probability of a successful healing encounter, as cognitive and affective factors are a dominating influence.

The cognitive dimension of pain experience is known to include a learned component. The underlying mechanism remains under active investigation, but it is likely to include the mechanism of Hebbian neuroplasticity, the mode of CNS processing that provides long-term memory storage of highly relevant information *(16)*. This process may involve the induction of long-term potentiation or depression. The formation of a pain memory may be a maladaptive form of neuroplasticity or learning. In a use-dependent manner, persistent excitation, disinhibition or central sensitization occurring in the pain neuromatrix may provoke and sustain pain memories formed through neuroplastic mechanisms. One (or more) of these mechanisms is likely involved in the transformation of acute to chronic pain *(68)*.

Functional neuroimaging literature supports a model of neuroplasticity in chronic pain in humans wherein cortical somatotopy that underlies the maladaptive neuro-plasticity of chronic pain, (central sensitization?) can be therapeutically modified by modulating patterns of sensory input. Some degree of clinical improvement in chronic pain has been reported *(55,69)*. Conditioning afferent inputs may be modulating neural plasticity, improving behavioral performance, and improving learning and functional recovery in disorders including stroke *(70)*. This approach offers promise as a new tool in neurorehabilitation.

There is good reason for optimism in pain research, as much has been learned over the last 50 years. However, difficult questions remain unanswered, not the least of which is the mechanism operating over the transformation of acute to chronic pain. At present, we have no integrated view of the dynamics of the entire pain system; advances in functional neuroimaging will help remedy this shortcoming by simultaneously imaging the brain, brainstem and spinal cord during states of pain. Insights into the complex mechanism of pain neuroplasticity will be a vital link in understanding acute and chronic pain, as it appears to generate and maintain the perception of pain. There are multiple mechanisms underlying placebo analgesia, clarification of their role could enhance the use of placebo as a therapy. Increased understanding of CNS nociceptive processing and pain perception will continue to evolve, buoyed by the significant contributions from breakthroughs in modern research techniques ranging from neuroanatomy, functional neuroimaging and neurorehabilitation. One day, when these and other questions are answered, many will benefit from the advances in knowledge and scholarship acquired through basic and clinical pain research.

REFERENCES

1. Merskey HBN. 1994. Classification of Chronic Pain. Seattle WA: IASP Press.
2. Innes SI. Psychosocial factors and their role in chronic pain: a brief review of development and current status. Chiropr Osteopath 2005;13(1):6.
3. Peyron R, Laurent B, Garcia-Larrea L. Functional imaging of brain responses to pain. A review and meta-analysis (2000). Neurophysiol Clin 2000;30(5):263–288.
4. Head H, Holmes G. Sensory disturbances from cerebral lesions. Brain 1911;34: 102–254.
5. Penfield W, Boldrey G. Somatic motor and sensory representation in the cerebral cortex of man studied by electrical stimulation. Brain 1937;60:389–443.
6. Melzack R. Phantom limbs and the concept of a neuromatrix. Trends Neurosci 1990;13(3):88–92.
7. DeLeo JA. Basic science of pain. J Bone Joint Surg Am 2006;88(Suppl 2):58–62.
8. Berthoud HR, Neuhuber WL. Functional and chemical anatomy of the afferent vagal system. Auton Neurosci 2000;85(1–3):1–17.
9. Ammons WS, Blair RW, Foreman RD, Vagal afferent inhibition of spinothalamic cell responses to sympathetic afferents and bradykinin in the monkey. Circ Res 1983;53(5):603–612.
10. Multon S, Schoenen J. Pain control by vagus nerve stimulation: from animal to man...and back. Acta Neurol Belg 2005;105(2):62–67.
11. Budgell B, Polus B. The effects of thoracic manipulation on heart rate variability: a controlled crossover trial. J Manipulative Physiol Ther 2006;29(8):603–610.
12. Haker E, Egekvist H, Bjerring P. Effect of sensory stimulation (acupuncture) on sympathetic and parasympathetic activities in healthy subjects. J Auton Nerv Syst 2000;79(1):52–59.
13. Melzack R, Wall PD. Pain mechanisms: a new theory. Science 1965;150(699):971–979.
14. Rexed B. The cytoarchitectonic organization of the spinal cord in the cat. J Comp Neurol 1952;96: 415–495.
15. McMahon SB, Wall KM. 2006. Melzack's Textbook of Pain, 5th edition. Philadelphia: Elsevier/Churchill Livingstone.

16. Bliss, TV, Lomo T. Long-lasting potentiation of synaptic transmission in the dentate area of the anaesthetized rabbit following stimulation of the perforant path. J Physiol 1973;232(2):331–356.

17. Ikeda H, Heinke B, Ruscheweyh R, et al. Synaptic plasticity in spinal lamina I projection neurons that mediate hyperalgesia. Science. 2003 Feb 21;299(5610):1237–40.

18. Narita M, Kuzumaki N, Narita M, et al. Chronic pain-induced emotional dysfunction is associated with astrogliosis due to cortical delta-opioid receptor dysfunction. J Neurochem. 2006 Jun;97(5):1369–78.

19. Le Bars D, Villanueva L, Bouhassira D, et al. Diffuse noxious inhibitory controls (DNIC) in animals and in man. Patol Fiziol Eksp Ter. 1992 Jul-Aug;(4):55–65. Review.

20. Weiss N, L.H., Greenspan JD, Ohara S, Lenz FA. Studies of human ascending pain pathways. Thalamus Relat Res 2005;3(1):71–86.

21. Fields HL. Neurophysiology of pain and pain modulation. Am J Med 1984;77(3A):2–8.

22. Porreca F, Ossipov MH, Gebhart GF. Chronic pain and medullary descending facilitation. Trends Neurosci 2002;25(6):319–25.

23. Staud R, Robinson ME, Price DD. Isometric exercise has opposite effects on central pain mechanisms in fibromyalgia patients compared to normal controls. Pain 2005;118(1–2):176–184.

24. Pielsticker A, Haag G, Zaudig M, et al. Impairment of pain inhibition in chronic tension-type headache. Pain. 2005 Nov;118(1–2):215–23. Epub 2005 Oct 3.

25. Millan MJ. Descending control of pain. Prog Neurobiol 2002;66(6):355–474.

26. Casey KL. Forebrain mechanisms of nociception and pain: analysis through imaging. Proc Natl Acad Sci USA 1999;96(14):7668–7674.

27. Petrovic P, Kalso E, Petersson KM, et al. Placebo and opioid analgesia– imaging a shared neuronal network. Science. 2002 Mar 1;295(5560):1737–40. Epub 2002 Feb 7.

28. Takeshige C, et al., Descending pain inhibitory system involved in acupuncture analgesia. Brain Res Bull 1992;29(5):617–634.

29. Skyba DA, Radhakrishnan R, Rohlwing JJ, et al. Joint manipulation reduces hyperalgesia by activation of monoamine receptors but not opioid or GABA receptors in the spinal cord. Pain. 2003 Nov;106(1–2):159–68.

30. Stroman, PW, Nance PW, Ryner LN. BOLD MRI of the human cervical spinal cord at 3 tesla. Magn Reson Med 1999;42(3):571–576.

31. Borsook D, Burstein R, Becerra L. Functional imaging of the human trigeminal system: opportunities for new insights into pain processing in health and disease. J Neurobiol 2004;61(1):107–125.

32. Liu WC, Feldman SC, Cook DB, et al. fMRI study of acupuncture-induced periaqueductal gray activity in humans. Neuroreport. 2004 Aug 26;15(12):1937–40.

33. Tracey I. Nociceptive processing in the human brain. Curr Opin Neurobiol 2005;15(4):478–487.

34. Zambreanu L, Wise RG, Brooks JC, et al. A role for the brainstem in central sensitisation in humans. Evidence from functional magnetic resonance imaging. Pain. 2005 Apr;114(3):397–407.

35. Sandkuhler J. The organization and function of endogenous antinociceptive systems. Prog Neurobiol 1996;50(1):49–81.

36. Loeser JD. 2001. Bonica's Management of Pain, 3rd edition. Philadelphia: Lippincott, Williams & Wilkins.

37. Apkarian AV, Bushnell MC, Treede RD, et al. Human brain mechanisms of pain perception and regulation in health and disease. Eur J Pain. 2005 Aug;9(4):463–84. Epub 2005 Jan 21. Review.

38. Mackey SC, Maeda F. Functional imaging and the neural systems of chronic pain. Neurosurg Clin N Am 2004;15(3):269–288.

39. Treede RD, Kenshalo DR, Gracely RH, et al. The cortical representation of pain. Pain. 1999 Feb;79(2–3):105–11. Review.

40. Jones AK, et al. In vivo distribution of opioid receptors in man in relation to the cortical projections of the medial and lateral pain systems measured with positron emission tomography. Neurosci Lett 1991;126(1):25–28.

41. Jones AK, Watabe H, Cunningham VJ, et al. Cerebral decreases in opioid receptor binding in patients with central neuropathic pain measured by [11C]diprenorphine binding and PET. Eur J Pain. 2004 Oct;8(5):479–85.

42. Pert CB, Snyder SH. Opiate receptor: demonstration in nervous tissue. Science 1973;179(77):1011–1014.

43. Hughes J, Smith TW, Kosterlitz HW, et al. Identification of two related pentapeptides from the brain with potent opiate agonist activity. Nature. 1975 Dec 18;258(5536):577–80.

44. Levine JD, Gordon NC, Fields HL. The mechanism of placebo analgesia. Lancet 1978;2(8091):654–657.

45. Zubieta JK, Smith YR, Bueller JA, et al. Regional mu opioid receptor regulation of sensory and affective dimensions of pain. Science. 2001 Jul 13;293(5528):311–5.

46. Mayer DJ, Price DD. Central nervous system mechanisms of analgesia. Pain 1976;2(4):379–404.

47. Mason P. Deconstructing endogenous pain modulations. J Neurophysiol 2005;94(3):1659–1663.

48. Kumar K, Toth C, Nath RK. Deep brain stimulation for intractable pain: a 15-year experience. Neurosurgery 1997;40(4):736–746;discussion 746–747.

49. Brown JA. Motor cortex stimulation. Neurosurg Focus 2001;11(3):E5.

50. Kaas J. 2000. The reorganization of somatosensory and motor cortex after peripheral nerve or spinal cord injury in primates. In Neuroplasticity and Regeneration, S. FJ, Ed. New York: ElsevierScience. pp. 173–179.

51. Flor H, Birbaumer N. Phantom limb pain: cortical plasticity and novel therapeutic approaches. Curr Opin Anaesthesiol 2000;13(5):561–564.

52. Flor H. Remapping somatosensory cortex after injury. Adv Neurol 2003;93:195–204.

53. Napadow V, Kettner N, Ryan A, et al. Somatosensory 17.cortical plasticity in carpal tunnel syndrome– a cross-sectional fMRI evaluation. Neuroimage. 2006 Jun;31(2):520–30. Epub 2006 Feb 3.

54. Flor H. The modification of cortical reorganization and chronic pain by sensory feedback. Appl Psychophysiol Biofeedback 2002;27(3):215–227.

55. Napadow V, Liu J, Li M, et al. Somatosensory cortical plasticity in carpal tunnel syndrome treated by acupuncture. Hum Brain Mapp. 2007 Mar;28(3):159–71.

56. de Leeuw R, et al. The contribution of neuroimaging techniques to the understanding of supraspinal pain circuits: implications for orofacial pain. Oral Surg Oral Med Oral Pathol Oral Radiol Endod 2005;100(3):308–314.

57. Rainville P, Duncan GH, Price DD, et al. Pain affect encoded in human anterior cingulate but not somatosensory cortex. Science. 1997 Aug 15;277(5328):968–71.

58. Brooks J, Tracey I. From nociception to pain perception: imaging the spinal and supraspinal pathways. J Anat 2005;207(1):19–33.

59. Augustine JR. Circuitry and functional aspects of the insular lobe in primates including humans. Brain Res Brain Res Rev 1996;22(3):229–244.

60. Baliki M, Al-Amin HA, Atweh SF, et al. Attenuation of neuropathic manifestations by local block of the activities of the ventrolateral orbito-frontal area in the rat. Neuroscience. 2003;120(4):1093–104.

61. Saab CY, Willis WD. The cerebellum: organization, functions and its role in nociception. Brain Res Brain Res Rev 2003;42(1):85–95.

62. Neugebauer V, Li W, Bird GC, et al. The amygdala and persistent pain. Neuroscientist. 2004 Jun;10(3):221–34. Review.

63. Giesecke T, Gracely RH, Williams DA, et al. The relationship between depression, clinical pain, and experimental pain in a chronic pain cohort. Arthritis Rheum. 2005 May;52(5):1577–84.

64. Critchley HD. Neural mechanisms of autonomic, affective, and cognitive integration. J Comp Neurol 2005;493(1):154–166.

65. Rodgers BL, Cowles KV. A conceptual foundation for human suffering in nursing care and research. J Adv Nurs 1997;25(5):1048–1053.

66. Ulrich-Lai YM, Xie W, Meij JT, et al. Limbic and HPA axis function in an animal model of chronic neuropathic pain. Physiol Behav. 2006 Jun 15;88(1–2):67–76. Epub 2006 May 2.

67. Gracely RH, Geisser ME, Giesecke T, et al. Pain catastrophizing and neural responses to pain among persons with fibromyalgia. Brain. 2004 Apr;127(Pt 4):835–43. Epub 2004 Feb 11.

68. Sandkuhler J. Learning and memory in pain pathways. Pain 2000;88(2):113–118.

69. Flor H, Elbert T, Knecht S, Wienbruch C, et al. Phantom-limb pain as a perceptual correlate of cortical reorganization following arm amputation. Nature. 1995 Jun 8;375(6531):482–4.

70. Hummel FC, Cohen LG. Drivers of brain plasticity. Curr Opin Neurol 2005;18(6):667–674.

4

Neuroimaging for the Evaluation of CAM Mechanisms

Vitaly Napadow, Rupali P. Dhond, and Norman W. Kettner

Contents

Summary

Complementary and alternative medicine (CAM) research is entering a new era where state-of-the-art neuroimaging modalities are able noninvasively to measure brain response in humans to both simple and complex CAM stimuli. While the neurophysiological mechanisms of action for many CAM treatments and pain are not well understood and controversy regarding their clinical efficacy remains, neuroimaging research can begin to decode any specific treatment-related mechanisms, if indeed they exist. This chapter will briefly outline the pain neuromatrix and modern neuroimaging techniques such as functional magnetic resonance imaging (fMRI), positron emission tomography (PET), electroencephalography (EEG), and magnetoencephalography (MEG). We will also summarize neuroimaging results for several CAM treatments, though the focus will be on acupuncture, which has been most extensively researched with neuroimaging. Acupuncture is an ancient healing modality that originated in China and has been in use for over 2000 years. Importantly, acupuncture needling often evokes complex somatosensory sensations and may modulate the cognitive/affective perception of pain, suggesting that many effects are mediated by the brain and extending central nervous system (CNS) networks. Other CAM modalities evaluated with neuroimaging include meditation and biofeedback. We will also discuss future directions for CAM neuroimaging research, as this is a very dynamic and evolving field which may ultimately shed light on the mechanisms of action for several CAM treatments.

Key Words: acupuncture; functional MRI, fMRI; PET; MEG; EEG; brain; neurophysiology

From: *Contemporary Pain Medicine: Integrative Pain Medicine: The Science and Practice of Complementary and Alternative Medicine in Pain Management*
Edited by: J. F. Audette and A. Bailey © Humana Press, Totowa, NJ

1. INTRODUCTION

Throughout the long history of CAM, empirical clinical observations guided the evolution of procedures, including acupuncture, herbal remedies, spinal manipulation, meditation, and others. Treatment protocols were passed down through texts and oral history. The "scientific method" has only recently been applied to the study of acupuncture and other CAM techniques with the motivation of elucidating their underlying neurophysiological mechanisms of action and ultimately determining their clinical efficacy. Within the last 20 years, the explosive growth of CAM techniques has been paralleled by the emergence of a CAM research culture. The National Institutes of Health initiated a historically significant development to this end, when it established a Center for Complementary and Alternative Medicine in 1992.

Today, CAM researchers embrace a wide range of scientific techniques with sophisticated research designs. For example, studies may include monitoring changes in animal gene expression during acupuncture intervention to randomized controlled clinical trials of spinal manipulation in low back pain. One of the most powerful research approaches in modern times has been the use of functional neuroimaging technologies developed over the last 20 years. The primary benefit of these techniques is their capacity to monitor brain activity. These technologies are minimally invasive or noninvasive and may be used to study neural activity in animals and humans. Depending on the technique used, neuronal activity may be resolved directly or indirectly with good to excellent temporal and spatial resolution. These technologies include positron emission tomography (PET), single photon emission computed tomography (SPECT), functional magnetic resonance imaging (fMRI), optical imaging, electroencephalography (EEG), and magnetoencephalography (MEG). Data obtained from these techniques have provided new insight on central nervous system (CNS) processing of both acute and chronic pain.

Functional neuroimaging can provide information about which areas within the brain are active. Typically, 3-D data sets allow for baseline and task related correlation of regional neural activity in the cortex, subcortex, cerebellum, and brainstem and eventually within the spinal cord. This view of the functional and integrated circuitry offers a unique tool for exploring the functional neural activity of the CNS. An example of successful adoption of neuroimaging in CAM research comes from fMRI studies of brain response to acupuncture. It was in the mid-1990s, only a few years after its development, that fMRI was first employed to study the CNS neural correlates of acupuncture stimulation. Since then, several laboratories around the world have utilized functional neuroimaging techniques to study acupuncture and its CNS effects in healthy adults and clinical patients. This new era of investigations utilizing functional neuroimaging promises to extend our understanding of acupuncture interactions (and other CAM techniques) with related functional systems beyond the CNS, such as the endocrine, immune, or the autonomic system.

Parallel to the ongoing study of the CNS correlates of acupuncture, there has been an increasing body of neuroimaging data elucidating the CNS processing underlying acute and chronic pain perception. The multidimensional aspects of pain perception (discriminative, affective, cognitive) will require the identification of each of their influences on the pain state. Functional neuroimaging tools can best provide this integrative perspective.

The role of neuroplasticity in pain perception is another research horizon for functional neuroimaging research in CAM. Pain is a highly filtered perception with bidirectional modulation of its amplitude by mechanisms within the CNS. The perception of pain is under constant modulation—either diminishing or increasing depending on a myriad of peripheral and central neural inputs. Chronic pain may be the result of persistent maladaptive neuroplasticity in these peripheral and central circuits. Hence, the questions that naturally arise include the following: Is it possible to reduce or resolve chronic pain by modifying this maladaptive altered state of CNS activity? Are CAM techniques useful to this end? Do they act on descending inhibitory pathways in the CNS thus dampening afferent barrage? To what degree is the placebo response involved in CAM techniques? These and many other questions are currently being addressed in many neuroimaging laboratories around the world.

The objectives of this chapter are to provide a review of the current state of knowledge regarding the CNS neural circuitry underlying CAM and it's modulation of pain processing, including the placebo response. The techniques of functional neuroimaging will be described and their role in the field of pain medicine will be reviewed. The status of functional neuroimaging will then be discussed with a focus on acupuncture—the CAM modality studied most rigorously by neuroimaging. Recent neuroimaging data suggest that therapeutic acupuncture may involve endogenous anti-nociceptive networks as well as autonomic nervous system (ANS) modulation. Higher-order cognitive and affective control centers may also play a role by modifying pain encoding. Although most acupuncture neuroimaging studies have been conducted in healthy adult subjects, the potential for acupuncture therapy in chronic pain populations has prompted neuroimaging research in disease models such as carpal tunnel syndrome (CTS) and fibromyalgia. Furthermore, neuroimaging the specific versus non-specific (placebo) effects of acupuncture may promote its acceptance as a viable clinical treatment. In closing, future directions for CAM functional neuroimaging research will be proposed with the hopes of motivating additional research to further the ever-expanding boundaries of CAM research.

2. NEUROIMAGING MODALITIES

Today there are multiple neuroimaging techniques that allow us to observe structure and/or function within the living brain. For example, magnetic resonance imaging (MRI) may be used to non-invasively acquire high-resolution images of brain structure. A special version of this technique, functional magnetic resonance imaging (fMRI), may be used to assess which areas of the brain are active. PET, like fMRI, makes use of hemodynamic (i.e., blood flow) measures to monitor brain function and is minimally invasive due to its use of radioactivity. Both fMRI and PET have been consistently used to understand *where* processing occurs in the brain. Techniques such as EEG and MEG are used for mapping the brain's electrical activity on a millisecond timescale so are best used to understand *when* during task performance brain areas may be most active. Together, these technologies may be used to investigate which areas of the brain are active and when they are active, thus, providing us with valuable insight into the functional mechanisms by which acupuncture exerts its effects.

2.1. MRI/fMRI and PET: Where in the Brain

FMRI is the most commonly applied method of functional neuroimaging (Figure 1A). It relies on the hemodynamic "blood oxygenation level dependent" (BOLD) effect that reflects the ratio between oxygenated and deoxygenated hemoglobin *(1,2)*. This

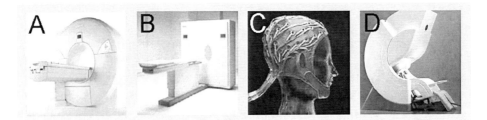

Fig. 1. Modern neuroimaging modalities. **A:** MRI scanner: The subject lies on the table that slides into the magnet bore. This system allows for both high resolution structural imaging of the brain and functional MRI scanning to monitor brain activity (Siemen's 3T Magnetom Trio). **B:** PET scanner: Subjects are intravenously administered radiolabeled markers while lying on the scanner bed. Blood flow within the brain is monitored by mapping the movement of radiolabeled markers. **C:** EEG cap: The cap has multiple electrodes to measure difference in electrical potentials at the scalp generated by currents within the brain. **D:** MEG scanner: A subject sits in the chair and places their head in the helmet. SQUID sensors in the helmet are used to measure the small magnetic fields around the head which are generated by neurons in the brain. (306 channel Elekta-Neuromag).

contrast is used to infer which areas of the brain are active and may be used to map response within superficial as well as deep areas of the brain. This includes limbic, cerebellar, and even brainstem areas all putatively involved in therapeutic acupuncture. BOLD fMRI has high spatial resolution ($1–3\,mm^3$) and does not involve harmful radiation but has limited temporal resolution due to the delay and temporal spread of the hemodynamic response which is thought to peak 4–5 seconds after neuronal activity *(3)*.

Another imaging tool, PET (and a close relative, SPECT), may be used to monitor regional cerebral blood flow (rCBF), regional cerebral blood volume (rCBV), and regional cerebral metabolic rate (rCMR) using radionuclides (Figure 1B). PET may also be used to map specific neuroreceptors using radiopharmaceuticals such as ^{18}F-fluoroethylspiperone for dopaminergic D2 receptors and ^{11}C-carfentanil for opiate receptors, both of which may play a role in therapeutic acupuncture. Unfortunately, the use of such radioactive tracers limits the number of scans an individual may have at any given time. Furthermore, while the spatial resolution in PET can be as good as 8 mm^3, the temporal resolution, being on the order of minutes, is too low to investigate neuronal mechanisms of the brain in real-time *(4)*.

2.2. EEG and MEG: When in the Brain

EEG monitors changes in electrical potentials measured at the scalp surface (Figure 1C). These potentials may be generated by cortical as well as deep structures within the brain and may arise from either neuronal and/or glial cell populations *(5)*. MEG, however, measures changes in weak magnetic fields outside of the head (Figure 1D). The recorded field mainly reflects postsynaptic potentials in dendrites of pyramidal cells within the neocortex *(6)*. MEG is less sensitive to deep than superficial sources because the strength of the neuronal magnetic field decreases as a function of the distance from the source. Although EEG and MEG are good for determining *when* cells may be active they have relatively limited spatial resolution (>1 cm) due to an ill-posed inverse problem.

Most EEG and MEG somatosensory studies utilize paradigms in which trials of sensory stimuli are given repeatedly. Thus, when averaging trials, brain responses that are time locked to the stimulus become visible against background noise. These

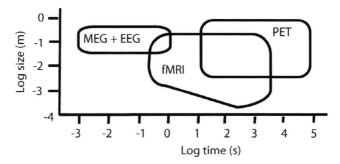

Fig. 2. Relative spatial vs. temporal resolution of neuroimaging modalites. fMRI and PET are most often used to localize brain activity, while procedures such as MEG and EEG have high temporal resolution.

averaged responses are called somatosensory evoked potentials (SEPs) when recorded with EEG (somatosensory evoked fields SEFs in MEG studies). Signals occurring ~0–20 ms indicate signal transmission in the spinal cord and subcortical structures [for review see *(7)*]. By ~20 ms, the sensory signal has reached contralateral primary somatosensory cortex (SI) and may be observed as a negative deflection at parietal electrode sites—often referred to as the EEG N20 (or N1). It is followed by a positive peak at 30 ms, termed the P30 or P1, which also has SI generators. In MEG data, these components are often called the M20 and M30, respectively. Later components, at ~40–60 ms, may have strong contributions from secondary somatosensory cortex (SII), while longer latency components may have even more distributed sources including prefrontal areas. Spectral analysis is another common EEG/MEG analysis method that is often used to quantify signals on the basis of the amount of 'frequency power' present in different frequency bands (i.e., alpha, beta, gamma, theta, delta etc.). However, even today the precise functional significance of these oscillatory bands remains debatable. Alpha oscillations, putatively related to attention, were among the first "brain waves" to be characterized and can be modulated even by the simple act of opening and closing one's eyes *(8)*. Data suggest that alpha activity may in some cases be related to attention *(9)*, while recently activity in the gamma band range has been linked to local binding of stimulus features in visual cortex *(10)*. Activity within the beta and alpha frequency ranges has also been linked to somatomotor function *(11)*.

2.3. Summary of Neuroimaging Modalities

Modern neuroimaging technologies allow us to spatiotemporally map brain networks supporting acupuncture effects in humans. Techniques such as fMRI and PET are most useful for telling us which brain networks are activated and are better for localizing subcortical (e.g., limbic, cerebellar, and brainstem etc.) activity. However, because of their excellent temporal resolution, EEG/MEG are best suited for determining the temporal sequence of activity within active brain networks *(12)*. Figure 2 summarizes the relative spatiotemporal resolution of these different neuroimaging modalities.

3. PAIN NEUROMATRIX

Functional neuroimaging techniques (PET, SPECT, fMRI, M/EEG) provide visualization and quantification of the central supraspinal neurophysiological processing associated with nociception and the perception of pain. Experimental and clinical models using inflammatory or neuropathic pain have been investigated in both animals and humans. Functional magnetic resonance imaging (fMRI) in particular is a valid diagnostic tool for pain evaluation and is evolving from a research laboratory tool into clinical use for the diagnosis and monitoring of pain treatment *(13)*. The functional neuroimaging literature has already provided major contributions to the understanding of the multidimensional nature of pain perception in health and disease *(14)*. These techniques will continue to be used to investigate the relative impact of such variables as affect, attention, memory, and behavior on the complex and multidimensional pain experience. This effort will be especially important in the study of chronic pain, which has proven very difficult to evaluate with neuroimaging tools. The evolution of functional neuroimaging techniques will also contribute to the continued development of research in CAM interventions for both experimental and clinical pain.

Efforts to map the neural networks comprising the supraspinal pain system have resulted in models for experimental study. It was Ronald Melzack who coined the term *pain neuromatrix* to describe the cortical and subcortical neural circuits involved in the multidimensional pain experienced by phantom limb patients *(15)*. The degree of involvement in the supraspinal targets varies significantly across functional neuroimaging pain studies. Supraspinal sites activated by pain processing typically include the brainstem targets such as the rostroventral medulla, parabrachial nucleus, and mesencephalic periaqueductal gray. The pain experience also activates the cerebellum, medial, lateral, and posterior thalamus, hypothalamus, basal ganglia, amygdala, and several areas of the cortex. The cortical regions that are activated include the anterior cingulate (ACC), insula, frontal, prefrontal, motor, and primary somatosensory (S1) and secondary somatosensory (S2) cortex *(14,16,17)*. There is converging evidence from experimental, clinical and functional neuroimaging studies that these supraspinal targets process different aspects of the multidimensional pain experience. The somatosensory cortices are important in sensory evaluative and discrimination and provide for the recognition of pain intensity and its localization. The limbic and para-limbic cortices (insula, ACC) process the emotional and cognitive components of pain perception. A key challenge facing the field of pain neuroimaging will be to measure the contributions of these various pain dimensions to the overall pain experience in clinical pain.

Functional and dynamic nociceptive processing occurs in multiple other neural systems that ultimately contribute to the generation of pain perception. These systems include motor, affective, endocrine, autonomic, behavioral, and descending facilitatory and inhibitory pathways. Each of these neural inputs contributes to the pain experience. In addition, each has the potential to leave a neural fingerprint as an imaging pattern using modern neuroimaging techniques. The elucidations of these interacting inputs are important goals for future neuroimaging research in the fields of experimental and clinical pain. If neuroimaging techniques are successful to this end, they will yield valuable insights into acute and chronic pain mechanisms, which should ultimately translate into therapeutic success.

Neuroimaging of pain can also be applied before and after an intervention that attempts to provide analgesia. Furthermore, neuroimaging of the intervention itself can also provide valuable insight as to how an intervention may modulate the pain experience. Thus, the many tools of neuroimaging can also be used to study different CAM modalities, such as acupuncture.

4. NEUROIMAGING ACUPUNCTURE EFFECTS IN THE BRAIN

Acupuncture is an ancient healing modality that originated in China and has been in use, in one form or another, for more than 2000 years. As acupuncture can be characterized by a complex somatosensory and cognitive stimulus, a potential component of its mechanism of action is the central nervous system. Unfortunately, the neurophysiological mechanisms by which it exerts its effects are not well understood and controversy regarding its clinical efficacy remains. Modern neuroimaging modalities provide a means to safely monitor brain activity and thus may be used to help map the neurophysiological basis of acupuncture.

4.1. Acupuncture Modulates a Distributed Network of Brain Areas

While the most likely form of acupoint specificity lies in the somatotopic response in the primary somatosensory cortex (i.e., the SI homunculus), some fMRI data suggest that acupuncture given at traditional vision-related acupoints elicits activity primarily within the visual (occipital) cortex *(18,19)*. However, such acupoint specificity has been controversial and difficult to replicate *(20,21)*. Other studies suggest that modulation of the pain neuromatrix is specific to acupoints compared to non-acupoints *(22)*. However, which locations on the body are considered acupoints and which are considered non-acupoints has been ever-changing in the >2000- year history of acupuncture. Many of the acupoints investigated in acupuncture fMRI studies (e.g., large intestine-4, stomach-36, gall bladder-34, liver-3) have been chosen because they are considered potent and have a wide clinical applicability. However, acupoints may also be locations with increased somatosensory innervation and, thus, more efficient locations to induce *deqi** (a deep aching sensation thought to be a key therapeutic component of acupuncture stimulation) sensations. EEG studies investigating SEPs at acupoints versus non-acupoints also suggest that although responses are largely similar, existing amplitude and latency differences may be due to increased innervation at acupoints *(23,24)*. Thus, differences in brain response for stimulation at different points on the body may be due to variation in both sensory perception as well as cognitive/evaluative processing.

With respect to acupoint stimulation much of the published fMRI and PET neuroimaging data suggests that stimulation of different acupoints can elicit overlapping response within multiple cortical, subcortical/limbic and brainstem areas *(26–31)*. This includes primary and secondary somatosensory cortices (SI, SII) that support initial localization and early qualitative characterization of somatosensory stimuli. Limbic brain regions (e.g., hypothalamus, amygdala, cingulate, hippocampus) are also recruited. The hippocampus and amygdala putatively support learning and memory while the amydala may also play a dominant role in affective encoding (i.e., mood) *(32)*. Both structures are directly connected to the brainstem as well as the hypothalamus that modulates neuroendocrine and homeostatic function. Coordinated interaction between the amygdala/hippocampus and the hypothalamus may affect arousal and motivational state within the nervous system. Furthermore, many acupuncture studies demonstrate modulation of anterior and posterior insula, and the prefrontal cortex (PFC). The anterior insula has been implicated in the sensory-discriminative dimension of visceral pain *(33)* and may also play a role in therapeutic acupuncture *(31)*. Finally, the prefrontal cortex, which has multiple distributed connections with the limbic system, is likely to play an important role in expectancy related modulation of pain processing (34).

Collectively, neuroimaging data strongly suggest that cortico-limbic brain networks process acupuncture stimuli and may play an important role in acupuncture efficacy. These networks also support endogenous anti-nociceptive mechanisms and are part of the "pain neuromatrix." Primary somatosensory areas also play a role in pain perception and long-term modulation of SI activity may foster reversal of the maladaptive plasticity seen in chronic pain states. Furthermore, modulation of areas within this "acupuncture network" may contribute to stress reduction by shifting autonomic nervous system (ANS) balance, and modulating affective and cognitive dimensions of pain processing. Finally, acupuncture has been demonstrated to modulate cortical areas also believed to support directed attention, which has short-term effects and would mainly play a role during acupuncture stimulation. These topics are addressed in more detail below.

4.2. Acupuncture Modulates Endogenous Anti-Nociceptive Brain Networks

Data from animal research suggests that acupuncture analgesia may be largely supported by endogenous opioidergic and/or monoaminergic anti-nociceptive networks (35). Endogenous analgesia manifests at least partially through inhibition of afferent pain signaling by brainstem modulation (36). Specifically, the periaqueductal gray (PAG) may activate off cells in the rostroventral medulla (RVM), which inhibits afferent pain signaling at the level of the dorsal horn (37). In humans, PAG activity may be triggered or facilitated by "top-down" pain signaling from higher centers including the PFC and ACC. These areas along with limbic regions including the hippocampus and amygdala are activated during pain and are associated with the pain neuromatrix. Importantly, brainstem activity may also modulate opioidergic and/or monoaminergic transmission within the pain neuromatrix thereby decreasing the subjective/conscious experience of pain.

Neuroimaging data demonstrate that multiple areas supporting endogenous anti-nociception are also modulated by acupuncture. Furthermore, some fMRI studies have demonstrated acupuncture stimulation-associated signal decrease in limbic structures including the amygdala (Figure 3) (27,28,30,38). The amygdala plays an important role in pain perception and a decrease in amygdala activity may correspond to decreased affective pain processing. An fMRI study of transcutaneous electrical acupoint stimulation (TEAS) found greater limbic deactivation in high compared to low acupuncture analgesia responders (Figure 4) (39). However, TEAS is different from insertive electroacupuncture in many ways, and results from these studies may not apply to acupuncture. EEG studies also support possible limbic involvement in acupuncture. High-frequency TEAS at large intestine-4 was associated with processing in the ACC and decreased theta frequency power (40). Unfortunately, neither EEG nor fMRI studies have shed light on whether acupuncture's analgesic effects are supported by opioidergic and/or monoaminergic neurotransmission.

While many of the above studies have mapped brain response to acupuncture stimulation, other studies have explored the direct effects of acupuncture stimulation, e.g., how brain response to a pain stimulus is altered by acupuncture. For example, Harris et al. have demonstrated that both verum and sham acupuncture have been found to reduce fMRI pain responses in the thalamus and insula of fibromyalgia patients (41); PET data using carfentanil in this same population also supports μ-opioid receptor involvement in acupuncture and/or sham analgesia. Other studies in healthy adults also

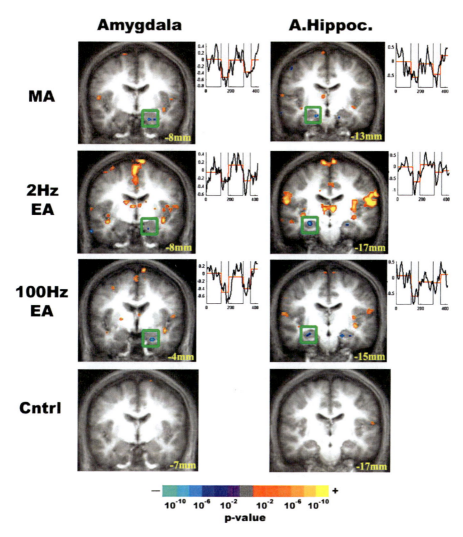

Fig. 3. Acupuncture-related fmri activity decreases in limbic areas. Both manual and electro-acupuncture at ST-36 induces fMRI signal decrease in the amygdala and anterior hippocampus. This decrease was not seen for superficial tactile control stimulation (adapted from Napadow et al. *(30)*).

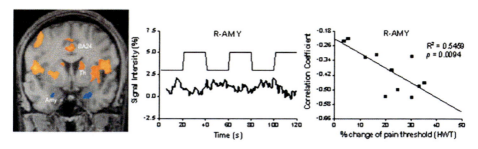

Fig. 4. Amygdala deactivations correlate with decreased pain ratings. 100-Hz TEAS at ST-36 induced fMRI signal decrease in the amygdala. A negative correlation was found between TEAS response in the amygdala and post-TEAS analgesia (adapted from Zhang et al. *(39)*).

demonstrate similar fMRI signal reduction to pain within the sensory thalamus, ACC, and premotor cortex after acupuncture stimulation at either real or sham (non-classical) acupoints *(42)*.

In general, acupuncture analgesia that occurs in immediate response to needling may be supported by spinal gating mechanisms and/or diffuse noxious inhibitory control (DNIC) *(43)*. With respect to non-painful needling at the affected site, the gate-control theory proposes that incoming somatosensory signals carried by large diameter Aβ-fibers can inhibit transmission of pain signals carried by smaller diameter pain fibers at the level of the spinal cord *(44)*. Furthermore, EEG studies have demonstrated that EA may result in modulation of median nerve SEPs due to sensory interference *(23,45)*. In contrast, the diffuse noxious inhibitory control (DNIC) hypothesis proposes that painful acupuncture needling may serve as a counter-irritant that attenuates perception of the original pain sensation *(46,47)*. Intentionally painful acupuncture is less common in clinical practice (especially in Western countries) and DNIC effects are not likely to play a major role in clinical acupuncture efficacy (see 43 for discussion). Furthermore, the time course of both DNIC and sensory gating effects is relatively short-lived (minutes), while clinically relevant acupuncture analgesic effects have been found to peak hours, if not days, after stimulation *(48)*.

4.3. Acupuncture Alters Sensorimotor Cortex Processing and Cortical Somatotopy in Chronic Pain and Stroke Patients

Pain is often accompanied by maladaptive plasticity in primary somatosensory cortex associated with the affected body part *(49–51)*. The reasons for this are not fully understood but may be correlated with decreased movement and increased pain and/or paresthesias arising from the affected area. Studies with carpel tunnel syndrome (CTS) patients demonstrate that pain coincides with sensorimotor hyperactivation and an overlapping or blurred representation of adjacent fingers within the primary somatosensory cortex *(51)*. Our group also found that following a five-week course of acupuncture treatment, there was clinical improvement, partial release from hyper-activation, and more somatotopically separated finger representations (Figures 5, 6) *(52)*. As maladaptive neuroplasticity may contribute to the maintenance of a centrally mediated chronic pain state, future studies should explore acupuncture's role in correcting maladaptive plasticity in the brain.

Another disease population which has received attention from acupuncture neuroimaging groups has been chronic stroke. While preliminary, the results of these investigations have found that both acupuncture and somatosensory stimuli to the contralesional side produce hyperactivation in ipsilesional primary sensorimotor cortex and SII *(53)*. Another fMRI study revealed that after acupuncture intervention (verum or sham), patients exhibited changes in motor cortex activity associated with the stroke-affected hand that were positively correlated with changes in somatosensory-motor function of the affected upper limb. There was a trend toward greater increases in motor cortex activity in patients treated with verum acupuncture than sham acupuncture *(41)*. A SPECT study found contralesional acupoint stimulation increased rCBF in regions surrounding the ischemic lesion *(54)*. While these studies are preliminary, they do suggest potential mechanisms for acupuncture efficacy in chronic stroke.

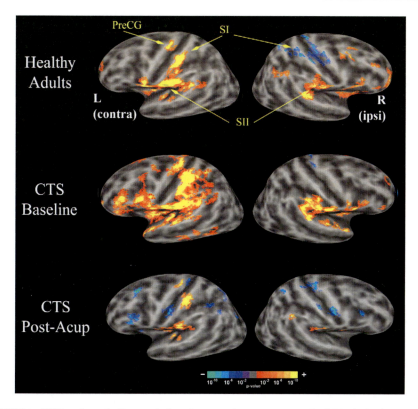

Fig. 5. fMRI in CTS patients before and after therapeutic acupuncture. In CTS the brain demonstrates hyperactivation to innocuous stimulation of the third finger (median nerve innervated) of the affected hand. This hyperactivation occurs within the contralateral hemisphere in primary somatosensory cortex (SI) and precentral gyrus (PreCG). Ipsilateral SI demonstrates less inhibition. After a 5-week course of acupuncture treatment, CTS patients demonstrated less hyperactivation, and more focused SI finger representation (adapted from Napadow et al. *(52)*).

4.4. Acupuncture May Modulate Brain Regions Supporting Autonomic Nervous System (ANS) Activity

Therapeutic acupuncture may also modulate ANS function. In general, it is hypothesized that enhanced parasympathetic (or reduced sympathetic) activity may decrease stress responses and promote immunological homeostasis through altered brainstem and hypothalamic-neuroendocrine function *(55)*. Previous data have demonstrated that acupuncture may be associated with an immediate stimulus-induced and/or a post-stimulation sympathovagal shift toward parasympathetic dominance as assessed by heart-rate variability (HRV) *(56–59)*. On the other hand, skin sympathetic nerve activity has been found to shift toward the sympathetic during stimulation *(60)*. Again, the strength of stimulation may play a significant role in how noxious the stimulus is perceived and in what direction the sympathovagal system shifts. The neural correlates of acupuncture autonomic modulation are also beginning to be explored. A preliminary study found that activity in hypothalamic and brainstem regions correlated with modulation of HRV parameters by EA at stomach-36 *(61)*.

Increased vagal stimulation by therapeutic acupuncture may also initiate fast "neural" and slow "diffusible" components of the cholinergic anti-inflammatory pathway *(62)*. In

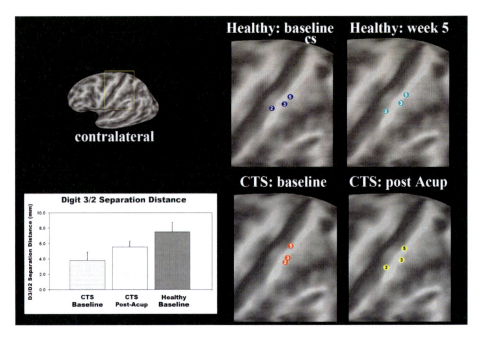

Fig. 6. Effects of acupuncture treatment on CTS Patients. Compared to healthy adults, carpal tunnel syndrome patients demonstrated more closely separated somatotopic representations for the second and third fingers (both median nerve innervated). After acupuncture treatment, the second and third finger representations moved further apart, toward the separation seen in healthy adults. Bar graphs calculated from individual subjects' ROI analysis, Image patches with cluster center-of-mass from group analysis (adapted from Napadow et al. *(52)*).

general, the cholinergic anti-inflammatory pathway is driven by brainstem and hypothalamic activity which may down-regulate macrophage activation and suppress synthesis of tumor necrosis factor (TNF) and other peripheral pro-inflammatory cytokines. Although more research remains to be done, it is possible that this pathway plays a role in acupuncture efficacy *(62,63)*. Furthermore, while neuroimaging studies have noted hypothalamic response to acupuncture stimulation in healthy adults *(27,28)*, recent fMRI data support greater involvement of the hypothalamus in acupuncture response for CTS patients (Figure 7) *(64)*. The amygdala, which influences ANS activity through its connections to the hypothalamus, is also a component of acupuncture processing in these same patients (Figure 7). In fact, a functional connectivity analysis found a close link between fMRI response in the amygdala and hypothalamus, suggesting cooperative activity in these two areas.

4.5. Acupuncture Modulates Activity Within Brain Networks Supporting Attention and Higher-Cognition

Acupuncture modulates multiple areas of cortex including PFC, ACC, and insula. These areas have also been demonstrated to support higher-order cognition including directed attention *(65)*, but their precise role in acupuncture analgesia remains unclear. Previously, it was believed that acupuncture analgesia might simply be based on attentional modulation of pain signaling. To address this issue many EEG studies tested the effects of acupuncture versus anesthetics on experimental pain stimuli. For example,

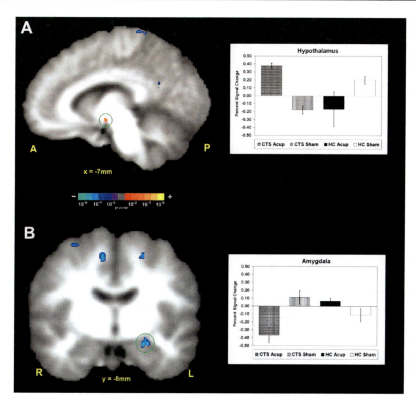

Fig. 7. FMRI analysis of brain response to verum acupuncture for CTS patients and healthy controls (HC), controlling for effects of sham acupuncture. (CTS.acup – CTS.sham) – (HC.acup – HC.sham). A positive interaction was found in the hypothalamus (**A**), while a negative interaction was found in the amygdala (**B**). Bar plots demonstrated that the greatest %-signal change in the interaction was by the subgroup: CTS patients with verum acupuncture stimulation (adapted from Napadow et al. *(64)*).

one study compared the effects of fentanyl, nitrous oxide (NO), and low frequency EA stimulation on experimental pain and found that all three treatments decreased the amplitude of the P250 pain component *(66)*. The authors suggested that acupuncture analgesia might be based on attentional mechanisms. However, a more recent study comparing low frequency EA with desflurane anesthesia on noxious abdominal stimulation was unable to find any significant effects of EA *(67)*. Such variability in findings may be due to differences in the acupoints stimulated and the pain model used. Another EEG study compared effects of verum versus sham EA in subjects given propofol anesthesia. A significant decrease was found in the P260 pain SEP after real but not sham EA *(68)*. The authors argued that acupuncture analgesia is not related to changes in attention since both groups were sedated. Thus, results are somewhat conflicting and whether modulation of these areas is related to acupuncture specific analgesia mechanisms remains questionable. Furthermore, acupuncture analgesia that occurs in the context of acute experimental pain may be mediated by different mechanisms than when it occurs in the clinical pain setting (i.e. chronic pain treated with multiple intervention sessions).

4.6. Neuroimaging Acupuncture Specific Versus Placebo Effects in the Brain

Before acupuncture can be widely established as a treatment for pain management, its specific and nonspecific (e.g., placebo) effects must be dissociated. However, finding an appropriate placebo or sham intervention for acupuncture is complicated by a lack of understanding of the "verum" mechanism of acupuncture *(69)*.

Research on the brain circuitry underlying the placebo effect has yielded some interesting results. Early work with naloxone suggests that placebo analgesia is partially mediated by opioidergic *(70)* limbic and brainstem networks *(71)* which may be activated during sustained pain and modulated by sensory and affective dimensions of pain perception *(72,73)*. In a recent fMRI investigation of experimental pain, Wager et al. explored how expectancy for pain relief modulates the cortical and subcortical pain neuromatrix *(74)*. Decreased pain rating during covert placebo (i.e., subjects were given an "analgesic cream") was accompanied by *decreased* brain activity in the insula, ACC and thalamus while the anticipation of pain was associated with increased activity in the prefrontal cortex. The authors hypothesized that placebo analgesia may arise from changes in the expectation of pain within higher cognitive centers such as the prefrontal cortex and ACC. A similar study with PET used noxious thermal stimuli with covert placebo (saline) and active treatment (opioid receptor agonist remifentanil) administered intravenously *(75)*. In both conditions, analgesia was accompanied by changes in rostral ACC activity that correlated with activity in the brainstem PAG and pons. Increased activity was noted in orbitofrontal regions. The authors suggested that the prefrontal cortex and ACC might support top down regulation of pain. Although both studies support involvement of limbic regions in placebo analgesia there are some differences. For example, ACC response during placebo analgesia resulted in decreased fMRI activity *(74)* but increased rCBF *(75)*. Such discrepancies are hard to explain but may be due to differences in task conditions and/or simply the imaging modality used.

Overall, the data demonstrate that placebo analgesia recruits subcortical and cortical opioid sensitive brain regions including the PAG, rostral ACC, thalamus, insula, amygdala, and in some studies PFC. However, to understand how acupuncture specific effects differ from placebo it is necessary to study expectancy in the context of verum (real) and sham acupuncture. Recently, Pariente et al. used PET to explore brain response to verum, covert (Streitberger needle) and overt sham needling *(31)*. They found that verum acupuncture induced greater brain response in the ipsilateral insula compared to covert sham. Subjects were reportedly unable to distinguish between verum and covert sham interventions. However, verum acupuncture induced greater increases in brain response within ipsilateral insular cortex than covert sham. Verum acupuncture and covert sham both differed from overt sham in dorsolateral PFC (DLPFC), rostral ACC (rACC), and midbrain activation. The authors hypothesized that activity within the insular cortex may support acupuncture specific effects while modulation of the DLPFC, rACC and midbrain may be related to expectancy. However, there were no analgesic effects of any treatment on experimental or ongoing pain.

In a study of experimental pain processing, Kong et al. determined that analgesia induced through the use of a placebo acupuncture needle was associated with *increased* activity within multiple pain processing regions including bilateral rostral ACC, lateral PFC, right anterior insula, supramarginal gyrus and the left inferior parietal lobe (Figure 8) *(76)*. Furthermore, pain ratings correlated negatively with response within

FMRI Activation During Encoding of Pain

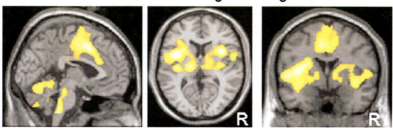

Brain Regions Involved in Pain Analgesia

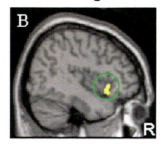
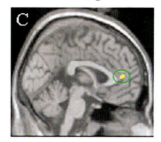

Fig. 8. Neuroimaging pain and placebo analgesia in the brain. A: fMRI signal changes evoked by contrasting pretreatment high pain with pretreatment low pain stimuli. Brain regions including the bilateral insular/opercular cortices, ACC/MPFC, cerebellum, and brainstem showed activation. (A1: sagittal view, A2: axial, A3: coronal) B,C: Representative regions revealed by the contrast of the post-treatment and pretreatment difference (post - pre) on the control side subtracted from the same difference on the placebo side [placebo (post - pre) - control (post - pre)]. B shows activation in right anterior insula *(20–24,46)*, and C shows activation in bilateral rACC *(2,10,44)* (adapted from Kong et al. *(76))*.

bilateral PFC, rostral ACC, cerebellum, right fusiform, parahippocampus and pons. These results differ from those found by Wager et al. *(74)* that showed *decreased* activity within similar brain regions for a placebo condition. The authors concluded that placebo needling may evoke different types of brain responses than those typically seen in studies utilizing creams/pills, thus, differences in brain response with comparison to Wager et al. may be due to conditioning. However, the study did not directly image the acupuncture intervention, nor compare sham with a verum treatment.

To further investigate the specific and non-specific effects of acupuncture, it may be most useful to map brain networks supporting both positive *and negative* expectancy conditions for both verum and placebo treatments. In particular, a finding that verum acupuncture given in the guise of "placebo acupuncture" has significantly greater analgesic effects than placebo/sham needling would lend strong support for the existence of acupuncture specific analgesic effects.

4.7. Choosing the Appropriate Sham/Placebo for Acupuncture Neuroimaging

Choosing an appropriate control is challenging and although several control modalities are available, it is unclear which ones most effectively mimic verum treatment. One approach is to use a "placebo needle" to enact sham acupuncture. Placebo needles mimic the sensation of needle *insertion* and appear to penetrate the skin but actually consist of a blunt tip that retracts into a hollow shaft, like a stage-dagger *(77,78)*.

Placebo needles are certainly necessary when subjects are able to view the procedure that is taking place. In PET and fMRI studies, where subjects lie supine in the scanner and cannot see the intervention performed, sham acupuncture may just as easily consist of simulating an insertion with any sharp-tipped object (e.g., a toothpick in a guidetube *(79)* and inducing poking sensations with any blunt tipped object (e.g., von Frey monofilament). This latter approach has been taken by several research groups *(28–30,38)*. Unfortunately, how well any of these sham treatments actually mimic the sensory experience of verum needle *manipulation* (e.g., twisting, lifting-and-thrusting) remains uncertain and the intensity of *deqi* sensations is likely not equivalent between verum acupuncture and any sham intervention [for discussion see *(80)*]. In general, however, studies should be consistent in their use of control and employ only one form of placebo/sham throughout.

5. NEUROIMAGING COGNITIVE ANALGESIA (PLACEBO, HYPNOSIS, BIOFEEDBACK, MEDITATION)

Hypnosis analgesia has also been explored by neuroimaging. Several authors have found ACC modulation of hypnotic analgesia with PET *(81–83)*. While the ACC is heterogeneous, the pregenual and rostral subregions can interact with medial and lateral prefrontal cognitive brain regions to monitor and induce executive inhibitory control over afferent pain stimuli. In fact, this hypothesis has also been supported by a structural MRI study which demonstrated a larger rostrum in the corpus collosum for subjects deemed highly hypnotizable *(84)*. This structure carries interhemispheric connecting fibers between right and left prefrontal (orbitofrontal, dorsolateral prefrontal etc.) and cingulate cortices.

Self-regulation of brain activity through biofeedback can also affect the endogenous pain inhibitory network. Studies have shown that subjects can be trained to control volitionally heart rate *(85)*, skin conductance *(86)*, and even brain activity as monitored by alpha-wave EEG *(87)* and, more recently, fMRI *(88)*. However, these changes have not seemed to correlate well with clinical effects and biofeedback may be most efficacious in subjects with low susceptibility to hypnosis *(89)*. However, investigators have also explored brain activity biofeedback with real-time fMRI during pain stimuli and have found that subjects were able to learn to control activation in the rACC *(90)*. A deliberate increase or decrease in fMRI signal in the rACC corresponded to a change in perception of a thermal pain stimulus. Furthermore, chronic pain patients could be trained to control activation in rACC and thereby decrease their level of ongoing chronic pain (Figure 9). This study suggests an application of non-invasive real-time fMRI for therapy in chronic pain patients. Furthermore, the ACC has again been implicated as a key brain region for executive control of pain.

Meditation has also been explored to control clinical pain. Meditation involves a state change of consciousness and may increase alpha wave power in occipital, parietal, and temporal brain regions as measured by MEG *(91)* and gamma power as measured by EEG *(92,93)*. Long-term meditation practice may also help preserve regions of the brain, including the prefrontal cortex and right anterior insula *(94)*. In regard to pain specifically, meditation may also diminish laser pain evoked MEG response in SI and SII, as well as fMRI activity in several affect modulating brain regions including the insula and cingulate cortices *(91)*. A recent study also found that long-term meditators have a diminished thalamic response to experimental pain

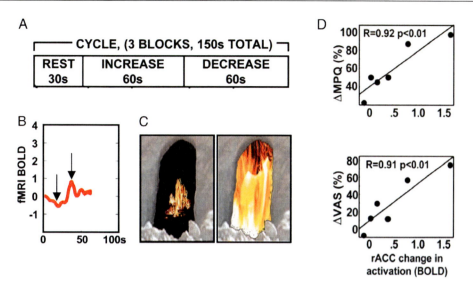

Fig. 9. Brain biofeedback using realtime-fMRI has shown promise in mitigating pain in chronic pain patients. Subjects were trained using the paradigm in (**A**) and visual feedback in (**C**), to modify fMRI signal in the ACC (**B**). The degree to which subjects were able to decrease fMRI signal in the ACC correlated with improvement in pain rating by VAS (Visual Analog Scale) and MPQ (McGill Pain Questionnaire) scales (**D**) (adapted from deCharms, PNAS, 2005) .

stimuli compared with age-matched non-meditators, even though the psychophysical rating of the pain stimulus was similar for both groups (95). The authors suggest that these results are consistent with the notion that while the sensory experience of pain in meditators is as intense as controls (sensory-discriminative), they are less distressed by the pain (affective). This study also found that after the non-meditators trained for 5 months with meditation techniques, their response to experimental pain also decreased in the thalamus, prefrontal cortex, and ACC. These results should be confirmed by other groups, but are a promising step toward deciphering the neural substrates of meditation's effects on the brain.

6. FUTURE DIRECTIONS FOR CAM NEUROIMAGING RESEARCH

There are a number of challenges that CAM neuroimaging researchers must overcome in order to understand the therapeutic mechanisms behind any given technique. One important question is finding an appropriate placebo control. For some interventions (e.g., acupuncture, surgery etc.), a true double-blinded study is impossible, and even a single-blind study is difficult given that we do not know exactly what it is that we should be controlling for.

In the specific case of acupuncture, previous research studies have investigated the effects of stimulating only one or two acupoints simultaneously, although an actual treatment session typically involves needling at many acupoints. Furthermore, variability in needling technique, deqi sensations, stimulation paradigm as well as scanner and data analysis parameters may all account for many of the reported differences in brain response. Thus, it may be useful to devise a standardized reporting system to describe details of needling depth, manipulation style (lift-thrust, rotating, etc.) and stimulus duration. This could be extended to include qualitative ratings of individual deqi responses. Recently, efforts in standardizing the reporting of research clinical trials were made with the publication of "Standards for Reporting Interventions in Controlled Trials in Acupuncture" (STRICTA) *(96)*. Similar standardization should be incorporated to neuroimaging studies. Studies would then be able to be more readily compared by meta-analyses. Facilitating data sharing can only benefit the field of acupuncture research by increasing access to information from around the world.

Collectively, neuroimaging data demonstrate that acupuncture modulates a widely distributed network of brain areas including limbic, paralimbic, prefrontal and brainstem regions. Future studies involving PET may help determine if modulation is linked to opioidergic and/or monoaminergic transmission within these areas. Concurrent physiological measurements (e.g., electrocardiography, pupilometry, and electro-dermal activity) during neuroimaging may help correlate acupuncture related changes in ANS function to brain activity. It is important to remember that the brain is not necessarily the main component of acupuncture mechanism for all conditions. Hence, neuroimaging studies should also be performed in conjunction with monitoring of peripheral effects, local to the needle. Studies that evaluate both central and peripheral effects of needle stimulation in a well chosen disease model may go a long way towards answering which effects are crucial to clinical efficacy and which are simply epiphenomena.

In regard to other CAM interventions, relatively few neuroimaging studies exist, most likely due to the difficulty of incorporating some techniques into the restrictive scanner environment, e.g., chiropractic manipulation in motion-sensitive environments such as fMRI and PET. Excessive noise generated by fMRI can also be a major confounding factor in attempting adequately to simulate the typical CAM experience. However, with improving technologies and the continuing evolution of neuroimaging methods, we are likely on the cusp of an explosion in CAM mechanisms research that will hopefully lead to a better understanding of CAM modalities and of ourselves.

REFERENCES

1. Kwong KK, Belliveau JW, Chesler DA, Goldberg IE, Weisskoff RM, Poncelet BP, Kennedy DN, Hoppel BE, Cohen MS, Turner R, et al. Dynamic magnetic resonance imaging of human brain activity during primary sensory stimulation. Proc Natl Acad Sci USA 1992;89(12):5675–5679.
2. Ogawa S, Tank DW, Menon R, Ellermann JM, Kim SG, Merkle H, Ugurbil K. Intrinsic signal changes accompanying sensory stimulation: functional brain mapping with magnetic resonance imaging. Proc Natl Acad Sci USA 1992;89(13):5951–5955.
3. Rosen BR, Buckner RL, Dale AM. Event-related functional MRI: past, present, and future. Proc Natl Acad Sci USA 1998;95(3):773–780.
4. Jacobs AH, Li H, Winkeler A, Hilker R, Knoess C, Ruger A, Galldiks N, Schaller B, Sobesky J, Kracht L, Monfared P, Klein M, Vollmar S, Bauer B, Wagner R, Graf R, Wienhard K, Herholz K, Heiss WD. PET-based molecular imaging in neuroscience. Eur J Nucl Med Mol Imaging 2003;30(7):1051–1065.
5. Nunez PL. Localization of brain activity with electroencephalography. Adv Neurol 1990;54:39–65.
6. Hamalainen MS. Magnetoencephalography: a tool for functional brain imaging. Brain Topogr 1992;5(2):95–102.
7. Niedermeyer E. Dipole theory and electroencephalography. Clin Electroencephalogr 1996;27(3): 121–131.
8. Berger H. On the electroencephalogram of man. Archiv. fur Psychiatrie Nervenkrankheiten 1929; 527–570.
9. Portin K, Salenius S, Salmelin R, Hari R. Activation of the human occipital and parietal cortex by pattern and luminance stimuli: neuromagnetic measurements. Cereb Cortex 1998;8(3):253–260.

10. Gray CM, Konig P, Engel AK, Singer W. Oscillatory responses in cat visual cortex exhibit inter-columnar synchronization which reflects global stimulus properties. Nature 1989;338(6213):334–337.
11. Salmelin R, Hari R. Spatiotemporal characteristics of sensorimotor neuromagnetic rhythms related to thumb movement. Neuroscience 1994;60(2):537–550.
12. Dale AM, Halgren E. Spatiotemporal mapping of brain activity by integration of multiple imaging modalities. Curr Opin Neurobiol 2001;11(2):202-208.
13. Borsook D, Becerra L. Functional imaging of pain and analgesia-a valid diagnostic tool? Pain 2005;117(3):247–250.
14. Apkarian AV, Bushnell MC, Treede RD, Zubieta JK. Human brain mechanisms of pain perception and regulation in health and disease. Eur J Pain 2005;9(4):463–484.
15. Melzack R. Labat lecture. Phantom limbs. Reg Anesth 1989;14(5):208–211.
16. Ingvar M. Pain and functional imaging. Philos Trans R Soc Lond B Biol Sci 1999;354(1387): 1347–1358.
17. Brooks J, Tracey I. From nociception to pain perception: imaging the spinal and supraspinal pathways. J Anat 2005;207(1):19–33.
18. Cho ZH, Chung SC, Jones JP, Park JB, Park HJ, Lee HJ, Wong EK, Min BI. New findings of the correlation between acupoints and corresponding brain cortices using functional MRI. Proc Natl Acad Sci USA 1998;95(5):2670–2673.
19. Li G, Cheung RT, Ma QY, Yang ES. Visual cortical activations on fMRI upon stimulation of the vision-implicated acupoints. Neuroreport 2003;14(5):669–673.
20. Gareus IK, Lacour M, Schulte AC, Hennig J. Is there a BOLD response of the visual cortex on stimulation of the vision-related acupoint GB 37? J Magn Reson Imaging 2002;5(3):227–232.
21. Cho ZH, Chung SC, Lee HJ, Wong EK, Min BI. Retraction. New findings of the correlation between acupoints and corresponding brain cortices using functional MRI. Proc Natl Acad Sci USA 2006a;103(27):10527.
22. Wu MT, Sheen JM, Chuang KH, Yang P, Chin SL, Tsai CY, Chen CJ, Liao JR, Lai PH, Chu KA, Pan HB, Yang CF. Neuronal specificity of acupuncture response: a fMRI study with electroacupuncture. Neuroimage 2002;16(4):1028–1037.
23. Yamauchi N, Okazari N, Sato T, Fujitani Y, Kuda K. The effects of electrical acupuncture on human somatosensory evoked potentials and spontaneous brain waves. Yonago Acta Med 1976;20(2):88–100.
24. Wei H, Kong J, Zhuang D, Shang H, Yang X. Early-latency somatosensory evoked potentials elicited by electrical acupuncture after needling acupoint LI-4. Clin Electroencephalogr 2000;31(3):160–164.
25. Vincent CA, Richardson PH, Black JJ, Pither CE. The significance of needle placement site in acupuncture. J Psychosom Res 1989;33(4):489–496.
26. Hsieh JC, Cheng FP, Tu CH, Tsai JS, Huang DF, Lee TY, Liu RS. Brain activation by acupuncture with "de-qi": a PET study. J Nuclear Med 1998;39(5 suppl.):205.
27. Wu MT, Hsieh JC, Xiong J, Yang CF, Pan HB, Chen YC, Tsai G, Rosen BR, Kwong KK. Central nervous pathway for acupuncture stimulation: localization of processing with functional MR imaging of the brain-preliminary experience. Radiology 1999;212(1):133–141.
28. Hui KK, Liu J, Makris N, Gollub RL, Chen AJ, Moore CI, Kennedy DN, Rosen BR, Kwong KK. Acupuncture modulates the limbic system and subcortical gray structures of the human brain: evidence from fMRI studies in normal subjects. Hum Brain Mapp 2000;9(1):13–25.
29. Yoo SS, The EK, Blinder RA, Jolesz FA. Modulation of cerebellar activities by acupuncture stimulation: evidence from fMRI study. Neuroimage 2004;22(2):932–940.
30. Napadow V, Makris N, Liu J, Kettner NW, Kwong KK, Hui KK. Effects of electroacupuncture versus manual acupuncture on the human brain as measured by fMRI. Hum Brain Mapp 2005b;24(3): 193–205.
31. Pariente J, White P, Frackowiak RS, Lewith G. Expectancy and belief modulate the neuronal substrates of pain treated by acupuncture. Neuroimage 2005;25(4):1161–1167.
32. Zald DH. The human amygdala and the emotional evaluation of sensory stimuli. Brain Res Brain Res Rev 2003;41(1):88–123.
33. Peyron R, Laurent B, Garcia-Larrea L. Functional imaging of brain responses to pain. A review and meta-analysis (2000). Neurophysiol Clin 2000;30(5):263–288.
34. Casey KL. Forebrain mechanisms of nociception and pain: analysis through imaging. Proc Natl Acad Sci USA 1999;96(14):7668–7674.
35. Pomeranz B. (2001). Acupuncture Analgesia-Basic Research. In Clinical Acupuncture: Scientific Basis. Stux G, Hammerschlag R, Eds. Berlin: Springer. pp 1–28.
36. McMahon S, Koltzenburg M, Eds. 2005. Wall and Melzack's Textbook of Pain. Churchill Livingstone.

37. Fields H. State-dependent opioid control of pain. Nat Rev Neurosci 2004;5(7):565–575.

38. Hui KK, Liu J, Marina O, Napadow V, Haselgrove C, Kwong KK, Kennedy DN, Makris N. The integrated response of the human cerebro-cerebellar and limbic systems to acupuncture stimulation at ST 36 as evidenced by fMRI. Neuroimage 2005;27(3):479–496.

39. Zhang WT, Jin Z, Cui GH, Zhang KL, Zhang K, Zeng YW, Luo F, Chen AC, Han JS. Relations between brain network activation and analgesic effect induced by low vs. high frequency electrical acupoint stimulation in different subjects: a functional magnetic resonance imaging study. Brain Res 2003;982(2):168–178.

40. Chen AC, Liu FJ, Wang L, Arendt-Nielsen L. Mode and site of acupuncture modulation in the human brain: 3D (124-ch) EEG power spectrum mapping and source imaging. Neuroimage 2006;29(4): 1080–1091.

41. NCCAM_Clearinghouse. 2005. P.O. Box 7923. Gaithersburg, MD. 1-888-644-6226. Single copies of the CD are available.

42. Cho Z, Oleson T, Alimi D, Niemtzow R. Acupuncture: the search for biologic evidence with functional magnetic resonance imaging positron emission tomography techniques. J Alter Complement Med 2002;8(4):399–401.

43. Carlsson C. Acupuncture mechanisms for clinically relevant long-term effects-reconsideration and a hypothesis. Acupunct Med 2002;20(2-3):82–99.

44. Melzack R, Wall PD. Pain mechanisms: a new theory. Science 1965;150(699):971–979.

45. Abad-Alegria F, Melendo JA, Prieto M, Martinez T. Somatosensory evoked potential elicited by acupoint's stimulus. Clin Electroencephalogr 1995;26(4):219–224.

46. Le Bars D, Dickenson AH, Besson JM. Diffuse noxious inhibitory controls (DNIC). I. Effects on dorsal horn convergent neurones in the rat. Pain 1979a;6(3):283–304.

47. Le Bars D, Dickenson AH, Besson JM. Diffuse noxious inhibitory controls (DNIC). II. Lack of effect on non-convergent neurones, supraspinal involvement and theoretical implications. Pain 1979b;6(3):305–327.

48. Price DD, Rafii A, Watkins LR, Buckingham B. A psychophysical analysis of acupuncture analgesia. Pain 1984;19(1):27–42.

49. Flor H. Phantom-limb pain: characteristics, causes, and treatment. Lancet Neurol 2002;1(3):182–189.

50. Maihofner C, Handwerker HO, Neundorfer B, Birklein F. Patterns of cortical reorganization in complex regional pain syndrome. Neurology 2003;61(12):1707–1715.

51. Napadow V, Kettner N, Ryan A, Kwong KK, Audette J, Hui KK. Somatosensory cortical plasticity in carpal tunnel syndrome–a cross-sectional fMRI evaluation. Neuroimage 2006, June;31(2): 520–530.

52. Napadow V, Liu J, Li M, Kettner N, Ryan A, Kwong KK, Hui KKS, Audette J. Somatosensory cortical plasticity in carpal tunnel syndrome treated by acupuncture. Human Brain Mapp. 2007, March;28(3):159–171.

53. Li G, Jack Jr. CR, Yang ES. An fMRI study of somatosensory-implicated acupuncture points in stable somatosensory stroke patients. J Magn Reson Imaging 2006.

54. Lee JD, Chon JS, Jeong HK, Kim HJ, Yun M, Kim DY, Kim DI, Park CI, Yoo HS. The cerebrovascular response to traditional acupuncture after stroke. Neuroradiology 2003;45(11):780–784.

55. Czura CJ, Tracey KJ. Autonomic neural regulation of immunity. J Intern Med 2005;257(2):156–166.

56. Nishijo K, Mori H, Yosikawa K, Yazawa K. Decreased heart rate by acupuncture stimulation in humans via facilitation of cardiac vagal activity and suppression of cardiac sympathetic nerve. Neurosci Lett 1997;227(3):165–168.

57. Haker E, Egekvist H, Bjerring P. Effect of sensory stimulation (acupuncture) on sympathetic and parasympathetic activities in healthy subjects. J Auton Nerv Syst 2000;79(1):52–59.

58. Huang ST, Chen GY, Lo HM, Lin JG, Lee YS, Kuo CD. Increase in the vagal modulation by acupuncture at neiguan point in the healthy subjects. Am J Chin Med 2005;33(1):157–164.

59. Li Z, Wang C, Mak AF, Chow DH. Effects of acupuncture on heart rate variability in normal subjects under fatigue and non-fatigue state. Eur J Appl Physiol 2005;94(5-6):633–640.

60. Knardahl S, Elam M, Olausson B, Wallin BG. Sympathetic nerve activity after acupuncture in humans. Pain 1998;75:19–25.

61. Napadow V, Dhond R, Purdon P, Kettner N, Makris N, Kwong K, Hui K. 2005a. Correlating acupuncture fMRI in the human brainstem with heart rate variability. 27th Annual International IEEE EMBS Conference, Shanghai, China.

62. Tracey KJ. The inflammatory reflex. Nature 2002;420(6917):853–859.

63. Cho ZH, Hwang SC, Wong EK, Son YD, Kang CK, Park TS, Bai SJ, Kim YB, Lee YB, Sung KK, Lee BH, Shepp LA, Min KT. Neural substrates, experimental evidences and functional hypothesis of acupuncture mechanisms. Acta Neurol Scand 2006b;113(6):370–377.
64. Napadow V, Kettner N, Liu J, Li M, Kwong KK, Vangel M, Makris N, Audette J, Hui KK. Hypothalamus and amygdala response to acupuncture stimuli in carpal tunnel syndrome. Pain 2007;130(3):254–266.
65. Smith EE, Jonides J. Storage and executive processes in the frontal lobes. Science 1999;283(5408):1657–1661.
66. Chapman CR, Colpitts YM, Benedetti C, Kitaeff R, Gehrig JD. Evoked potential assessment of acupunctural analgesia: attempted reversal with naloxone. Pain 1980;9(2):183–197.
67. Chernyak G, Sengupta P, Lenhardt R, Liem E, Doufas AG, Sessler DI, Akca O. The timing of acupuncture stimulation does not influence anesthetic requirement. Anesth Analg 2005;100(2): 387–392.
68. Meissner W, Weiss T, Trippe RH, Hecht H, Krapp C, Miltner WH. Acupuncture decreases somatosensory evoked potential amplitudes to noxious stimuli in anesthetized volunteers. Anesth Analg 2004;98(1):141–147, (table of contents).
69. Hammerschlag R, Zwickey H. Evidence-based complementary and alternative medicine: back to basics. J Altern Complement Med 2006;12(4):349–350.
70. Levine DW, Simmons BP, Koris MJ, Daltroy LH, Hohl GG, Fossel AH, Katz JN. A self-administered questionnaire for the assessment of severity of symptoms and functional status in carpal tunnel syndrome. J Bone Joint Surg Am 1993;75(11):1585–1592.
71. Hoffman GA, Harrington A, Fields HL. Pain and the placebo: what we have learned. Perspect Biol Med 2005;48(2):248–265.
72. Zubieta JK, Bueller JA, Jackson LR, Scott DJ, Xu Y, Koeppe RA, Nichols TE, Stohler CS. Placebo effects mediated by endogenous opioid activity on mu-opioid receptors. J Neurosci 2005;25(34): 7754–7762.
73. Zubieta JK, Yau WY, Scott DJ, Stohler CS. Belief or need? Accounting for individual variations in the neurochemistry of the placebo effect. Brain Behav Immun 2006;20(1):15–26.
74. Wager TD, Rilling JK, Smith EE, Sokolik A, Casey KL, Davidson RJ, Kosslyn SM, Rose RM, Cohen JD. Placebo-induced changes in FMRI in the anticipation and experience of pain. Science 2004;303(5661):1162–1167.
75. Petrovic P, Ingvar M. Imaging cognitive modulation of pain processing. Pain 2002;95(1-2):1–5.
76. Kong J, Gollub RL, Rosman IS, Webb JM, Vangel MG, Kirsch I, Kaptchuk TJ. Brain activity associated with expectancy-enhanced placebo analgesia as measured by functional magnetic resonance imaging. J Neurosci 2006;26(2):381–388.
77. Streitberger K, Kleinhenz J. Introducing a placebo needle into acupuncture research. Lancet 1998;352(9125):364–365.
78. Park H, Park J, Lee H. Does Deqi (needle sensation) exist? Am J Chin Med 2002;30(1):45–50.
79. Sherman KJ, Hogeboom CJ, Cherkin DC, Deyo RA. Description and validation of a noninvasive placebo acupuncture procedure. J Altern Complement Med 2002;8(1): 11–19.
80. Tsukayama H, Yamashita H, Kimura T, Otsuki K. Factors that influence the applicability of sham needle in acupuncture trials: two randomized, single-blind, crossover trials with acupuncture-experienced subjects. Clin J Pain 2006;22(4):346–349.
81. Rainville P, Carrier B, Hofbauer RK, Bushnell MC, Duncan GH. Dissociation of sensory and affective dimensions of pain using hypnotic modulation. Pain 1999;82(2):159–171.
82. Faymonville ME, Laureys S, Degueldre C, DelFiore G, Luxen A, Franck G, Lamy M, Maquet P. Neural mechanisms of antinociceptive effects of hypnosis. Anesthesiology 2000;92(5):1257–1267.
83. Faymonville ME, Roediger L, Del Fiore G, Delgueldre C, Phillips C, Lamy M, Luxen A, Maquet P, Laureys S. Increased cerebral functional connectivity underlying the antinociceptive effects of hypnosis. Brain Res Cogn Brain Res 2003;17(2):255–262.
84. Horton JE, Crawford HJ, Harrington G, Downs H, III. Increased anterior corpus callosum size associated positively with hypnotizability and the ability to control pain. Brain 2004;127(Pt 8): 1741–1747.
85. Manuck SB. The voluntary control of heart rate under differential somatic restraint. Biofeedback Self Regul 1976;1(3):273–284.
86. Zeier H. Arousal reduction with biofeedback-supported respiratory meditation. Biofeedback Self Regul 1984;9(4):497–508.
87. Nowlis DP, Kamiya J. The control of electroencephalographic alpha rhythms through auditory feedback and the associated mental activity. Psychophysiology 1970;6(4):476–484.

88. Weiskopf N, Veit R, Erb M, Mathiak K, Grodd W, Goebel R, Birbaumer N. Physiological self-regulation of regional brain activity using real-time functional magnetic resonance imaging (fMRI): methodology and exemplary data. Neuroimage 2003;19(3):577–586.

89. Wickramasekera I. How does biofeedback reduce clinical symptoms and do memories and beliefs have biological consequences? Toward a model of mind-body healing. Appl Psychophysiol Biofeedback 1999;24(2):91–105.

90. deCharms RC, Maeda F, Glover GH, Ludlow D, Pauly JM, Soneji D, Gabrieli JD, Mackey SC. Control over brain activation and pain learned by using real-time functional MRI. Proc Natl Acad Sci USA 2005;102(51):18626–18631.

91. Kakigi R, Nakata H, Inui K, Hiroe N, Nagata O, Honda M, Tanaka S, Sadato N, Kawakami M. Intracerebral pain processing in a Yoga Master who claims not to feel pain during meditation. Eur J Pain 2005;9(5):581–589.

92. Lehmann D, Faber PL, Achermann P, Jeanmonod D, Gianotti LR, Pizzagalli D. Brain sources of EEG gamma frequency during volitionally meditation-induced, altered states of consciousness, and experience of the self. Psychiatry Res 2001;108(2):111–121.

93. Lutz A, Greischar LL, Rawlings NB, Ricard M, Davidson RJ. Long-term meditators self-induce high-amplitude gamma synchrony during mental practice. Proc Natl Acad Sci USA 2004;101(46): 16369–16373.

94. Lazar SW, Kerr CE, Wasserman RH, Gray JR, Greve DN, Treadway MT, McGarvey M, Quinn BT, Dusek JA, Benson H, Rauch SL, Moore CI, Fischl B. Meditation experience is associated with increased cortical thickness. Neuroreport 2005;16(17):1893–1897.

95. Orme-Johnson DW, Schneider RH, Son YD, Nidich S, Cho ZH. Neuroimaging of meditation's effect on brain reactivity to pain. Neuroreport 2006;17(12):1359–1363.

96. MacPherson H, White A, Cummings M, Jobst KA, Rose K, Niemtzow RC. Standards for reporting interventions in controlled trials of acupuncture: the STRICTA recommendations. J Altern Complement Med 2002;8(1):85–89.

5

Integrating Dry Needling with New Concepts of Myofascial Pain, Muscle Physiology, and Sensitization

Jay P. Shah

CONTENTS

Summary

Myofascial trigger points are a commonly overlooked cause of chronic neuromusculoskeletal pain and dysfunction. Examination for trigger points requires good palpation skills and understanding of the common referral patterns of myofascial pain. The unique neurobiology of muscle pain and the concepts of peripheral and central sensitization provide new insights into the pathophysiology of myofascial pain. Acupuncture dry needling is an effective technique for treating myofascial pain particularly when local twitch responses are elicited. Uncovering the biochemical profile of active myofascial trigger points and determining the local biochemical effects of needle insertion may help elucidate mechanisms behind the initiation and amplification of myofascial pain and how dry needling works.

Key Words: acupuncture, myofascial pain, dry needling, sensitization, myofascial trigger points, nociceptor, dorsal horn

1. INTRODUCTION

Musculoskeletal (MSK) pain is the most common manifestation of chronic pain. Use of the term *neuro*musculoskeletal pain is preferable for this form of chronic pain to convey accurately the notion that the perpetuation of pain depends upon fundamental and in some cases irreversible changes in the nervous system. Neuroplasticity is a normal adaptive change in the function and/or structure of the nervous system in response to a nociceptive signal. However, in chronic pain, these neuroplastic changes

From: *Contemporary Pain Medicine: Integrative Pain Medicine: The Science and Practice of Complementary and Alternative Medicine in Pain Management*
Edited by: J. F. Audette and A. Bailey © Humana Press, Totowa, NJ

become maladaptive and can fundamentally alter one's pain threshold, pain intensity, and affective interpretation of pain.

The most common type of MSK pain is believed to be myofascial pain, or pain that arises from discrete hyperirritable palpable nodules in taut bands of muscle called myofascial trigger points (MTrP) (see Figure 1) *(1)*. The presence of this type of muscle tissue pain generator is still somewhat controversial given the lack of an objective test to verify its presence and, at this point, diagnosis depends upon the systematic palpation of the soft tissue by an experienced examiner following a thorough medical history. An active MTrP causes pain at rest and may often cause general motor dysfunction (stiffness and restricted range of motion). Gerwin et al. concisely summarized the diagnostic criteria for myofascial pain *(2)*:

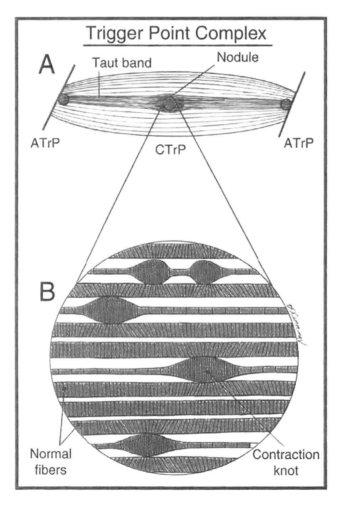

Fig. 1. Schematic of a trigger point complex in longitudinal section. The central trigger point (CTrP) and attachment trigger point (ATrP) regions can exhibit abnormal tenderness. The contraction knots are believed to cause the taut band and make a trigger point feel nodular. (Simons DG, Travell JG, Simons LS. 1999. Travell and Simons' Myofascial Pain And Dysfunction: The Trigger Point Manual. Vol 1. Upper Half of Body. Baltimore: Williams and Wilkins. Original is Figure 2.25 on page 70 of text.)

1. Localized pain in a taut band of muscle
2. Local twitch response to cross fiber stimulation of the taut band
3. Pain to deep palpation that is recognized pain
4. Referred pain to a characteristic distant region based on myofascial referral maps
5. Restricted movement in joints related to muscle
6. Weakness that is not caused by neurological compromise
7. Autonomic dysfunction

A latent MTrP often causes motor dysfunction without pain. Otherwise, latent MTrPs have all the characteristics of active MTrPs, although usually to a lesser degree. Normal muscle does not contain taut bands or MTrPs *(3)*.

There is no standard of care for the treatment of soft tissue pain, in part, because both clinical and basic science research in this area still lags behind research on other painful conditions such as arthritis and neuropathic pain. Dry needling is a treatment technique that has its roots in acupuncture and has been found in clinical studies to be as effective as lidocaine injection in inactivating a myofascial trigger point (MTrP) and providing symptomatic relief *(4)*. Recent experimental data demonstrates that active MTrPs have a unique biochemical milieu that changes with acupuncture dry needling and this data provides important clues about the unique physiology of acupuncture points and the therapeutic effects of acupuncture stimulation *(5)*.

2. MYOFASCIAL TRIGGER POINTS VERSUS ACUPUNCTURE POINTS

In 1977, Melzack theorized that classic acupuncture and trigger point stimulation techniques are generally painful and produce analgesia based on hyper-stimulation of the peripheral nociceptive system, inducing a self-regulating pain modulating effect. He went on to speculate:

> *...the close correlations between trigger points and acupuncture points for pain is remarkable since the distribution of both types of points are historically derived from such different concepts of medicine. Trigger points are firmly anchored in the anatomy of the neural and muscular systems, while acupuncture points are associated with an ancient conceptual but anatomically non-existent system of meridians, which carry Yin (spirits) and Yang (blood). Despite the different origins, however, it is reasonable to assume that acupuncture points for pain relief, like trigger points are derived from the same kind of empirical observation: that pressure at certain points is associated with particular pain patterns, and brief, intense stimulation of the points by needling sometimes produces prolonged relief of pain. These considerations suggest a hypothesis; that trigger points and acupuncture points for pain, though discovered independently and labeled differently, represent the same phenomenon (6).*

Melzack noted a 71% correspondence between acupuncture points and Travell and Simons' MTrPs in terms of spatial location and referral patterns *(6)*. For example, the referral pattern of a common MTrP in the latissimus dorsi muscle tracks very closely together with the paired heart-small intestine meridian described in traditional Chinese medicine. A recent study by Birch has challenged the degree of spatial correspondence between acupuncture points and MTrPs and found a probable correspondence between MTrPs and *a shi* points, which are a different class of acupuncture points. However, his argument is based on an assumption that MTrPs should only be compared to acupuncture points that have a pain indication, which is a misunderstanding of the basic insight of Melzack's, which is based on spatial location alone *(7)*. The actual degree of correspondence notwithstanding, acupuncture meridians, *a shi* points and Travell and Simons' grid of MTrPs may represent a guide or map of where to examine for common "active" acupuncture points, or points that when palpated or needled can influence the health and pain levels of an organism. An overview of the unique neurobiology of muscle pain and what makes a point "active," whether an acupuncture point or MTrP is needed to better understand this relationship.

3. THE UNIQUE NEUROBIOLOGY OF MUSCLE

Muscle pain has several unique characteristics when compared to cutaneous pain with important physiological consequences:

—Activation of muscle nociceptors causes an aching, cramping pain that is difficult to localize and refers to deep somatic tissues.
—Muscle pain activates unique cortical structures *(8)*.
—Muscle pain is inhibited more strongly by descending pain-modulating pathways.
—Activation of muscle nociceptors is much more effective at inducing neuroplastic changes in dorsal horn neurons *(9)*.

In what follows, we will elucidate what is known about the unique neurobiology of muscle nociception to help understand the biological basis of the development of "active" MTrPs and by extension acupuncture points.

3.1. Sensitization/Activation of Muscle Nociceptors

Muscle nociceptors can be activated mechanically, by deforming the axonal membrane of the nerve ending, or by chemical activation, from the release of sensitizing or pain producing substances from the surrounding tissues and immune cells (see Table 1) *(10)*. It is the latter mechanism of chemical activation that is of clinically greater interest, especially in chronic pain where often there is little gross swelling evident. Endogenous substances such as bradykinin (BK), prostaglandins (PG), and serotonin (5-HT) are not only very effective at sensitizing and/or activating muscle nociceptors but also cause vasodilation. Therefore, it is likely that the release of these substances will also lead to mechanoreceptor activation by distorting the normal tissue relationships. A sensitized muscle nociceptor lowers its normally high stimulation threshold into the innocuous range such that it will respond to everyday stimuli like light pressure and muscle movement *(11)*. Furthermore, at sufficient concentrations, BK and 5-HT can directly activate muscle nociceptors.

The nociceptor endings contain neuropeptides such as substance P (SP) and calcitonin gene-related peptide (CGRP) that, when released, produce vasodilation and plasma extravasation around the nociceptor and the release of sensitizing substances from the surrounding tissue. Whenever the nociceptor is activated by a noxious stimulus, the stored neuropeptides are released, which directly influence the local microcirculation by stimulating vasodilation and increasing the permeability of the microvasculature. More importantly, the secretion of the neuropeptides in sufficient quantity leads to a cascade of events, including the release of histamine from mast cells, BK from kallidin, 5-HT from platelets, and PGs from endothelial cells. The cumulative effect is the increased production and release of sensitized substances in a localized region of edema in the muscle tissue. Therefore, the muscle nociceptor is not merely a passive structure designed to record potentially noxious stimuli. Rather, muscle nociceptors play an active role in the

Table 1
Chemical Sensitivities of Muscle Nociceptors*

Biochemical	Source	Effect on muscle nociceptor
Acid and potassium	Damaged cells, ischemia	Sensitization/activation
Serotonin	Platelets, mast cells	Sensitization/activation
Bradykinin	Kallidin	Sensitization/activation
Histamine	Mast cells	Sensitization/activation
Prostaglandins	Arachidonic acid, endothelial cells	Sensitization
Leukotriene D4	Arachidonic acid, tissue cells	Desensitization
Substance P	Primary afferent fiber	Sensitization
Cytokines	Damaged cells, myocytes, immune cells, mast cells	Desensitization sensitization/activation

*Adapted from references 10 and 11.

maintenance of normal tissue homeostasis by balancing the vasoconstrictive activity of the sympathetic nervous system and sensing the peripheral biochemical milieu. With tissue injury the secretion of SP and CGRP increases, leading to vasodilation, plasma extravasation, localized swelling and the release of sensitizing substances that can alter the responsiveness of the nociceptor. The sensitization of muscle nociceptors is clearly involved in animal models of muscle pain and may play a key role in the exquisite tenderness found when firm pressure is applied over an active MTrP (11).

It is now known that the activation of a nociceptive ending is not primarily due to a nonspecific damage of the nerve ending by a strong stimulus. Rather, it is due to the binding of specific substances (e.g., BK, PG, 5-HT, etc.) to their paired receptors on muscle nociceptors (see Figure 2) (11). Receptor responsiveness is dynamic. For example, the BK receptor changes when the tissue is pathologically altered. Ordinarily, BK binds to the B2 receptor, but with tissue inflammation a different BK receptor (B1) is synthesized in the cell body of the ending (in the dorsal root ganglion) and inserted into the nociceptor terminal membrane. Unlike the B2 receptor, which is constitutively expressed, the B1 receptor is inducible and is involved in sensitization of the peripheral nociceptor. Induction and binding of the B1 receptor can also lead to the production of pro-inflammatory mediators, including tumor necrosis factor-alpha (TNF-α) and Interleukin-1beta (IL-1β). Stimulation of B2 receptors leads to only transient increases in calcium concentration and as a result, the nociceptor is less prone to sensitization. However, the B1 receptor is considered less susceptible to desensitization mechanisms and its stimulation results in sustained elevations of calcium concentration, which can lead to sustained peripheral sensitization (12,13).

This is an example of an adaptive peripheral neuroplastic change. However, if the change persists after the inflammation has subsided, it becomes maladaptive and may herald the transition from acute to chronic pain. One can imagine, then, that the degree to which muscle nociceptors in a MTrP become sensitized and/or activated will vary according to the balance of sensitizing substances in the muscle tissue and the threshold of their respective receptors. There may be a spectrum of nociceptor irritability based on this balance that distinguishes a normal muscle from a muscle with a latent MTrP from one with an active MTrP.

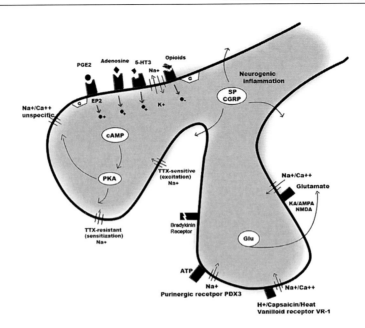

Fig. 2. Schematic drawing of a muscle nociceptor. Membrane receptor molecules for serotonin, bradykinin, prostaglandins, etc. and the intracellular events that increase the sensitivity of the nerve ending are illustrated. (Mense S. The Pathogensis of Muscle Pain. Current Pain and Headache Reports 2003; 7:419–425. Copyright by Current Science, Inc. Original is Figure 1 on page 420 of article.)

3.2. Central Sensitization

The pain and dysfunction from MTrPs may not be caused only by changes in the sensitization of the peripheral nociceptors but also by alteration in the responsiveness of the dorsal horn. A chronic active MTrP may be the nidus of on-going noxious input that sensitizes dorsal horn neurons potentially leading to increased pain or the spread of pain to other segments via central sensitization. Conversely, a sensitized central nervous system may lead to a lowering of the activation threshold of the peripheral nociceptors in a MTrP, which in turn can lead to the transition from a latent to an active MTrP (see Chapter 2). A review of basic muscle pain neurophysiology is helpful in understanding how central sensitization develops.

The primary peripheral sensing apparatus in muscle involves the group III (thinly myelinated, low-threshold fibers, morphologically identical to Aδ fibers in the skin) and group IV (unmyelinated, high-threshold fibers, identical to C fibers in the skin) afferent nerve fibers. These fibers cause aching, cramping pain when stimulated with micro-neural techniques.

The central projections of these fibers share several important characteristics:

a) *reduced spatial resolution* due to a lower innervation density of muscle tissue compared to the skin, thus making it more difficult to localize muscle pain;

b) *convergence of sensory input* from skin, muscle, periosteum, bone and viscera into lamina IV and V of the dorsal horn onto the wide dynamic range neuron, making it difficult to distinguish the origin of the pain compared to cutaneous nociception;

c) *divergence of sensory input* into the dorsal horn with sustained noxious input leads to the opening of previously ineffective connections (this is especially true of group IV fibers in animal models, which then begin to respond to lower levels of stimulation, i.e., mechanical allodynia) *(11)*.

Compared to normal muscle and muscle with latent MTrPs, a muscle with active MTrPs is more tender and mechanically sensitive, suggesting that peripheral nociceptors are already sensitized. Once sensitized, the group IV afferents will fire at lower thresholds, even though they are normally high-threshold nociceptors. For example, in animal models, injection of bradykinin into muscle will cause the group IV afferents to respond to much lower levels of stimulation (i.e., they become sensitized) *(14)*. Muscle tenderness is mainly due to the sensitization of muscle nociceptors by protons, BK, prostaglandins, and serotonin. Presumably, then, peripheral sensitization by these substances contributes to the tenderness seen in active MTrPs and may contribute to the pain that individuals with active MTrPs describe. For example, in an active MTrP, the stretch of muscles with normal movement may now be sufficient to activate nociceptors that normally are high threshold and would not respond to this type of mechanical activation, thus causing pain.

With the lowering of the activation threshold, the peripheral nociceptors in muscle will fire more readily and can induce central sensitization. In animal models of pain, a nociceptive input from skeletal muscle is much more effective at inducing neuroplastic changes in the spinal cord than is input from the skin *(9)*. Experimentally induced myositis in animal models causes a marked expansion of the response of second-order neurons in the muscle's target area of the dorsal horn. Hoheisel et al. found that noxious input from the gastrocsoleus (L5) muscle after a localized inflammatory reaction was created, also activated second-order neurons in the L3 segment. This segment would ordinarily not be activated by noxious stimulation of the gastrocsoleus in non-inflamed muscle *(15)*. The expansion of the receptive field in the dorsal horn is a result of a central sensitization—i.e., the L3 dorsal horn neurons have become hyperexcitable via previously ineffective afferent inputs due to the continuous nociceptive drive from this L5 muscle and now the L3 segment responds to an input from muscle that it previously did not *(11)*.

The expansion of the receptive field in the spinal cord with myositis-induced excitation is clinically relevant because it can help explain the unusual referral patterns seen in MPS. For example, MTrPs in the suboccipital muscles may refer to the frontal region of the head and MTrPs in the piriformis may cause sciatica (see Chapter 1). In addition, this observed phenomenon in animal models of muscle pain could begin to explain the spread of muscle pain to other segments that many patients experience over time with chronic myofascial pain syndrome (MPS). It also can explain the hyperalgesia many patients report because many of these neurons are hyperexcitable. How do these myositis-induced changes in the spinal cord occur? In what follows, we will show that the changes represent a type of rewiring of the nervous system in response to sustained peripheral drive of an irritable muscle nociceptor (e.g., a MTrP).

3.3. Synaptic Connections in the Dorsal Horn

There are at least two functional types of synaptic connections in the dorsal horn. One is an *effective* synapse—where action potentials arriving at the pre-synaptic portion of the synapse exert a strong influence on the post-synaptic or 2nd order neuron. There are a much larger number of *ineffective* synapses between primary afferents and second-order neurons—ineffective because they don't influence the post-synaptic neuron in a way that will cause it to fire under normal circumstances. These ineffective synapses are multi-segmental, and there is anatomical evidence that deep somatic afferents can ramify and enter the dorsal horn at up to six to seven segments (see Chapter 2).

The excitatory amino acid glutamate is the pre-synaptic transmitter for nociceptive information in dorsal horn neurons and can act on N-methyl-D-aspartate (NMDA) and the alpha-amino-3-hydroxy-5-methyl-4-isoxazolepropionic acid (AMPA) receptors at the post-synaptic site. Under normal conditions, only the AMPA channel is active— so, if one sustains a blow to a muscle, then a short train of nociceptive impulses from the injured muscle will cause the pre-synaptic site in the dorsal horn to release glutamate. This causes a brief activation of the AMPA receptor and post-synaptic neuron. An ineffective synapse doesn't have AMPA channels and so even though the train of impulses may reach segments of the dorsal horn that are normally thought to be outside the myotome of the injured muscle, the second-order neurons will not fire at these levels. However, with an intense or prolonged noxious input, SP will start to co-release with glutamate. If this noxious barrage continues and sufficient quantities of SP are released, the NMDA channel will become responsive to glutamate and open up, allowing the entry of calcium into the cell. The rush of calcium ions into the second-order neuron activates enzymes, leading to a cascade of events that eventually causes the *de novo synthesis* of AMPA receptors in what were previously ineffective synapses. In this way, the release of SP in the dorsal horn in sufficient quantities will increase the efficacy of synaptic connections in the spinal cord, allowing the multi-segmental spread of noxious input. This explains how action potentials emanating from nociceptors in an L5 muscle can then excite neurons in the L3 segment *(11)*.

4. MYOFASCIAL TRIGGER POINTS AND DRY NEEDLING

Myofascial pain associated with MTrPs is a common cause of non-articular musculoskeletal pain. In a community-based chronic pain clinic, Gerwin et al. found that MTrPs were the primary source of pain in 74% of 96 patients with musculoskeletal pain *(16)*. Similarly, Fishbain et al. found that MTrPs were the primary source of pain in 85% of 283 patients consecutively admitted to a comprehensive pain center *(17)*. Myofascial trigger points should be considered in the differential diagnosis of any musculoskeletal condition and are often an overlooked cause of pain in individuals with co-existing joint or visceral disease, including cervical disc lesions, hip osteoarthritis, temporomandibular joint disorders, pelvic pain, headaches and epicondylitis *(18–22)*.

The author's preference for treatment of MTrPs is to use a 32-gauge acupuncture needle for dry needling. An acupuncture needle has a rounded tip compared to the beveled edge of a hypodermic needle and is therefore less painful and less traumatic to tissue. Furthermore, it affords the clinician superior proprioceptive feedback that is very helpful in guiding the needle toward the active MTrPs, which are often firm and initially resistant to needle passage.

In clinical practice, identifying the precise location of the MTrP during injection or dry needling is more important than the type of anesthetic solution injected. The local twitch response (LTR) is a valuable clinical indicator that confirms the accurate location of the MTrP. Furthermore, it is essential to elicit local twitch responses while needling to obtain the desired clinical effect *(4)*. Lewit determined that the effects of dry needling are primarily due to the mechanical stimulation of a MTrP. In his study, treating MTrPs with an acupuncture dry needling technique resulted in immediate pain relief in nearly 87% of the treated sites. Lewit also found that pain relief was permanent in over 31% of the subjects (20% experienced several months, 22% several weeks and 11% several days of pain relief). Only 14% of subjects had no pain relief *(23)*. There is evidence that needling MTrPs in one muscle group may eliminate MTrPs in muscles that belong to the referred pain area of the treated MTrPs *(24)*. How does dry needling work? In order to answer that question, a better understanding of the pathophysiology of MTrPs is needed.

5. UNCOVERING THE BIOCHEMICAL MILIEU OF MYOFASCIAL TRIGGER POINTS

A team at the National Institutes of Health designed a clinical protocol to assess the local biochemical milieu of MTrPs. A novel 32-gauge microdialysis needle was fabricated that is capable of collecting small volumes ($\sim$0.5 µl), at sub-nanogram levels of solutes <75 kDa, from muscle tissue. With such a device it was possible to study the local muscle biochemical milieu in subjects with and without pain and with and without MTrPs at GB-21 in the upper trapezius muscle. This is the most common MTrP in the body and has a unique referral pattern of pain (Figure 3). Furthermore, this needle has the same size, shape and handling characteristics of an acupuncture needle and allows simultaneous sampling of the local biochemical milieu of muscle before, during and after a local twitch response is elicited with the same needle *(5)* (Figure 4).

Three subjects were selected based on history and physical examination to be in each of 3 groups (total 9 subjects): Group 1—*Normal* (no neck pain, no MTrP); Group 2—*Latent* (no neck pain, MTrP present); Group 3—*Active* (neck pain, MTrP present). Samples were obtained continuously with the microdialysis needle at regular intervals, including at the time of needle insertion, elicitation of a local twitch response, and post twitch.

The main outcome measures were concentration levels of protons (pH), substance P (SP), calcitonin gene-related peptide (CGRP), bradykinin, serotonin, norepinephrine, tumor necrosis factor-alpha (TNF-α), and Interleukin -1beta (IL-1β) determined by analysis of samples.

Overall the amounts of SP, CGRP, bradykinin, serotonin, norepinephrine, TNF-α, and IL-1β were significantly higher in the *Active* group than either of the other two groups ($p < 0.01$). The pH was also significantly lower in the *Active* group than the other two groups ($p < 0.03$). In the *Active* group, the amounts of SP and CGRP were significantly lower at the end of sampling (post twitch) than at baseline ($p < 0.02$) (Figures 5, 6).

Subjects with active MTrPs and greater pain levels (i.e., lower pressure pain sensitivities) had lower pH levels in the vicinity of their MTrPs. A positive correlation has previously been shown between pain and local acidity *(25)*. In a rat model, Sluka et al. found that repeated injections of acidic saline into one gastrocnemius muscle produced *bilateral*, long-lasting mechanical hypersensitivity (i.e., hyperalgesia) of the paw *(26)*. Sluka found that the degree of nociceptor activation correlated with increasing acidity of the saline injected. The hyperalgesia was reversed by spinally administered µ- or ∂-opioid receptor agonists *(27)* or N-methyl-D-aspartate (NMDA) or non-NMDA ionotropic glutamate receptor antagonists *(28)*. This model demonstrates secondary mechanical hyperalgesia is maintained by neuroplastic changes in the CNS. Furthermore, the persistent mechanical hyperalgesia was not caused by muscle tissue

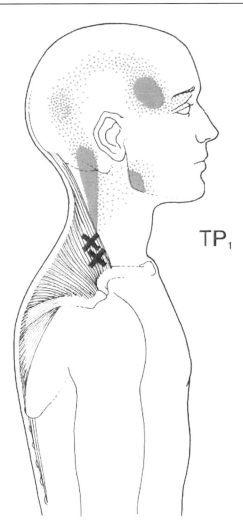

Fig. 3. Referred pain pattern and location of (X) of central trigger point 1, identical to GB-21, in the upper trapezius muscle. (Simons DG, Travell JG, Simons LS. 1999. Travell And Simons' Myofascial Pain and Dysfunction: The Trigger Point Manual. Vol 1. Upper Half of Body. Baltimore: Williams and Wilkins. Original is Figure 6.1 on page 279 of text.)

damage and did not require continuous nociceptive input from the site of injury. That is, the hyperalgesia persisted even after the cessation of acid administration *(25)*.

Therefore, an acidic milieu alone (without muscle damage) is sufficient to cause profound changes in the properties of nociceptors, axons, and dorsal horn neurons (i.e., the pain matrix). This model elegantly demonstrated that secondary mechanical hyperalgesia is maintained by neuroplastic changes in the central nervous system. Mechanical hyperalgesia is a hallmark of a MTrP. An acidic pH is well known to stimulate the production of bradykinin during local ischemia and inflammation and may further explain the cause of pain in patients with an active MTrP.

Significantly elevated levels of SP and CGRP were also found in the vicinity of the active MTrPs. As mentioned in the previous section, prolonged nociceptor activation is known to greatly increase the amount of SP that is transported orthodromically from

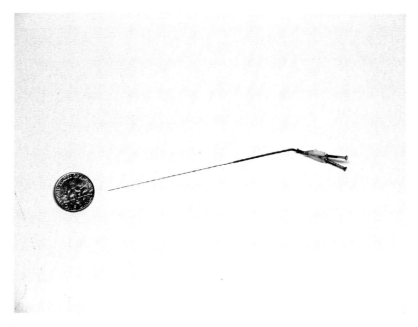

Fig. 4. Microdialysis needle. This 32-gauge device has the size, shape, and handling properties of an acupuncture needle and, likewise, is designed to be minimally invasive. (Shah JP, Phillips TM, Danoff JV, Gerber LH. An in vivo microanalytical technique for measuring the local biochemical milieu of human skeletal muscle. J Appl Physiol 2005 Nov;99(5):1977–84. Epub 2005 Jul 21. Original is Figure 2 on page 1978 of article.)

the dorsal root ganglion into the dorsal horn of the spinal cord and this process can lead directly to neuroplastic changes. However, in this study, it was demonstrated that the neuropeptides SP and CGRP were transported antidromically along the primary afferent axon and secreted in the peripheral muscle tissue leading to concentrations that were significantly elevated in the subjects with active MTrPs. SP causes mast cell degranulation with the release of serotonin (in addition to histamine) and up regulation of pro-inflammatory cytokines such as TNF-α. Increases in TNF-α can in turn stimulate the production of norepinephrine.

In support of this effect of the elevated TNF-α, significantly elevated levels of serotonin and norepinephrine were found in subjects with active MTrPs. The increased levels of norepinephrine may be associated with increased sympathetic activity in the motor end plate region of the MTrP. In one study, intra-arterial injection of phentolamine, an α–adrenergic antagonist, decreased the spontaneous electrical activity from the locus of a myofascial trigger spot in rabbit skeletal muscle (29). It is believed that this locus in the rabbit animal model is equivalent to the human MTrP. This finding supports the hypothesis that the autonomic nervous system is involved in the pathogenesis of MTrPs.

Interestingly, both SP and CGRP concentrations dropped significantly after the one local twitch response was elicited. The sudden drop in concentration of these analytes may be due to a local increase in blood flow following the LTR or some direct effect on the ability of the nociceptors to secrete neuropeptides, perhaps via mechanical hyperpolarization of the nerve ending. This effect also leads to the question of whether the commonly observed (at least temporary) decrease in pain after the

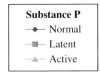

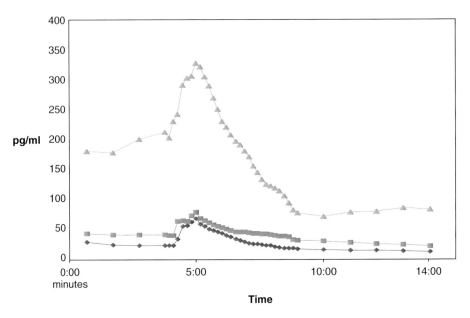

Fig. 5. Concentration of Substance P (SP) over time. A local twitch response (LTR) was elicited at 5 minutes in subjects in the Active and Latent groups. Only in the Active group was this followed by a rapid decline in SP to a concentration below that compared to initial needle insertion

release of a MTrP is causally related in some way to the change in concentration of these neuropeptides. Physiologically, the LTR may also induce chemical changes in the local environment of the nociceptor and thereby interfere with the responsiveness of the nociceptor membrane channels, raising its firing threshold and reducing pain transmission.

These experimental findings pose additional questions as to whether MTrPs are local phenomena, dependent upon a process of segmental sensitization initiated by some form of local trauma, which ultimately persists; or whether individuals who develop active MTrPs have a more systemic neuroendocrine dysregulation that would lead to sites remote from active or latent MTrPs to have similar biochemical profiles to the MTrP itself. These remote sites should be evaluated to help distinguish whether MTrPs have unique biochemical profiles or are associated with a more widespread phenomenon. To answer this question an unaffected muscle without MTrPs, the gastrocnemius, was identified and sampled for its biochemical milieu in subjects with active, latent, and absent MTrPs in the upper trapezius in a new series of subjects using the same paradigm as aforementioned.

Preliminary unpublished findings confirmed that at needle insertion in the upper trapezius muscle the concentrations of the analytes such as SP, CGRP, serotonin, bradykinin, TNF-α and so on were significantly higher in the *Active* group when compared to the *Latent* and *Normal* groups. Significant differences in analyte levels at

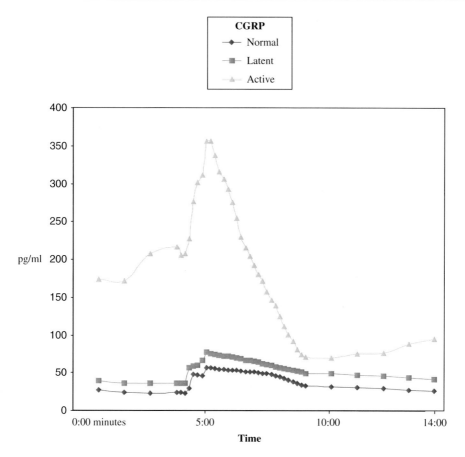

Fig. 6. Concentration of calcitonin gene-related peptide (CGRP) over time. A local twitch response (LTR) was elicited at 5 minutes in subjects in the Active and Latent groups. Only in the Active group was this followed by a rapid decline in CGRP to a concentration below that compared to initial needle insertion

needle insertion were demonstrated between the area sampled in the trapezius (active MTrP) and the normal, non-painful gastrocnemius in the same subject, suggesting that the vicinity of the active MTrP exhibits a unique biochemical milieu of substances associated with pain and inflammation. Further studies and analyses are on going.

6. CONCLUSION

Myofascial trigger points are a common cause of neuromusculoskeletal pain and dysfunction. Active myofascial trigger points function as dynamic foci of peripheral nociception that can initiate, accentuate, and maintain central sensitization and chronic pain states. Continuous nociceptive input from myofascial trigger points can increase excitability of dorsal horn neurons (causing allodynia and hyperalgesia) and open ineffective synapses—resulting in new receptive fields and referral of pain.

Until now, the distinction between active and latent myofascial trigger points depended solely upon the palpation skills and clinical acumen of the examiner and the subjective responses of the patient. Active and latent myofascial trigger points share the same physical findings—i.e., a hyperirritable nodule in a taut band of muscle. As a result clinicians must rely on historical factors such as the description of pain at rest and provocative tests, attempting to reproduce the patient's pain and referral pattern with deep palpation. In clinical practice, the diagnosis of myofascial pain is confirmed retrospectively if, after identification and treatment of the myofascial trigger points, the patient's pain is eliminated or reduced. However, given the lack of high quality randomized controlled studies using standard treatment protocols for MPS, the benefit an individual patient may receive by local treatment is often attributed to the placebo effect.

The application of a minimally invasive micro-analytical technique to sample the biochemical milieu of active versus latent MTrPs demonstrates that there is now objective data to confirm the clinical distinction between subjects with active myofascial trigger points from those with either latent myofascial trigger points or muscle without myofascial trigger points in the upper trapezius. Furthermore, the biochemical milieu of the *Active* group is distinguished by elevated concentrations of a variety of biochemicals (inflammatory mediators, neuropeptides, catecholamines cytokines, etc.) that can sensitize and/or activate muscle nociceptors, thereby providing an enhanced explanatory model of why they have pain.

In essence, then, by learning to carefully examine and distinguish between active and latent myofascial trigger points when evaluating patients with chronic pain and dysfunction one can, in effect, identify the presence of a facilitated nervous system. This which involves changes both in the peripheral nociceptor and centrally in the dorsal horn leading to central sensitization and pathological neuroplastic changes in pain processing.

This data also supports that acupuncture dry needling may be an effective technique for deactivating myofascial trigger points. Uncovering the biochemical profile of active myofascial trigger points and determining the local effects of needle insertion may help elucidate mechanisms behind the initiation and amplification of myofascial pain, allowing targeted pharmacologic treatments. It may also explain how acupuncture dry needling and other physical modalities work at the local level.

REFERENCES

1. Simons DG. Myofascial pain syndromes: One term but two concepts; a new understanding. Invited editorial. J Musculoskeletal Pain 1995;3(1).
2. Gerwin RD, Shannon S, Hong CZ et al. Interrater reliability in myofascial trigger point examination. Pain 1997;69(1–2):65–73.
3. Simons DG, Travell JG, Simons LS. Travell and Simons' Myofascial Pain and Dysfunction: the Trigger Point Manual. Volume 1. Upper Half of Body. Baltimore: Williams and Wilkins. 1999.
4. Hong CZ. Lidocaine injection versus dry needling to myofascial trigger point. The importance of the local twitch response. Am J Phys Med Rehabil 1994;73(4):256–263.
5. Shah JP, Phillips TM, Danoff JV, Gerber LH. An in vivo micro analytical technique for measuring the local biochemical milieu of human skeletal muscle. J Appl Physiol 2005;99(5):1977–1984 [Epub 2005 Jul 21].
6. Melzack R. Trigger points and acupuncture points for pain: correlations and implications. Pain 1977; 3(1):3–23 (Review).
7. Birch S. Trigger point-acupuncture point correlations revisited. J Altern Complement Med 2003;9(1):91–103.
8. Svensson P, Minoshima S, Beydoun A, Morrow TJ, Casey KL. Cerebral processing of acute skin and muscle pain in humans. J Neurophysiol 1997;78(1):450–460.
9. Wall PD, Woolf CJ. Muscle but not cutaneous C-afferent produces prolonged increases in the excitability of the flexion reflex in the rat. J Physiol 1984;356:443–458.
10. Mense S. The pathogenesis of muscle pain. Curr Pain Headache Rep 2003;7:419–425.

11. Mense S, Simons DG. Muscle Pain: Understanding its Nature, Diagnosis and Treatment. Baltimore: Lippincott, Williams and Wilkins, 2001.
12. Marceau F, Sabourin T, Houle S, Fortin JP, Petitclerc E, Molinar G, Adam A. Kinin receptors: functional aspects. Int Immunopharmacol 2002;2:1729–1739.
13. Calixto JB, Cabrini DA, Ferreira J, Campos MM. Kinins in pain and inflammation. Pain 2000;87:1–5.
14. Hoheisel U, Mense S, Simons DG. Yu XM. Appearance of new receptive fields in rat dorsal horn neurons following noxious stimulation of skeletal muscle: a model of referral of muscle pain? Neurosci Lett 1993;153:9–12.
15. Hoheisel U, Koch K, Mense S. Functional reorganization in the rat dorsal horn during an experimental myositis. Pain 1994;59:111–118.
16. Gerwin RD. A study of 96 subjects examined both for fibromyalgia and myofascial pain. J Musculoskeletal Pain 1995;3(Suppl. 1):121.
17. Fishbain DA, Goldberg M, Meagher BR, Steel R, Rosomoff H. Male and female chronic pain patients categorized by DSM-III psychiatric diagnostic criteria. Pain 1986;26(2):181–197.
18. Hsueh TC, Yu S, Kuan TS, Hong CZ. Association of active myofascial trigger points and cervical disc lesions. J Formos Med Assoc 1998;97(3):174–180.
19. Bajaj P, Graven-Nielsen T, Arendt-Nielsen L. Trigger points in patients with lower limb osteoarthritis. J Musculoskeletal Pain 2001;9(3):17–33.
20. Kleier DJ. Referred pain from a myofascial trigger point mimicking pain of endodontic origin. J Endod 1985;11(9):408–411.
21. Ling FW, Slocumb JC. Use of trigger point injections in chronic pelvic pain. Obstet Gynecol Clin North Am 1993;20(4):809–815.
22. Mennell J. Myofascial trigger points as a cause of headaches. J Manipul Physiol Ther 1989;12(4): 308–313.
23. Lewit K. The needle effect in the pain relief of myofascial pain. Pain 1979;6:83–90.
24. Carlson CR, Okeson JP, Falace DA, et al. Reduction of pain and EMG activity in the masseter region by trapezius trigger point injection. Pain 1993;55:397–400.
25. Issberner U, Reeh PW, Steen KH. Pain due to tissue acidosis: a mechanism for inflammatory and ischemic myalgia? Neurosci Lett 1996;208:191–194.
26. Sluka KA, Kalra A, Moore SA. Unilateral intramuscular injections of acidic saline produce a bilateral, long-lasting hyperalgesia. Muscle Nerve 2001;24:37–46.
27. Sluka KA, Rohlwing KA, Bussey JJ, Eikenberry RA, Wilken JM. Chronic muscle pain induced by repeated acid injection is reversed by spinally administered μ- and δ-, but not κ-, opioid receptor agonists. J Pharmacol Exp Ther 2002;302:1146–1150.
28. Skyba DA, King EW, Sluka KA. Effects of NMDA and non-NMDA ionotropic glutamate receptor antagonists on the development and maintenance of hyperalgesia induced by repeated intramuscular injection of acidic saline. Pain 2002;98:69–78.
29. Chen JT, Chen SM, Kuan TS, et al. Phentolamine effect on the spontaneous electrical activity of active loci in a myofascial trigger spot of rabbit skeletal muscle. Arch Phys Med Rehabil 1998;79:790–794.

6

Potential Role of Fascia in Chronic Musculoskeletal Pain

Helene M. Langevin

Summary

Many empirically developed physical therapy techniques as well as alternative manual therapies (e.g., Rolfing, myofascial release) are aimed at treating fascia and other "unspecialized" connective tissues; however, compared with muscles, joints, and the nervous system, very little research has been devoted to the role of fascia in chronic musculoskeletal pain. One possible reason for this discrepancy is the lack of an integrative pathophysiological model linking connective tissue to known musculoskeletal pain mechanisms *(1)*. This chapter examines the potential role of fascia in musculoskeletal pain, especially regarding how connective tissue remodeling may interact with other factors such as fear of movement, muscle activity patterns and central nervous system plasticity.

Key Words: pain, musculoskeletal, connective tissue, fascia, remodeling, fibrosis, movement, plasticity, fibroblasts

1. DYNAMIC FIBROBLASTS AND PLASTIC CONNECTIVE TISSUE

A hallmark of connective tissue is its mutability, plasticity, or remodeling in response to varying levels of mechanical stress *(2)*. Connective tissue can become more or less stiff due to changes in its composition and architecture. The viscoelastic properties of connective tissue (e.g., stiffness, damping) are determined by its architecture, molecular

From: *Contemporary Pain Medicine: Integrative Pain Medicine: The Science and Practice of Complementary and Alternative Medicine in Pain Management*
Edited by: J. F. Audette and A. Bailey © Humana Press, Totowa, NJ

composition (mainly collagen, elastin and glycosaminoglycans) and water, all of which are mutually interdependent *(3–5)*. Water content, for example, is dependent on both the concentration of negatively charged glycosaminoglycans (GAGs) that bind large amounts of water and on the organization, strength, and stiffness of the collagen fiber network, which resists tissue swelling *(3)*.

Fibroblasts secrete the main structural components of connective tissue (collagen, GAGs, and elastin) and therefore play a key role in determining the composition of the matrix. Fibroblasts also are able to perceive and respond to mechanical forces because they are linked to the extracellular matrix at specialized membrane complexes called focal adhesions or focal contacts *(6)*. These protein complexes essentially form a mechanical link between the cell's internal cytoskeleton and the extracellular matrix *(7)*. Mechanical stimuli applied to whole tissue, such as stretching, cause direct, local mechanical deformation of the cytoskeleton. When connective tissue is stretched, fibroblasts respond within minutes by expanding, flattening and actively reorganizing their cytoskeleton *(8)* (Figure 1). This active cellular response has been shown to involve specific intracellular signaling (Rho and Rac) as well as lamellipodia formation, actin redistribution and actomyosin contractility *(9,10)*. Mechanical deformation of cultured fibroblasts has been shown to directly influence the synthesis of key matrix components via cytoskeletal mechanotransduction mechanisms *(11)*. In other words, the amount of matrix protein secreted by fibroblasts is influenced by

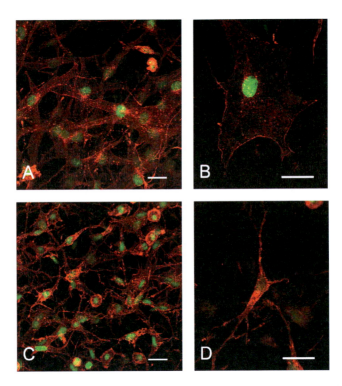

Fig. 1. Response of mouse subcutaneous tissue fibroblasts to tissue stretch ex vivo. **A,B:** Mouse subcutaneous tissue was incubated under stretch for 30 minutes immediately following excision, then fixed and stained with phalloidin, a specific stain for polymerized actin (red) and SYTOX nuclear stain (green). **C,D:** Control tissue incubated 30 minutes without stretch Fibroblast cell bodies became larger and flatter in the plane of the tissue in response to tissue stretch Scale bars, 40 μm.

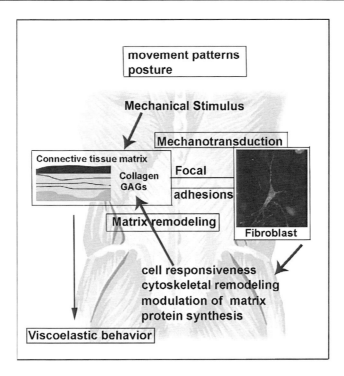

Fig. 2. Diagrammatic representation of relationships among tissue movement, cellular mechanotransduction, matrix remodeling, and tissue biomechanical properties.

the fibroblasts' mechanical environment. Changes in extracellular matrix composition due to mechanotransduction-mediated cellular effects, therefore, can have an important influence on the connective tissue's viscoelastic properties (Figure 2). Because changes in the tissue's viscoelastic properties (e.g., stiffness, damping) affect the degree of cellular deformation occurring when subsequent external forces are applied to the tissue *(7,12)*, fibroblasts actively influence the mechanical forces that act upon them over time. In vivo, an ongoing remodeling of connective tissue underlies physiological responses to changing levels of activity and movement patterns (e.g., immobilization, beginning a new exercise or occupation), as well as tissue repair following injury *(13)*.

Fibroblasts can also respond to chronic mechanical stimulation and injury by synthesizing increased amounts of alpha actin over several days and developing a more robust contractile apparatus, thus differentiating into smooth muscle-like cells known as myofibroblasts *(14)*. It also was recently shown that stimulation of connective tissue with specific pharmacological agonists could induce a measurable tissue contraction. *(15)* Fibroblasts, therefore, are dynamic cells that are likely to play a complex active role in determining connective tissue tension via cytoskeletal reorganization, active contraction/relaxation, and modification of matrix viscoelastic properties.

2. FIBROSIS: THE DARK SIDE OF CONNECTIVE TISSUE PLASTICITY

While connective tissue remodeling is essential for both normal and functional adaptation to changes in activity levels and response to injury, it can alternatively be harmful if it causes excessive collagen and matrix deposition. Decreased stress due to immobilization or hypomobility can cause connective tissue atrophy, architectural disorganization, fibrosis, adhesions, and contractures *(16–20)*. Chronic degenerative changes can be accompanied by either increased tissue water (decreased collagen network integrity causing decreased resistance to swelling pressure), or decreased tissue water due to decreased GAG content *(21–23)*. Immobilization-induced atrophy tends to cause decreased collagen, GAG, and water content *(24,25)*, while fibrosis tends to result in collagen bundle accumulation and disorganization, increased interfibrillar contacts and restricted gliding of fibers relative to each other *(5,16,24,26–29)*. Collagen cross-links have been shown to increase in number and strength with increasing duration of immobilization *(30)*. Factors determining whether connective tissue remodeling will be appropriate or pathological include the amount of mechanical stress, the adequacy of tissue perfusion and oxygenation, and the presence of inflammation and cytokines such as TGFß-1 that promote fibrosis *(31,32)*. Regardless of its precipitating cause, connective tissue fibrosis is detrimental, as it leads to increased tissue stiffness and movement impairment.

3. CONNECTIVE TISSUE/MUSCLE INTERACTIONS

In muscle, plasticity of perimuscular and intramuscular connective tissue plays an important role in how muscle responds to mechanical stress. It has been shown, for example, that during the early phase of immobilization, loss of muscle length is primarily due to shortening of muscle-associated connective tissue, which is only later followed by actual shortening of muscle fibers *(33)*. The poorly understood phenomena of myofascial trigger points, taut muscle bands, and muscle spasm may also contribute to connective tissue remodeling and fibrosis. Although there is some controversy as to the definition and nature of these entities, and whether or not they are related to each other *(34–36)*, decreased tissue pH and increased levels of inflammatory cytokines were recently reported in painful myofascial trigger points *(37)*. Thus, the presence of painful muscle contraction or tender foci within muscle and/or perimuscular fascia may add to the factors promoting hypomobility and tissue fibrosis.

4. LINK BETWEEN PAIN, FEAR, AND MOVEMENT

Most episodes of acute musculoskeletal pain resolve with resumption of normal activities. In some cases, however, pain becomes recurrent or chronic. A number of studies *(38–40)* suggest that psychological factors such as emotional distress and pain-related behavior may play a key role in the development of recurrence and/or chronicity. A key component of pain-related behavior is fear of pain with consequent decrease in physical activity *(41)*. While rest may be initially important in the face of acute injury, it is increasingly recognized that timely resumption of physical activity is critical to successful rehabilitation *(42)*. However, after an episode of acute musculoskeletal pain, patients often remain sedentary because of fear that movement will cause pain. Such behavior is particularly detrimental, since decreased recreational activity leads to deconditioning, which further impacts emotional well-being *(43,44)*.

In addition, a growing body of evidence supports the notion that both pain and fear affect not only how much, but also the manner in which, patients with pain actually move. In chronic low back pain, for example, abnormal trunk muscle activity during postural perturbation, impaired control of trunk and hip movement during quiet standing, and abnormal postural compensation for respiration all have been documented

(45–47). Several models have been proposed to explain such abnormal movement patterns, including the "pain-spasm-pain" model (reflex sustained co-contraction of agonists and antagonist muscles) *(48)* and "pain adaptation" (slowing and decreased range of motion due to selective increased activation of antagonists) *(49)*. Recent experiments suggest that, in normal individuals, fear of pain by itself can cause altered muscle activation patterns *(50)*. Thus, patients with chronic musculoskeletal pain appear to have a constellation of motion-limiting muscle activation patterns that may be initiated or aggravated by emotional factors. In chronic musculoskeletal pain, decreased tissue movement is a potential key factor in the development of connective tissue fibrosis and the perpetuation of chronic pain.

5. RELATIONSHIP BETWEEN CONNECTIVE TISSUE PLASTICITY AND NEUROPLASTICITY

Connective tissue is richly innervated with mechano-sensory and nociceptive neurons *(51)*. Modulation of nociceptor activity has been shown to occur in response to changes in the innervated tissue. Tissue levels of protons, inflammatory mediators (prostaglandins, bradykinin), nerve growth factors (NGFs) and hormones (adrenaline) *(52–54)* all have been shown to influence sensory input to the nervous system. Conversely, nociceptor activation has been shown to modify the innervated tissue; release of Substance P from sensory C-fibers in the skin can enhance the production of histamine and cytokines from mast cells, monocytes and endothelial cells *(55,56)*. Increased TGFβ-1 production, stimulated by tissue injury and histamine release, is a powerful driver of fibroblast collagen synthesis and tissue fibrosis *(31,57,58)*. Thus, activation of nociceptors, and the subsequent cascade of local tissue response eventually leading to neurogenic inflammation and cytokine release (see Chapter 2), can by itself contribute to the development or worsening of fibrosis and inflammation, causing even more tissue stiffness and movement impairment.

6. CENTRAL NERVOUS SYSTEM SENSITIZATION

Ongoing pain is associated with *w*idespread neuroplastic changes at multiple levels within the nervous system *(59–61)*, including primary afferent neurons *(54)*, spinal cord dorsal horn *(62,63)*, brainstem, *(64)*, thalamus, limbic system and cortex. Recent neuroimaging data (see Chapter 4) have uncovered distinct "brain networks" involved in acute versus chronic pain, with chronic pain specifically involving regions related to cognition and emotions *(65)*. At the level of the somatosensory cortex, functional reorganization of somatosensory areas has been documented in chronic pain *(66)*. Indeed, current models increasingly view chronic pain as a multilevel response of the neuroaxis called the "pain neuromatrix" that includes both sensory and motor components *(67–69)*.

7. PATHOPHYSIOLOGICAL MODEL LINKING BEHAVIOR, CONNECTIVE TISSUE, AND NEUROPLASTICITY

In the hypothetical model shown in Figure 3, progression to chronic pain first involves changes in the amount and pattern of body movements, leading to connective tissue remodeling and locally increased tissue stiffness. Peripheral and central nervous system sensitization will then contribute to tissue inflammation with enhanced afferent, nociceptive drive to the CNS followed by increased emotional distress, pain-related fear, and decreased movement. In patients with musculoskeletal pain, local connective tissue fibrosis may occur due to one or several of the following factors: (1) decreased activity, (2) changes in muscle activation patterns causing muscle co-contraction, muscle spasm, or myofascial trigger points, and (3) neurally mediated inflammation. Connective tissue remodeling may play an important role in the pathophysiology of musculoskeletal pain because (1) plasticity in response to changing mechanical loads is one of connective tissue's fundamental properties, and (2) pathological remodeling (fibrosis) due to changes in tissue movement is well documented in other types of connective tissues (e.g., ligaments, joint capsules).

In both the connective tissue and nervous system, plasticity responses are characterized by changes over time and the potential for reversibility. The hypothetical mechanism shown in Figure 3 is compatible with the complex natural history of musculoskeletal pain, including temporal variability (i.e., waxing and waning of symptoms and disability) and potential for "feed-forward" acute exacerbation of symptoms (i.e., acute flare-ups). An acute flare-up of pain may be triggered by any situation causing locally increased inflammatory cytokines, decreased tissue pH or oxygen content. In fibrosed connective tissue and muscle, blood and lymphatic flow may be chronically compromised by the disorganized tissue architecture and thus vulnerable to unusual muscle activity (e.g., beginning a new work activity or sport), or to conditions causing further decrease in perfusion such as prolonged sitting. Once local activation of nociceptors is initiated, peripheral and central nervous system sensitization mechanisms amplify both the tissue inflammation (via release of inflammatory neurotransmitters such as substance P) and the perceived pain. This leads to emotional distress, fear of movement, and, when persistent, deconditioning and its adverse long-term consequences; therefore, each exacerbation of pain potentially leads to greater movement restriction and fibrosis, setting the patient up for more painful episodes.

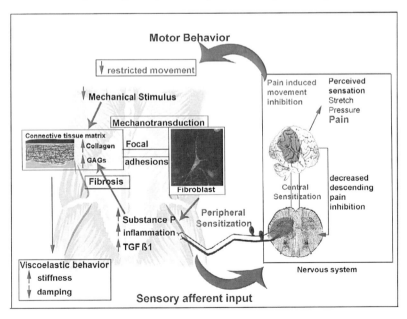

Fig. 3. Pathophysiological model for chronic musculoskeletal pain incorporating connective tissue remodeling, neuroplasticity, and emotional and motor behavior.

8. EFFECT OF TREATMENTS AND PLACEBOS

In addition to its role in the pathological consequences of immobility and injury, the dynamic and potentially reversible nature of connective tissue plasticity may be key to the beneficial effects of widely used physical therapy techniques, as well as several treatments considered within the realm of complementary and alternative medicine (CAM). Many of these therapies involve the external application of mechanical forces (e.g., massage, chiropractic manipulation, acupuncture), changes in specific movement patterns (e.g., movement therapies, tai chi, yoga) or more general changes in activity levels (e.g., increased recreational and therapeutic exercise) (Figure 4). Connective tissue remodeling also may be important in the therapeutic effect of pharmacological treatments commonly used for musculoskeletal pain via direct effects on tissues (anti-inflammatories), reduction of muscle spasm (muscle relaxants), and/or pain-induced fear of movement (analgesics, anxiolytics). The effect of placebos in musculoskeletal pain may also involve decreased fear of pain with consequent increased physical activity and the subsequent beneficial connective tissue remodeling effects. Improving our understanding of the physiological basis of these therapeutic techniques is key to developing more effective treatment strategies with minimal adverse effects. While manual or movement-based treatments have the advantage of not causing drug-induced side effects (e.g., gastritis, sedation), these treatments can potentially worsen pain if applied forces actually cause inflammation due to excessive tissue stretching or pressure.

A paradoxical aspect of connective tissue remodeling is that it potentially underlies both beneficial and harmful effects of mechanical forces, including those used thera-peutically. Application of direct tissue stretch to ligaments and joint capsules needs to be gauged carefully to avoid causing excessive tissue inflammation *(13)*. Indeed, understanding how much force (or movement) is beneficial, and how much can be

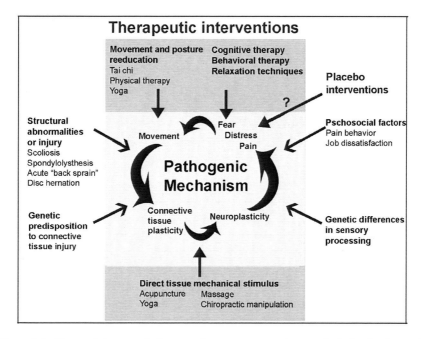

Fig. 4. Potential effects of therapeutic interventions on proposed musculoskeletal pain mechanism.

harmful is one of the greatest challenges of these clinical modalities and at this stage of understanding is often relegated into the realm of the art of medicine rather that to science. This scientific model suggests that behavior modification and movement reeducation may be most effective in the early stages of musculoskeletal pain before extensive tissue fibrosis has occurred and that combining these approaches with carefully applied direct tissue stretch may be necessary in cases of long-standing hypomobility with pronounced fibrosis and stiffness. Understanding the underlying pathophysiology will help optimize the selection of the best treatment or treatment combination. Some techniques such as yoga may act on multiple levels, causing direct tissue stretching as well as movement reeducation and relaxation.

In summary, plasticity of fascia and interstitial connective tissue may play an important role in both normal adaptive responses to changes in activity level, as well as maladaptive responses to pain and hypomobility. Treatments involving behavioral modification, movement reeducation, and direct mechanical stimulation of connective tissue all can potentially reverse connective tissue fibrosis, leading to increased mobility. The hypothetical model presented in this chapter is aimed at stimulating further research and encouraging integrative approaches to treatment.

REFERENCES

1. Langevin HM, Sherman KJ, Pathophysiological model for chronic low back pain integrating connective tissue and nervous system mechanisms. Med Hypotheses, 2007;68(1):74–80.
2. Tillman LJ, Cummings GS. 1992. Biologic Mechanisms of Connective Tissue Mutability, in Dynamics of Human Biologic Tissues Contemporary Perspectives in Rehabilitation. Volume 8. Currier DP, Nelson RM, Eds. F.A. Davis: Philadelphia, pp. 1–44.
3. Mow VC, Ratcliffe A. 1997. Structure and Function of Articular Cartilage and Meniscus, in Basic Orthopaedic Biomechanics. Mow VC, Hayes WC, Eds. Lippincott-Raven: Philadelphia, pp. 113–177.
4. Guilak F, Sah R, Setton LA. 1997. Physical Regulation of Cartilage Metabolism, in Basic Orthopaedic Biomechanics. Mow VC, Hayes WC, Eds. Lippincott-Raven: Philadelphia, pp. 179–207.
5. Woo S, Livesay GA, Runco TJ, Young EP. 1997. Structure and Function of Tendons and Ligaments, in Basic Orthopaedic Biomechanics. Mow VC, Hayes WC, Eds. Lippincott-Raven: Philadelphia, pp. 209–252.
6. Giancotti, FG, Ruoslahti E. Integrin signaling. Science 1999;285(5430):1028–1032.
7. Chicurel ME, Chen CS, Ingber DE. Cellular control lies in the balance of forces. Curr Opin Cell Biol 1998;10(2):23–29.
8. Langevin HM, et al., Dynamic fibroblast cytoskeletal response to subcutaneous tissue stretch ex vivo and in vivo. Am J Physiol Cell Physiol 2005;288(3):C747–C756.
9. Langevin HM, et al. Subcutaneous tissue fibroblast cytoskeletal remodeling induced by acupuncture: Evidence for a mechanotransduction-based mechanism. J Cell Physiol, 2006;207(3):767–774.
10. Langevin HM, et al. Fibroblast spreading induced by connective tissue stretch involves intracellular redistribution of alpha- and beta-actin. Histochem Cell Biol 2006;125(5):487–495.
11. Chiquet M. Regulation of extracellular matrix gene expression by mechanical stress. Matrix Biol 1999;18(5):417–426.
12. Brand RA. What do tissues and cells know of mechanics? Ann Med 1997;29(4):267–269.
13. Cummings GS, Tillman LJ. 1992. Remodeling of Dense Connective Tissue in Normal Adult Tissues, in Dynamics of Human Biologic Tissues Contemporary Perspectives in Rehabilitation. Volume 8. Currier DP, Nelson RM, Eds. F.A. Davis: Philadelphia, pp. 45–73.
14. Gabbiani G. The myofibroblast in wound healing and fibrocontractive diseases. J Pathol 2003;200(4):500–503.
15. Schleip R, Klingler W, Lehmann-Horn F. Active fascial contractility: Fascia may be able to contract in a smooth muscle-like manner and thereby influence musculoskeletal dynamics. Med Hypotheses 2005;65(2):273–277.
16. Savolainen J, Vaananen K, Vihko V, et al. Effect of immobilization on collagen synthesis in rat skeletal muscles. Am J Physiol 1987;252(5 Pt 2):R883–R888.

17. Uebelhart D, Bernard J, Hartmann DJ, et al. Modifications of bone and connective tissue after orthostatic bedrest. Osteoporos Int 2000;11(1):59–67.
18. Williams PE, Catanese T, Lucey EG, et al. The importance of stretch and contractile activity in the prevention of connective tissue accumulation in muscle. J Anat 1988;158:109–114.
19. Woo SLY, Mathews JV, Akeson WH, et al. Connective tissue response to immobility. Correlative study of biomechanical and biochemical measurements of normal and immobilized rabbit knees. Arthritis Rheum 1975;18(3): 257–264.
20. Akeson WH, Amiel D, Woo SL. Immobility effects on synovial joints the pathomechanics of joint contracture. Biorheology 1980;17(1–2):95–110.
21. Armstrong CG, Mow VC. Variations in the intrinsic mechanical properties of human articular cartilage with age, degeneration, and water content. J Bone Joint Surg Am, 1982;64(1):88–94.
22. Lyons G, Eisenstein SM, Sweet MB. Biochemical changes in intervertebral disc degeneration. Biochim Biophys Acta 1981;673(4):443–453.
23. Jenkins JPR, Hickey DS, Zhu XP, et al. MR imaging of the intervertebral disc: a quantitative study. Br J Radiol 1985;58(692):705–709.
24. Akeson WH, Amiel D, Mechanic GL, et al. Collagen cross-linking alterations in joint contractures: changes in the reducible cross-links in periarticular connective tissue collagen after nine weeks of immobilization. Connect Tissue Res 1977;5(1):15–19.
25. Akeson WH, Woo SLY, Amiel D, et al. The connective tissue response to immobility: biochemical changes in periarticular connective tissue of the immobilized rabbit knee. Clin Orthop Relat Res 1973;93:356–362.
26. Finsterbush, A, Friedman B. Early changes in immobilized rabbits knee joints: a light and electron microscopic study. Clin Orthop 1973;92:305–319.
27. Giannelli G, De Marzo A, Marinosci F, et al. Matrix metalloproteinase imbalance in muscle disuse atrophy. Histol Histopathol 2005;20(1):99–106.
28. Han XY, Wang W, Myllyla R, et al., mRNA levels for alpha-subunit of prolyl 4-hydroxylase and fibrillar collagens in immobilized rat skeletal muscle. J Appl Physiol 1999;87(1):90–96.
29. Kovacs EJ, DiPietro LA, Fibrogenic cytokines and connective tissue production. FASEB J 1994;8(11):854–861.
30. Grodin AJ, Cantu RI. 1993. Soft Tissue Mobilization, in Rational Manual Therapies. Basmajian JV, Nyberg R, Eds. Baltimore: Williams & Wilkins, pp. xii and 484.
31. Leask A, Abraham DJ, TGF-beta signaling and the fibrotic response. FASEB J 2004;18(7):816–827.
32. Hunt TK, Banda MJ, Silver IA. Cell interactions in post-traumatic fibrosis. Ciba Found Symp 1985;114:127–149.
33. Williams PE, Goldspink G. Connective tissue changes in immobilised muscle. J Anat 1984;138 (Pt 2):343–350.
34. Hong CZ, Simons DG. Pathophysiologic and electrophysiologic mechanisms of myofascial trigger points. Arch Phys Med Rehabil 1998;79(7):863–872.
35. Bohr T. Problems with myofascial pain syndrome and fibromyalgia syndrome. Neurology 1996;46(3):593–597.
36. Travell JG. 1990. Chronic myofascial pain syndromes. Mysteries of the History. In Advances in Pain Research and Therapy. Friction JR, Awad E, Eds. New York: Raven Press Ltd. pp. 129–137.
37. Shah JP, Phillips TM, Danoff JV, et al. An in-vivo microanalytical technique for measuring the local biochemical milieu of human skeletal muscle. J Appl Physiol 2005.
38. Hurwitz EL, Morgenstern H, Yu F. Cross-sectional and longitudinal associations of low-back pain and related disability with psychological distress among patients enrolled in the UCLA Low-Back Pain Study. J Clin Epidemiol 2003;56(5):463–471.
39. Dionne CE. Psychological distress confirmed as predictor of long-term back-related functional limitations in primary care settings. J Clin Epidemiol 2005;58(7):714–718.
40. Pincus T, Burton KA, Vogel S, et al. A systematic review of psychological factors as predictors of chronicity/disability in prospective cohorts of low back pain. Spine 2002;27(5):E109–E120.
41. Swinkels-Meewisse IEJ, Roelofs J, Oostenclorp RAB, et al. Acute low back pain: pain-related fear and pain catastrophizing influence physical performance and perceived disability. Pain 2006;120:36–43.
42. van Tulder MW, Koes B, Malmivaara A. Outcome of non-invasive treatment modalities on back pain: an evidence-based review. Eur Spine J 2006;15(Suppl 1):S64–S81.
43. Hurwitz EL, Morgenstern H, Chiao C. Effects of recreational physical activity and back exercises on low back pain and psychological distress: findings from the UCLA Low Back Pain Study. Am J Public Health 2005;95(10):1817–1824.

44. Grotle M, Vollestad NK, Veierod MB, et al. Fear-avoidance beliefs and distress in relation to disability in acute and chronic low back pain. Pain 2004;112(3):343–352.

45. Reeves NP, Cholewicki J, Milner TE. Muscle reflex classification of low-back pain. J Electromyogr Kinesiol 2005;15(1):53–60.

46. Grimstone SK, Hodges PW. Impaired postural compensation for respiration in people with recurrent low back pain. Exp Brain Res 2003;151(2):218–224.

47. Mok, NW, Brauer SG, Hodges PW. Hip strategy for balance control in quiet standing is reduced in people with low back pain. Spine 2004;29(6):E107–E112.

48. Roland MO. A critical review of the evidence for a pain-spasm-pain cycle in spinal disorders. Clin Biomech 1986;1(2):102–109.

49. Lund JP, Donga R, Widmer CG, et al. The pain-adaptation model: a discussion of the relationship between chronic musculoskeletal pain and motor activity. Can J Physiol Pharmacol 1991;69(5):683–694.

50. Moseley GL, Nicholas MK, Hodges PW. Does anticipation of back pain predispose to back trouble? Brain 2004;127(Pt 10):2339–2347.

51. Willis WD, Coggeshall RE. 1991. Sensory Mechanisms of the Spinal Cord, 2nd edition. Volume XIV. New York: Plenum Press, p 575.

52. Koltzenburg M. The changing sensitivity in the life of the nociceptor. Pain 1999;(Suppl 6):S93–S102.

53. Waldmann R, Champigny G, Bassilana F, et al. A proton-gated cation channel involved in acid-sensing. Nature 1997;386(6621):173–177.

54. Woolf CJ, Salter MW. Neuronal plasticity: increasing the gain in pain. Science 2000;288(5472):1765–1769.

55. Bessou P, Laporte Y. Etude des recepteurs musculaires innerves par les fibres afferents du groupe III (fibres myelinisees fines) chez le chat. Arch Ital Biol 1961;99:293–321.

56. Ansel JC, Kaynard AH, Armstrong CA, et al. Skin–nervous system interactions. J Invest Dermatol 1996;106(1):198–204.

57. Barnard JA, Lyons RM, Moses HL. The cell biology of transforming growth factor beta. Biochim Biophys Acta 1990;1032(1):79–87.

58. Sporn MB, Roberts AB. TGF-beta: problems and prospects. Cell Regul 1990;1(12):875–882.

59. Ji RR, Woolf CJ. Neuronal plasticity and signal transduction in nociceptive neurons: implications for the initiation and maintenance of pathological pain. Neurobiol Dis 2001;8(1):1–10.

60. Boal RW, Gillette RG. Central neuronal plasticity, low back pain and spinal manipulative therapy. J Manipulative Physiol Ther 2004;27(5):314–326.

61. Coderre TJ, Katz J, Vaccarino AL, et al. Contribution of central neuroplasticity to pathological pain: review of clinical and experimental evidence. Pain 1993;52(3):259–285.

62. Bolay H, Moskowitz MA. Mechanisms of pain modulation in chronic syndromes. Neurology 2002;59(5 Suppl 2):S2–S7.

63. Ikeda H, Heinke B, Ruscheweyh R, et al. Synaptic plasticity in spinal lamina I projection neurons that mediate hyperalgesia. Science 2003;299(5610):1237–1240.

64. Gebhart GF. Descending modulation of pain. Neurosci Biobehav Rev 2004;27(8):729–737.

65. Apkarian AV, Bushnell MC, Treede RD, et al. Human brain mechanisms of pain perception and regulation in health and disease. Eur J Pain 2005;9(4):463–484.

66. Flor H, Cortical reorganisation and chronic pain: implications for rehabilitation. J Rehabil Med 2003(41 Suppl):66–72.

67. Melzack R. From the gate to the neuromatrix. Pain 1999;(Suppl 6):S121–S126.

68. Moseley GL. A pain neuromatrix approach to patients with chronic pain. Man Ther 2003;8(3):130–140.

69. Khalsa PS. Biomechanics of musculoskeletal pain: dynamics of the neuromatrix. J Electromyogr Kinesiol 2004;14(1):109–120.

7 Biochemical and Nutritional Influences on Pain

Steve Parcell

Contents

Summary

This chapter is meant to be an introduction to how plant extracts, vitamins, functional foods, minerals, nutraceuticals, and therapeutic diets might be utilized to improve symptoms in chronic pain. Emphasis will be placed on physiological processes and conditions where some form of nutritional intervention will have a high probability of being efficacious. An in-depth treatise on all pain mechanisms will not occur, as this will be covered elsewhere. Also, an exhaustive review of the clinical studies for or against specific treatments will not be undertaken.

Inflammation, cytokines, neurohormones, and oxidative stress all play important roles in persistent pain conditions. Many aspects of immune and neuroendocrine function may be modified by dietary factors such as phenols, saponins, sterols, and antioxidants. Inflammation may be controlled at different levels. Omega-3 fatty acid supplementation can modify the eicosanoid cascade, tipping the balance toward an

From: *Contemporary Pain Medicine: Integrative Pain Medicine: The Science and Practice of Complementary and Alternative Medicine in Pain Management*
Edited by: J. F. Audette and A. Bailey © Humana Press, Totowa, NJ

anti-inflammatory profile. Lowering insulin and neurotoxin levels may also help to reduce inflammation by modulation of PLA2 activity. Flavanoids, such as rutin and quercetin, and retinoids, such as vitamin A, additionally help to inhibit PLA2 activity. Some examples of chronic pain conditions that may be amenable to dietary interventions include osteoarthritis, rheumatoid arthritis, fibromyalgia, autoimmune diseases, migraine headache, chronic abdominal pain, Crohn's disease, and arthralgia. Dietary interventions for pain include increasing fruit and vegetable intake, consumption of grass-fed beef and DHA eggs, lowering lectin consumption, adding functional foods such as soy and green tea, and elimination of food allergens. Lowering inflammatory cytokines and modifying the eicosanoid cascade with n-3 fats may attenuate systemic inflammation. Neuroendocrine perturbations, notably of cortisol and growth hormone, exist in many chronic pain states. Vital neurohormones such as melatonin and serotonin may be lower in chronic pain patients in connection with plasma amino acid imbalances. Metabolic deficits in mitochondrial function and glycemic control should also be addressed in order to reduce systemic inflammation and oxidative stress. Acid-base disturbances, primarily of dietary origin, may contribute to the progression of osteoporosis, which can lead to painful fractures and disability. The cartilage destruction seen in osteoarthritis is the result of an imbalance between catabolic and anabolic activity and may be modified by various antioxidants, as well as glucosamine, Chondroitin, and SAMe. Evidence indicates that obesity and insulin resistance contribute to chronic inflammation, providing good rationale for aggressive lifestyle and diet intervention in obese patients with chronic pain conditions. Targeted clinical nutritional interventions may effectively inhibit synthesis of inflammatory prostaglandins and cytokines. Though the subject of treating pain with nutritional factors is rarely discussed in medical textbooks, published data on the use of nutritional interventions in the treatment of various chronic inflammatory conditions does exist. Many opportunities to improve our treatment of chronic pain conditions through dietary changes exist and will be further elaborated on in the chapter "Nutrition and Supplements" that follows.

Key Words: nutrition, supplements, nutraceutical, naturopathy, inflammatory cascade, inflammation, fatty acids

1. INTRODUCTION

The term *nutraceutical* was coined by the Foundation for Innovation in Medicine in 1991 and is defined as "any substance that may be considered a food or part of a food and provides medical or health benefits, including the prevention and treatment of disease." It will be used here to refer to any supplement or food component other than vitamins, plant extracts, or minerals. For instance, soy isoflavones and plant sterols are nutraceuticals, whereas Panax ginseng extract is not. Substances like green tea fall into both categories because they are both a functional food and an herbal extract. There is no universally accepted definition of functional foods. Although functional foods remain undefined under current US food regulations, they are usually understood to be any potentially healthful food or food ingredient that may provide a health benefit beyond the traditional nutrients it contains. The term *functional* implies that the food has some identified value leading to health benefits, including reduced risk for disease, for the person consuming it.

Increasingly the scientific and medical community is becoming cognizant of the tremendous impact diet and lifestyle can have on health. For example, the American Heart Association (AHA) and the National Heart, Lung, and Blood Institute (NHLBI) have stated emphatically that the metabolic syndrome in adults should be treated first with diet and lifestyle therapy, rather than medications. The metabolic syndrome comprises a group of metabolic risk factors occurring in one person, including abdominal obesity, hypercholesterolemia, hypertension, insulin resistance, and pro-thrombotic and pro-inflammatory states (1). In reference to the metabolic syndrome, the executive summary from the AHA and the NHLBI states: "Lifestyle interventions deserve prime consideration for risk reduction across a lifetime; these interventions include weight control, increased physical activity, and a diet designed to reduce the risk for atherosclerotic cardiovascular disease (ASCVD)." *(1)*.

Conventionally, pain syndromes have been treated in a reactionary manner. In other words, a patient first experiences pain and is then treated with an analgesic or anti-inflammatory medication. When treating pain from a prevention-based mindset, however, treatment is proactive and requires knowledge of the patient in order to address the underlying cause of the painful symptoms. Proactive treatment also requires the clinician to adopt a mindset of early detection. In addition to a detailed physical and medical history, non-standard lab work may be necessary. Examples include measuring cytokine levels, urine neurotransmitter metabolites, C-reactive protein, red blood cell fatty acids, and markers of gut inflammation, such as eosinophil protein X.

In chronic pain, the goal is to bring cytokines under control, modify the eicosanoid cascade, and reestablish normal sleep and hormone secretion patterns. Herbal, vitamin, and nutraceutical treatments for pain include agents that work as cyclooxygenase (COX), nuclear factor kappa beta (NF-Kb), or lipoxygenase (LOX) inhibitors. High doses must be given to achieve results comparable to conventional non-steroidal anti-inflammatory drugs (NSAIDS). In addition, there are few natural substances, other than morphine derivatives, that are powerful analgesics. It is relatively impractical to attempt to treat acute pain in this way because nutritional or herbal interventions take time to begin to work and must be dosed fairly high. For instance, the herbal COX and NF-Kb inhibitors take approximately three days to show effects. In chronic pain, however, immune, neurological, and endocrine mechanisms are often perturbed, and these imbalances, which feed into and exacerbate the chronic pain cycle, may be responsive to nutritional interventions.

When tackling the problem of chronic pain, a functional approach is clinically useful. The term *functional medicine* refers to more than "holistic" or "alternative" medicine and has been defined as a science-based field of health care that is "anchored by an examination of the core clinical imbalances that underlie various disease conditions. Those imbalances arise as environmental inputs such as diet, nutrients (including air and water), exercise, and trauma are processed by one's body, mind, and spirit through a unique set of genetic predispositions, attitudes, and beliefs. The fundamental physiological processes include communication, both outside and inside the cell; bioenergetics, or the transformation of food into energy; replication, repair, and maintenance of structural integrity, from the cellular to the whole-body level; elimination of waste; protection and defense; and transport and circulation."*(2)* Most naturopathic physicians practice functional medicine because it is a core part of their training and philosophy. Increasingly, however, complementary and alternative medicine (CAM)-based medical doctors, chiropractors, and osteopathic physicians are also practicing functional medicine.

2. FATTY ACIDS

It is first crucial to have a working understanding of the importance of fatty acids in the human diet and how they affect inflammation. Fats supply approximately 30% of daily caloric needs and are composed of three fatty acids linked to a glycerol backbone. These are called triacylglycerols and are the storage form of fatty acids in the body. Upon hydrolysis, free fatty acids are released from the triacylglycerol molecule. Fatty acids are hydrocarbon chains with a methyl and a carboxyl end. Dietary fatty acids can vary in length from 4 to 22 carbons. Fatty acids with chain lengths of 16–18 make up the bulk of those in the diet and the body. In addition to chain length, fatty acids are also distinguished by degree of saturation and location of double bonds. There are three types of fatty acids: saturated, monounsaturated, and polyunsaturated (see Figure 1). Saturated fatty acids have no double bonds, which make the molecule straighter, giving them a higher melting point and making them more resistant to oxidation. Fatty acids with a single double bond are called monounsaturated fatty acids. Polyunsaturated fatty acids have more than one double bond between carbon atoms, causing kinks in the molecule. These kinks prevent the molecules from stacking together well, resulting in lower melting points than the saturated fatty acids.

Polyunsaturated *trans* fatty acids are polyunsaturated fats that have been partially saturated with a process called hydrogenation. This causes a different positioning of the hydrogen atoms in the middle of the molecule. The hydrogen atoms in the middle are in a "trans" as opposed to "cis" position that makes this a "trans" fatty acid. The effect is to straighten out the molecules so they can pack together more closely and make the oil less liquid, more solid and have a longer shelf life. Trans fats are present in many food products, including vegetable shortening, margarines, baked goods, snack foods, fried foods, salad dressings, and many processed foods. Low levels are also found in dairy products, lamb and beef fat, because small amounts of trans fat are produced

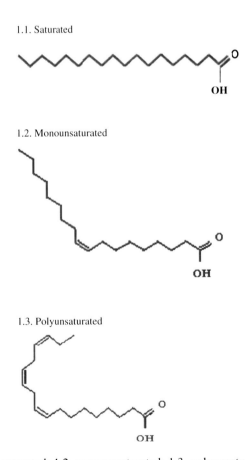

1.1. Saturated

1.2. Monounsaturated

1.3. Polyunsaturated

Fig. 1. Fatty acids: 1.1, saturated; 1.2, monounsaturated; 1.3, polyunsaturated.

in the gastrointestinal tract of ruminants. These fats cannot be used by the body to produce useful mediators because the molecules have unnatural shapes that are not recognized by enzymes. *Trans* fatty acids may also have a detrimental effect on the brain and nervous system. Neural tissue consists mainly of lipids and fats. Myelin is composed of 30% protein and 70% fat. Oleic acid and docosahexaenoic (DHA) are two of the principal fatty acids in myelin. DHA is also critical for brain function. Loss in DHA concentrations in brain cell membranes correlates to a decline in structural and functional integrity of this tissue. Researchers have linked suboptimal DHA status in the brain with early-onset Alzheimer's disease, cognitive decline, aggression, and low IQ in children *(3)*. Studies demonstrate that *trans* fatty acids in the diet can be incorporated into brain cell membranes, as well as the myelin sheath *(4)*. These synthetic fats replace the natural DHA in the membrane and inhibit DHA synthesis via delta 6 desaturase *(5)*, which affects the electrical activity of the neuron. *Trans* fatty acid molecules alter the ability of neurons to communicate and may cause neural degeneration and diminished mental performance *(3)*. *Trans* fatty acids have also been reported to raise LDL cholesterol and increase the risk of cardiovascular disease *(6)*. Though found in nature, *trans* fatty acid intake has increased dramatically in the last 60 years due to increased use of hydrogenated vegetable oils in the diet.

2.1. Essential Fatty Acids

The essential fatty acids include the omega-3 and omega-6 fatty acids and linoleic and linolenic acids. They are polyunsaturated fatty acids that cannot be synthesized in the body and must, therefore, be obtained from the diet. Arachidonic acid (AA) is an omega-6 fatty acid that gains notoriety due to being the substrate for the inflammatory series two eicosanoids (PGE2). When linoleic acid is present in sufficient quantities in the diet, arachidonic acid is formed.

Over the past 20 years, data has accumulated on the metabolism of polyunsaturated fatty acids (PUFAs) in general and on omega-3 fatty acids in particular. It is now known that omega-3 fatty acids are essential for normal growth and development. They are also believed to play an important role in the prevention and treatment of coronary artery disease, hypertension, diabetes, cancer, arthritis, and other inflammatory and autoimmune disorders *(7)*. N-6 fatty acids are important for anti-inflammatory series

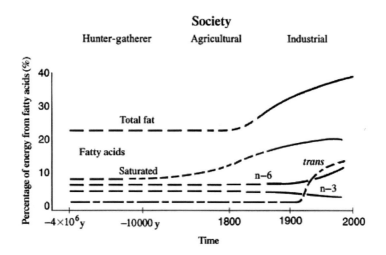

one eicosanoid synthesis, via Dihomo-gamma-linolenic acid (DGLA) and are found in abundance in plant oils. N-3 fatty acids are used as substrates for series three eicosanoids (PGE3).

Data from Paleolithic nutrition experts and modern-day hunter-gatherer populations indicate that human beings evolved consuming a diet that was much lower in saturated fat than our modern diet *(7)*. This fact is clinically significant because the human genome has not changed appreciably since this time. This "Paleo" diet contained approximately equal amounts of n-6 and n-3 PUFAs (1–2:1) and much lower amounts of *trans* fatty acids than does today's diet *(7)*. The current Western diet is very high in n-6 fatty acids (the ratio of n-6 to n-3 fatty acids is 20–30:1). Yehuda and colleagues *(8)* have also done much work on the subject of optimal n-6 to n-3 fatty acid ratio. This group developed the "SR-3" (specific ratio of n-6 to n-3), which they found to be 4:1. The majority of researchers agree with this ratio. Unfortunately, intake of the n-3 fatty acids is much lower today due to the decrease in fish consumption and the

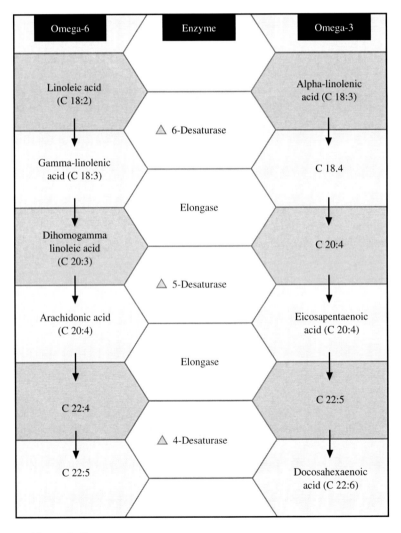

Fig. 2. Fatty acid metabolism.

industrial production of animal feeds rich in grains containing n-6 fatty acids. This leads to the production of meat rich in n-6 and poor in n-3 fatty acids *(4)*. The same is true for cultured fish and eggs. Even cultivated vegetables contain fewer n-3 fatty acids than do plants in the wild *(8)*.

Vegetable oils do not contain any arachidonic acid, eicosahexaenoic acid (EPA) or DHA. Only foods of animal origin (particularly eggs, meat and organ meats) contain arachidonic acid and DHA. This is particularly true of commercial grain-fed beef. The relatively new "DHA eggs" contain less AA than regular eggs. Fatty meats contain the most AA, whereas fatty cold water fish contain the most DHA and EPA. Omega-6 fats are easily converted into AA, the parent fatty acid in the eicosanoid cascade (see Figure 2). Omega-3 fats are converted into the beneficial EPA and DHA *(7)*.

3. INFLAMATORY MEDIATORS

3.1. Eicosanoids

Metabolism of natural 20-carbon polyunsaturated fatty acids like AA and EPA results in the biosynthesis of lipid-derived mediators with potent physiological effects. These include the prostaglandins (PG), prostacyclins (PGI2), thromboxanes (TXA), leukotrienes (LTB), and lipoxins. These substances are known collectively as eicosanoids because they contain 20 carbon atoms (Greek *eikosi* = 20). The two crucial rate-limiting steps for prostaglandin (PG) synthesis is phospholipase A_2 (PLA_2) which regulates the release of arachidonic acid (AA) from membrane phospholipids, and cyclooxygenase (COX), which converts AA to the intermediate PG precursor PGH_2 *(9)*. The process of all eicosanoid production begins with the enzyme PLA2. This enzyme cleaves off either linoleic or linolenic acid from cell membrane phospholipids.

These fatty acids then serve as substrates for the synthesis of eicosanoids (see Figure 3). It should be noted that only n-6 and n-3 fatty acids serve as eicosanoid substrates. Fatty acids are incorporated into the cell membrane either directly through diet, e.g., arachidonic acid (AA) in eggs and meat, or through de novo synthesis from the parent essential fatty acid such as linoleic acid. The n-6 fatty acids produce Series 1 (generally "good") and Series 2 (generally "bad") eicosanoids, whereas the n-3 fatty acids produce Series 3 (all "good") eicosanoids. Series 2 eicosanoids play a role in swelling and inflammation at sites of injury, causing pain (see Table 1). Of course, during the acute stage of injury this is an important protective mechanism, allowing the body to immobilize the affected site in order to prevent further injury and facilitate healing *(10)*. The Series 2 prostaglandins also appear to play a role in inducing labor, regulating temperature, lowering blood pressure, and controlling platelet aggregation and clotting *(10)*. The Series 3 prostaglandins are formed at a slower rate and work to attenuate excessive Series 2 production.

Cyclo-oxygenase is present in different forms: cyclo-oxygenase 1 (COX-1) and cyclo-oxygenase 2 (COX-2). The two isoforms are encoded by different genes and have unique patterns of expression. COX-1 is essential for the maintenance of normal physiologic states in many tissues including the kidney, gastrointestinal tract, and platelets. For example, COX-1 activation in the gastric mucosa leads to production of the prostaglandin, PGI2 (prostacyclin), which protects the gastric mucosa. Inhibition of COX-1 is thought to be the main way in which NSAIDs induce gastrointestinal damage.

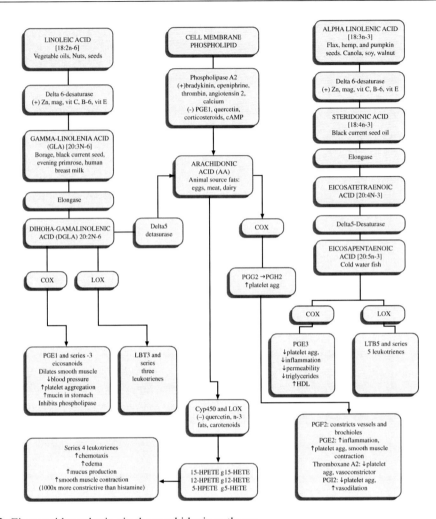

Fig. 3. Eicosanoid synthesis via the arachidonic pathway.

Thromboxane A2, which is primarily synthesized in platelets through COX-1 activity, causes platelet aggregation, vasoconstriction, and smooth muscle proliferation *(9)*. Activation of COX-1 is observed during the early phase of PG biosynthesis occurring within several minutes of stimulation, whereas COX-2-dependent PG generation proceeds over several hours in parallel with the induction of COX-2 expression *(9)*.

Although the expression of COX-1 may be regulated, it is usually expressed constitutively. Similarly, although COX-2 expression may be constitutive, particularly in the cells of the reproductive tract and in the nervous system, its expression is usually tightly regulated, particularly by cytokines, growth factors, and tumor-promoting agents. These observations have implicated COX-2 in PG generation and in chronic inflammation *(11)*.

Cyclo-oxygenase 2, readily induced by pro-inflammatory stimuli, increases production of proinflammatory eicosanoids. Upregulation of COX-2 mRNA and protein occurs during inflammation and has been shown to result in a great increase in PGE2 production *(12)*. COX-2 has been observed in osteoarthritic cartilage and has also been

Table 1
Series 1 and Series 2 Eiosanoids*

Series 1	Series 2
Vasodilation	Vasoconstriction
Enhance immune function	Immune suppression
Decrease cellular proliferation	Increase cellular proliferation
Dilate airways	Constrict airways
Inhibit platelet aggregation	Increase platelet aggregation
Increase endurance	Decrease endurance
Increase oxygen delivery	Decrease oxygen delivery
Decrease pain	Increase pain perception
Decrease inflammation	Increase inflammation

*The n-6 fatty acids produce Series 1 (generally "good") and Series 2 (generally "bad") eicosanoids, whereas the n-3 fatty acids produce Series 3 (all "good") eicosanoids. Series 2 eicosanoids play a role in swelling and inflammation at sites of injury, causing pain (from ref. 10).

observed in the synovial tissue of patients with osteoarthritis, but not that of normal patients (13). Prostaglandin E2 is involved with inflammation, pyresis, and hyperalgesia. Its levels can increase ten- to twenty-fold through inflammation, particularly in macrophages, monocytes, synoviocytes, chondrocytes, fibroblasts and endothelial cells. COX-2 has many other functions besides its role in inflammation. In vascular endothelium, for instance, it mediates production of PGI2, a vasodilator and inhibitor of both platelet aggregation and proliferation of vascular smooth muscle cells (13).

As mentioned above, the key initial regulatory step for the AA cascade is the cleaving of either linoleic or linolenic acid from cell membrane phospholipids by PLA2. Phospholipase A2 belongs to a family of enzymes that cleave membrane phospholipids to release AA, as discussed above. Several different isoforms of PLA2 have been described. These include a large-molecular-weight cytosolic PLA2, which is calcium-dependent and selective for AA and small-molecular-weight, calcium-dependent enzymes that are not selective for AA. In addition, a number of PLA2 enzymes have been described which are activated by a mechanism that does not require calcium. These include a calcium-independent enzyme found in cardiac myocytes that is selective for arachidonic acid and an enzyme in macrophage-like cells that is not (14). Flavanoids such as rutin and quercetin and retinoids such as vitamin A have been shown to inhibit phospholipase A2 (15,16). Research is emerging that reveals insulin's role in stimulating PLA2 (17). Dietary restriction of high glycemic carbohydrates and other interventions to control insulin response, such as chromium and EPA or DHA supplementation, could play an important role in preventing the elaboration of the inflammatory response. Other stimulators of PLA2 include methylmercury (18), pesticides (14), various biotoxins, calcium, (19) aspartic acid (aspartame) (20), and glutamic acid (MSG) (21).

Use of NSAIDs as an anti-inflammatory therapy acts by inhibiting cyclooxygenases (COX-1, COX-2), but has no effect on PLA2 or the production of leukotrienes or platelet activating factor (PAF). Additionally, two COX-2 inhibitors have recently been pulled from the market due to unexpected side effects. Inhibitors of PLA2 therefore offer the potential to block production of a more complete set of inflammatory substances through blockade at the onset of the cascade of reactions that follow arachidonic acid release.

3.2. Neurotoxins

Other activators of the inflammatory cascade include lipid-soluble neurotoxins such as heavy metals and biotoxins from bacteria, viruses and fungi. These toxins can lead to over expression of PLA2, leading to endemic inflammation and pain (22). Various methods exist to lower body burden of these neurotoxic factors and include heavy metal chelation, phospholidipid exchange with phosphatidylcholine, dietary intervention (detox diets), and various supplements intended to modulate phase-one and phase-two hepatic detoxification. Phase-one reactions comprise oxidation, reduction and dehalogenation, whereas phase-two reactions involve conjugation with sulphur (sulfonation), glucuronic acid (gluconidation), glutathione, acetyl CoA (N-Acetylation) and methyl groups (methylation). Neurotoxins cause damage by disrupting sodium and calcium channel receptors, disrupting enzyme reactions important for glucose production, impairing cell membrane function, and stimulating PLA2. Neurotoxins can also turn on NF-Kb thus increasing production of interleukin 1b (IL-1b), interluekin 6 (IL-6), and tumor necrosis factor alpha (TNF-α) (22).

3.3. Cytokines

In addition to eicosanoids, cytokines are released during inflammation (23). Cytokines are very small, soluble proteins that are released from immune cells and act to mediate and regulate immune cell activity and the inflammatory cascade. Mitogens, injury, viruses, lipopolysaccharides, and other antigens can all act as activators of the immune system (24,25). These activating factors bind to specific protein kinases on the cell surface and activate nuclear transcription factors such as nuclear factor kappa B (NF-kB), which ultimately leads to the genetic expression and synthesis of cytokines (23-25). It follows that inflammatory cytokines may be blocked by the inhibition of cell surface protein kinases and subsequent inhibition of NF-kB or by blocking the specific cellular receptors for cytokines.

Cytokines generally act over short distances, are short-acting, and are potent at very low concentrations. Cytokines bind to specific cell membrane receptors, which then signal the cell to alter its expression of certain genes and consequently transcription of various proteins. Cell responses to cytokines include increasing or decreasing expression of membrane proteins (including cytokine receptors), cell growth and proliferation, and secretion of effector molecules (24,25).

Proinflammatory cytokines have beneficial or negative effects depending on the context and the amount that is produced. During acute infection, they are generally beneficial, whereas in chronic inflammatory states such as osteoarthritis they are generally harmful (26). Cytokine levels may persist beyond what is necessary or optimal, causing tissue destruction and pathology. Interleukin 1 (IL-1), interleukin 6 (IL-6), and tumor necrosis factor alpha (TNF-α) are cytokines that play important roles in the inflammatory response (23) and pathological processes such as in rheumatoid arthritis (RA) and osteoarthritis (OA). IL-1 and TNF are able to up-regulate the production of each other in a feed-forward manner, and are potent stimulants of oxidant molecule production such as nitric oxide, hydrogen peroxide, and superoxide radicals. Free radical mediated oxidative stress is implicated in numerous disease states, including atherosclerosis, aging, tumor promotion, carcinogenesis, and inflammation. The negative effects of free radicals include cell death, lipid peroxidation, and DNA damage *(23)*.

Both RA and OA provide us with good models for cytokine overexpression. Articular cartilage consists of a highly structured extracellular matrix composed primarily of type II collagen and proteoglycans that account for the tensile strength and load-bearing capacity of the joint. Chondrocytes are embedded within this matrix; these cells participate in the degradation of the extracellular matrix as well as in the synthesis of new matrix proteins. Under normal conditions, these processes are maintained in balance by various cytokines and growth factors. In RA and OA these processes are tipped in favor of net cartilage destruction *(26)*.

In RA, the first signs of joint disease appear in the synovial lining layer, with proliferation of synovial fibroblasts and their attachment to the articular surface at the joint margin. Subsequently, macrophages, T cells and other inflammatory cells are recruited into the joint, where they produce a number of mediators, including IL-1. This mediator contributes to the chronic sequelae of the disease by promoting bone and cartilage destruction and stimulating the release of TNF-α. The concentration of IL-1 in plasma is significantly higher in patients with RA than in healthy individuals, and plasma IL-1 levels correlate with RA disease activity. In addition, synovial fluid levels of IL-1 are correlated with various radiographic and histologic features of RA *(27)*.

This imbalance is fundamental to the study of chronic pain and inflammation and provides a unifying theory for all chronic disease states. Chronic diseases in which elevated or imbalanced cytokines may play a role include rheumatoid arthritis, osteoarthritis, fibromyalgia, psoriasis, eczema and cancer. Inflammation may also be a contributory factor in many neuropathic pain conditions, such as sciatica, peripheral neuralgia, and trigeminal neuralgia. Proinflammatory cytokines and oxidants may be involved with sensitization of nociceptors, producing hyperalgesia, and neuropathic pain may be reduced with anti-cytokine treatment *(23)*. Hyperalgesia and nerve injury-induced degeneration have been significantly reduced with supplementation of N-acetyl-cysteine (NAC) *(23)*. NAC is the rate-limiting substrate for synthesis of the endogenous antioxidant glutathione. This data points to a possible role of dietary antioxidants in pain mitigation, which will be discussed further below.

TNF-α is one of a group of proinflammatory cytokines that appears rapidly after infection and injury. TNF-α has widespread effects. It causes loss of lean and adipose tissue, raises body temperature, reduces appetite, and stimulates production of a diverse range of immunomodulatory cytokines and oxidant molecules *(28)*. TNF-α plays an important part in the pathology of inflammatory diseases such as rheumatoid arthritis and inflammatory bowel disease. This cytokine is the major inflammatory mediator in arthritis, invoking multiple responses and regulating numerous genes implicated in inflammation *(25)*. It is found at high levels in the synovial fluids of patients with both RA and OA *(29)*.

Inhibition of stromelysin mRNA induction by the reactive oxygen species scavenger NAC suggests that reactive oxygen species are involved in stromelysin induction by TNF-α. Stromelysin is one member of a family of matrix metalloproteinases (MMPs) consisting of collagenases, stromelysins, gelatinases, and membrane-type MMPs, which can degrade extracellular matrix *(30)*. Oxidant by-products are used by phagocytes to combat infections during immune responses but are also a source of oxidative damage in degenerative diseases of aging.

Osteoarthritic cartilage is more susceptible to stimulation by TNF-α due to up-regulation of TNF-α receptors on the chondrocytes of patients with OA *(29)*. TNF-α inhibits transcription of cartilage-specific type-II, -IX, and -XI collagens in humans and thus contributes to cartilage loss in joint diseases *(31)*. In the context of osteoarthritis, TNF-α also promotes tissue destruction through stimulating the release of degradative enzymes called metalloproteinases (MMPs) *(30)*. This results in the net effect of TNF-*a* inhibiting cartilage synthesis and actively promoting cartilage destruction. Inhibition of its action is a major target for suppressing inflammation.

IL-1 is also believed to play a central role in the cartilage destruction inherent to both RA and OA. In RA, IL-1 stimulates the release of various species of MMPs by synovial fibroblasts and chondrocytes. Different members of the MMP family target different components of the cartilage matrix. Collagenase degrades collagen; collagenase-3, also known as MMP-13, degrades type-II collagen *(27)*. Stromelysins degrade proteoglycans and activate latent collagenases, whereas gelatinases further degrade collagen that has already been clipped by collagenase *(27,32)*.

Interleukin 1 also stimulates the production of nitric oxide (NO) and PGE2 from chondrocytes and inhibits the synthesis of key matrix proteins of type-II collagen, again contributing to the pathology of both RA and OA *(27)*. Much like TNF-α, IL-1 can simultaneously inhibit cartilage formation and promote tissue destruction.

In addition, NO produced by cartilage and the synovial membrane is implicated in the pathogenesis of OA and RA. In inflamed joints, NO is synthesized in response to proinflammatory cytokines and is involved in joint destruction. Most data indicate that NO is at least partially responsible for IL-1-induced suppression of glycosamino-glycan and collagen synthesis and may be a mediator of IL-1-induced expression of degradative enzymes *(33)*. Under certain conditions, NO may have anabolic and protective effects on the maintenance of cartilage health. In certain tissues, notably in skin and muscle, NO has been found to have a stimulatory role in extracellular matrix repair. In antimicrobial defense and in bacterial arthritis specifically, NO is an important protective molecule *(33,34)*. Production of NO in arthritis-affected cartilage and synovium is a consistent feature of human arthritis. Niacinamide, a niacin analog, has been shown to inhibit excessive NO production in articular cartilage through inhibition of poly-ADP-ribose synthetase (PARS) *(34)*.

The nuclear factor kappa B (NF-κb) family of transcriptional factors regulates the expression of a wide spectrum of genes critically involved in host defense and inflammation. Its production is regulated by the intracellular redox state *(24,26)*. Therefore, its expression may be stimulated by excessive oxidative stress. As a transcription factor, NF-Kb contributes to the gene expression and production of IL-1, IL-6 TNF-α, lymphotoxin, granulocyte monocyte colony stimulating factor (GM-CSF), interferon gamma (IFN-γ), and inducible nitric oxide synthase (iNOS) *(24)*.

GM-CSF plays a key role in proliferation and differentiation of hematopoetic cells, acting on bone marrow to increase the number of neutrophils and monocytes and early erythroid and eosinophilic progenitor cells. In granulocytes GM-CSF stimulates the release of arachidonic acid metabolites and subsequent increased generation of reactive oxygen species (free radicals) *(35)*.

Lymphotoxin, also known as TNF-β, is a tumor necrosis factor family member that is released by lymphocytes. Lymphotoxin is distinct from TNF-α though they both share common receptors and biological activities as described above *(36)*.

T cells and natural killer (NK) cells secrete interferon gamma (IFN-γ) when activated by an antigen or the transcription factor NF-Kb. The major functions of IFN-γ are to activate macrophages and increase expression of antigens. IFN-γ has a role in many different types of immune responses such as delayed type hypersensitivity, inflammation, antibody production and viral infection. The synthesis of IFN-γ is inhibited by 1-alpha, 25-dihydroxy vitamin D3, dexamethasone, and cyclosporin A *(35)*.

Inducible nitric oxide synthase (iNOS) is found in a variety of cell types, including macrophages, hepatocytes, synoviocytes, and smooth muscle cells. Cytokines such as interferon-gamma (IFN-γ), tumor necrosis factor (TNF), and interleukin-1 and -2 cause an increase in iNOS production and activity levels *(32)*. After cytokine induction, iNOS facilitates a significant increase in NO production over a long period of time. In chronic disease states, up-regulated NO production is implicated in the net cartilage destruction that occurs in RA and OA *(32,33,37)*. In addition, some cytokines such as IL-1 and TNF-α activate NF-Kb demonstrating an autoregulatory feedback loop *(26)*.

Cytokines play an important role in the pathogenesis of RA and OA, which can serve as useful models for many other chronic pain conditions. Numerous opportunities may exist for modulating cytokine levels with diet, functional foods, individual nutrients and plant extracts. The following are some specific immunomodulating strategies that may be employed.

3.3.1. NUTRITIONAL CYTOKINE INHIBITION STRATEGIES: ANTIOXIDANTS

Many of the vitamins and foods which are beneficial for chronic pain patients have antioxidant activity. Pro-inflammatory cytokines such as IL-1, TNF, and TGF-β can be modified by a diet high in antioxidants *(38)*. Impaired antioxidant defenses and increases in reactive oxygen and nitrogen species are postulated to be causative factors in aging-related functional decline and in neurodegenerative diseases. Indeed, a lower serum antioxidant level has been recognized as a risk factor for rheumatoid arthritis *(39)*. Many of the events basic to immune regulation are sensitive to the balance between oxidants and antioxidants. Critical steps in signal transduction such as protein phosphorylation and binding of transcription factors (such as NF-Kb) to DNA are modulated by the intracellular redox state *(26)*.

Many of the basic events of cellular regulation are sensitive to the balance between oxidants and antioxidants. Critical steps in signal transduction such as protein phosphorylation and binding of transcription factors to DNA are modulated by the intracellular redox status. Increasing evidence suggests that inflammatory processes are linked to oxidative damage in the central nervous system (CNS) *(38)*.

Several studies have examined antioxidants and their effects in aged animals and humans. A diet high in antioxidant activity when fed to rats for periods as short as 2 weeks can reverse the age-related onset of some neurological deficits *(38)*. Much of the evidence supporting the beneficial role of fruits and vegetables to health comes from epidemiological literature. The traditional common diet of the Mediterranean region, a diet high in fruits, virgin olive oil and vegetables, is associated with a significant (17%) reduction in overall mortality in the elderly from these regions *(40)*. However, in vivo evidence that increased intake of fruits and vegetables actually reduces markers of oxidative stress in humans has now been reported *(41)*. An 8-week dietary intervention was conducted on 246 women randomly assigned to receive one of three diets, with varying intake of fruits and vegetables, from on average 3 up to 9.2 servings per day.

The urinary marker of oxidative stress 8-isoprostane F2-α(8-iso-PGF2-α) was used to assess in vivo reductions in lipid peroxidation. A significant reduction in the excretion of 8-iso-PGF2-α was seen in a dose-dependent manner by all diets. The greatest reductions were seen in those with the highest baseline values for 8-iso-PGF2-α. Therefore measuring levels of this marker may help to identify the best candidates for this type of dietary intervention.

4. DIETARY SUPPLEMENTS

The following is a discussion of some of the dietary compounds that may impact immune function and inflammation, and could be employed as therapeutic agents in the treatment of chronic pain. A detailed account of the chemistry, metabolism, mechanism of action, and scientific evidence is beyond the scope of this chapter.

4.1. Soy

An isoflavone found in soybeans, genistein, inhibits IL-2 synthesis, IL receptor expression, and leukotriene production. Genistein also inhibits the production of nitric oxide from macrophages and acts as an immunosuppressive agent. Soybean isoflavones also have antioxidant properties, which reduce free radical production and oxidative stress. Additional constituents of soy are saponins (see below) and n-3 polyunsaturated fatty acids *(23)*. Not often discussed is the fact that soy also contains many "antinutrients" such as lectins (discussed below), goitrogens (inhibits iodine incorporation into thyroxine), and phytic acid and tannins, both of which inhibit mineral absorption. In addition, soybeans also contain hemagglutinin, a clot-promoting substance that causes red blood cells to clump together and trypsin inhibitors, which inhibit protein digestion. Researchers are also studying the phytoestrogenic effects of the soy isoflavones as endocrine disruptors and in cancer. As of this writing, however, most of the data falls in favor of moderate soy consumption. Fermentation destroys the antinutrients but not the phytoestrogens. Therefore products like miso and tempeh are better tolerated and possibly "safer." Any soybean product that is concentrated will contain more phytoestrogens. Two good examples are soymilk and especially soy protein powder. Most of the work on soy phytoestrogens favors a protective role against cardiovascular disease, cancer and osteoporosis. Some scientists however remain concerned about the role of phytoestrgens as endocrine disrupters *(42)*.

4.2. Niacinamide and PARS Inhibition

Niacinamide is related to niacin. The primary mechanism of action of niacinamide relates to its ability to suppress the cytokine-mediated induction of NO synthase and through inhibition of the nuclear DNA repair enzyme poly (ADP-ribose) synthetase (PARS) *(34)*. Nitric oxide reacts with superoxide, forming peroxynitrite, a potent trigger for DNA single-strand damage, which then activates PARS. Both NO overproduction and PARS activation are implicated in the pathogenesis of OA *(33,34)*. PARS also appears to modulate the course of inflammation by regulating the expression of a number of genes, including the gene for intercellular adhesion molecule 1, collagenase and the inducible nitric oxide synthase *(43)*. In arthritis, PARS activation may trigger a futile energy-consuming cycle, depleting NAD^+, slowing the rate of glycolysis, electron transport and ATP formation and causing cell death of the chondrocyte *(43)*. This feed-forward cycle plays an important role in chronic inflammation and destruction of articular cartilage. Therapeutic levels of niacinamide are not available in food.

4.3. N-acetylcysteine (NAC)

N-acetylcysteine is a powerful antioxidant, providing cysteine, the rate-limiting step in glutathione (GSH) synthesis. NAC also controls oxidative stress-mediated damage in rheumatic diseases by modulation of ROS-dependent signal transduction pathways such as the production of cytokines and activation of PARS *(30,44)*. NAC is very similar in structure and in activity to the disease modifying anti-rhuematic drug bucillamine and is a known inhibitor of NF-Kb *(45)*. The human body can synthesize glutathione from sulfur-containing amino acids (SAAs) such as NAC, methionine and cysteine *(46)*. Glutathione deficiency can be induced by protein-deficient diets that are also low in SAAs such as a strict vegan diet *(46)*. Low GSH levels in elderly subjects have also been reported *(47)* and theorized to accelerate the aging process. GSH can also bind to and detoxify a number of neurotoxins.

4.4. Plant Sterols

Plant sterols may reduce joint pain and stiffness by reducing IL-4 and IL-6 *(48)*. Researchers found that mice fed phytosterol-enriched diets had higher anti-inflammatory IL-10, lower proinflammatory IL-6, and lower TNF-α production. In contrast, the ability to mount an effective immune response was as strong as or even improved in the phytosterol-treated mice compared to controls *(49)*, allaying concerns that sterols could be immunosupressive. Plant sterols given to rats demonstrated potent anti-inflammatory properties similar to cortisone. A proprietary blend of sterols and sterolins was reported capable of reducing the secretion of pro-inflammatory cytokines *(49,50)*.

Phytosterols are non-toxic, do not result in clinically relevant immune suppression, and are rarely associated with adverse reactions. Plant oils contain the highest concentration of phytosterols, nuts and seeds contain moderate amounts, and fruits and vegetables generally contain the lowest phytosterol concentrations *(48)*. One contraindication for use is the rare condition called sitosterolemia where serum sterol levels are elevated. Plant sterols are available in concentrated pill form at a standardized dose, making the use of sterols more precise than if food sources were used.

4.5. Phenols and Polyphenols

Mono and poly phenols are members of the flavonoid family of plant-derived chemicals. Resveratrol, in red and white wine and catechins in tea, are polyphenols that inhibit IL-1β, TNF-α, and IL-6. Resveratrol has also been reported to suppress activation of NF-Kb *(51,52)*. The mechanism may be due to inhibition of cell surface protein kinases leading to suppressed activation of toxins, free radicals and similar stimulatory factors *(53)*.

Red wine may be beneficial for patients with chronic painful inflammatory conditions. Research indicates that both alcohol and resveratrol (the main bioactive polyphenol) in red wine have a synergistic effect on the immune system. *(51)* Resveratrol is found in larger quantities in red wine over white wine. Major biological activities of resveratrol relating to nociception include free radicl scavenging, alteration of eicosanoid synthesis, and blocking of protein kinases and NF-kB activation *(53,54)*.

However, the study of resveratrol thus far has been in vitro and has not involved humans. In addition, the amount of red wine that needs to be consumed for effectiveness of resveratrol is unknown; yet, clearly excessive quantities could do more harm than good. So at this point resveratrol remains a promising anti-inflammatory agent but further clinical studies are needed to better understand its safe use.

Green tea is another excellent dietary source of polyphenols. The most abundant of the polyphenolic compounds in green tea is epigallocatechin gallate (EGCG); other catechins such as epicatechin (EC), epigallocatechin (EGC) and epicatechin gallate (ECG) are also present (55). Green tea-derived EGCG has been described as the most powerful antioxidant of plant origin, and the consumption of green tea leads to a significant increase in the antioxidant activity of plasma. When condensed, these form tannins such as found in black tea and grape skins and seeds. Green tea polyphenols have anti-inflammatory properties, which may be due to their ability to inhibit TNF synthesis by the inhibition of kinases in signaling cascades (40). They are also inhibitors of MMPs (55). The monomeric polyphenols catechin and epicatechin have been shown to completely counteract IFN-γ induced NF-Kb activation (26). Pretreatment of macrophages with catechin and epicatechin decreased IFN-γ-induced NO production significantly compared to IFN-γ-treated controls (56). Catechins possess two actions, one anti-inflammatory and one antiproteolytic, both of which may be helpful for arthritis patients. Human intervention studies are needed to prove efficacy in arthritis. The low toxicity, low cost, and collateral benefits of green tea on other biochemical parameters make it worth a closer look.

Procyanidins are high molecular weight polymers of phenol units such as the catechin and epicatechins found in green tea. Significant concentrations of procyanidins occur in cocoa, berries, tea, *Ginkgo biloba*, apples, and grapes. Standardized nutraceuticals are also available such as pycnogenol (pine bark extract) and grape seed extract (26). Procyanidins extracted from *Pinus maritima* (pine bark extract) have been shown to have several biological effects including NO radical scavenging, inhibition of inducible nitric oxide synthase (iNOS) activity, and iNOS mRNA expression (57). The author has seen a number of cases where patients experienced relief from arthritis with pine bark extract.

4.6. Plant Saponins

Triterpenoid and steroidal saponins, referred to collectively as saponins, are natural detergents found in many edible and inedible plants and most notably legumes. Food sources include soybeans, peas, tea, ginseng, chickpeas, alfalfa sprouts, and fenugreek. Saponins have been shown to have immunomodulatory, antioxidant, and anti-inflammatory activity in animal and in vitro models (58,59). Saponins are also found in medicinal plants such as various species of ginseng and are very likely to play a role in their bioactivity. For instance, ginosides extracted from ginseng protect against free radical damage to cultured endothelial cells, reduce oxidative damage to heart muscle and demonstrate superoxide dismutase (SOD) activity (59). The saponins from *Panax notoginseng* have been shown to decrease phospholipase A2 activity (60). Tea leaf saponins inhibit the activity of hyaluronidase and leukotrienes D4 (46). Soybean saponins may inhibit the release of PGE, NO, TNF-α and monocyte chemotactic protein-1 (MCP-1) in a dose-dependent manner and suppress NF-Kb activation. Soybean saponins have also been shown to down-regulate the expression of COX-2 and iNOS at mRNA/protein levels (61).

4.7. Herbal Extracts

Plants have been widely used as folk medicines in Asia for more than 2 millennia. Numerous plants have potent anti-inflammatory activity via transcription factor and cytokine inhibition. Though a full review of useful plants goes beyond the scope of this chapter, a few can be mentioned to spark interest. The plant Andrographis (*Andrographis paniculate*), which is a rich source for andrographolide, has long been used as a folk remedy for alleviation of inflammatory disorders in China, India, Japan, and Korea. It currently is a prescribed medicine for treatment of laryngitis, diarrhea, and rheumatoid arthritis in China. Andrographis prevents NF-Kb oligonucleotide binding to p50, inhibiting nuclear NF-Kb transcriptional activity, and attenuates inflammation in various in vitro and in vivo models *(62)*. The culinary herb rosemary (*Rosmarinus officinalis*) contains carnosol, rosemarinic acid and carnosolic acid, all of which have anti-inflammatory activity. Carnosol, in particular, inhibits NF-Kb, and iNOS. The relative amount of carnosol in dry ground rosemary leaves is 3.8–4.6% *(63)*. Luduxin, a hops [*Humulus lupulus*] extract, and oleanolic acid (an isomer of usolic acid) also show promise for inhibition of PGE2 synthesis.

4.8. Therapeutic Intervention with n-3 Fats

Increased dietary intake of n-3 fats displaces n-6 fat from the cell membrane. As a result, ingestion of EPA and DHA from fish or fish oil leads to *(1)* decreased production of Series-2 eicosanoids; *(2)* decreased concentrations of thromboxane A_2, a potent platelet aggregator and vasoconstrictor; *(3)* decreased formation of leukotriene B_4, an inducer of inflammation and a powerful inducer of leukocyte chemotaxis and adherence; *(4)* increased concentrations of thromboxane A3, a weak platelet aggregator and vasoconstrictor; *(5)* increased concentrations of prostacyclin 3 (PGI3), leading to an overall increase in total prostacyclin by increasing PGI3 without decreasing PGI2 (both PGI2 and PGI3 are active vasodilators and inhibitors of platelet aggregation); and *(6)* increased concentrations of leukotriene B_5, a weak inducer of inflammation and a chemotactic agent *(7)*.

Fish oil has been shown to exert an anti-inflammatory influence in animal models of inflammation *(16,60,61)* and produces anti-inflammatory effects in rheumatoid arthritis *(64)*, Crohn's disease *(65)*, and psoriasis *(66)*.

Dietary supplementation of n-3 PUFA may have the beneficial effect of slowing and reducing inflammation in the pathogenesis of degenerative joint disease and other inflammatory states. Loading the cell membrane with EPA and DHA with subsequent displacement of AA from the cell membrane is a key nutritional strategy for treating chronic inflammatory conditions. By loading the cell membrane with EPA and DHA, pro-inflammatory Series-2 ecosanoids and Series-4 leukotrienes are suppressed while synthesis of anti-inflammatory Series-3 ecosanoids and Series-5 leukotrienes are increased *(7,67–70)*. This shifts the balance of the eicosanoid production to a less inflammatory profile. Compliance with dietary fish oil treatment can be monitored through assessing red blood cell membrane fatty acid composition.

Dietary fish oil supplementation decreases production of the proximate cytokines IL-1 and TNF by peripheral blood mononuclear cells *(71)*. Fish oil may have a biphasic effect on immune function. Fish oil intake decreases cytokine secretion in individuals who are high producers, whereas fish oil intake increases secretion in low producers. Some patients do not respond to the TNF-α-lowering effects of fish oil.

Table 2
Summary of Effects of n-3 Fatty Acids on Joint Health

Reduction, in a dose-dependent manner, of the endogenous and IL-1-induced release of
proteoglycan breakdown products from articular cartilage and strong inhibition of proteolytic
activity (72,73).
Alteration of cell membrane fluidity and influence on the activities of membrane associated
enzymes and receptors.
Inhibition of MMPs mRNA expression (72).
Inhibition of COX2, 5-lipoxygenase (LOX), 5-lipoxygenase-activating protein, TNF-α ,
IL-1alpha, and IL-1 beta mRNA without disruption of proteins involved in normal tissue
homeostasis (72,74).

Polymorphisms in TNF-α and lymphotoxin genes could explain why some patients
are non-responders (28). Increased lipid peroxidation and free radical formation is
one potential adverse effect. Supplementation with lipid soluble antioxidants such as
vitamin E helps prevent this. See Table 2 for a summary of the mechanisms by which
n-3 fats affect metabolism of cells within the synovial joint tissues.

5. GENETIC POLYMORPHISMS

A polymorphism is defined as an alternate form of a gene present in >1% of the
population. Some polymorphisms have been shown to alter cofactor binding and affect
a large percentage of the population. Up to one-third of the mutations possible in a
gene can cause an increase in the Michaelis constant (K_m). Increases in the K_m cause
decreased enzyme binding affinity for the vitamin-derived coenzyme (75). This, in
turn, lowers the reaction rate. High-dose vitamin therapy may increase intracellular
cofactor concentrations and mechanistically work by activating a defective enzyme
and partially restoring function leading to alleviation of symptoms.

There are more than 30,000 human genes. Of the 3,870 enzymes cataloged in the
ENZYME database (76), 860 (22%) use a cofactor (75). The cofactors are vitamin and
mineral derived. The recent availability of genetic testing for polymorphisms gives the
practitioner the ability to test for some of the more common ones. Highly individualized
nutritional protocols can then be implemented.

Readers are referred to Ames et al for in-depth information on the polymorphisms
and various cofactors, vitamins, and enzymes involved. In the context of hyperalgesia
and chronic pain, which this chapter is dedicated to, a few common polymorphism-
induced enzymatic defects deserve mention.

5.1. B-Vitamins

Human methylenetetrahydrofolate reductase (MTHFR) uses NADP (niacin),
folate, and FAD (riboflavin) cofactors to catalyze the conversion of 5,
10-methylenetetrahydrofolate to 5-methyltetrahydrofolate (75). The latter is the
predominant circulatory form of folate and the main carbon donor for the remethylation
of homocysteine to methionine. The 677C-T polymorphism results in a smaller pool of
5-methyltetrahydrofolate and an accumulation of homocysteine, which is well known
to be associated with an elevated risk of cardiovascular disease. A higher frequency
of the 677C-T polymorphism has also been associated with migraine (77), diabetic

nephropathy *(78)*, and other conditions. There are reports of a significant reduction in migraine attack frequency with high-dose riboflavin treatment (400 mg/d) *(79)*. High-dose folate or a special form of folate called 5-methyltetrahydrofolate is the treatment of choice for this polymorphism.

5.2. Glutathione

Glucose-6-phosphate 1-dehydrogenase (G6PD) is an X-linked cytosolic enzyme that generates NADPH in the oxidative branch of the pentose phosphate pathway. NADPH is a key electron donor in biochemical reactions and important in the defense against oxidizing agents, possibly through the maintenance of reduced glutathione concentrations. G6PD deficiency is the single most common metabolic disorder, with an estimated 400 million persons thought to be affected worldwide. Red blood cells, in particular, are susceptible to lysis, mediated by oxidative stress because of their lack of mitochondria and subsequent reliance on G6PD and one other pentose phosphate pathway enzyme for the production of NADPH. Defects in G6PD usually result in reduced enzymatic activity and a lower ratio of NADPH to NADP. Although some G6PD defects do not affect cofactor binding, many G6PD defects result in an increased K_m for NADP (niacin) and directly alter the NADP binding site. Since patients with this polymorphism are more sensitive to oxidative stress, they may benefit from clinical interventions designed to raise glutathione levels with supplementation of such agents as selenium, N-acetyl-cysteine (NAC), oral reduced glutathione, and intravenous glutathione. Antioxidant therapy with ascorbate, tocopherols, carotenoids or poly or mono phenols may also be employed *(75)*.

5.3. Tumur Necrosis Factor

There are various isoforms of the gene that codes for tumor necrosis factor (TNF) that seem to influence not only baseline TNF levels, but also may affect how these patients respond to N-3 fat supplementation.

TNF production varies widely between healthy persons. This variation results because polymorphisms in the promoter regions of genes influence the amount of TNF produced after an inflammatory stimulus. For example, persons homozygous for the TNF-308 *(TNF*2)* allele had 7 times the rate of malaria-related mortality and serious neurological symptoms of persons heterozygous or homozygous for the more common *TNF*1* allele *(28)*.

Data by Grimble et al. suggest that the sensitivity of a person to the suppressive effects of n-3 PUFAs on TNF production is linked to the baseline level of production of the cytokine from the person before supplementation and to genetic variation encoded by, or associated with, the TNF polymorphisms. They found that fish oil could enhance TNF production in subjects that were in the lowest level of TNF prior to fish oil supplementation. A possible explanation for this paradoxical effect could be that fish oil can alter pro-inflammatory cytokine production in either direction by replacing arachidonic acid in the cell membrane. Such an effect would decrease PGE2 and LTB4 production and increase the formation of PGE3 and LTB5. These eicosanoids have lower bioactivities than do PGE2 and LTB4. Thus, the overall effect on TNF production (inhibition or stimulation) will depend on the balance among the different stimulatory and inhibitory eicosanoids produced from arachidonic and eicosapentaenoic acids *(28)*.

6. ACID–BASE BALANCE

The healthy pH range for arterial blood is 7.35 to 7.45, and carbon dioxide-laden venous blood is 7.31 to 7.41. The healthy intracellular pH is 7.4 ± 0.1. Even minor variation from these values is biologically costly. An acidic tilt to cellular pH adversely alters cellular metabolism leading to impaired ATP production, increased free radical production, increased interstitial fluid, nitrogen wasting, and, interestingly, suppression of growth hormone (80). A 500–900% increase in osteoclast-mediated rat bone resorption was seen with just a 0.2 pH unit change (81) and a study with fasting humans showed that a venous pH drop from 7.37 to 7.33 causes significant release of calcium from bone (82).

Bone minerals serve as an extensive buffer in the control of plasma pH (83). Research has documented that urinary calcium excretion is associated with bone loss and parallels total acid excretion (80). Upon significant depletion of buffering mineral salts, compensation for total acid load is reduced, resulting in decreased intracellular and first-morning pH (84). First-morning pH has been promoted as a useful clinical marker for cellular and systemic acid-alkaline balance and should be maintained at 6.5 to 7.5 for optimal health (80,84).

Though a link between osteoporosis and metabolic acidosis was established many years ago (85), it is still not a common practice among physicians to address acid–base balance in this patient population. Osteoporosis may cause loss of height, stooped posture, a kyphotic curve (kyphosis), and severe pain and disability. It commonly affects the thoracic and thoracolumbar regions of the spine. The structural deterioration of bone increases the risk for fracture in the hip, spine, and wrist. Bone is sensitive to small changes in pH. In vitro studies demonstrate that a one-tenth drop in pH can greatly increase osteoclastic activity, inhibit osteoblastic activity, and induce bone and mineral loss (86).

The main source of net acid load is protein, especially when in excess of 60 grams/day. Other sources of net acid load are phosphoric acid, SAA supplementation, sulfate, excessive intake of long-chain fatty acids (>15-20% of total daily calories), stress, hormones, and delayed-type hypersensitivity reactions. Buffering elements in the form of organic anions are obtained in the diet from fruits, vegetables, pulses (lentils, peas), herbs, and spices. Certain organic acids such as citrate, malate, succinate, and fumarate are also base forming, explaining why lemons and limes are alkalinizing (80).

It appears that chronic excess in metabolic acids is the rule rather than the exception in North America (80,84,87). According to Brown et al modern diets cause a net acid load excess that is two to four times higher than the 50 mEq that the body should obtain on an ideal diet (80,84,87,88). Only 12% of the United States population eats the recommended 2–4 servings of fruit and 3–5 servings of vegetables per day (80). (80) Among children, only 7% consume two servings of fruit and vegetables per day (89). A study was done on vegetarian and animal protein diets containing the same amount of protein. Researchers found that urinary pH was significantly lower and urinary calcium higher in the animal protein group. Osteoporosis in uncommon in cultures that eat an alkaline-rich diet such as the Mayan, African, and Chinese (80).

7. THE ROLE OF GUT IMMUNE FUNCTION AND INTESTINAL PERMEABILITY

A healthy intestinal environment participates in a wide range of supportive roles, from formation and absorption of nutrients to neutralization of toxins and protection from antigens and pathogens. Small intestinal bacterial overgrowth and increased gut permeability are possible initiating or exacerbating factors in rheumatoid arthritis *(90)*, arthralgia *(91)* and food allergy. *(92)* The barrier function of the gastrointestinal tract has been shown to be impaired following stress, infection or inflammation *(92)*.

7.1. Bowel Bacterial Overgrowth

Approximately 20% of all patients with inflammatory bowel disease have joint inflammation *(93)*, and intestinal inflammation occurs in approximately 67% of patients with RA, *(90–94)* particularly when joint disease is active *(91)*. Because gut inflammation is known to increase intestinal permeability, it is possible that an increased uptake of intestinal bacterial components across the inflamed mucosa leads to systemic distribution of these bacterially derived factors *(95)*, resulting in joint inflammation and/or arthralgia.

A high frequency of small bowel bacterial overgrowth *(96)* is seen in RA, particularly with anaerobes *(97)*. There is evidence that antibiotic therapy relieves clinical symptoms in patients with RA, and animal and human experiments support this notion *(98)*. Additionally, cell wall fragments of the human commensal *Eubacterium aerofaciens*, the main resident of gut flora, can cause both acute and chronic arthritis in rats after a single intraperitoneal injection of cell wall fragments *(99)*. Also known as "leaky gut," increased intestinal permeability allows intraepithelial pathogens and intact proteins that have escaped enzymatic digestion to cross the gastrointestinal barrier and enter peripheral circulation. The stage is then set for homologous amino acid sequence-mediated molecular mimicry. In this scenario, T-cells cross-react between the amino acid sequence on the foreign antigen and the self-antigen, causing autoimmunity *(95)*. Autoimmune disease occurs when the body loses the ability to discriminate between self and non-self proteins. This loss of tolerance may ultimately result is tissue destruction by the immune system and the clinical features of disease. Most autoimmune diseases are thought to develop via the interaction of an environmental factor (antigen) or factors with a specific hereditary component such as those genes that code for the human leucocyte antigens (HLA) (see Figure 4) *(95)*.

Healthy epithelial mucosal cells normally do not allow passage of more than approximately 2% of intact dietary proteins *(100)*. Passage of viable bacteria from the gastrointestinal tract to extra-intestinal sites has been shown to occur with intestinal bacterial overgrowth, immune deficiencies, and increased permeability of the intestinal barrier *(95–101)*. Unhydrolyzed dietary peptides have also been shown to enter the peripheral circulation, particularly with increased intestinal permeability, NSAID use, ethanol, acetic acid and dietary lectins derived from legumes and cereal grains *(95,100)*.

7.2. Lectins

Sometimes referred to as anti-nutrients, lectins are found in cereal grains and legumes. Lectins are glycoproteins that influence the structure and function of both enterocytes and lymphocytes *(95,102)*. Common foods that contain lectins include peanuts, soy, barley, lentils, rice, mung beans, lima beans, kidney beans, split peas,

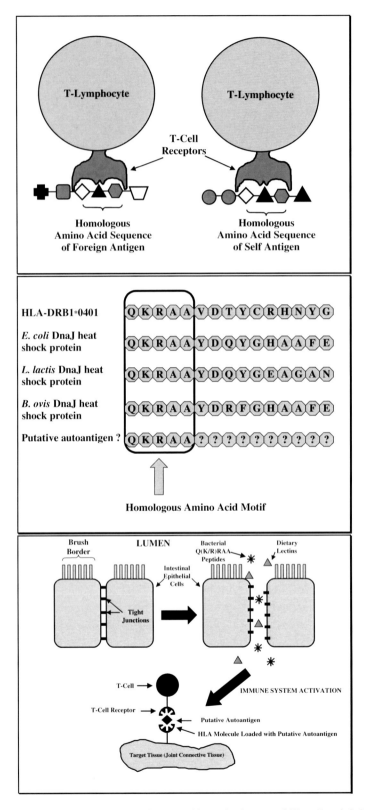

Fig. 4. Mechanisms of autoimmunity and increased intestinal permeability. Special thanks to Loren Cordain, PhD.

potatoes, and wheat *(95)*. Wheat-germ agglutinin, a lectin derived from dietary wheat products, is heat-stable and resistant to digestive proteolytic breakdown in both rats and human subjects *(102)*. Lectins may contribute to increased intestinal permeability, bacterial overgrowth, immune reactivity, and arthritis *(95)*.

Lectins can bind surface glycans on gut brush-border epithelial cells causing damage to the base of the villi, which includes disarrangement of the cytoskeleton, increased endocytosis, and shortening of the microvilli These structural changes on intestinal epithelial cells elicit functional changes, including increased intestinal permeability, allowing undigested peptides and bacteria to enter the circulation *(95)*. Interestingly, high-wheat-gluten diets have been shown to induce unfavorable jejunal mucosal architectural changes in normal subjects *(103)*. Lectins are resistant to proteolytic breakdown, and therefore the intestinal lumen concentrations can be high. Lectins transported through the gut wall can greatly exceed that of other dietary antigens, and absorbed dietary lectins can be presented by macrophages to competent lymphocytes of the immune system *(95,102,104)*.

7.2.1. LECTINS AND RHEUMATOID ARTHRITIS

Dietary lectins may also be implicated in RA because they can cause the preferential overgrowth of gut bacteria such as *Escherichia coli* and *Lactobacillus lactis*. These bacteria are associated with the expression of RA because they contain an amino acid sequence (Q(K/R)RAA) which is also found in the gene products of the human leukocyte antigens (HLA) system in a high percentage of patients with RA *(95,105)*. Dietary lectins may indirectly increase the symptoms of RA by facilitating movement of bacterial antigens with arthrogenic properties to the periphery and directly increasing gut permeability. Because dietary lectins are able to cross the gastrointestinal barrier rapidly and enter the circulation intact, they may also be able to interact directly with synovial tissues *(95)*. It is generally assumed that cooking eliminates lectin activity; however, it has been demonstrated that residual lectin activity is present in kidney beans even when cooked at 85°F for 6 hours or at 90°F for 3 hours *(106)*. See Table 3 for a summary of the actions of dietary lectins on the gastrointestinal and immunological function.

Table 3
The Influence of Dietary Lectins on All Aspects of Gastrointestinal and Immunological Function (from Cordain et al *(95)*)*

Stimulate production of inflammatory cytokines

Cause abnormal ICAM expression on T-cells

Stimulate IFN causing HLA class-II expression

Stimulate T-cell proliferation

Upregulate HLA class-II expression on epithelial cells

Increase gut permeability

Bind surface glycan on gut brush border cells causing damage to microvilli

Cause overgrowth of gut bacteria including those with the Q(K/R)RAA susceptibility moiety

*Abbreviations: Intercellular adhesion molecule (ICAM); human leukocyte antigen (HLA); Interferon (IFN).

7.3. Diet and Crohn's Disease

In Crohn's disease, approximately 20% of patients experience arthralgia together with gut inflammation *(107)*. Elemental diets have been shown to be as effective as corticosteroids in treating the disease, and most subjects (> 80%) achieve disease remission with these drastic dietary changes. Elemental diets are defined as protein-free diets consisting of essential amino acids, trace elements, glucose, and vitamins. A controlled study of elemental diets in the treatment of RA demonstrated improvements in grip strength and Ritchie score (a score of joint tenderness to pressure) that relapsed following food re-introduction *(108)*.

7.4. Diet and Rheumatoid Arthritis

Removal of gluten-containing grains not only eliminates celiac disease, but also symptoms of arthritis, and such diets may be of benefit for a subset of patients with RA or idiopathic arthralgia *(95)*. It has been demonstrated that some arthritic patients have elevated gliadin antibody levels *(109)*, and gluten-free diets have been shown to be effective in reducing arthritic symptoms in celiac patients, supporting the notion that wheat-containing diets can increase intestinal permeability, allowing luminal antigens access to the circulation. Additionally, both fasting *(110)* and grain-free diets *(111)* have been shown to alleviate symptoms of RA, supporting the concept that damage to intestinal physiology by dietary substances may allow both dietary and bacterial antigens to enter the circulation, causing persistent immune system stimulation.

Dairy products have been implicated in the etiology of RA *(112)*. Elevated serum IgG antibodies to milk, wheat or both dietary proteins have been observed in patients with RA. Bovine serum albumin (BSA), a milk protein, may be the causative factor in milk products because it contains an amino acid sequence homologous with human collagen *(113)*. Blood from RA patients has demonstrated reactivity to synthetic peptides containing the BSA residues, and exogenous BSA peptides can bind to RA HLA-DR moieties *(114)*. Case studies have shown that elimination of milk and dairy products from the diets of patients with RA improved symptoms, and the disease was markedly exacerbated on re-challenge *(115)*.

The interaction among dietary lectins, enterocytes, and lymphocytes facilitates the translocation of both dietary and gut-derived bacterial antigens into the circulation, which in turn causes persistent antigenic stimulation. In susceptible individuals this antigenic stimulation may ultimately result in the expression of overt RA via molecular mimicry in which foreign peptides are similar enough in structure to cause T-lymphocytes and antibodies to cross-react with endogenous proteins such as proteoglycans in cartilage *(95)*. The translocation of bacteria and bacterial products across the gut wall may be involved in autoimmune disease, and a prolonged systemic inflammatory response *(95,116)*. Proinflammatory cytokines such as TNF-α are released both systemically and locally in the gut. Additionally, TNF-α has been shown to increase the permeability of intercellular gap junctions *(116)*.

7.5. Glutamine

Administration of glutamine has been shown to reduce septic complications and to significantly reduce impairment in gut barrier function and bacterial translocation seen in models of critical illness and gut injury. Glutamine is regarded as conditionally essential in conditions of stress, including trauma, sepsis, and ischemia-reperfusion injury because the body's requirements for glutamine may exceed supply. Glutamine plays a key role in metabolism for rapidly dividing cells such as enterocytes and cells of the immune system. Glutamine also acts as a key precursor for intestinal synthesis of the antioxidant glutathione and stimulates intestinal synthesis of polyamines, which play a major role in the control of enterocyte proliferation and repair. Atrophy of the small intestinal mucosa that follows prolonged total parenteral nutrition can be prevented or reversed by addition of glutamine to intravenous feeding regimens. Finally, glutamine depletion may lead to increased gut permeability and bacterial translocation in both animals and humans *(116)*.

8. FOOD ALLERGY

Though still a subject of some contention among the medical community, food allergy, generally defined as an immunological reaction to food, may contribute to recurrent abdominal pain (RAP) *(117)*. There is little disagreement that acute IgE-mediated hypersensitivity to foods qualifies as food allergy. Less clear has been the role of IgG in the clinical diagnosis and pathophysiology of food allergy. IgG reactions are known as delayed-type hypersensitivity reactions and are less severe than the anaphylactic, or immediate-type hypersensitivity reactions mediated by IgE. IgG sensitivities are typically tested for via the serum radioallergosorbent test (RAST). These tests, while not known to be highly accurate, have demonstrated usefulness in a clinical setting for the treatment of delayed-type hypersensitivity reactions *(118)*.

8.1. Food Allergy Diagnosis

The gold standard for diagnosis of food allergy is the double-blind placebo-controlled food challenge test *(119)*; however, because this test is so cumbersome it is seldom done. The open food challenge test is often done instead. In the open challenge, individual foods are eliminated and then "challenged" to reproduce symptoms.

Symptoms of food allergy can include diarrhea, constipation, gastroesophageal reflux, abdominal pain, and fatigue. On endoscopy, histologic abnormalities such as lymphonodular doudenitis and esophagitis are sometimes seen. It has been reported that up to 33% of children suffering from recurrent abdominal pain have food allergy, as determined though open challenge. Because intestinal T lymphocytes and mast cells play a coordinating role in inflammatory cytokine production, addressing food allergy could improve clinical outcomes in some patients with gastrointestinal disorders *(117)*.

8.2. Food Allergy and Rheumatoid Arthritis

Many patients with RA have been noted to suffer from increased intestinal permeability, especially when experiencing symptoms *(95)* and RA has been linked to allergies and food sensitivities *(120)*. In many people, RA worsens when they eat foods to which they are allergic or sensitive and improves by avoiding these foods *(115,121,122)*. In one study, the vast majority of RA patients had elevated levels of antibodies to milk, wheat, or both, suggesting a high incidence of allergy to these substances in this patient population *(112)*. It has been reported that one-third of people with RA may be able to control their disease completely through allergy elimination *(123)*.

8.3. Food Allergy and Inflammation

Allergy can affect cytokines, histamine, and other inflammatory mediators. Kaufman first reported the association between ingestion of allergenic foods and musculoskeletal syndromes in susceptible people in 1953 *(124)*. In addition to the early work of Kaufman, Zussman et al. also reported cases of exacerbation of musculoskeletal problems with certain food ingestions *(125)*. Of 1,000 consecutive adults with allergic complaints, 20% had rheumatic complaints, and 27 had rheumatic symptoms exacerbated by ingestion of specific foods. Ratner et al studied 15 women and eight men with rheumatoid or psoriatic arthritis *(126)*. The patients were instructed to remove dairy products and beef from their diet. Seven patients became asymptomatic within 3–4 weeks after starting the diet, and these patients had an exacerbation of symptoms after reintroducing dairy products into their diet. The other 16 patients did not improve. The seven patients who improved were all women, seronegative, and lactase deficient, suggesting a diet free of dairy products and beef is of value in lactase-deficient women with seronegative rheumatoid arthritis or psoriatic arthritis.

9. CORTISOL/DHEA IMBALANCES

Suboptimal or low cortisol has a negative effect on immunity and inflammation. Whereas high cortisol is well known to be associated with hyperglycemia, sarcopenia, osteoporosis, central obesity and suppressed immune function, the clinical significance of low-normal levels is less well appreciated. In 1990 Neeck et al. reported that patients with RA had impaired diurnal variation in serum cortisol that varied with fluctuations in disease activity *(127)*. A 1992 study *(128)* reported that patients with RA had lower diurnal plasma cortisol levels compared to controls, and that RA patients failed to increase cortisol normally following surgery despite having normal responses to cortisol releasing factor (CRF). This is consistent with the notion that hypothalamic dysfunction and mild adrenocortical insufficiency are implicated in this disease and possibly other autoimmune conditions.

Phosphatidylserine may prevent stress-induced elevations in cortisol *(129)*, and certain plant substances (Holy basil, ginseng, cordyceps, and Rhodiola) have been shown to normalize hypothalamic-pituitary-adrenal (HPA) axis dysfunction as well. However, few dietary interventions exist for raising cortisol. Freeze-dried adrenal extract may be employed, as it may contain cortisol, but quality concerns and lack of standardization present drawbacks to this approach. Prescription oral hydrocortisone provides a better alternative as popularized by William Jefferies in his book *The Safe Uses of Cortisol*. Because cortisol is synthesized from the parent compound cholesterol, low total cholesterol could contribute to low cortisol levels. Increasing dietary saturated fat intake raises cholesterol. There also are reports of plant sterols having the ability to raise dehydroepiandrosterone (DHEA) and normalize the cortisol response *(48)*.

10. ADULT HUMAN GROWTH HORMONE DEFICIENCY (AGHD)

Human growth hormone (HGH) plays an important role in muscle accretion, creating a feeling of well being, lipolysis, weight maintenance, glucose control, and tissue repair. Suboptimal growth hormone secretion may occur as a co-morbid factor in chronic inflammatory diseases, chronic corticosteroid use, and fibromyalgia (FMS) *(130)*. The most common cause of AGHD is pituitary adenoma *(131)*. Other causes of AGHD include surgery or radiotherapy for the treatment of other non-pituitary pathologies, cranial irradiation, and head trauma. Typical signs of AGHD include increased fat mass, particularly central adiposity, decreased lean body mass, and reduced exercise capacity and muscle strength, particularly in active individuals. Other common symptoms include thin, dry skin with cool extremities, impaired sense of psychological well being, depressed mood, social anxiety, and fatigue.

The diagnosis of AGHD is based on a growth hormone stimulation test through a variety of methods (insulin tolerance test, arginine stimulation, L-DOPA, or glucagon test). Most patients with AGHD demonstrate a reduced serum insulin-like growth factor-I (IGF-I) concentration, increased low-density lipoprotein (LDL)-cholesterol concentration, and reduced bone mineral density *(131)*.

10.1. Fibromyalgia

Some of the clinical features of fibromyalgia (FM) are similar to the ones described in AGHD. Shared features in these two syndromes include muscle weakness, fatigue, decreased exercise capability, and feeling of social isolation. Insulin-like growth factor (IGF)-1 level is frequently reduced in these patients, suggesting that this could be caused by impaired HGH secretion. Maximal HGH secretion occurs during stage-4 sleep, and this stage is reduced in patients with FM. Researchers have found a marked decrease in HGH secretion at night in association with reduced length of stage III–IV sleep in FMS patients. Data show that patients with FM exhibited a marked decrease in HGH secretion but normal pituitary responsiveness to exogenously administered growth hormone releasing hormone (GHRH), suggesting hypothalamic dysfunction in the control of GH secretion *(132)*.

10.2. Human Growth Hormone

While the safety and efficacy of exogenously administered human growth hormone (HGH) has yet to be determined, using nutritional factors conservatively to raise HGH could be considered. The amino acids arginine, ornithine, and glutamine have all been shown to raise nighttime release of HGH, though results are mixed. Arginine is effective intravenously, but if given orally, must be consumed at very high doses (2–5 g). Glutamine also must be given at doses of 2–6 g to be effective for stimulating HGH release. The compound acetyl-L-carnitine (ALCAR) may also work synergistically with ornithine to effectively raise HGH release at night at more manageable dose levels. Parr published a case report using 500 mg of ALCAR and 2–30 mg of ornithine to improve quality of sleep and raise IGF-1 concentrations *(133)*. The author has also tried this with mostly positive results. The aforementioned treatments must be given at least 2 hours away from food and with water only. A transdermal preparation is also available that works as an analogue of Growth Hormone Releasing Hormone. It is given five days out of seven two to three times a day and will raise urinary HGH while lowering IGF-1.

11. NEUROHORMONES AND NEUROTRANSMITTERS

Dysregulation of certain neurohormones/neurotransmitters has been implicated as a contributing factor in several chronic pain conditions, such as migraine headache and fibromyalgia. Serotonin is a neurotransmitter synthesized by enzymes that act on tryptophan and/or 5-HTP. Serotonin is stored in pre-synaptic vesicles and released to transmit electrochemical signals across the synapse. Serotonin is a therapeutic target for diseases like depression, compulsive disorders, anxiety, and migraines. Serotonin acts, in most cases, as an inhibitory neurotransmitter and modulates neuron voltage potentials to inhibit glutamate activity and neurotransmitter firing. Other biologically active neurotransmitters include epinephrine, norepinephrine, dopamine, melatonin, beta-phenylethylamine (PEA), gamma-aminobutyric acid (GABA), histamine, and glutamate.

11.1. Serotonin

Serotonin is synthesized through the substrate amino acid tryptophan. The catecholamines (dopamine, norepinephrine, and epinephrine) and PEA are synthesized from the substrate amino acid, phenylalanine. Food protein sources like eggs, meat, or whey protein contain many amino acids including tryptophan and phenylalanine, but the amount of precursors that cross the blood–brain barrier after eating these foods is relatively small. Diets that are restrictive in either the amount or variety of the foods they include, such as vegetarian, low-calorie, or low-protein, are the most likely to limit neurotransmitter production. Melatonin is a neurohormone produced by the pineal gland and synthesized from serotonin under the regulation of norepinephrine. Melatonin levels follow a precise circadian pattern with high levels at night and low to undetectable levels during the day. This fluctuation controls the body's sleep-wake cycle. Decreased levels of melatonin during the night can cause difficulty falling asleep and reduce the restfulness of sleep.

It has been hypothesized that excessive serotonin coupled with low melatonin may be the biochemical trigger for the headache phase of migraine. Migraine is caused by primary dysfunction of cerebral neurons with secondary involvement of extracranial and intracranial blood vessels. The pineal gland, which contains 90% of the serotonin in the CNS and most of the melatonin, may act as the intermediate trigger factor in migraine (134).

Pineal serotonin, when released into the CSF will increase the activity of cerebral neurons but decrease the activity of the serotonergic neurons of the raphe nuclei, which normally act to inhibit the trigeminovascular system (135). Resulting hyperactivity of the trigeminovascular system leads to dilation and inflammation of the cerebral vessels near the trigeminal nerve, which can result in headache. Melatonin may counteract this hyperactivity by increasing the activity of the raphe nuclei. Decreases in plasma and urine melatonin in migraine patients have been reported and a small trial demonstrated that IV infusion of melatonin relieved headache in 100% (6 out of 6) of patients (136).

11.2. Fibromyalgia

Fibromyalgia syndrome (FMS) is a form of non-articular rheumatism characterized by chronic (>3 months), widespread musculoskeletal pain, insomnia, stiffness, and pressure hyperalgesia at characteristic soft tissue sites, referred to as tender points. Deficiency of serontenergic neuronal functioning is among the potential mechanisms postulated to explain this baffling disorder (137). Serotonergic system dysregulation may contribute to hypothalamic pituitary axis (HPA) hyperactivation (138–141), which has been hypothesized to cause the sleep disturbances common in this syndrome. Various groups have reported a flattened, yet elevated diurnal cortisol curve that does not respond to dexamethasone suppression (139). Reduced sensitivity to adreno-corticotropin-hormone (ACTH) at the adrenal level or reduced glucocorticoid receptor function has also been proposed to explain the decreased sensitivity to negative feedback control.

11.2.1. TRYPTOPHAN

Serotonin (5-hydroxytryptamine, 5-HT) is a neurotransmitter that plays a major role in the regulation of mood, emotion, cognition and motor functions, as well as circadian and neuroendocrine rhythms *(139,140)*. Serotonin plays a pivotal role in the regulation of HPA axis function. In particular, 5-HT is involved in the stimulation of ACTH secretion during stress. Both tryptophan and 5-HT raise serotonin levels in both the central and enteric nervous systems. Most studies of serotonin in the serum of FMS patients reveal lower levels than in controls *(137–139)*, but the relevance of these findings remains unclear. Studies exploring tryptophan (TRP) in fibromyalgia revealed lower than normal levels. Reduced tryptophan could result in decreased 5-HT synthesis, thus impairing descending antinociceptive mechanisms within the CNS *(138)*.

11.2.2. SUBSTANCE P

Substance P (SP) is a neuropeptide strongly involved in the process of nociception. Decreased serotonin activity and increased SP activity influence circadian rhythm and sleep, as well as pain perception. A negative correlation between levels of SP and both tryptophan and its metabolite 5-hydroxyindoleacetic acid (5-HIAA) has been demonstrated. 5-HT is synthesized from its precursor TRP and metabolized to 5-HIAA. In a study on 51 FM patients, high levels of 5-HIAA and lower SP levels were associated with improved sleep and reduced nociception, whereas low 5-HIAA and high substance P levels correlated with increased nociception and strong sleep disturbances *(141)*. This is not too surprising since earlier experiments demonstrated that if animals were pretreated with serotonergic agonists before infusion of SP, the receptive field of nociception is reduced *(142)*. Decreased levels of 5-HT may influence pain perception and sleep through a negative feedback loop with SP. Elevated levels of SP have been found in cerebrospinal fluid of patients with FMS. Decreased serotonergic activity and increased SP activity may cause a pain amplification syndrome in FMS *(139)*. Capsaicin from red pepper is an effective topical SP inhibitor. In animal models of magnesium deficiency (9% of the RDA), SP levels are increased. *(143)*.

12. MAGNESIUM (Mg)

Magnesium is an essential mineral to include in the clinical armamentarium and has important implications for many pain conditions. It is needed for bone, protein, and fatty acid formation, hematopoesis, muscle contraction, clot formation, and synthesizing ATP. The secretion and action of insulin also require magnesium. Sleep latency, dyssomnia, and HPA axis dysfunction are all features of FMS and chronic fatigue syndrome (CFS) that may respond to magnesium supplementation. Ample evidence strongly supports the use of magnesium for migraine headache and other pain conditions such as angina, PMS, and in kidney stone prevention. Magnesium depletion has been associated with hypofunction of the biological clock in humans. A marker for this is a decrease in melatonin and its metabolites in serum and urine *(144,145)*.

Photophobia, nervous excitability, anxiety, headaches, and dyssomnia are all features of Mg depletion *(144,145)*. Magnesium status directly influences biological clock function by causing dysfunction of the suprachiasmatic nuclei and pineal gland.

Calcium, magnesium, potassium and sodium all play homeostatic roles in muscle tone and contraction. Suboptimal or frank deficiencies of any of these minerals can cause muscle tetany, hypertonicity and faciulations. Chronic muscle hypertonicity, in turn, is one cause of myalgia. Red blood cell magnesium is more sensitive than serum magnesium. Chelated forms such as magsesium citrate and glycinate are better tolerated than non-chelated forms such as magnesium oxide. Magnesium may also be given intravenously, allowing for more rapid repletion without gastrointestinal side effects.

13. CHOLINESTERASE

Several reports have provided evidence for the critical importance of the cholinergic system in pain inhibitory pathways. Since the first observation 40 years ago that the cholinesterase inhibitor physostigmine increased the pain threshold in humans a vast body of literature has accumulated on the antinociceptive action of cholinesterase inhibitors and cholinomemetic drugs *(146)*.

Chinese club moss (*Huperzia serrata*) contains the alkaloid huperzine A, which is a potent and selective inhibitor of acetylcholineesterase. Huperzine A has been shown to be neuroprotective and enhance cognitive function. Its role in the treatment of Alzheimer's disease is currently underway *(147)*. Since huperzine A is also a nootropic and neuroprotective agent, it could be a treatment to consider in painful neurodegenerative diseases, especially in those patients with a positive history of exposure to neurotoxic agents. *Nootropic* is a term coined to describe the first substance found to have beneficial effects in the treatment of memory loss, age-related memory decline, and lack of concentration. That substance was piracetam (branded Nootropil).

14. MITOCHONDRIA AND ATP

The mitochondria generate more than 90% of the cell's supply of ATP *(148)* Compromised. mitochondrial function or mitochondrial uncoupling can result in altered muscle function as well as nervous, immune and cardiac dysfunction. Fibromyalgia patients may have mitochondrial uncoupling and low levels of high-energy phosphates, suggesting suboptimal levels of ATP *(149,150)*. Histological changes such as Type-I and Type-II fiber atrophy have also been observed in FMS *(148)*. Indeed, mitochondrial complex I gene variants (mitochondrial DNA mutations) are also associated with Multiple Sclerosis (MS) *(151)*. L-carnitine or ALCAR is neuroprotective and may promote neuron survival *(152)*. L-carnitine and ALCAR convert to each other via the enzyme carnitine acetyltransferase. Carnitine is an essential cofactor in the transport of long-chain acetyl-CoA through the inner mitochondrial membrane for beta-oxidation and is considered to be a treatment that improves mitochondrial function. Though an in-depth discussion of mitochondrial uncoupling and its treatment is beyond the scope of this chapter, two other mitochondrial nutrients deserve mention.

Coenzyme Q10 (CoQ10) and alpha lipoic acid (ALA) are both antioxidants that serve a key role mitochondrial function by helping drive the ATP turbine. Coenzyme Q10 is critically important for mitochondrial oxidative phosphorylation, shuttling electrons from complexes I and II to complex III while also providing potent antioxidant protection for the inner membrane OXPHOS complex. It is a conditionally essential nutrient, and (in skeletal muscle) CoQ10 deficiencies are always associated with mitochondrial pathology. Coenzyme Q10 has been shown to benefit symptoms of neurodegeneration. Alpha lipoic acid is an essential cofactor (prosthetic group) for two mitochondrial enzyme complexes centrally involved in bioenergetics. Lipoic acid has been an effective treatment for both diabetic peripheral neuropathy and cardiac autonomic neuropathy; ALA also improves burning mouth syndrome. Further opportunities exist to optimize mitochondrial function by addressing the mitochondrial phospholipid membrane with phospatidylserine *(148).*

15. INFLAMMATION AND OBESITY

There is a link between chronic inflammation, obesity, and insulin resistance. This was first recognized a decade ago with the discovery that TNF-α was over-expressed in the adipose tissue of rodent models of obesity. Since then it has been demonstrated that TNF-α is over-expressed in adipose and muscle tissue in obese individuals. Once insulin binds to its receptor on a cell, phosphorylation occurs, triggering downstream activation of a family of second messengers known as insulin receptor substrates (IRS). The inhibition of downstream signaling is thought to be the main mechanism through which cytokines cause insulin resistance. TNF-α blocks the action of insulin through inhibitory phosphorylation of serine residues on IRS-1. This reduces the ability of IRS-1 to respond to insulin receptor-mediated downstream signaling. Thus, it appears that obesity begets obesity because adipocytes promote inflammation, and inflammation promotes insulin resistance *(153).*

In obesity, macrophages accumulate in white adipose tissue and produce inflammatory molecules such as TNF-α, IL-6 and MMPs *(153).* This finding could provide insight into the pathophysiology of FMS in those patients who are overweight. Hyperlipidemia should be treated aggressively, as increased serum fatty acid levels and metabolism can initiate inflammatory cascades and contribute to impaired insulin signaling. Recent studies have demonstrated that free fatty acids induce insulin resistance in skeletal muscle by blocking insulin activation of insulin receptor substrate-1 (IRS-1)-associated phosphatidylinositol 3-kinase (PI3-kinase) *(154).*

Recently, the intersection of metabolism, immunity, and inflammation has been elucidated in an excellent review. *(153)* The following summarizes these findings:

- Obesity stresses the endoplasmic reticulum (ER) by inducing changes in tissue architecture that increases lipid synthesis and intracellular nutritional demands. This overloads the functional capacity of the ER and activates two important inflammatory signaling pathways, such as the IκB kinase complex (IKK).
- Increased glucose delivery to adipocytes causes nearby endothelial cells to take up glucose, overloading mitochondrial capacity. Excess reactive oxygen species (ROS) are byproducts of increased glucose metabolism in both adipocytes and endothelial cells. This initiates an inflammatory cascade mediated by proinflammatory cytokines causing oxidative stress.
- Adipocytes produce their own inflammatory molecules, mainly IL-6, TNF-α, and MMPs, thus sharing the functional attributes of macrophages.
- Insulin stimulates PLA2, which in turn unleashes AA from the plasma membrane, leading to the synthesis of proinflammatory series-two prostaglandins *(17).*

Ideally, obese patients in chronic pain should be placed on a medically supervised weight optimization program to reduce mechanical stress on joints, lower inflammation, and reduce the risk of obesity-linked diseases.

16. DEFECTS IN AMINO ACID HOMEOSTASIS

Patients with fibromyalgia have demonstrated significantly lower plasma concentrations of the three branched chain amino acids (BCAAs) and phenylalanine than normal controls *(137,155)*. Suboptimal L-tryptophan status has also been observed in fibromyalgia and may result in low serotonin levels, contributing to increased nociception and dysregulation of the central nervous system *(155)*. Serotonin is involved in emotional, cognitive and motor functions as well as control of circadian and neuroendocrine rhythms *(156)*. Researchers have hypothesized that amino acid deficiencies may be the result of defective intestinal amino acid transport mechanisms. It is hypothesized that the relative deficiency in the BCAAs may play a role in the pathophysiology of fibromyalgia, since the BCAAs supply energy to the muscle and regulate protein synthesis in the muscles. The BCAAs L-leucine and L-isoleucine are also involved in the synthesis of oxytocin *(157)*, providing a good opportunity for follow-up intervention trials using these amino acids.

The neuropeptide oxytocin is known to have antinociceptive, analgesic, as well as anxiolytic and antidepressant effects. In a controlled study on 39 FMS patients, depressed patients demonstrated low levels of oxytocin compared to the non-depressed patients and the controls. Low levels of oxytocin were also seen in patients with high pain, stress, and depression scores. A negative correlation was found between depression, anxiety, and oxytocin concentration, whereas a positive correlation was seen between happiness and oxytocin *(157)*.

17. THE ENDOGENOUS ANALGESIA SYSTEM (EAS)

The EAS is a neural pathway that projects caudally from medullary nuclei to the dorsal horn of the spinal column. When stimulated by therapeutic measures such as opiates or acupuncture, the EAS suppresses activation of second-order pain-receptive neurons in the dorsal horn, and thereby alleviates pain. Enhancing the activation of the EAS may allow lower dose opiate therapy, thus reducing dependence and side effects. The amino acid DL-phelyalanine (DLPA) and serotonergic agents may be useful as adjuvant agents with opiate therapy. DLPA has analgesic properties possibly due to its ability to inhibit enkephalinase, an enzyme that degrades endogenous opiates. Supplemental tryptophan and 5-HT, by enhancing serotonin synthesis, could also potentiate dorsal horn serotonin release *(158)*. Agents such as hyperforin (St. John's Wort) that act as serotonin reuptake inhibitors may also be useful as adjuvant therapy.

18. SULFUR COMPOUNDS

Sulfur is the sixth most abundant macromineral in breast milk and the third most abundant mineral based on percentage of total body weight. The sulfur-containing amino acids (SAAs) are methionine, cysteine, cystine, homocysteine, homocystine, and taurine. Dietary SAA analysis and protein supplementation may be indicated for vegan athletes, children, or patients with HIV, because of an increased risk for SAA deficiency in these groups. Organic sulfur, much like SAAs, can be used to increase synthesis of S-adenosylmethionine (SAMe), glutathione (GSH), taurine, and N-acetylcysteine (NAC). Nutritional substances that can donate sulfur may be effective for the treatment of allergies, pain syndromes, athletic injuries, and bladder disorders. Other sulfur compounds such as SAMe, dimethylsulfoxide (DMSO), taurine, glucosamine or chondroitin sulfate, and reduced glutathione may also have clinical applications in the treatment of a number of pain related conditions such as depression, fibromyalgia, and arthritis *(46)*.

18.1. Glucosamine and Chondroitin

Glucosamine sulfate (GS) and chondroitin sulfate (CS) are increasingly being used to reduce symptoms of osteoarthritis. GS is an aminomonosaccharide (a combination of glutamine and glucose) combined with a sulfate group. Used to treat osteoarthritis (OA), GS is concentrated in joint cartilage where it is a substrate for cartilage glycosaminoglycan (GAG) synthesis *(46)*. GS supplements are derived from chitin, a substance found in the shells of shrimp, lobsters, and crabs. Synthetic glucosamine sulfate is also available for those with shellfish allergies or who wish to avoid shellfish products. Glucosamine is currently sold as the sulfate, hydrochloride, N-acetyl, or chlorhydrate salt. Most of the clinical studies have used either the sulfate or chloride salt. Reviews of clinical trials and meta-analyses support the efficacy of glucosamine in both the prevention of OA and in treatment of its symptoms *(159–163)*. Chondroitin sulfate (CS) is a member of the polysaccharide group called glycosaminoglycans (GAGs). CS is made up of linear repeating units of D-galactosamine and D-glucuronic acid and is found in human cartilage, bone, skin, cornea, and the arterial wall. Sources used in nutritional supplements include bovine and pork cartilage, shark cartilage, and whale septum. Whereas glucosamine sulfate is thought to promote the formation and repair of cartilage, chondroitin sulfate is believed to promote water retention and elasticity in cartilage and inhibit enzymes that break down cartilage. When administered, chondroitin exhibits a tropism for GAG-rich tissues such as the eyes, joints, lumbar disks, and epiphysis at the ends of long bones. Studies have shown efficacy for chondroitin in decreasing pain due to knee OA. Another sulfur compound, methylsulfonylmethane (MSM), though potentially useful for allergy and interstitial cystitis, is largely marketed for use in arthritis where little data supports its use *(46)*.

18.2. SAMe

S-Adenosylmethionine (SAMe) was first discovered in Italy in 1952 and is moderately effective for reducing symptoms of musculoskeletal pain and depression. It is produced endogenously from methionine and adenosine triphosphate (ATP). SAMe is an important methyl group donor, playing an essential role in many biochemical reactions involving enzymatic transmethylation. Such reactions play an important role in the biosynthesis of phospholipids that are important for the integrity of cell membranes. The exact mechanism of SAMe in reducing pain due to OA is unknown, but evidence suggests that it may play a role in reducing inflammation or increasing proteoglycan synthesis. Alternately, it may work by having a more generalized analgesic effect. Whether SAMe is a COX-2 inhibitor also remains unknown. In vitro studies using human articular chondrocytes have revealed SAMe-induced increases in proteoglycan synthesis and proliferation rates in rabbits. SAMe may work by reducing inflammatory mediators thereby reducing pain *(164)*.

REFERENCES

1. Grundy SM, Cleeman JI, Daniels SR, Donato KA, Eckel RH, Franklin BA, Gordon DJ, Krauss RM, Savage PJ, Smith SC, Jr., Spertus JA, Costa F. Diagnosis and management of the metabolic

syndrome: an American Heart Association/National Heart, Lung, and Blood Institute Scientific Statement. Circulation 2005;112(17):2735–2752.

2. No authors listed. What is Functional Medicine. In; 2005 http://www.functionalmedicine.org/about/ whatis.asp date accessed 1/16/2006.

3. McCann JC, Ames BN. Is docosahexaenoic acid, an n-3 long-chain polyunsaturated fatty acid, required for development of normal brain function? An overview of evidence from cognitive and behavioral tests in humans and animals. Am J Clin Nutr 2005;82(2):281–295.

4. Grandgirard A, Bourre JM, Julliard F, et al. Incorporation of trans long-chain n-3 polyunsaturated fatty acids in rat brain structures and retina. Lipids 1994;29(4):251–258.

5. Larque E, Perez-Llamas F, Puerta V, et al. Dietary trans fatty acids affect docosahexaenoic acid concentrations in plasma and liver but not brain of pregnant and fetal rats. Pediatr Res 2000; 47(2):278–283.

6. Mensink RP, Katan MB. Effect of dietary trans fatty acids on high-density and low-density lipoprotein cholesterol levels in healthy subjects. N Engl J Med 1990;323(7):439–445.

7. Simopoulos AP. Essential fatty acids in health and chronic disease. Am J Clin Nutr 1999;70 (3 Suppl):560S-569S.

8. Yehuda S, Carasso RL. Modulation of learning, pain thresholds, and thermoregulation in the rat by preparations of free purified alpha-linolenic and linoleic acids: determination of the optimal omega 3-to-omega 6 ratio. Proc Natl Acad Sci USA 1993;90(21):10345–10349.

9. Murakami M, Kambe T, Shimbara S, Kudo I. Functional coupling between various phospholipase A2s and cyclooxygenases in immediate and delayed prostanoid biosynthetic pathways. J Biol Chem 1999;274(5):3103–315.

10. Fallon S. Tripping lightly down the prostaglandin pathways. Price-Pottenger Nutr Found Health J 1999;574–763.

11. Reilly MP, Lawson JA, FitzGerald GA. Eicosanoids and isoeicosanoids: indices of cellular function and oxidant stress. J Nutr 1998;128(2 Suppl):434S-438S.

12. Molloy ES, McCarthy GM. Eicosanoids, osteoarthritis, and crystal deposition diseases. Curr Opin Rheumatol 2005;17(3):346–450.

13. Taking stock of coxibs. Drug Ther Bull 2005 Jan;43(1):1–6.

14. Tithof PK, Olivero J, Ruehle K, Ganey PE. Activation of neutrophil calcium-dependent and - independent phospholipases A2 by organochlorine compounds. Toxicol Sci 2000;53(1):40–47.

15. Fawzy AA, Vishwanath BS, Franson RC. Inhibition of human non-pancreatic phospholipases A2 by retinoids and flavonoids. Mechanism of action. Agents Actions 1988;25(3–4):394–400.

16. Lindahl M, Tagesson C. Flavonoids as phospholipase A2 inhibitors: importance of their structure for selective inhibition of group II phospholipase A2. Inflammation 1997;21(3):347–356.

17. Simonsson E, Ahren B. Phospholipase A2 and its potential regulation of islet function. Int J Pancreatol 2000;27(1):1–11.

18. Shanker G, Mutkus LA, Walker SJ, Aschner M. Methylmercury enhances arachidonic acid release and cytosolic phospholipase A2 expression in primary cultures of neonatal astrocytes. Brain Res Mol Brain Res 2002;106(1–2):1–11.

19. Gijon MA, Spencer DM, Siddiqi AR, Bonventre JV, Leslie CC. Cytosolic phospholipase A2 is required for macrophage arachidonic acid release by agonists that do and do not mobilize calcium. Novel role of mitogen-activated protein kinase pathways in cytosolic phospholipase A2 regulation. J Biol Chem 2000;275(26):20146–20156.

20. Lazarewicz JW, Wroblewski JT, Costa E. *N*-methyl-D-aspartate-sensitive glutamate receptors induce calcium-mediated arachidonic acid release in primary cultures of cerebellar granule cells. J Neurochem 1990;55(6):1875–1881.

21. Rodriguez De Turco EB, Jackson FR, DeCoster MA, Kolko M, Bazan NG. Glutamate signalling and secretory phospholipase A2 modulate the release of arachidonic acid from neuronal membranes. J Neurosci Res 2002;68(5):558–567.

22. Toggas SM, Krady JK, Thompson TA, Billingsley ML. Molecular mechanisms of selective neuro-toxicants: studies on organotin compounds. Ann NY Acad Sci 1993;679:157–177.

23. Tall JM, Raja SN. Dietary constituents as novel therapies for pain. Clin J Pain 2004;20(1):19–26.

24. Tak PP, Firestein GS. NF-kappaB: a key role in inflammatory diseases. J Clin Invest 2001;107(1):7–11.

25. Vilcek J, Lee TH. Tumor necrosis factor. New insights into the molecular mechanisms of its multiple actions. J Biol Chem 1991;266(12):7313–7316.

26. Moini H, Rimbach G, Packer L. Molecular aspects of procyanidin biological activity: disease preventative and therapeutic potentials. Drug Metabol Drug Interact 2000;17(1–4):237–259.

27. Abramson SB, Amin A. Blocking the effects of IL-1 in rheumatoid arthritis protects bone and cartilage. Rheumatology (Oxford) 2002;41(9):972–980.

28. Grimble RF, Howell WM, O'Reilly G, et al. The ability of fish oil to suppress tumor necrosis factor alpha production by peripheral blood mononuclear cells in healthy men is associated with polymorphisms in genes that influence tumor necrosis factor alpha production. Am J Clin Nutr 2002;76(2):454–459.

29. Westacott CI, Sharif M. Cytokines in osteoarthritis: mediators or markers of joint destruction? Semin Arthritis Rheum 1996;25(4):254–272.

30. Morin I, Li WQ, Su S, Ahmad M, Zafarullah M. Induction of stromelysin gene expression by tumor necrosis factor alpha is inhibited by dexamethasone, salicylate, and N-acetylcysteine in synovial fibroblasts. J Pharmacol Exp Ther 1999;289(3):1634–1640.

31. Reginato AM, Sanz-Rodriguez C, Diaz A, Dharmavaram RM, Jimenez SA. Transcriptional modulation of cartilage-specific collagen gene expression by interferon gamma and tumour necrosis factor alpha in cultured human chondrocytes. Biochem J 1993;294 (Pt 3):761–769.

32. Pelletier JP, Mineau F, Ranger P, Tardif G, Martel-Pelletier J. The increased synthesis of inducible nitric oxide inhibits IL-1ra synthesis by human articular chondrocytes: possible role in osteoarthritic cartilage degradation. Osteoarthritis Cartilage 1996;4(1):77–84.

33. Lotz M. The role of nitric oxide in articular cartilage damage. Rheum Dis Clin North Am 1999;25(2):269–282.

34. Cuzzocrea S, Sautebin L, Costantino G, Rombola L, Mazzon E, Caputi AP. Regulation of prostaglandin production by inhibition of poly (ADP-ribose) synthase in carrageenan-induced pleurisy. Life Sci 1999;65(12):1297–1304.

35. Ibelgauft H. Cytokines Online Pathfinder Encyclopedia. In: Horst Ibelgauft; 2002.

36. No authors listed. Disease Database. http://www.diseasesdatabase.com/umlsdef.asp?glngUser Choice=33430; 2005.

37. Chan PS, Caron JP, Rosa GJ, Orth MW. Glucosamine and chondroitin sulfate regulate gene expression and synthesis of nitric oxide and prostaglandin E(2) in articular cartilage explants. Osteoarthritis Cartilage 2005;13(5):387–394.

38. Gemma C, Mesches MH, Sepesi B, Choo K, Holmes DB, Bickford PC. Diets enriched in foods with high antioxidant activity reverse age-induced decreases in cerebellar beta-adrenergic function and increases in proinflammatory cytokines. J Neurosci 2002;22(14):6114–6120.

39. Heliovaara M, Knekt P, Aho K, Aaran RK, Alfthan G, Aromaa A. Serum antioxidants and risk of rheumatoid arthritis. Ann Rheum Dis 1994;53(1):51–53.

40. Willett WC. Diet, nutrition, and avoidable cancer. Environ Health Perspect 1995;103(Suppl 8): 165–170.

41. Thompson HJ, Heimendinger J, Sedlacek S, et al. 8–Isoprostane F2alpha excretion is reduced in women by increased vegetable and fruit intake. Am J Clin Nutr 2005;82(4):768–776.

42. McLachlan JA, Simpson E, Martin M. Endocrine disrupters and female reproductive health. Best Pract Res Clin Endocrinol Metab 2006;20(1):63–75.

43. Szabo C. Role of poly(ADP-ribose)synthetase in inflammation. Eur J Pharmacol 1998;350(1):1–19.

44. Kroger H, Miesel R, Dietrich A, et al. Suppression of type II collagen-induced arthritis by N-acetyl-L-cysteine in mice. Gen Pharmacol 1997;29(4):671–674.

45. Tsuji F, Miyake Y, Aono H, Kawashima Y, Mita S. Effects of bucillamine and N-acetyl-L-cysteine on cytokine production and collagen-induced arthritis (CIA). Clin Exp Immunol 1999;115(1):26–31.

46. Parcell S. Sulfur in human nutrition and applications in medicine. Altern Med Rev 2002;7(1):22–44.

47. Lang CA, Naryshkin S, Schneider DL, Mills BJ, Lindeman RD. Low blood glutathione levels in healthy aging adults. J Lab Clin Med 1992;120(5):720–725.

48. No authors listed. Monograph. Plant sterols and sterolins. Altern Med Rev 2001;6(2):203–206.

49. Nashed B, Yeganeh B, Hayglass KT, Moghadasian MH. Antiatherogenic effects of dietary plant sterols are associated with inhibition of proinflammatory cytokine production in Apo E–KO Mice. J Nutr 2005;135(10):2438–2444.

50. Bouic PJ, Etsebeth S, Liebenberg RW, Albrecht CF, Pegel K, Van Jaarsveld PP. Beta-Sitosterol and beta-sitosterol glucoside stimulate human peripheral blood lymphocyte proliferation: implications for their use as an immunomodulatory vitamin combination. Int J Immunopharmacol 1996;18(12):693–700.

51. Badia E, Sacanella E, Fernandez-Sola J, et al. Decreased tumor necrosis factor-induced adhesion of human monocytes to endothelial cells after moderate alcohol consumption. Am J Clin Nutr 2004;80(1):225–230.

52. Carluccio MA, Siculella L, Ancora MA, et al. Olive oil and red wine antioxidant polyphenols inhibit endothelial activation: antiatherogenic properties of Mediterranean diet phytochemicals. Arterioscler Thromb Vasc Biol 2003;23(4):622–629.

53. Palmieri L, Mameli M, Ronca G. Effect of resveratrol and some other natural compounds on tyrosine kinase activity and on cytolysis. Drugs Exp Clin Res 1999;25(2–3):79–85.

54. Fremont L. Biological effects of resveratrol. Life Sci 2000;66(8):663–673.

55. Adcocks C, Collin P, Buttle DJ. Catechins from green tea (Camellia sinensis) inhibit bovine and human cartilage proteoglycan and type II collagen degradation in vitro. J Nutr 2002;132(3): 341–346.

56. Park YC, Rimbach G, Saliou C, Valacchi G, Packer L. Activity of monomeric, dimeric, and trimeric flavonoids on NO production, TNF-alpha secretion, and NF-kappaB-dependent gene expression in RAW 264.7 macrophages. FEBS Lett 2000;465(2–3):93–97.

57. Virgili F, Kobuchi H, Packer L. Procyanidins extracted from Pinus maritima (Pycnogenol): scavengers of free radical species and modulators of nitrogen monoxide metabolism in activated murine RAW 264.7 macrophages. Free Radic Biol Med 1998;24(7–8):1120–1129.

58. Ahn KS, Noh EJ, Zhao HL, Jung SH, Kang SS, Kim YS. Inhibition of inducible nitric oxide synthase and cyclooxygenase II by Platycodon grandiflorum saponins via suppression of nuclear factor-kappaB activation in RAW 264.7 cells. Life Sci 2005;76(20):2315–2328.

59. Wang ZF, Xiao JS, Yan SZ, Wan ZB. Protective effects of panaxadiol saponins on cardiac functions in burned rats. Zhongguo Yao Li Xue Bao 1995;16(4):345–834.

60. Li SH, Chu Y. Anti-inflammatory effects of total saponins of Panax notoginseng. Zhongguo Yao Li Xue Bao 1999;20(6):551–554.

61. Kang JH, Sung MK, Kawada T, et al. Soybean saponins suppress the release of proinflammatory mediators by LPS-stimulated peritoneal macrophages. Cancer Lett 2005;230(2):219–227.

62. Xia YF, Ye BQ, Li YD, et al. Andrographolide attenuates inflammation by inhibition of NF-kappa B activation through covalent modification of reduced cysteine 62 of p50. J Immunol 2004;173(6):4207–4217.

63. Lo AH, Liang YC, Lin-Shiau SY, Ho CT, Lin JK. Carnosol, an antioxidant in rosemary, suppresses inducible nitric oxide synthase through down-regulating nuclear factor-kappaB in mouse macrophages. Carcinogenesis 2002;23(6):983–991.

64. Calder PC. Polyunsaturated fatty acids and inflammation. Biochem Soc Trans 2005;33(Pt 2): 423–427.

65. Belluzzi A, Brignola C, Campieri M, Pera A, Boschi S, Miglioli M. Effect of an enteric-coated fish-oil preparation on relapses in Crohn's disease. N Engl J Med 1996;334(24):1557–1560.

66. Mayser P, Mrowietz U, Arenberger P, et al. Omega-3 fatty acid-based lipid infusion in patients with chronic plaque psoriasis: results of a double-blind, randomized, placebo-controlled, multicenter trial. J Am Acad Dermatol 1998;38(4):539–547.

67. Calder PC. n-3 polyunsaturated fatty acids and cytokine production in health and disease. Ann Nutr Metab 1997;41(4):203–234.

68. Calder PC. Immunoregulatory and anti-inflammatory effects of n-3 polyunsaturated fatty acids. Braz J Med Biol Res 1998;31(4):467–490.

69. Cleland LG, James MJ, Proudman SM. The role of fish oils in the treatment of rheumatoid arthritis. Drugs 2003;63(9):845–853.

70. James MJ, Cleland LG. Dietary n-3 fatty acids and therapy for rheumatoid arthritis. Semin Arthritis Rheum 1997;27(2):85–97.

71. Endres S, Ghorbani R, Kelley VE, et al. The effect of dietary supplementation with n-3 polyunsaturated fatty acids on the synthesis of interleukin-1 and tumor necrosis factor by mononuclear cells. N Engl J Med 1989;320(5):265–271.

72. Curtis CL, Hughes CE, Flannery CR, Little CB, Harwood JL, Caterson B. n-3 fatty acids specifically modulate catabolic factors involved in articular cartilage degradation. J Biol Chem 2000;275(2):721–724.

73. Curtis CL, Rees SG, Little CB, et al. Pathologic indicators of degradation and inflammation in human osteoarthritic cartilage are abrogated by exposure to n-3 fatty acids. Arthritis Rheum 2002;46(6):1544–1553.

74. Curtis CL, Rees SG, Cramp J, et al. Effects of n-3 fatty acids on cartilage metabolism. Proc Nutr Soc 2002;61(3):381–389.
75. Ames BN, Elson-Schwab I, Silver EA. High-dose vitamin therapy stimulates variant enzymes with decreased coenzyme binding affinity (increased K(m)): relevance to genetic disease and polymorphisms. Am J Clin Nutr 2002;75(4):616–658.
76. Swiss Institute of Bioinformatics. ENZYME. Enzyme nomenclature database. . In: Release 27.0, October 2001, updates up to 1 Feb 2002. Internet: accessed 2 February 2002;2001.
77. Kowa H, Yasui K, Takeshima T, Urakami K, Sakai F, Nakashima K. The homozygous C677T mutation in the methylenetetrahydrofolate reductase gene is a genetic risk factor for migraine. Am J Med Genet 2000;96(6):762–764.
78. Shpichinetsky V, Raz I, Friedlander Y, et al. The association between two common mutations C677T and A1298C in human methylenetetrahydrofolate reductase gene and the risk for diabetic nephropathy in type II diabetic patients. J Nutr 2000;130(10):2493–2497.
79. Schoenen J, Jacquy J, Lenaerts M. Effectiveness of high-dose riboflavin in migraine prophylaxis. A randomized controlled trial. Neurology 1998;50(2):466–470.
80. Brown S. Acid alkaline balance and its affect on bone health. International journal of Integrative Medicine 2000;2(6).
81. Arnett TR, Dempster DW. Effect of pH on bone resorption by rat osteoclasts in vitro. Endocrinology 1986;119(1):119–124.
82. Grinspoon SK, Baum HB, Kim V, Coggins C, Klibanski A. Decreased bone formation and increased mineral dissolution during acute fasting in young women. J Clin Endocrinol Metab 1995;80(12):3628–3633.
83. Lemann J, Jr., Lennon EJ. Role of diet, gastrointestinal tract and bone in acid-base homeostasis. Kidney Int 1972;1(5):275–279.
84. Remer T, Manz F. Estimation of the renal net acid excretion by adults consuming diets containing variable amounts of protein. Am J Clin Nutr 1994;59(6):1356–1361.
85. Wachman A, Bernstein DS. Diet and osteoporosis. Lancet 1968;1(7549):958–959.
86. Arnett TR, Spowage M. Modulation of the resorptive activity of rat osteoclasts by small changes in extracellular pH near the physiological range. Bone 1996;18(3):277–279.
87. Remer T. Influence of diet on acid-base balance. Semin Dial 2000;13(4):221–226.
88. Remer T. Influence of nutrition on acid-base balance—metabolic aspects. Eur J Nutr 2001;40(5):214–220.
89. Krebs-Smith SM, Cook A, Subar AF, Cleveland L, Friday J, Kahle LL. Fruit and vegetable intakes of children and adolescents in the United States. Arch Pediatr Adolesc Med 1996;150(1):81–86.
90. Katz KD, Hollander D. Intestinal mucosal permeability and rheumatological diseases. Baillieres Clin Rheumatol 1989;3(2):271–284.
91. Smith MD, Gibson RA, Brooks PM. Abnormal bowel permeability in ankylosing spondylitis and rheumatoid arthritis. J Rheumatol 1985;12(2):299–305.
92. Heyman M. Gut barrier dysfunction in food allergy. Eur J Gastroenterol Hepatol 2005;17(12):1279–1285.
93. Hazenberg MP, Klasen IS, Kool J, Ruseler-van Embden JG, Severijnen AJ. Are intestinal bacteria involved in the etiology of rheumatoid arthritis? Review article. Apmis 1992;100(1):1–9.
94. Sartor RB. Importance of intestinal mucosal immunity and luminal bacterial cell wall polymers in the aetiology of inflammatory joint diseases. Baillieres Clin Rheumatol 1989;3(2):223–245.
95. Cordain L, Toohey L, Smith MJ, Hickey MS. Modulation of immune function by dietary lectins in rheumatoid arthritis. Br J Nutr 2000;83(3):207–217.
96. Henriksson AE, Blomquist L, Nord CE, Midtvedt T, Uribe A. Small intestinal bacterial overgrowth in patients with rheumatoid arthritis. Ann Rheum Dis 1993;52(7):503–510.
97. Benno P, Alam M, Henriksson K, Norin E, Uribe A, Midtvedt T. Abnormal colonic microbial function in patients with rheumatoid arthritis. Scand J Rheumatol 1994;23(6):311–315.
98. Trentham DE, Dynesius-Trentham RA. Antibiotic therapy for rheumatoid arthritis. Scientific and anecdotal appraisals. Rheum Dis Clin North Am 1995;21(3):817–834.
99. Kool J, Gerrits-Boeye MY, Severijnen AJ, Hazenberg MP. Immunohistology of joint inflammation induced in rats by cell wall fragments of *Eubacterium aerofaciens*. Scand J Immunol 1992;36(3):497–506.
100. Travis S, Menzies I. Intestinal permeability: functional assessment and significance. Clin Sci (Lond) 1992;82(5):471–488.
101. Berg RD. Bacterial translocation from the gastrointestinal tract. J Med 1992;23(3–4):217–244.

102. Pusztai A. Dietary lectins are metabolic signals for the gut and modulate immune and hormone functions. Eur J Clin Nutr 1993;47(10):691–669.

103. Doherty M, Barry RE. Gluten-induced mucosal changes in subjects without overt small-bowel disease. Lancet 1981;1(8219):517–520.

104. Banwell JG, Howard R, Kabir I, Costerton JW. Bacterial overgrowth by indigenous microflora in the phytohemagglutinin-fed rat. Can J Microbiol 1988;34(8):1009–1013.

105. Auger I, Roudier J. A function for the QKRAA amino acid motif: mediating binding of DnaJ to DnaK. Implications for the association of rheumatoid arthritis with HLA-DR4. J Clin Invest 1997;99(8):1818–1822.

106. Grant G, More LJ, McKenzie NH, Pusztai A. The effect of heating on the haemagglutinating activity and nutritional properties of bean (Phaseolus vulgaris) seeds. J Sci Food Agric 1982;33(12): 1324–1326.

107. Riordan AM, Hunter JO, Cowan RE, et al. Treatment of active Crohn's disease by exclusion diet: East Anglian multicentre controlled trial. Lancet 1993;342(8880):1131–1134.

108. Kavanaghi R, Workman E, Nash P, Smith M, Hazleman BL, Hunter JO. The effects of elemental diet and subsequent food reintroduction on rheumatoid arthritis. Br J Rheumatol 1995;34(3):270–273.

109. Lepore L, Pennesi M, Ventura A, et al. Anti-alpha-gliadin antibodies are not predictive of celiac disease in juvenile chronic arthritis. Acta Paediatr 1993;82(6–7):569–573.

110. Kjeldsen-Kragh J, Haugen M, Borchgrevink CF, et al. Controlled trial of fasting and one-year vegetarian diet in rheumatoid arthritis. Lancet 1991;338(8772):899–902.

111. Lunardi C, Bambara LM, Biasi D, et al. Food allergy and rheumatoid arthritis. Clin Exp Rheumatol 1988;6(4):423–424.

112. O'Farrelly C, Price R, McGillivray AJ, Fernandes L. IgA rheumatoid factor and IgG dietary protein antibodies are associated in rheumatoid arthritis. Immunol Invest 1989;18(6):753–764.

113. Perez-Maceda B, Lopez-Bote JP, Langa C, Bernabeu C. Antibodies to dietary antigens in rheumatoid arthritis—possible molecular mimicry mechanism. Clin Chim Acta 1991;203(2–3):153–165.

114. Chicz RM, Urban RG, Gorga JC, Vignali DA, Lane WS, Strominger JL. Specificity and promiscuity among naturally processed peptides bound to HLA-DR alleles. J Exp Med 1993;178(1):27–47.

115. Panush RS. Possible role of food sensitivity in arthritis. Ann Allergy 1988;61(6 Pt 2):31–35.

116. Clark EC, Patel SD, Chadwick PR, Warhurst G, Curry A, Carlson GL. Glutamine deprivation facilitates tumour necrosis factor induced bacterial translocation in Caco-2 cells by depletion of enterocyte fuel substrate. Gut 2003;52(2):224–230.

117. Husby S, Hoost A. Recurrent abdominal pain, food allergy and endoscopy. Acta Paediatr 2001;90(1):3–4.

118. Dixon HS. Treatment of delayed food allergy based on specific immunoglobulin G RAST testing. Otolaryngol Head Neck Surg 2000;123(1 Pt 1):48–54.

119. Bock SA, Sampson HA, Atkins FM, et al. Double-blind, placebo-controlled food challenge (DBPCFC) as an office procedure: a manual. J Allergy Clin Immunol 1988;82(6):986–997.

120. Aguero Garcia L. Not Available. Medicamenta (Madr) 1949;7(Pt. 2):200–202; see also page 170.

121. Darlington LG, Ramsey NW. Review of dietary therapy for rheumatoid arthritis. Br J Rheumatol 1993;32(6):507–514.

122. Darlington LG, Ramsey NW, Mansfield JR. Placebo-controlled, blind study of dietary manipulation therapy in rheumatoid arthritis. Lancet 1986;1(8475):236–238.

123. Diets for rheumatoid arthritis. Lancet 1991;338(8776):1209–1210.

124. Kaufman W. Food-induced, allergic musculoskeletal syndromes. Ann Allergy 1953;11(2):179–184.

125. Zussman BM. Food hypersensitivity simulating rheumatoid arthritis. South Med J 1966;59(8): 935–939.

126. Ratner D, Schneeyour A, Eshel E, Teitler A. Does milk intolerance affect seronegative arthritis in lactase-deficient women? Isr J Med Sci 1985;21(6):532–534.

127. Neeck G, Federlin K, Graef V, Rusch D, Schmidt KL. Adrenal secretion of cortisol in patients with rheumatoid arthritis. J Rheumatol. 1990;17(1):24–29.

128. Chikanza IC, Chrousos G, Panayi GS. Abnormal neuroendocrine immune communications in patients with rheumatoid arthritis. Eur J Clin Invest 1992;22(10):635–637.

129. Hellhammer J, Fries E, Buss C, et al. Effects of soy lecithin phosphatidic acid and phosphatidylserine complex (PAS) on the endocrine and psychological responses to mental stress. Stress 2004;7(2): 119–126.

130. Bennett R. Growth hormone in musculoskeletal pain states. Curr Pain Headache Rep 2005;9(5): 331–338.

131. Monson JP. Long-term experience with GH replacement therapy: efficacy and safety. Eur J Endocrinol 2003;148(Suppl 2):S9–S14.

132. Leal-Cerro A, Povedano J, Astorga R, et al. The growth hormone (GH)-releasing hormone-GH-insulin-like growth factor-1 axis in patients with fibromyalgia syndrome. J Clin Endocrinol Metab 1999;84(9):3378–3381.

133. Parr TB. A new technique to elevate night time growth hormone release and a potential growth hormone feedback control loop. Med Hypotheses 2001;56(5):610–613.

134. Toglia JU. Melatonin: a significant contributor to the pathogenesis of migraine. Med Hypotheses 2001;57(4):432–434.

135. Anton-Tay F, Chou C, Anton S, Wurtman RJ. Brain serotonin concentration: elevation following intraperitoneal administration of melatonin. Science 1968;162(850):277–278.

136. Claustrat B, Brun J, Geoffriau M, Zaidan R, Mallo C, Chazot G. Nocturnal plasma melatonin profile and melatonin kinetics during infusion in status migrainosus. Cephalalgia 1997;17(4): 511–517 (discussion 487).

137. Maes M, Verkerk R, Delmeire L, Van Gastel A, van Hunsel F, Scharpe S. Serotonergic markers and lowered plasma branched-chain-amino acid concentrations in fibromyalgia. Psychiatry Res 2000;97(1):11–20.

138. Neeck G. Neuroendocrine and hormonal perturbations and relations to the serotonergic system in fibromyalgia patients. Scand J Rheumatol Suppl 2000;113:8–12.

139. Neeck G. Pathogenic mechanisms of fibromyalgia. Ageing Res Rev 2002;1(2):243–255.

140. Tsigos C, Chrousos GP. Hypothalamic-pituitary-adrenal axis, neuroendocrine factors and stress. J Psychosom Res 2002;53(4):865–871.

141. Schwarz MJ, Spath M, Muller-Bardorff H, Pongratz DE, Bondy B, Ackenheil M. Relationship of substance P, 5-hydroxyindole acetic acid and tryptophan in serum of fibromyalgia patients. Neurosci Lett 1999;259(3):196–198.

142. Murphy RM, Zemlan FP. Differential effects of substance P on serotonin-modulated spinal nociceptive reflexes. Psychopharmacology (Berl) 1987;93(1):118–121.

143. Kramer JH, Mak IT, Phillips TM, Weglicki WB. Dietary magnesium intake influences circulating pro-inflammatory neuropeptide levels and loss of myocardial tolerance to postischemic stress. Exp Biol Med (Maywood) 2003;228(6):665–673.

144. Durlach J, Pages N, Bac P, Bara M, Guiet-Bara A. Importance of magnesium depletion with hypofunction of the biological clock in the pathophysiology of headaches with photophobia, sudden infant death and some clinical forms of multiple sclerosis. Magnes Res 2004;17(4):314–326.

145. Durlach J, Pages N, Bac P, Bara M, Guiet-Bara A. Magnesium depletion with hypo- or hyper-function of the biological clock may be involved in chronopathological forms of asthma. Magnes Res 2005;18(1):19–34.

146. Nicolodi M, Galeotti N, Ghelardini C, Bartolini A, Sicuteri F. Central cholinergic challenging of migraine by testing second-generation anticholinesterase drugs. Headache 2002;42(7):596–602.

147. Wang R, Tang XC. Neuroprotective effects of huperzine A. A natural cholinesterase inhibitor for the treatment of Alzheimer's disease. Neurosignals 2005;14(1–2):71–82.

148. Kidd PM. Neurodegeneration from mitochondrial insufficiency: nutrients, stem cells, growth factors, and prospects for brain rebuilding using integrative management. Altern Med Rev 2005;10(4): 268–293.

149. Bengtsson A, Henriksson KG. The muscle in fibromyalgia—a review of Swedish studies. J Rheumatol Suppl 1989;19:144–149.

150. Park JH, Phothimat P, Oates CT, Hernanz-Schulman M, Olsen NJ. Use of P-31 magnetic resonance spectroscopy to detect metabolic abnormalities in muscles of patients with fibromyalgia. Arthritis Rheum 1998;41(3):406–413.

151. Vyshkina T, Banisor I, Shugart YY, Leist TP, Kalman B. Genetic variants of Complex I in multiple sclerosis. J Neurol Sci 2005;228(1):55–64.

152. Ishii T, Shimpo Y, Matsuoka Y, Kinoshita K. Anti-apoptotic effect of acetyl-l-carnitine and l-carnitine in primary cultured neurons. Jpn J Pharmacol 2000;83(2):119–124.

153. Wellen KE, Hotamisligil GS. Obesity-induced inflammatory changes in adipose tissue. J Clin Invest 2003;112(12):1785–1788.

154. Yu C, Chen Y, Cline GW, et al. Mechanism by which fatty acids inhibit insulin activation of insulin receptor substrate-1 (IRS-1)-associated phosphatidylinositol 3-kinase activity in muscle. J Biol Chem 2002;277(52):50230–50236.

155. van West D, Maes M. Neuroendocrine and immune aspects of fibromyalgia. Biodrugs 2001;15(8):521–531.

156. Yunus MB, Dailey JW, Aldag JC, Masi AT, Jobe PC. Plasma tryptophan and other amino acids in primary fibromyalgia: a controlled study. J Rheumatol 1992;19(1):90–94.

157. Anderberg UM, Uvnas-Moberg K. Plasma oxytocin levels in female fibromyalgia syndrome patients. Z Rheumatol 2000;59(6):373–379.

158. Russell AL, McCarty MF. DL-phenylalanine markedly potentiates opiate analgesia-an example of nutrient/pharmaceutical up-regulation of the endogenous analgesia system. Med Hypotheses 2000;55(4):283–288.

159. Neil KM, Caron JP, Orth MW. The role of glucosamine and chondroitin sulfate in treatment for and prevention of osteoarthritis in animals. J Am Vet Med Assoc 2005;226(7):1079–1088.

160. Poolsup N, Suthisisang C, Channark P, Kittikulsuth W. Glucosamine long-term treatment and the progression of knee osteoarthritis: systematic review of randomized controlled trials. Ann Pharmacother 2005;39(6):1080–1087.

161. Reiter S. Evidence-based evaluation of study results of symptomatic glucosamine therapy. Z Rheumatol 2005;64(7):456–466.

162. Simanek V, Kren V, Ulrichova J, Gallo J. The efficacy of glucosamine and chondroitin sulfate in the treatment of osteoarthritis: are these saccharides drugs or nutraceuticals? Biomed Pap Med Fac Univ Palacky Olomouc Czech Repub 2005;149(1):51–56.

163. Towheed TE, Maxwell L, Anastassiades TP, et al. Glucosamine therapy for treating osteoarthritis. Cochrane Database Syst Rev 2005(2):CD002946.

164. Najm WI, Reinsch S, Hoehler F, Tobis JS, Harvey PW. S-adenosyl methionine (SAMe) versus celecoxib for the treatment of osteoarthritis symptoms: a double-blind cross-over trial [ISRCTN36233495]. BMC Musculoskelet Disord 2004;5:6.

8   Exercise Testing and Training in Patients with (Chronic) Pain

Harriët Wittink and Tim Takken

CONTENTS

DEFINITION AND BACKGROUND
MECHANISM OF ACTION
INTRODUCTION TO EXERCISE TESTING
EXERCISE TRAINING AND THE PATIENT WITH CHRONIC PAIN
CONCLUSION

"Those movements which do not alter respiration are not called exercise."
Galen (~200 A.D.)

Summary

A vast body of literature supports the idea that exercise training is an important modality in the treatment and rehabilitation of the chronic pain patient. Exercise testing and prescription should therefore be incorporated in the therapeutic armamentarium of health care professionals working with chronic pain patients. In this chapter we present the scientific basis of the positive effects regular exercise can have on pain, mood, sleep, function, and fitness. Moreover, specific guidelines for exercise testing and prescription for the chronic patient are provided.

Key Words: exercise physiology, aerobic capacity, exercise testing, submaximal, aerobic, anaerobic, frequency, intensity, time

1. DEFINITION AND BACKGROUND

Exercise physiology arose mainly in early Greece and Asia Minor, although the topics of exercise, sports, games, and health were of interest to even earlier civilizations. The greatest influence on Western medical traditions came from the Greek physicians of antiquity, including Herodicus (fifth century B.C.), Hippocrates (460–377 B.C.), and Claudius Galenus or Galen (A.D. 131–201). Proper diet and physical training has been recommended since Herodicus's day. Galen wrote descriptions about the forms, kinds, and varieties of "swift" and vigorous exercises, including their proper quantity and duration *(1)*. In the first century A.D., the Roman satirist Juneval famously observed

From: *Contemporary Pain Medicine: Integrative Pain Medicine: The Science and Practice of Complementary and Alternative Medicine in Pain Management*
Edited by: J. F. Audette and A. Bailey © Humana Press, Totowa, NJ

"Orandum est, ut sit mens sana in corpore sano," or "A sound mind in a sound body is something to be prayed for."

In Venice in 1539, the Italian physician Hieronymus Mercurialis published *The Art of Gymnastics Among the Ancients.* This text was heavily influenced by Galen and other early Greek and Latin authors and profoundly affected subsequent writings about gymnastics (physical training and exercise), not only in Europe (influencing the Swedish and Danish gymnastics systems), but also in early America (the 19th -century gymnastics-hygiene movement). By the middle of the 19th-century American physicians had the opportunity to either teach in medical school and conduct research, or become associated with departments of physical education and hygiene. There, they would oversee programs of physical training for students and athletes *(1)*. The first formal exercise physiology laboratory in the United States was established in 1891 at Harvard University.

Exercise physiology is now defined as the branch of physiology that studies how the body adapts to physical movement. It is "the identification of physiological mechanisms underlying physical activity, the comprehensive delivery of treatment services concerned with the analysis, improvement, and maintenance of health and fitness, rehabilitation of heart disease and other chronic diseases and/or disabilities, and the professional guidance and counsel of athletes and others interested in athletics, sports training, and human adaptability to acute and chronic exercise" *(2)*.

2. MECHANISM OF ACTION

The human body is made for movement. This statement is supported by the fact that human movement influences cardiovascular, respiratory, musculoskeletal, renal, gastrointestinal, genitourinary, nervous, lymphatic, endocrine, and immune systems at the cellular, organ, and systemic levels. In fact, not moving enough causes people to become ill. Epidemiological data have established that physical inactivity increases the incidence of at least 17 unhealthy conditions, almost all of which are chronic diseases or considered risk factors for chronic diseases *(3)*.

Chronic conditions related to inactivity include coronary heart disease (CHD), hypertension, Type II diabetes, colon cancer, depression and anxiety, osteoporotic hip fractures, and obesity. Increasing adiposity, or obesity, is itself a direct cause of Type II diabetes, hypertension, CHD, gallbladder disease, osteoarthritis, and cancer of the breast, colon, and endometrium *(3,4)*.

Exercise is one key management strategy used by physical therapists to address impairments (problems with body function or structure such as pain or weakness), activity limitations (difficulties an individual may have in executing activities such as walking, sitting, and standing), and participation restrictions (problems an individual may experience in life situations such as working, playing sports or socializing) in patients with chronic pain *(5)*. Exercise testing (see Section 3) can identify impairments or deficits in muscle endurance, strength and aerobic capacity as related to the patient's desired physical activity level in order to target these for treatment.

Multiple meta-analyses on the effects of exercise on various painful conditions report exercise to have a positive effect on pain, aerobic capacity and physical function. The mechanisms behind these effects are not completely clear and are most likely due to multiple factors. Exercise may also influence pain in a number of nonspecific ways, e.g., through its influences on body mass, mood, sleep, motivation, deconditioning, skill acquisition, self-efficacy, or social contact *(6,7)*. Possible mechanisms that contribute to these effects are discussed below.

2.1. Pain

A number of studies have been conducted to examine whether pain perception is altered during and following exercise, and several reviews have been published on this topic *(8,9)*. Most studies have investigated whether decreased sensitivity to pain (hypoalgesia) occurs following aerobic exercise with less research investigating whether hypoalgesia occurs after other modes of exercise (e.g., resistance or isometric exercise). A number of investigators have reported the development of hypoalgesia during and following exercise under experimental and clinical conditions *(8)*.

Hypoalgesia occurs consistently following high-intensity exercise (i.e., a high workload > 200 W or 60–75% of maximal oxygen uptake) *(9)*. Most of these studies have used normal (usually college-aged) subjects. Studies on the effects of exercise on pain threshold in patients with chronic pain, however, are scarce. A recent study found that pain ratings from an experimentally induced pressure pain stimulus was reduced after aerobic exercise (25 minutes at 50–70% of peak VO_2) in patients (N = 8) with minimal to moderate disability from chronic low back pain *(10)*. The analgesic effect lasted for more than 30 minutes following the aerobic exercise intervention. In contrast, pain thresholds were found to decrease in subjects with chronic fatigue syndrome (CFS), while the same exercise intervention caused an increase in the pain threshold of normal control subjects *(11)*. The authors of this study hypothesized that increased perception of pain and/or fatigue after exercise may be indicative of a dysfunction of the central anti-nociceptive mechanism in CFS patients.

The mechanisms for analgesia following exercise are poorly understood. The most commonly tested hypothesis to explain exercise-induced analgesia has been that the observed hypoalgesia that results from strenuous exercise is secondary to activation of the endogenous opioid system. However, results from studies that have investigated the role that the endogenous opioid system plays in the analgesic response to exercise are mixed. Hypoalgesia following exercise does appear to be mediated in part by the endogenousopioid system; however, an elevation in pain threshold can also occur following pre-injection with opioid antagonists, providing evidence for a non-opioid based mechanism. The role of the endocannabinoid system as an alternative neuromodulatorysystem in pain perception is currently a topic of much investigation. The endocannabinoid system has been shown to suppress pain at both central and peripheral sites *(12)*. Preliminary evidence shows that exercise of moderate intensity activates the endocannabinoid system *(13)*, suggesting a new mechanism for exercise-induced analgesia and possibly other physiological and psychological adaptations to exercise.

2.2. Aerobic Capacity

Aerobic capacity is a measure of the ability and efficiency of the body to take oxygen up and to use it as a fuel by turning it into energy (adenosine triphosphate or ATP, section 3). The higher the oxygen uptake for a given activity, the higher the aerobic energy output demanded. Aerobic fitness is expressed in liters/minute (L/min) and often adjusted for bodyweight milliliters/kilogram/minute (mL/kg/min). Physical activities are coded in metabolic equivalent (MET) intensity levels. One MET is defined as the resting metabolic rate obtained during quiet sitting and equals an oxygen uptake of 3.5 mL/kg/min. The oxygen cost for physical activities ranges from 0.9 MET for sleeping to 18 METs (running at 10.9 mph) *(14)*.

The level of a person's aerobic capacity thus directly affects the amount and intensity of physical activity this individual is able to perform. Practical experience has shown that one cannot tax more than about 30–40% of one's aerobic capacity during an eight-hour day without developing subjective or objective symptoms of fatigue *(15)*.

A common hypothesis is that aerobic capacity is reduced in patients with chronic pain as a result of physical inactivity, although studies on this topic do not consistently support this conclusion *(16)*. Physical inactivity, or disuse, will lead to deconditioning over time. The "deconditioning syndrome" *(17,18)* was postulated in the mid 1980s to be the primary factor that contributed to a chronic pain patient's intolerance to physical activity. The theory was that pain leads to inactivity (disuse), which in turn leads to deconditioning, which further contributes to loss of function and activity avoidance, causing greater deconditioning and disability in a downward spiralling, vicious cycle. More recently, disuse has been presented as one factor among many that perpetuates chronic pain in theoretical pain research models *(19,20)*. Reconditioning, to reverse the physiological effects of disuse, is a frequently used approach in pain rehabilitation to increase activity levels and reduce disability. In addition, exercise can provide behavioral cues that physical activity levels can be increased without a concomitant increase in pain. Greater levels of exercise have been associated with improvements in mood and functioning in patients with chronic conditions over a 2-year study period *(21)*.

2.3. Physical Function

Aerobic training of sufficient intensity and duration will increase aerobic capacity, and thus the capacity for physical activities. This change may not be sufficient to alter the level of physical function in a particular individual; therefore, other indices of fitness, including muscle strength, endurance, and flexibility that may have a more direct or additive effect on functional capacity should be considered. Matching the body's capacity to the individual's need to perform physical activities is important to prevent injury. For example, focused training to develop greater strength of the muscles of the back and trunk could protect from or minimize injury in a work environment that involves heavy lifting. Endurance training may prevent fatigue and maintain motor control in individuals who have jobs that require repetitive activity. In work environments that demand frequent bending, improved flexibility may be the critical factor to reduce injury risk. Often a combination of improved strength, endurance, and flexibility will enhance the capacity of a pain patient's ability to return to work safely. Strength and flexibility exercises have also been shown to improve circulation to the back structures and mood, which would favorably influence sensitivity to pain *(7,22,23)*.

2.4. Mood

Depressed chronic pain patients report greater pain intensity, less life control, and more use of passive–avoidant coping strategies. They also describe greater interference from pain and exhibit more pain behaviors than chronic pain patients without depression *(24)*. The prevalence of major depression in patients with chronic low back pain is three to four times greater than in the general population *(25,26)* Quasi-experimental and randomized controlled trials (RCTs) demonstrate that both resistance training and aerobic exercise can reduce symptoms of depression *(27,28)*, although there is still a lack of good quality research on clinical populations *(7)*. Aerobic exercise is associated with reductions in state anxiety *(29)*. More recent evidence suggests that resistance training may reduce state anxiety, but more so in subjects with a high baseline level of state anxiety *(30)*. Low to moderate aerobic exercise appears to improve mood states in patients with low back pain *(31)*.

2.5. Sleep

Sleep disturbance is a prevalent complaint in patients with chronic pain *(32)*. Twenty percent of American adults (42 million people) report that pain or physical discomfort disrupts their sleep a few nights a week or more *(33)*. Epidemiological studies show that exercise is perceived as helpful in promoting sleep and suggest that regular physical activity may be useful in improving sleep quality and reducing daytime sleepiness *(34)*. Although only moderate effect sizes have been noted, meta-analyses have shown that exercise increases total sleep time and delays REM sleep onset (10 min), increases slow-wave sleep (SWS) and reduces REM sleep (2–5 min) *(35,36)*. Menefee et al. *(32)* found that higher overall sleep quality and lower sleep latency primarily were related to higher ratings of physical functioning and shorter duration of pain in patients with chronic pain. Their data suggest that physical functioning, duration of pain, and age may be more important than pain intensity and depressed mood in contributing to decreased overall sleep quality and sleep latency. The contribution of physical functioning was particularly strong. This suggests that increasing the level of physical functioning may contribute to better sleep quality in patients with chronic pain.

2.6. Exercise and the Brain

Regular physical exercise benefits the nervous system, as well as the musculoskeletal and cardiovascular systems. In humans, exercise may improve mood and cognition, and the data suggests that regular exercise can also promote maintenance of cognitive function with aging. When mice are provided access to a running wheel, the amount of neurogenesis in their hippocampi is increased and they exhibit improved performance in learning and memory tasks. Exercise results in an increase in the level of brain-derived neurotrophic factor (BDNF) in the hippocampus, suggesting a role for BDNF in the beneficial effects of exercise on brain function and plasticity. BDNF is a member of the structurally and functionally homologous neurotrophin family. It is the most widely distributed trophic factor in the brain, and participates in neuronal growth, maintenance, and use-dependent plasticity mechanisms such as long-term potentiation and learning *(37)*. There is a reciprocal relationship between BDNF and serotonergic signaling, in which BDNF enhances serotonin production and release, and serotonergic signaling stimulates BDNF production *(38)*. Research has also provided evidence that circulating insulin-like growth factor-1 (IGF-1) plays an important role in the stimulation of hippocampal neurogenesis by physical exercise *(38)*. Two additional effects of exercise on the brain that may contribute to its ability to promote neuronal plasticity and ward off neurodegenerative disease are enhancement of serotonergic signaling *(39)* and stimulation of angiogenesis *(40)*. Different forms of training in rats, e.g., aerobic and motor skill, had differential effects on the vasculature and synaptic connectivity of the brain. The aerobic group was found to have a higher density of capillaries in the cerebellum than the animals trained on motor skills or the inactive control animals. The animals in the motor skill group showed a larger number of synapses in the cerebellum than the other groups *(41)*. Subsequent studies have shown that fitness training can also enhance vascularization of other regions of the brain, such as the motor cortex, in primates as well as rats. It has been suggested that increases in vascularization serves an important function in providing a greater reserve capacity to respond in situations requiring increased oxygen *(40)*.

2.7. Exercise and the Immune System

Over the past several decades a variety of studies have demonstrated that exercise induces considerable physiological change in the immune system.

Various types of psychological and physiological stressors, including physical activity, influence the immune system. It is well known that physical activity can influence neuropeptide levels both in the central nervous system as well as in peripheral blood. The consensus among exercise immunologists is that moderate exercise enhances immune function and may reduce the incidence of infections, while long-term exhaustive endurance exercise results in immunosuppression and an increased susceptibility to infections *(42)*.The reported changes of immune function in response to exercise have been suggested to be partly regulated by the activation of different neuropeptides. The most common neuropeptides mentioned in this context are the endogenous opioids activated by long-term aerobic exercise. Other neuropeptides, such as serotonin, substance P and vasoactive intestinal peptide (VIP), could also be of interest, as well as several neuroendocrine hormones, including growth hormone (GH), prolactin, and adrenocorticotrophin (ACTH) *(43)*.

The identification of receptors for neuropeptides and steroid hormones on cells of the immune system has created a new dimension in this endocrine–immune interaction. It has also been shown that immune cells are capable of producing neuropeptides, creating a bidirectional link between the nervous and immune systems *(43)*.

3. INTRODUCTION TO EXERCISE TESTING

The maximal oxygen consumption $(VO_{2peak})^*$ attained during a graded maximal exercise to volitional exhaustion is considered the single best indicator of aerobic exercise capacity by the World Health Organization *(44)*. VO_{2peak} reflects the maximal oxygen flux through the mitochondria of the exercising muscle. Based on the Fick principle, VO_{2peak} is the product of cardiac output (heart rate x stroke volume) and the mixed arterio-venous oxygen difference *(45)*. Thus VO_{2peak} is dependent on cardiac function and the ability of the muscles to extract (utilize) oxygen from the circulation. However, measurement of VO_{2peak} is not always possible in the clinical setting, because of the need for an expensive respiratory gas analysis system. Other methods of estimating VO_{2peak} include submaximal tests (see Section 3.3) that can be used as viable alternatives to measure change in aerobic capacity with exercise.

---

*Maximal exercise tests in patients are usually terminated when the subject despite strong verbal encouragement from the experimenters, is unwilling or unable to continue. The appropriate term to use is therefore peak oxygen consumption (VO_{2peak}), which represents the highest oxygen uptake during an exercise test to volitional exhaustion.

3.1. Energy Pathways

Broadly speaking, two general exercise forms can be distinguished: short-term intensive bouts of exercise or anaerobic exercise capacity, and the long-term endurance type of activity or aerobic exercise capacity. All physical activity involves muscular contractions powered by energy. The currency of energy expenditure is adenosine triphosphate (ATP). The phosphorolysis of ATP to adenosine diphosphate (ADP) and inorganic phosphate releases the energy. The amount of ATP stored in muscle at any time is small and must be resynthesized continuously if exercise continues for more than a few seconds. The synthesis of ATP requires a substrate for energy. Carbohydrate and fat act as substrates under usual conditions and in the presence of ADP, adenosine monophosphate (AMP), creatine phosphate (CP), and inorganic phosphate. Synthesis takes place by different aerobic or anaerobic enzyme pathways. Only carbohydrates (glycogen) use the anaerobic pathway for the generation of energy, whereas glycogen, fat, and protein can be used aerobically. These aerobic and anaerobic ATP-production pathways in humans are displayed in Table 1.

3.2. Maximal Exercise Testing in Pain Patients

Not much is known about the validity of exercise testing in patients with chronic pain, given that historically, exercise testing was mostly done in athletes, healthy subjects or subjects with cardiac and pulmonary conditions. One study (46) compared treadmill, bicycle, and upper extremity ergometry (UBE) exercise testing in a small (N = 30) sample of patients with chronic low back pain (CLBP). Respiratory gas exchange analysis was used to determine oxygen uptake and a three-lead electrocardiogram

Table 1
Pathways for Energy Production in the Muscle

Oxidative Phosphorylation:

$Glycogen_{(n)} + 6O_2 + 37Pi + 37\ ADP \rightarrow glycogen_{(n-1)} + 6\ CO_2 + 42\ H_2O + 37\ ATP$

$Glucose + 6\ O_2 + 36\ Pi + 36\ ATP \rightarrow 6\ CO_2 + 42\ H_2O + 36\ ATP$

$C_{16}H_{32}O_2$ (Fatty acids; palmitate) $+ 23\ O_2 + 129\ (ATP + Pi) \rightarrow 129\ ATP + 16\ CO_2 + 145\ H_2O$

Glycolysis:

$Glycogen_{(n)} + 3\ Pi + 3ATP \rightarrow glycogen_{(n-1)} + 2\ lactate + 2\ H_2O + 2\ ATP$

$Glucose + 2ATP + 2\ NAD^+ + e^- + H^+ \rightarrow Pyruvate + NADH + H^+$

Creatine Kinase reaction

$ADP + PCr + H^+ \leftrightarrow ATP + Cr$

Adenylate kinase / AMP deaminase reactions

$2ADP \leftrightarrow ATP + AMP\ /\ AMP + H_2O \rightarrow NH_3 + IMP + 2\ Pi$

ATP hydrolysis reaction

$ATP \rightarrow ADP + Pi + Energy$

O_2 = oxygen, Pi = inorganic phosphate; ADP= adenosine triphosphate; CO_2 = carbondioxide; H_2O = water; ATP = adenosinetriphosphate; PCr = creatine phosphate; H^+ = hydrogen; Cr = creatine; AMP = adenosinemonophosphate; NH_3 = ammonia; IMP = inosinemonophosphate; NAD^+ = Nicotinamide adenine dinucleotide; e– = electron. Table modified after reference (3).

(ECG) was used to determine heart rates at each minute of testing. Subjects were encouraged to "do as much as you can." The tests that were used were the modified Bruce treadmill test, the Åstrand-Ryhming bicycle test and a UBE test in which the workload was started at 20 W and increased by 10 W every 3 min. Patients were asked to maintain a cycling rate of 60 rotations per minute (rpm) throughout the UBE test.

Seventy percent of the patients with CLBP reported that arm fatigue was the reason to stop UBE testing, and leg fatigue was the major reason (56.7%) for the patients to stop bicycle testing. Peripheral fatigue may play an important role in the aerobic testing of patients with CLBP. This peripheral fatigue may be a reflection of a loss of muscle endurance as the result of prolonged inactivity. Despite this, the testing response for patients with CLBP was remarkably similar to that of normal subjects. Peak and predicted VO_{2peak} showed gender differences consistent with published results for normal subjects. Significantly higher heart rates, VO_{2peak} and predicted VO_{2peak} mL/kg/min were achieved by the modified Bruce treadmill test in this sample of patients than with the bicycle or UBE tests, despite pain.

3.3. Submaximal Exercise Testing in Pain Patients

It is important to understand that the most accurate way to measure VO_{2peak} in a *single individual* is through direct measurement of maximal oxygen uptake. In a chronic pain population this is neither practical nor feasible in a clinical setting. A variety of (submaximal) tests have been developed estimating aerobic capacity when direct measurement is not possible [for review see reference *(47)*]. These tests usually involve running/walking for a given time or distance, such as the 12-min walk/run test *(48)*, the shuttle test *(49)*, various step tests *(50,51)* and the 2-km walk test *(52)*. Longer distances and shorter test times are associated with higher levels of aerobic fitness. Other tests estimate VO_{2peak} by submaximal testing and extrapolation to maximal heart rate by treadmill walking or bicycling against a predetermined load with measurement of heart rates *(53,54)*.

These tests were mostly developed for testing aerobic fitness in healthy people and were validated by comparing actual measured VO_{2peak} to predicted VO_2 or to the test performance. The validity of a number of these tests was established for patients with cardiac or pulmonary problems *(55,56)*, but little has been done to validate these tests in patients with chronic pain. Modified versions exist of several exercise tests to accommodate sicker patients *(57–59)*, but little is known about the validity of these tests in patients with pain.

3.3.1. WALKING TESTS

Walking tests have become more popular in clinical settings. Since the introduction of the Balke 15-min walking test in 1963 *(60)*, many investigators have used such tests in research and clinical practice. Cooper originally developed a 12-min run test *(61)*. In the years after Cooper's publication, a variety of modifications to this test have been made. One of these modifications for patients is the 6-min walk test *(62)*. The 6-min walk test is a simple, relatively quick, inexpensive and safe test *(63)*. The 6-min walk test is used for different purposes. It has been used as a replacement of the symptom-limited cardiopulmonary exercise test for diagnostic purposes *(64)*. Other studies have used it to establish a prognosis for outcome, or used it as an objective measure to evaluate the efficacy of therapy *(65,66)*.

Solway et al. *(67)* recommend the 6-min walk test as the test of choice when using a functional walk test for clinical or research purposes. Most of the research with this test has been done in groups of patients with cardiac or chronic obstructive pulmonary disease *(63)*, but there is the suggestion in the literature that the 6-minute walk test might also be a proper instrument to determine the functional capacity of patients with rheumatic disease *(68)*.

The 6-min walk test is also gaining in acceptance as a functional test in the assessment of patients with chronic pain (see Table 2). Mannercorpi et al. *(69)* report excellent intra-rater reliability for the 6-min walk test in patients with fibromyalgia and showed that the 6-min walk test is sensitive enough to detect differences between patients with fibromyalgia and healthy controls.

Two studies have examined the relationship between the 6-min walk test and VO_{2peak} in patients with chronic pain. Correlations ranged from r = 0.328 (N = 28) before to r = 0.420 (N = 20) after an exercise program for fibromyalgia patients *(70)*. The Pearson correlation in patients with CLBP (N = 30) of the 6-min walk test was r = 0.46 (p = 0.02) with treadmill VO_{2peak} (mL/kg/min) *(71)*.The correlation of the 6-min walk test was r = 0.62 (p = 0.001), with bicycle VO_{2peak} (mL/kg/min); however, correlations with predicted VO_{2peak} were poor and non-significant.

It thus appears that in patients with chronic pain, the 6-min walk test has little relationship with aerobic fitness but has relevance as a physical performance test. This is further underscored by significant correlations of the 6-min walk distance with the Fibromyalgia Impact Questionnaire total (r = -0.494, p < 0.01) and physical impairment (r = –0.403, p <0.05) scores *(70)* and with the SF-36 Physical Functioning scale (r = 0.43, p <0.05) *(71)*.

Gibbons et al. *(74)* showed that some familiarity with the test is required. Reliability is optimized when the administration of walk tests was standardized according to the guidelines of the American Thoracic Society *(75)* and one practice walk is performed. The guidelines of the American Thoracic Society also provide standardized verbal

Table 2
Six-Minute Walk Test in Patients with Pain-Related Diseases

Author	Subjects	Reliability	Validity
Wittink et al. *(71)*	CLBP		Correlation with treadmill VO_{2peak} R = 0.46 Correlation with bicycle VO_{2peak} R = 0.62
Mannercorpi et al. *(69)*	Fibromyalgia	Coefficient of variation 2.9%	
King et al. *(72)*	Fibromyalgia	Test retest (ICC = 0.73)	Correlation with VO_{2peak} R = 0.657
Pankoff et al. *(70,73)*	Fibromyalgia		Correlation with VO_{2peak} R = 0.33 Correlation with W_{max} R = 0.42

ICC = intra-class correlation; VO_{2peak} = peak oxygen uptake; W_{max} = peak workload.

Table 3
Prediction Equations for the Six-minute Walk Test in Healthy Subjects

Author	Subject's age (yr)	Track length	Prediction equation (distance in meters)
Troosters et al. (76)	50–85	50-m	Distance = 218 + (5,14 x length [cm] – 5,32 × age [years]) – (1,80 × weight [kg]) + 51,31 × gender [1 = male, 0 = female]
Gibbons et al. (74)	20–80	20-m	Distance = 868.8 – (2.99 × age) – 74.7 × gender [male = 0; female = 1]
Enright and Sherill (77)	40–80	30-m	Male: Distance = (7.57 × length [cm]) – 5.02 × age [years] – (1.76 × weight [kg]) – 309 Female: Distance = (2.11 × length [cm]) – 2.29 × weight– (5.78 × age) + 667

encouragements to administer during the test. The covered distance in meters by the patients can be compared with several prediction equations obtained from data of healthy subjects. The achieved distance in meters can be calculated as a percentage of predicted distance using these equations. Several equations have been established (see Table 3) for various age groups and track lengths. It is recommended to use the equation with the most comparable age group.

3.4. Psychophysical Variables

During the exercise test every 2 min the patient will be asked, "How hard are you exercising with your arms/legs?" The patient has to answer on the following Borg 10-grade scale from 0 (nothing) to 10 (maximal). The same procedure is followed for dyspnea. The patient has to rate his breathlessness on the Borg 10-Grade Scale using the question, "What number describes your shortness of breath?" (Also see Section 4.1).

4. EXERCISE TRAINING AND THE PATIENT WITH CHRONIC PAIN

Evidence is growing that deconditioned muscle, inadequate motion, and periarticular stiffness may contribute to symptoms of osteoarthritis (79). Clinical trials have provided strong evidence for the efficacy of muscle conditioning and aerobic exercise to lessen symptoms in persons with osteoarthritis of the knee (80–82). Others have reported that exercise is an important tool for reducing pain, stiffness, and joint tenderness in rheumatoid arthritis patients (83,84) and patients with fibromyalgia (85). Exercise has been shown to be effective for short-term pain relief in patients with rotator cuff disease (RR 7.74 (1,97,30.32), and provides a longer term benefit with respect to functional measures (RR 2.45 (1.24, 4.86) (86). Exercise may be helpful for patients with chronic low back pain, enhancing return to normal daily activities and work (87,88). Supervised exercise therapy that consists of individually designed programs, including stretching or strengthening, may improve pain and function in chronic nonspecific low back pain *(89)*. In summary, exercise therapy encompasses a heterogeneous group of interventions, and although the previously cited studies found beneficial effects of exercise on pain and function, there continues to be uncertainty about the most effective exercise approach. In most studies there were insufficient data to provide useful guidelines on optimal exercise type or dosage.

As patients with chronic pain represent a heterogeneous population it is unlikely that all will benefit from the same exercise program. Exercise programs, therefore, need to be individually designed and tailored to the individual needs of the patient. More research is needed on alternative forms of exercise discussed in the Movement Therapies section of this textbook to better understand their effect on different chronic pain conditions.

4.1. Exercise and Safety

One of the most useful constructs to emerge in measuring the subjective response to physical exercise is a scale developed by Borg *(90)* for the rating of perception of effort. This perception scale quantifies the subjective sense of the intensity of effort, strain, discomfort or fatigue experienced during exercise *(91)*. The original category scale has been shown to correlate to heart rate, ventilation, and oxygen consumption in normal subjects *(92)*. Further, this correlation has been shown to be affected by psychological states (anxiety, depression, and personality traits) *(93)* and by different types of physical work (dynamic, static, eccentric, concentric, and isokinetic contractions) *(94)*. The RPE or rating of perceived exertion has been used in formulating an exercise prescription *(95)*.

A variety of central physiologic exercise responses contribute to the sense of effort, including heart rate, minute ventilation, respiratory rate, and oxygen consumption. The exercising body parts also contribute to the perception of exertion. Muscle cramps, twitches, aches, and tremors are reported that may be influenced by the elevation of local blood lactate concentration *(92)*, by the level of blood glucose *(96)*, and other possible local physiologic factors such as temperature *(97)*.

A ratio scale for RPE was also presented by Borg (Table 4) *(78)*. The major advantage to the use of this ratio scale is the ability to do parametric statistical testing. Borg and his colleagues *(98)* explored a possible relationship between RPE and leg muscle pain during a progressive maximal bicycle test in healthy non-pain subjects. They reported a moderate to high correlation between RPE and pain in this group of normal subjects ($r = 0.59$–0.91).

Patients with chronic back pain experience fatigue during exercise, which may often be excessive, perhaps due to aerobic deconditioning. However, they may rate their RPE based on their sensations of pain or based on their psychological state. The relationship of the RPE to a subjective rating of pain intensity was explored in patients with chronic low back pain *(99)*. Thirty-four patients with chronic low back pain provided RPE and pain scores at symptom-limited maximal exercise. Eighteen of these subjects stopped exercise due to pain (see Table 5) and 16 stopped due to fatigue. A surprising number of patients did not stop their peak exercise due to pain, but due to fatigue. This group achieved a higher VO_{2peak}, and a higher percent of predicted VO_{2peak}. It is suggested that when pain increases, it dominates all sensations so that fatigue is less obvious. When pain does not increase during progressive exercise, the RPE more accurately reflects fatigue, with typical RPE ratings of 18 out of 20.

Table 4
Borg 10-Grade Scale

Rating of perceived exertion / dyspnea

0	Nothing
0.5	Very, very weak (just noticeable)
1	Very weak
2	Weak (light)
3	Moderate
4	Somewhat strong
5	Strong (heavy)
6	
7	Very strong
8	
9	Very, very strong (almost maximum)
10	Maximum

From reference *(78)*.

In addition to assessing the change in pain rating during therapeutic exercise, adding an RPE to monitor changes in symptoms during exercise in patients with chronic low back pain gives important additional information, as there may be fundamental differences between those who stop exercise due to pain and those who stop exercise due to fatigue. In the latter, pain did not increase with exercise. In the former, pain increased and patients tended to overrate their RPE based on their actual oxygen consumption measurements, suggesting the possibility that their RPE reflected more psychological distress *(99)*. Another study investigated the efficacy of using ratings of perceived exertion (RPEs) to regulate exercise intensity in patients with chronic back pain while undergoing hydrotherapy *(100)*. At workloads below 55% of age-predicted maximum heart rate, great variability was found in the relationship between RPE and exercise intensity. However, for workloads between 55% and 85% of age-predicted maximum heart rate, RPE had a strong correlation with relative exercise intensity during hydrotherapy.

In addition to RPE and pain ratings, vital signs should be taken during exercise in all pain patients, as those with chronic pain are equally susceptible to cardiovascular or metabolic sources of exercise intolerance as any other population. In the absence of measures of oxygen consumption, heart rate, blood pressure, and respiratory rate

Table 5
Rating of Perceived Exertion (RPE) and Numeric Rating Scale (NRS) Scores in Chronic Low Back Pain Patients at Symptom-Limited Max Exercise: Comparison of Those Who Stopped Due to Pain (Pain Group) and Those Who Stopped Due to Fatigue (Fatigue Group)

	Pain group (n = 18)	*Fatigue group (n = 16)*
Initial pain (0–10 Scale)	4.19 ± 2.58	4.60 ± 2.38
End pain	7.26 ± 2.25	4.93 ± 1.83
Peak RPE (6–20 scale)	17.22 ± 1.77	18.00 ± 1.93

responses give valuable information about the amount of energy being used, and how much reserve capacity may still be available to the patient.

Patients who are planning to become much more physically active than before are advised to fill out the Physical Activity Readiness Questionnaire (PAR-Q; see http://www.csep.ca/forms.asp). This questionnaire screens patients between 15 and 69 years of age, using 7 simple questions, and helps determine if medical screening should be performed before they start with vigorous exercise training. Sedentary patients over 69 years of age should always undergo pre-exercise screening by a medical doctor.

4.2. Type of Exercise: Aerobic or Anaerobic

We have presented in an earlier section some of the work that has been done to investigate the effect of exercise on pain threshold; however, it appears that the predominant form of exercise studied has been aerobic training. Very little research has compared whether strength or aerobic exercise has a greater effect on raising pain threshold. The one study in the literature *(101)* comparing the effect of aerobic and strength conditioning on pain tolerance found that exercise incorporating aerobic fitness results in greater pain tolerance than strength training alone. Markedly increased pain tolerance for those undergoing aerobic training occurred between weeks 6 and 12 of the study. According to the authors, because the aerobic training effect on cardiovascular function also usually occurs after 6 weeks, they hypothesize that marked improvement in cardiovascular functioning is a relevant component in linking the role of aerobic work to pain tolerance.

4.3. Reconditioning Exercises

The primary goal of reconditioning exercise in chronic pain patients is to improve functional performance. A general weakening of all tissues takes place with disuse. Exercise treatment should be directed at reversing this process so the body can respond to the functional demands placed on it. This can be done effectively with high repetition, low-load exercise. Low loads prevent damage to the tissues, and high repetitions have been shown to be most effective in increasing metabolism in low-metabolic structures. This kind of exercise can be achieved with floor exercises, low-weight dumbbells, pulleys, or Nautilus®equipment. Placing stress on the low-metabolic structures can be done indirectly by muscle contractions. For instance, increasing the fluid exchange between the disc and the interstitial fluid surrounding the spine can be achieved by having the patient maximally flex and extend the lumbar spine repetitively. The patient can also be asked to perform a latissimus pull-down exercise with high repetitions. The contraction and relaxation of the muscle will have a pumping effect on the intervertebral disc, increasing its metabolic activity. Low-load, high-repetition exercise will increase muscle endurance. This is especially beneficial for postural muscles.

As the patient becomes stronger, the load can be increased and the number of repetitions decreased to increase the patient's muscle strength. The body will respond to the demands placed on it, but the challenge must not be punishing or damaging. The physical therapist must ensure that the exercise program matches the physical capacity of the patient's body.

The body responds to the demands placed on it by using a variety of homeostatic mechanisms. In the person with chronic pain, activity intolerance secondary to pain leads to physiologic and pathologic changes in almost all organ systems but specifically in those organ systems that are related to activity performance. Reconditioning the patient with chronic pain can restore health to many organ systems and specific tissues. This approach deals directly with pain as a symptom, changes the health status of the individual and has a profound effect on the perception of health status (and therefore on physical performance and quality of life) in individuals with persistent pain *(102)*.

4.4. Exercise Prescription and the Chronic Pain Patient

The aerobic challenge should follow the general guidelines for physical fitness development. The prescription is based on the FITT factors: Frequency of exercise, Intensity of exercise, Time (duration of exercise), and Type of exercise.

4.4.1. FREQUENCY

According to the Guidelines of the American College of Sports Medicine, exercise training should be executed 3 to 5 days a week to improve cardiorespiratory fitness and body composition *(103)*. For patients a minimum of two sessions per week on non-consecutive days is regarded as the lower limit to be effective. One session per week or less is not effective for improving cardiorespiratory fitness *(103)*.

4.4.2. INTENSITY

To be effective, a training stimulus should be above a certain basal intensity. This intensity is frequently prescribed using target heart rates. During aerobic exercise the target heart rate is calculated using the Karvonen formula *(104)*.

Exercise intensity = (exercise heart rate – resting heart rate)/(maximal hart rate – rest heart rate).

A rule of the thumb for an effective endurance training program is an intensity above 60% of the heart rate reserve, as calculated using the Karvonen formula.

In severely deconditioned patients the exercise intensity of the training can be reduced to 40–50% of the heart rate reserve *(103)*. However, the intensity should increase gradually towards the 60% of heart rate reserve. The maximal hart rate can be estimated from the following formulas: $HR_{max} = 220 - age$ or $HR_{max} = 210 - (0.65 \times age)$. Unfortunately these estimations are imprecise for individual patients and are not valid to use in children. Moreover RPE can be used as a surrogate for heart rate or VO_{2res} when no heart rate monitors are available. RPE values corresponding with the heart rate reserve intensities can be appreciated from Table 6.

4.4.3. TIME

The minimum duration of training should be 20 min per session. For deconditioned patients the session might be divided into two 10-min sessions over the day *(27)*. The duration of a session is dependent on the intensity of the activity; thus, lower-intensity activity should be conducted over a longer period of time, and individuals training at higher levels of intensity should train at least 20 min *(103)*.

4.4.4. TYPE OF EXERCISE

Any activity that uses large muscle groups, which can be maintained continuously, and is rhythmical and aerobic in nature (freely moving, freely breathing form, preferably one that is enjoyable to the patient) such a cycling, walking, steps, or swimming is

Table 6
Training Guidelines Based on Heart Rate, Oxygen Uptake, or Rating of Perceived Exertion

Intensity	$\%VO_{2res}\%\ HR_{res}$	$\%\ HR_{max}$	RPE6–20	RPE0–10
Very light	<20	<35	<10	<2
Light	20–39	35–54	10–11	3
Moderate	40–59	55–69	12–13	4–5
Heavy	60–84	70–89	14–16	6–7
Very heavy	>85	>90	17–19	8–9
Maximal	100	100	20	10

$\%VO_{2res}$ = percentage of VO_2 reserve, $\%\ HR_{res}$ = percentage of heart rate reserve. $\%HR_{max}$ = percentage of maximal heart rate, RPE = rating of perceived exertion. VO_{2res} and HR_{res} can be calculated using the subtraction of the resting value from maximal value during exercise. From reference (103).

recommended (103). Other alternative forms of exercise, such as Yoga and Tai Chi, have a growing literature to support their safety and benefit.

4.4.5. EVALUATION

It is known from the literature that the effects of exercise are mode specific (105). Therefore the training should include the preferred activities that the patient wants to include in their activities of daily life. Moreover, the evaluation of the program should be activity-specific. If the training included most frequently walking exercises, a walk or running test is the preferred testing mode of fitness, and conversely, when a cycling exercise is the dominant training mode a bicycle fitness test is the test of choice.

For the proper setting of the training intensity, a frequent exercise test evaluation is necessary. Every 6–8 weeks a test session should be incorporated in the training program to test effectiveness and to modify the intensity of the training program.

5. CONCLUSION

Exercise testing and prescription should be incorporated in the therapeutic management of the chronic pain patient. In this chapter we present a solid explanation as to why regular exercise can have positive effects on pain, mood, sleep, function, and fitness. Moreover, specific guidelines for exercise testing and prescription for the chronic pain patient are provided.

REFERENCES

1. Tipton C. Introduction: A view of the past. Exercise physiogy: roots and historical perspectives. In: Exercise physiology. Energy, nutrition and human performance. McArdle WD, Katch FI, Katch VL, Eds. Baltimore: Lipincott Williams & Wilkins, 2001: xvii–Ixii.
2. American Society of Exercise Physiologists. Exercise physiology. http://www.asep.org/. 2005.
3. Booth FW, Gordon SE, Carlson CJ, Hamilton MT. Waging war on modern chronic diseases: primary prevention through exercise biology. J Appl Physiol 2000;88(2):774–787.
4. Colditz GA. Economic costs of obesity and inactivity. Med Sci Sports Exerc 1999;31 (11 Suppl):S663–S667.
5. World Health Organization. 2001. The International Classification of Functioning, Disability and Health (ICF), 2nd edition. Geneva, Switzerland:WHO, Marketing and Dissemination.
6. Vuori IM. Dose–response of physical activity and low back pain, osteoarthritis, and osteoporosis. Med Sci Sports Exerc 2001;33(6 Suppl), (Review; 269 refs).

7. Lawlor DA, Hopker SW. The effectiveness of exercise as an intervention in the management of depression: systematic review and meta-regression analysis of randomised controlled trials. BMJ 2001;322(7289):763–767.
8. Koltyn KF. Analgesia following exercise: a review. Sports Med 2000;29(2):85–98.
9. Koltyn KF. Exercise-induced hypoalgesia and intensity of exercise. Sports Med 2002;32(8):477–487.
10. Hoffman MD, Shepanski MA, Mackenzie SP, Clifford PS. Experimentally induced pain perception is acutely reduced by aerobic exercise in people with chronic low back pain. J Rehabil Res Dev 2005;42(2):183–190.
11. Whiteside A, Hansen S, Chaudhuri A. Exercise lowers pain threshold in chronic fatigue syndrome. Pain 2004;109(3):497–499.
12. Dietrich A, McDaniel WF. Endocannabinoids and exercise. Br J Sports Med 2004;38(5):536–541.
13. Sparling PB, Giuffrida A, Piomelli D, Rosskopf L, Dietrich A. Exercise activates the endocannabinoid system. Neuroreport 2003;14(17):2209–2211.
14. Ainsworth BE, Haskell WL, Whitt MC, Irwin ML, Swartz AM, Strath SJ, O' Brien WL, Bassett DR, Jr, Schmitz KH, Emplaincourt PO, Jacobs DR, Jr., Leon AS. Compendium of physical activities: an update of activity codes and MET intensities. Med Sci Sports Exerc 2000 Sep;32(9 Suppl):S498–S504.
15. Astrand P, Rodahl K. 1986. Textbook of Work Physiology, Physiological Bases of Exercise, 3rd edition. New York:McGraw-Hill Book Company.
16. Verbunt JA, Seelen HA, Vlaeyen JW, van de Heijden GJ, Heuts PH, Pons K, et al. Disuse and deconditioning in chronic low back pain: concepts and hypotheses on contributing mechanisms. Eur J Pain 2003;7(1):9–21.
17. Mayer TG, Gatchel RJ, Kishino N, Keeley J, Capra P, Mayer H, et al. Objective assessment of spine function following industrial injury. A prospective study with comparison group and one-year follow-up. Spine 1985;10(6):482–493.
18. Mayer TG, Gatchel RJ, Kishino N, Keeley J, Mayer H, Capra P, et al. A prospective short-term study of chronic low back pain patients utilizing novel objective functional measurement. Pain 1986;25(1):53–68.
19. Verbunt JA, Seelen HA, Vlaeyen JW, van der Heijden GJ, Knottnerus JA. Fear of injury and physical deconditioning in patients with chronic low back pain. Arch Phys Med Rehabil 2003;84(8):1227–1232.
20. Vlaeyen JW, Linton SJ. Fear-avoidance and its consequences in chronic musculoskeletal pain: a state of the art. Pain 2000;85(3):317–332.
21. Stewart AL, Hays RD, Wells KB, Rogers WH, Spritzer KL, Greenfield S. Long-term functioning and well-being outcomes associated with physical activity and exercise in patients with chronic conditions in the Medical Outcomes Study. J Clin Epidemiol 1994;47(7):719–730.
22. Statens Beredning for Medicinsk Utvardering. Pain in the Back Pain in the Neck. Summary of Scientific Evidence. Stockholm:Statens Beredning for Medicinsk Utvardering, 2000.
23. Suni J. 2000. Health related fitness test battery for middle-aged adults with emphasis on musculoskeletal and motor tests. Finland:University of Jyväskylä.
24. Herr KA, Mobily PR, Smith C. Depression and the experience of chronic back pain: a study of related variables and age differences. Clin J Pain 1993;9(2):104–114.
25. Sullivan MJ, Reesor K, Mikail S, Fisher R. The treatment of depression in chronic low back pain: review and recommendations. Pain 1992;50(1):5–13.
26. Currie SR, Wang J. Chronic back pain and major depression in the general Canadian population. Pain 2004;107(1–2):54–60.
27. Dunn AL, Trivedi MH, O'Neal HA. Physical activity dose–response effects on outcomes of depression and anxiety. Med Sci Sports Exerc 2001;33(6 Suppl):S587–S597.
28. North TC, McCullagh P, Tran ZV. Effect of exercise on depression. Exer Sport Sci Rev 1990;18:379–415.
29. Petruzzello SJ, Landers DM, Hatfield BD. A meta analysis on the anxiety reducing effects of acute and chronic exercise. Sports Med 1991;11:143.
30. Focht BC. Pre-exercise anxiety and the anxiolytic responses to acute bouts of self-selected and prescribed intensity resistance exercise. J Sports Med Phys Fitness 2002;42(2):217–223.
31. Sculco AD, Paup DC, Fernhall B, Sculco MJ. Effects of aerobic exercise on low back pain patients in treatment. Spine J 2001;1(2):95–101.
32. Menefee LA, Frank ED, Doghramji K, Picarello K, Park JJ, Jalali S, et al. Self-reported sleep quality and quality of life for individuals with chronic pain conditions. Clin J Pain 2000;16(4):290–297.

33. 2000 National Sleep Foundation (NSF). Sleep in America poll. http://www.sleepfoundation.org/sleeplibrary/index.php?secid=&id=63 . 2000.

34. Sherrill DL, Kotchou K, Quan SF. Association of physical activity and human sleep disorders. Arch Intern Med 1998;158(17):1894–1898.

35. Driver HS, Taylor SR. Exercise and sleep. Sleep Med Rev 2000;4(4):387–402.

36. Kubitz KA, Landers DM, Petruzzello SJ, Han M. The effects of acute and chronic exercise on sleep. A meta-analytic review. Sports Med 1996;21(4):277–291.

37. Russo-Neustadt AA, Chen MJ. Brain-derived neurotrophic factor and antidepressant activity. Curr Pharm Des 2005;11(12):1495–1510.

38. Mattson MP, Duan W, Wan R, Guo Z. Prophylactic activation of neuroprotective stress response pathways by dietary and behavioral manipulations. NeuroRx 2004;1(1):111–116.

39. Lim BV, Jang MH, Shin MC, Kim HB, Kim YJ, Kim YP, et al. Caffeine inhibits exercise-induced increase in tryptophan hydroxylase expression in dorsal and median raphe of Sprague-Dawley rats. Neurosci Lett 2001;308(1):25–28.

40. Swain RA, Harris AB, Wiener EC, Dutka MV, Morris HD, Theien BE, et al. Prolonged exercise induces angiogenesis and increases cerebral blood volume in primary motor cortex of the rat. Neuroscience 2003;117(4):1037–1046.

41. Black JE, Isaacs KR, Anderson BJ, Alcantara AA, Greenough WT. Learning causes synaptogenesis, whereas motor activity causes angiogenesis, in cerebellar cortex of adult rats. Proc Natl Acad Sci USA 1990;87(14):5568–5572.

42. Shephard RJ. Sepsis and mechanisms of inflammatory response: is exercise a good model? Br J Sports Med 2001;35(4):223–230.

43. Jonsdottir IH. Special feature for the Olympics: effects of exercise on the immune system: neuropeptides and their interaction with exercise and immune function. Immunol Cell Biol 2000;78(5):562–570.

44. Shephard RJ, Allen C, Benade AJ, Davies CT, Di Prampero PE, Hedman R, et al. The maximum oxygen intake. An international reference standard of cardiorespiratory fitness. Bull World Health Organ 1968;38(5):757–764.

45. Fick A. Ueber die Messung des Blutquantums in den Herzventrikeln. 2 ed. Wurzburg: Sitx. der Physik-Med. Ges. 1870.

46. Wittink H, Michel TH, Kulich R, Wagner A, Sukiennik A, Maciewicz R, et al. Aerobic fitness testing in patients with chronic low back pain: which test is best? Spine 2000;25(13):1704–1710.

47. Noonan V, Dean E. Submaximal exercise testing: clinical application and interpretation. Phys Ther 2000;80(8):782–807.

48. Cooper KH. A means of assessing maximal oxygen intake. Correlation between field and treadmill testing. JAMA 1968;203(3):201–204.

49. Leger LA, Lambert J. A maximal multistage 20-m shuttle run test to predict VO2 max. Eur J Appl Physiol Occup Physiol 1982;49(1):1–12.

50. Francis KT. Fitness assessment using step tests. Compr Ther 1987;13(4):36–41.

51. Siconolfi SF, Garber CE, Lasater TM, Carleton RA. A simple, valid step test for estimating maximal oxygen uptake in epidemiologic studies. Am J Epidemiol 1985;121(3):382–390.

52. Oja P, Laukkanen R, Pasanen M, Tyry T, Vuori I. A 2-km walking test for assessing the cardiorespiratory fitness of healthy adults. Int J Sports Med 1991;12(4):356–362.

53. Astrand I. Aerobic work capacity in men and women with special reference to age. Acta Physiol Scand 1960;49:1–92.

54. Astrand PO, Ryhming I. A nomogram for calculation of aerobic capacity (physical fitness) from pulse rate during submaximal work. J Appl Physiol 1954;7:218.

55. Guyatt GH, Sullivan MJ, Thompson PJ, Fallen EL, Pugsley SO, Taylor, et al. The 6-minute walk: a new measure of exercise capacity in patients with chronic heart failure. Can Med Assoc J 1985;132(8):919–923.

56. Demers C, McKelvie RS. Reliability, validity, and responsiveness of the six-minute walk test in patients with heart failure. Am Heart J 2001;142(4):698–703.

57. Bradley J, Howard J, Wallace E, Elborn S. Reliability, repeatability, and sensitivity of the modified shuttle test in adult cystic fibrosis. Chest 2000;117(6):1666–1671.

58. Emtner M, Finne M, Stalenheim G. A 3-year follow-up of asthmatic patients participating in a 10-week rehabilitation program with emphasis on physical training. Archiv Phys MedRehabil 1998;79(5):539–544.

59. McInnis K, Balady G, Weiner D, Ryan T. Comparison of ischaemic and physiologic responses during exercise tests in men using the standard and modified Bruce protocols. Am J Cardiol 1992;69:84–89.

60. Balke B. A simple field test for the assessment of physical fitness. REP 63–6. Rep Civ Aeromed Res Inst USA 1963;53:1–8.

61. Cooper KH. A means of assessing maximal oxygen intake. Correlation between field and treadmill testing. JAMA 1968;203(3):201–204.

62. Butland RJ, Pang J, Gross ER, Woodcock AA, Geddes DM. Two-, six-, and 12-minute walking tests in respiratory disease. Br Med J Clin Res Ed 1982;284(6329):1607–1608.

63. Sadaria KS, Bohannon RW. The 6-minute walk test: a brief review of literature. Clin Exerc Physiol 2001;3:127–132.

64. Nixon PA, Joswiak ML, Fricker FJ. A six-minute walk test for assessing exercise tolerance in severely ill children. J Pediatr 1996;129(3):362–366.

65. Foley A, Halbert J, Hewitt T, Crotty M. Does hydrotherapy improve strength and physical function in patients with osteoarthritis—a randomised controlled trial comparing a gym based and a hydrotherapy based strengthening programme. Ann Rheum Dis 2003;62(12):1162–1167.

66. Guimaraes GV, Bellotti G, Bacal F, Mocelin A, Bocchi EA. Can the cardiopulmonary 6-minute walk test reproduce the usual activities of patients with heart failure? Arq Bras Cardiol 2002;78(6): 553–560.

67. Solway S, Brooks D, Lacasse Y, Thomas S. A qualitative systematic overview of the measurement properties of functional walk tests used in the cardiorespiratory domain. Chest 2001;119(1):256–270.

68. Minor MA, Kay DR. Arthritis. In: ACSM's exercise management for persons with chronic diseases and disabilities. Durstine JL, Ed. Champaign, Ill: Human Kinetics, 1997:149–154.

69. Mannerkorpi K, Svantesson U, Carlsson J, Ekdahl C. Tests of functional limitations in fibromyalgia syndrome: a reliability study. Arthritis Care Res 1999;12(3):193–199.

70. Pankoff B, Overend T, Lucy D, White K. Validity and responsiveness of the 6 minute walk test for people with fibromyalgia. J Rheumatol 2000;27(11):2666–2670.

71. Wittink HM. Physical fitness, function and physical therapy in patients with pain: clinical measures of aerobic fitness and performance in patients with chronic low back pain. In: Pain 1999—an updated review. Refresher Course Syllabus. Max M, Ed. Seattle:IASP press, 1999:137–145.

72. King S, Wessel J, Bhambhani Y, Maikala R, Sholter D, Maksymowych W. Validity and reliability of the 6 minute walk in persons with fibromyalgia. J Rheumatol 1999;26(10):2233–2237.

73. Pankoff BA, Overend TJ, Lucy SD, White KP. Reliability of the six-minute walk test in people with fibromyalgia. Arthritis Care Res 2000;13(5):291–295.

74. Gibbons WJ, Fruchter N, Sloan S, Levy RD. Reference values for a multiple repetition 6-minute walk test in healthy adults older than 20 years. J Cardiopulm Rehabil 2001;21(2):87–93.

75. Crapo RO, Casaburi R, Coates AL, Enright PL, et al. ATS statement: guidelines for the six-minute walk test. Am J Respir Crit Care Med 2002;166(1):111–117.

76. Troosters T, Gosselink R, Decramer M. Six minute walking distance in healthy elderly subjects. Eur Respir J 1999;14(2):270–274.

77. Enright PL, Sherrill DL. Reference equations for the six-minute walk in healthy adults. Am J Respir Crit Care Med 1998;158(5 Pt 1):1384–1387.

78. Borg G. Psychophysical scaling with applications in physical work and the perception of exertion. Scand J Work, EnvironHealth 1990;16(Suppl 1):55–58.

79. Felson DT, Lawrence RC, Hochberg MC, Mcalindon T, Dieppe PA, Minor MA, et al. Osteoarthritis: new insights. Part 2: treatment approaches. Ann Intern Med 2000;133(9):726–737.

80. Brosseau L, MacLeay L, Robinson V, Wells G, Tugwell P. Intensity of exercise for the treatment of osteoarthritis. Cochrane Database Syst Rev 2003;(2):CD004259.

81. Fransen M, McConnell S, Bell M. Exercise for osteoarthritis of the hip or knee. Cochrane Database Syst Rev 2003;(3):CD004286.

82. Roddy E, Zhang W, Doherty M. Aerobic walking or strengthening exercise for osteoarthritis of the knee? A systematic review. Ann Rheum Dis 2005;64(4):544–548.

83. Hakkinen A, Sokka T, Kotaniemi A, Hannonen P. A randomized two-year study of the effects of dynamic strength training on muscle strength, disease activity, functional capacity, and bone mineral density in early rheumatoid arthritis. Arthritis Rheum 2001;44(3):515–522.

84. Hakkinen A, Sokka T, Kautiainen H, Kotaniemi A, Hannonen P. Sustained maintenance of exercise induced muscle strength gains and normal bone mineral density in patients with early rheumatoid arthritis: a 5 year follow up. Ann Rheum Dis 2004;63(8):910–916.

85. Busch A, Schachter CL, Peloso PM, Bombardier C. Exercise for treating fibromyalgia syndrome. Cochrane Database Syst Rev 2002;(3):CD003786.

86. Green S, Buchbinder R, Hetrick S. Physiotherapy interventions for shoulder pain. Cochrane Database Syst Rev 2003;(2):CD004258.

87. van Tulder MW, Malmivaara A, Esmail R, Koes BW. Exercise therapy for low back pain. Cochrane Database Syst Rev 2000;(Issue 2):CD000335. 2000.

88. Hayden JA, van Tulder MW, Malmivaara AV, Koes BW. Meta-analysis: exercise therapy for nonspecific low back pain. Ann Intern Med 2005;142(9):765–775.

89. Hayden JA, van Tulder MW, Tomlinson G. Systematic review: strategies for using exercise therapy to improve outcomes in chronic low back pain. Ann Intern Med 2005;142(9):776–785.

90. Borg G. Perceived exertion as an indicator of somatic stress. Scand J Rehabil Med 1970;2(2):92–98.

91. Robertson RJ, Noble BJ. Perception of physical exertion: methods, mediators, and applications. Exerc Sport Sci Rev 1997;25:407–452.

92. Gamberale F. Perceived exertion, heart rate, oxygen uptake and blood lactate in different work operations. Ergonomics 1972;15(5):545–554.

93. Morgan WP. Psychological factors influencing perceived exertion. Med Sci Sports 1973;5(2):97–103.

94. Hollander DB, Durand RJ, Trynicki JL, Larock D, Castracane VD, Hebert EP, et al. RPE, pain, and physiological adjustment to concentric and eccentric contractions. Med Sci Sports Exerc 2003;35(6):1017–1025.

95. Smutok MA, Skrinar GS, Pandolf KB. Exercise intensity: subjective regulation by perceived exertion. Arch Phys Med Rehabil 1980;61(12):569–574.

96. Robertson RJ, Stanko RT, Goss FL, Spina RJ, Reilly JJ, Greenawalt KD. Blood glucose extraction as a mediator of perceived exertion during prolonged exercise. Eur J Appl Physiol Occup Physiol 1990;61(1–2):100–105.

97. Toner MM, Drolet LL, Pandolf KB. Perceptual and physiological responses during exercise in cool and cold water. Percept Mot Skills 1986;62(1):211–220.

98. Borg G, Ljunggren G, Ceci R. The increase of perceived exertion, aches and pain in the legs, heart rate and blood lactate during exercise on a bicycle ergometer. Eur J Appl Physiol Occup Physiol 1985;54(4):343–349.

99. Lin C, Michel TH, Steiner LA. 1999. The perception of exertion in chronic low back pain patients.

100. Barker KL, Dawes H, Hansford P, Shamley D. Perceived and measured levels of exertion of patients with chronic back pain exercising in a hydrotherapy pool. Arch Phys Med Rehabil 2003;84(9):1319–1323.

101. Anshel MH, Russell KG. Effect of aerobic and strength training on pain tolerance, pain appraisal and mood of unfit males as a function of pain location. J Sports Sci 1994;12:535–547.

102. Michel TH, Wittink HM. 2002. Pathophysiology of activity intolerance. In: Chronic pain management for physical therapists. Wittink HM, Michel TH, Eds. Boston: Butterworth-Heinemann, pp 101–127.

103. Pollock ML, Gaesser GA, Butcher, J.D., Despres J-P, Dishman RK et al. American College of Sports Medicine Position Stand. The recommended quantity and quality of exercise for developing and maintaining cardiorespiratory and muscular fitness, and flexibility in healthy adults. Med Sci Sports Exerc 1998;30(6):975–991.

104. Karvonen MJ, Kentala E, Mustafa O. The effects of training on heart rate. Annal Med Exp Biol Fenniae 1957;35:307–315.

105. Stromme SB, Ingjer F, Meen HD. Assessment of maximal aerobic power in specifically trained athletes. J Appl Physiol 1977;42(6):833–837.

III Therapeutic Techniques

9 Meditation and Chronic Pain

Joshua Wootton

CONTENTS

Summary

For many of us, the word *meditation* evokes a matrix of mental images associated with its spiritual heritage, whether our own or that of others—a solitary yogi in loincloth, Buddhist monks seated in the semi-lotus position, or even Roman Catholic priests praying in long robes and sandals. Although we in the West, until comparatively recently, have been largely dissociated from our meditative roots, meditation has found expression in every major religious tradition, including Christianity, Judaism, and Islam (1–3). Only in the last 30 years has it been pared from its spiritual underpinnings and applied to more generalized and secular considerations of physical and emotional well-being.

Now it is commonplace to see meditation taught on college campuses, in church and synagogue basements, and in hospitals and clinics—for the medically ill and the robust—as a means of improving and maintaining health. According to two recent national surveys, meditation was being sampled or practiced by seven to eight percent of the population in the United States during the one-year period studied (4,5). Despite this resurgence of interest, however, there remains considerable cultural mystery and even disagreement and misapprehension within the scientific community about the phenomenon (6). In this chapter, we will consider what meditation is and does, as well as why and how it can be an effective intervention in the reduction of medical symptoms, particularly in the management of chronic pain.

Key Words: meditation, relaxation response, mindfulness, musculoskeletal tension, autonomic nervous system, sympathetic response, parasympathetic response, stress reduction, stress-related disorders, mind–body techniques, biofeedback

From: *Contemporary Pain Medicine: Integrative Pain Medicine: The Science and Practice
of Complementary and Alternative Medicine in Pain Management*
Edited by: J. F. Audette and A. Bailey © Humana Press, Totowa, NJ

195

1. MEDITATION: DEFINED AND DISTINGUISHED

Any attempt to define meditation can easily prove a daunting experience, largely resulting from the impressive array of spiritual traditions and techniques represented. Even categorizing practices by their broadest traditions, like Hindu meditation or Buddhist meditation, can be misleading, because a variety of expressions of technique and purpose can be traced to each tradition and can differ in subtle and complex ways. The name of a particular school or teacher can be critical to understanding how one practice differs from another. Vipassana, often referred to as insight meditation, or simply mindfulness meditation in the United States, comes from the Theravada tradition of Buddhism and is usually traced to the teachings of the Burmese monk, Mahasi Sayadaw; however, transcendental meditation (TM) is derived exclusively from the teachings of the Maharishi Mahesh Yogi, who comes from the tradition of Vedic Hinduism *(2)*.

In Eastern meditation, there is an appreciation for the cultural context of a particular meditative practice: the spiritual tradition from which it was derived, the cosmology and philosophy it expresses, and the teacher and people for whom it is part of daily life. The attempt to condense the rich varieties of meditative experience to an essential form or paradigm of practice is a peculiarly Western idea *(7)*, likely born of two broad cultural idiosyncrasies: (1) The need to feel reassured that any investment we make will return the greatest possible benefit for our time and energy, and (2) the need to study and conduct scientific research to delineate and standardize anything that may benefit us, especially our health. The result has been phenomenal where the growth of scientific inquiry and the therapeutic application of meditation to life's problems are concerned. However, this culturally idiosyncratic view has also led us to view meditation as a form of therapy rather than a spiritual exercise, a distinction seldom made in the East. With the rise of the scientific study of meditation in the 1970s, methodological challenges in research have continually highlighted a frustrating feature of the inquiry, that there is no unified theory of what meditation is and how it works. Yet, in order to study meditation scientifically, some attempt must be made to describe the process involved more clearly. This has led, in turn, to attempts to define meditation operationally.

2. MEDITATION, OPERATIONALLY DEFINED

Shapiro was one of the first to suggest broad groupings of meditative practices, based upon their approach of consciously focusing attention in a non-analytical way, while avoiding the tendency to ruminate or think discursively *(8)*. He categorized three families of meditative technique: (1) those that focus on the *field* or background of perception and experience, making the meditator a passive observer; (2) those that focus on a pre-selected specific *object*, such as a sound or mantra; and (3) those that shift the focus between the field and the object. While this may seem to provide an operationally helpful set of distinctions where research is concerned, there can emerge differences of opinion concerning the category to which even the most popular forms of meditation belong. Mindfulness meditation, for example, is sometimes depicted as focusing on the field, and sometimes, shifting between field and object *(7,9,10)*.

This highlights a tendency of most proponents of a particular form or technique to contend that their practice cannot, in the end, be easily described or fit into a rigidly defined structure. Metaphors, like "awakening," "enlightening," and "purifying," do not easily lend themselves to mechanistic explanations. In fairness, some of the most impressive research in recent years has shifted the field of inquiry from mechanism to process *(6,11,12)*, permitting consideration of such Western concepts as ego development, self-actualization, and self-esteem. This is arguably closer to Eastern sensibility where the role of meditation is concerned. However, if the field of inquiry is directed more specifically to compare meditation with other interventions in order to determine which is more effective at reducing symptoms or to explain the effects of meditating on the physiology, then an operational definition becomes indispensable.

Cardoso and colleagues advanced an operational definition of meditation in an attempt to be more inclusive by being more phenomenological. They observed and described characteristics common to many forms of meditation without attempting to delineate specific techniques *(13)*. Their assertions include that for a particular form of meditation to be studied, it must (1) embrace a specific technique, capable of being taught or imparted by an instructor in a consistent fashion, regardless of the individual effects or future evolution of the result, from subject to subject; (2) result in relaxation of musculoskeletal tension; (3) result in "logic relaxation," that is, interruption or dispensation of the tendency to analyze, judge, or develop expectations of psychological and physiological effects; (4) enable the subject to apply the technique by him or herself, without developing dependence upon an instructor; and (5) involve the use of a "self-focus" skill, whether field or object, in order to avoid distraction by discursive thinking, torpor, sleep, or dissociation *(13)*.

Progress in advancing an operational definition of meditation has enabled scientists to address the underlying questions of health benefit by using the efficacy-effectiveness model of research, whereby meditation can be compared to other interventions and forms of therapy to assess its relative efficacy, while, at the same time, permitting the development of a model to explain the observation that not all forms of meditation are the same or exercise the same influence within the body *(9)*. Studies of the physiological activity and response associated with various techniques suggest that these patterns are specific to particular practices *(6,9,14)*. Even very early EEG studies revealed, for example, that the forms of meditation practiced by certain yogis lead to obliviousness toward the external world, while the mindfulness meditation of many Zen Buddhists leads to a keen attunement to the external world *(15)*.

3. INTEGRATING MEDITATION AND WESTERN MEDICINE

In the United States today, the two most widely researched meditative practices by a wide margin are transcendental meditation or TM *(16)*, often referred to as the "relaxation response" within the medical community, and mindfulness meditation *(3)*. Both have been successfully integrated into clinics and hospitals throughout the country; both conform to the operational definition proposed by Cardoso and his colleagues *(13)* and so lend themselves well to Western approaches of scientific research; and both are comparatively easy to apprehend and practice in a society typically unused to sitting quietly while suspending analytical thinking and judgment. They are, as well, the two forms of meditation currently being studied in multiple research projects supported by the National Center for Complementary and Alternative Medicine (NCCAM) of the National Institutes of Health (NIH) *(17)*.

3.1. Transcendental Meditation or Relaxation Response

While transcendental meditation originated within the Vedic tradition in India, it was brought to the United States by the Maharishi Mahesh Yogi in the 1970s and initially marketed as part of the self-actualization movement on college campuses. The form is characterized by the use of a mantra—a word, sound, or brief phrase—repeated silently to focus one's attention in a non-analytical way and prevent or reduce discursive or ruminative thinking *(8,17)*. During this form of meditation, the ordinary process of thinking becomes quiescent, with the mind settling into a less active state and the body attaining a state of deep restfulness, the endpoint being a state of relaxed or restful alertness *(18–20)*.

Among the first within the medical community to realize the potential for this technique and its application to the reduction of stress-related symptoms was Dr. Herbert Benson, a cardiologist and member of the faculty at Harvard Medical School. Benson has been a pioneer in the field of mind-body medicine—some would argue, its father—since the publication of his book, *The Relaxation Response* in 1975 *(21)*. He founded the Benson-Henry Institute for Mind Body Medicine *(22)* and has, for more than 35 years, worked to nurture a better understanding in medicine and medical research of the relationship between mind and body and the complex interactions between the two. Although introduced to the benefits of meditation through practitioners of TM, he and his colleagues have traced the origins of similar techniques and practices to almost every major religion—not only other Eastern spiritual traditions, like Tibetan Buddhism, but Christianity, Judaism, and Islam, as well—and outlined a basic, shared form of meditative practice, which he calls the "relaxation response" or RR.

Benson has fostered cooperation between Western science and such religious world leaders as the Dalai Lama and has also opened the door for the clinical application of meditation to the spectrum of stress-related illnesses, contributing 11 books and more than 175 scholarly articles to the scientific and popular literature *(22)*. The Mind/Body Institute tracks the research efforts of hundreds of scientists in their study of the positive impact of RR upon anxiety, cardiac health, headache, hypertension, irritable bowel syndrome, infertility, insomnia, menopause, chronic pain, premenstrual syndrome, and the reduction of symptoms in other medical conditions and illnesses. Benson's center in Boston, Massachusetts, offers group and individual treatment to patients suffering with these problems, as well as clinical training and supervision to healthcare providers who wish to integrate these techniques into their practice of medicine *(22,23)*.

3.2. Mindfulness Meditation

Mindfulness meditation originated within the tradition of Theravada Buddhism and is somewhat less mechanistic and more metaphorical than RR in its cultural apprehension, keeping its focus upon the field of perception rather than upon an object of concentration *(8)*. It is based upon the broader concept or state of being mindful, that is, having an increased awareness and acceptance of the present, rather than ruminating about the past or worrying about the future *(17)*. During meditation, the practitioner attempts to bring all of his or her attention to the internal experiences occurring moment to moment, whether bodily sensations, like the flow of breath, in and out, or the continual train of images, thoughts, and emotions *(24)*, in effect, focusing the attention upon what is being experienced, without analyzing or judging the experience.

Table 1
Key Differences Between Relaxation Response and Mindfulness Meditation

	Relaxation response	*Mindfulness meditation*
Origins of the form	Vedic Hinduism	Theravada Buddhism
Modern influence Usually Attributed to—	Maharishi Mahesh Yogi (India)	Mahasi Sayadaw (Burma)
Principal medical proponent and academic background	Herbert Benson, M.D., cardiologist	Jon Kabat-Zinn, Ph.D., biochemist
Institutional affiliation	Benson-Henry Institute for Mind Body Medicine, Harvard Medical School,Boston, Massachusetts	Center for Mindfulness, University of Massachusetts Medical School,Worcester, Massachusetts
Alternate names of technique	Relaxation response, RR, concentrative meditation, transcendental meditation, TM	Mindfulness meditation, insight meditation, vipassana
Principal template	Focusing attention on a single object, such as the repetition of a word, sound, or mantra	Focusing attention on the field or background of perception
Process	Focusing on an object to anchor the attention in the present moment— simply returning the focus to the object, without judgment or critical evaluation, when awareness that the attention has wandered occurs	Becoming an uncritical, non-judgmental observer of everything that passes through awareness, including images, thoughts, sensations, and emotions
End/beginning	Relaxed, restful alertness	Deep awareness of the present moment

The metaphorical nature of this form was emphasized when a team of neuroimaging specialists in the field of nuclear medicine described it as a process leading to "a subjective state characterized by a sense of no space, no time, and no thought…cognitively experienced as fully integrated and unified, such that there is no sense of self or other" (25, p. 283). The intent is to nurture the capacity of the practitioner to experience the thoughts and emotions of daily life with greater acceptance and a sense of balance, not as good or bad, true or false, healthy or sick, or important or trivial *(24,26,27)*.

The individual who brought mindfulness meditation and practice to the attention of the medical community in the United States and who, more than any other, is credited with the recent upsurge of research devoted to its influence is Dr. Jon Kabat-Zinn, founder of the Stress Reduction Program and Center for Mindfulness at the University of Massachusetts Medical Center and Medical School *(28)*. A biochemist by academic training, Kabat-Zinn relied upon his own Zen Buddhist practice to inform and shape the beginnings of his research and teaching, and since 1979 when the Stress Reduction Clinic was founded, his application of mindfulness to medical practice *(29)*. His program of mindfulness-based stress reduction (MBSR) is a patient-centered educational program that puts mindfulness meditation at the core of a full range of interventions such as sitting meditation, body scan, walking meditation, eating meditation, and mindful hatha yoga, directed toward the management and reduction of a broad range of physical and psychological symptoms *(30)*.

Although typically separated from its religious origins and cultural beliefs, the practice of mindfulness, according to its proponents, is more than a form of stress reduction because it elicits those dimensions of human experience described with metaphors like "heart," "spirit," "soul," "Tao," and "dharma" *(28)*, with the benefits of mindfulness extending into every area of life. Thousands of patients have completed the initial course in MBSR, and by the late 1990s, more than 240 hospitals and clinics in the United States were integrating stress reduction programs based upon mindfulness training into their care of patients *(31)*. The empirical literature suggests that mindfulness meditation and the MBSR program may lead to reduced symptoms in a variety of problematic medical conditions and illnesses, including chronic pain, stress-related disorders, anxiety, depression, binge eating, fibromyalgia, and psoriasis, as well as ancillary symptoms associated with some forms of cancer and multiple sclerosis *(24,28,30)*.

4. APPLICATIONS OF MEDITATION TO CHRONIC PAIN

Meditation, especially relaxation response and mindfulness meditation, has been applied in the medical setting to a variety of populations with chronic pain, generally reflecting statistically significant improvements in ratings of pain and related medical symptoms *(32–39)*. The basic physiological mechanisms through which this is accomplished have been well-reviewed *(3,17,32,40,41)*, but new studies continually suggest revisions in our understanding of how meditation works *(25,42,43)*, while highlighting new approaches to assessment *(44–46)*.

This increasingly minute focus on physiological processes sometimes brings science into seeming conflict with spirituality, but as the spiritual head of Tibetan Buddhism, His Holiness the Dalai Lama, reminds us, "Both science and the teachings of the Buddha tell us of the fundamental unity of all things" *(47)*. As an advocate of the scientific study of meditation, the Dalai Lama has long collaborated with Western researchers in attempting to understand the biological bases of beneficial changes occurring within the meditator. The tendency toward reductionism that results from applying too much emphasis upon lower level psychological and physiological mechanisms can be offset, to some degree, by reminding ourselves that, in its cultural and spiritual context, meditation remains a highly metaphoric phenomenon; while, subjectively and systemically, it can be seen more as an integrative process *(3,48)*, that is, less an "end" and more a "becoming." When applied to the symptom of chronic pain, the focus is less upon the end of being free from pain and more upon becoming better able to cope with and manage pain, thereby improving one's level of functioning.

5. MEDITATION AS DEEP RELAXATION AND BEYOND

The experience of acute pain has an immediate impact upon the sympathetic nervous system. Heart and respiratory rates, blood pressure, blood glucose levels, and muscle tension all increase, as the adrenal cortex activates the stress response with glucocorticoids that elicit the "fight or flight" response *(32)*. When pain goes unrelieved, however, and is unresponsive to medical care, enduring beyond its usefulness as a signal to action, then it may be said to have become chronic and indicative of changes in the way the brain processes pain *(49,50)*. The experience of chronic pain leads to changes in the subjective apprehension of pain, heightening responsiveness to pain stimuli and making the individual more susceptible to exacerbations with the trigger of psychological anticipation, giving rise to comorbid anxiety, fear, and ultimately, depression. In these circumstances, the threshold of pain is lowered, resulting from the depletion of serotonin and endorphin levels, while other hormonal responses, like the release of cortisol, are heightened and prolonged, increasing the deleterious impact of stress on the body *(32)*.

Meditation, by contrast, elicits a unique, wakeful or conscious hypometabolic integrated state in which the organism is even more deeply at rest than during sleep. Deep meditation can reduce cortisol secretion, oxygen consumption, and blood lactate levels and increase the secretion of hormones such as serotonin and melatonin *(7,19,48)*. Until relatively recently, the principal working hypothesis of how meditation, in particular the relaxation response and mindfulness meditation, exerts its therapeutic physiological influence was that, by reducing sympathetic arousal and increasing the activity of the parasympathetic nervous system, it moderates the impact of the fight or flight response *(17,23)*. With acute pain, the fight or flight response can motivate the organism toward preservation, but with chronic pain the response becomes obsolete, actually precipitating deterioration in normal pain processing and contributing toward exacerbations and persistence of pain, as well as poor pain tractability. By eliciting the relaxation response, meditation can be characterized as reasserting parasympathetic dominance, or, at least, balance, calming and relaxing the musculoskeletal system and adjusting the hormonal milieu and pain neurotransmission to a less urgent, excitatory, and preoccupying framework *(17,19,23,32,40)*.

Recent research has suggested more complex mechanisms through which meditation may affect chronic pain and has provided a number of correctives with regard to earlier hypotheses. Recent studies of the neural basis of meditation focusing on hypothalamic and autonomic nervous system changes, as well as autonomic cortical activity, have pointed to sharp increases in vasoconstrictor arginine vasopressin, resulting in decreased fatigue among meditators, as well as heightened arousal *(25)*. Research now indicates a mutual activation of the parasympathetic and sympathetic systems during meditation, as opposed to the original view of parasympathetic dominance, consistent with a balanced autonomic response that is, in turn, consistent with subjective descriptions of meditation as eliciting a sense of profound calmness, as well as alertness and attunement *(25,51–53)*.

Other recent electroencephalographic (EEG) studies have concluded that the long-term practice of meditation results in high-amplitude gamma synchrony, suggesting that meditation evokes temporal integrative mechanisms that may induce both short-term and long-term neural changes *(42)*. Similarly, advanced functional neuroimaging studies (fMRI) are beginning to provide a map of the brain during meditation that points to the activation of neural structures involved in attention and autonomic nervous system functioning *(44,46)*. The implication here is that both attention and affective processes may represent flexible skills that can be trained during meditation, thereby resulting in subjective changes in pain perception and the resulting affective response to pain *(43,45)*. With meditation, chronic pain can be influenced positively through a variety of mechanisms and neural pathways, including changes in the quality of neurotransmission, the generation of pain-blocking endorphins, the evocation of pain-blocking positive emotions, the selective redirection of attention away from the perception of pain, and adjustment of the spinal gateways to the brain *(40)*.

6. METHODOLOGICAL ISSUES IN THE STUDY OF MEDITATION

Further elucidation of the complex mechanisms involved in meditation is needed to explore thoroughly and validate our understanding of the ways in which meditation works and how it can be successfully applied to improving health and ameliorating chronic pain. Even the most recent studies tend to suffer from low numbers of subjects, lack of controls, and problems with factoring out confounding variables *(25)*. In the United States, most of the research has focused upon mindfulness meditation and the relaxation response, but while both techniques have yielded an impressive array of results, important differences between them have emerged that only begin to hint at how varied the neurophysiological mechanisms across the spectrum of meditative forms may be, as well as the differences between meditation and other forms of eliciting deep relaxation, such as guided imagery or visualization, hypnosis, biofeedback, and autogenic training, for example *(6,9)*.

Meditation is therefore difficult to standardize, quantify, and authenticate for research purposes; issues of adherence and compliance among subjects, choice of beginner versus advanced practitioners, and reliance largely upon self-report in many comparative or efficacy-effectiveness study designs all add to the methodological challenges involved in the scientific research of meditation *(3,9)*. True randomization of subjects exists in few studies, as meditators are typically a self-selected group. Selection bias and expectancy effects therefore represent powerful limitations in our ability to generalize conclusions to larger populations. Some researchers also point to a confounding longitudinal bimodal impact of meditation, with deep relaxation being elicited among beginners but with structurally more enduring hormonal and metabolic changes being detected among more experienced meditators *(7)*.

Where explanatory models of research are concerned, one recent, comprehensive meta-analytic review suggests that no clear, unified theory has yet emerged regarding the neurophysiological effects of meditative practice and that a major challenge in research will be differentiating among many forms of meditation and the early stages of sleep, which appear to exhibit similar alpha and theta enhancement during EEG studies *(44)*. Advances in neuroelectric and neuroimaging methods will likely make the distinctions clearer and illuminate the mechanisms implicated in the putative causal relationships between meditation and chronic pain, as well as other positive outcomes in health *(54)*. At present, however, the value of meditative practice and its relationship to medical symptom reduction is established more correlationally than causally *(3,25,44)*.

Another recent methodological review of the current status of research on meditation highlights four challenges to future scientific study: (1) not all practices are alike, whether in their expressed goals or in their neurophysiological results; (2) the variability of the delivery and personal mastery of the technique among subjects may represent a confounding influence within experimental groups; (3) compliance, which tends to insure uniformity of the intervention in most objective studies, actually says little about the quality and durability of the meditative state across subjects; and (4) the problem of true double-blinding and placebo-control. Meditative subjects cannot be blinded to their practice of meditation, and establishing a true placebo-control for meditation is both conceptually and practically difficult *(9)*. While the scientific study of meditation poses a daunting range of methodological issues, the overwhelming body of literature nevertheless continues to point to significant therapeutic benefits among meditators. The NIH's investment in pain research nearly tripled from $82 million in 1997 to $223 million in 2004, with an increasing proportion being devoted to research on mind-body techniques and complementary medicine *(17,54,55)*.

7. MEDITATION DISTINGUISHED FROM OTHER RELAXATION TECHNIQUES

While some providers and practitioners of mind-body techniques do not make distinctions among the wide variety of approaches to eliciting deep relaxation, meditation may differ in several important respects from other forms of therapeutic relaxation *(3,7)*. Most relaxation techniques *(1,32,56,57)*, such as structured breathing exercises, guided imagery or visualization, hypnosis, biofeedback, autogenic training, repetitive prayer, certain forms of repetitive exercise or activity (e.g., yoga, tai chi, and qi gong), will all, to a certain extent, elicit a hypometabolic state involving a parasympathetic response that will result in reduced heart rate, blood pressure, respiratory rate, and musculoskeletal tension *(1,32)*. In addition, they will all typically provide some measure of relief from chronic pain. What these techniques have in common, according to Benson, is that they all involve (1) the repetition of a word, sound, mantra, phrase, or muscular activity, and (2) the passive disregard of everyday thoughts or distractions, with the subject returning to his or her repetition, whenever he or she becomes aware of having been distracted *(1)*.

As a form of meditation, the relaxation response can be thought of as a concentrative technique but one in which the repeated word, sound, or mantra eventually occupies awareness without effort during meditative practice *(6)*. Mindfulness techniques differ from relaxation response in that any thoughts, images, feelings, or sensations may arise, as long as the meditator maintains the attentional stance of being a passive, detached observer without evoking judgment or analysis *(58)*. From the perspective of scientific study, the two approaches broadly overlap, with the former being characterized by a narrowing of focus and the latter by maintenance of a state of open receptivity. Concentrative techniques incorporate mindfulness by allowing the continual parade of thoughts, images, and feelings to come and go, without making them the focus of awareness; while mindfulness-based practices encourage a continual return to an attentive stance that is open, alert, and aware, without making thoughts, images, or feelings the objects of critical judgment (44).

Both relaxation response and mindfulness meditation, through a process of self-regulation or training the attention and awareness, elicit a shift in the subject's experience of himself or herself toward a perspective not centered on either the body or cognitive activity (3,44). By placing the focus on training attention and awareness, meditation is distinguished from other forms of eliciting deep relaxation, where the goal is often to exchange one set of mental contents for another, as in guided imagery or visualization, hypnosis, and autogenic training. Meditation also differs from those techniques by emphasizing alertness (25,51–53), a state of expanded self-awareness with a heightened sense of integrated cohesion (7). Meditation may also be distinguished from practices like repetitive exercise, yoga, tai chi, and qi gong, because the emphasis of the latter is on the additional elements of structured breathing, postures, and scripts for movement requiring bodily mastery that, especially in the early stages, may detract from training attention and awareness (3).

8. USING BIOFEEDBACK IN THE APPLICATION OF MEDITATION TO CHRONIC PAIN

Biofeedback may be considered a treatment in its own right or as a psychoeducational adjunct to other relaxation techniques. In its simplest form, it involves a therapist employing an electronic instrument or set of instruments to monitor a patient's bodily responses such as musculoskeletal tension, skin temperature, heart rate, blood pressure, electrodermal response, or EEG activity. This information is then communicated back to the patient in an easily comprehensible form, such as a visual display on a computer screen or a set of tones or auditory cues (59). Through this physiological feedback, the patient is given the opportunity to learn to control physiological processes, like blood pressure, for example, which he or she may have believed to be outside his or her control.

By learning to relax deeply, lower musculoskeletal tension and vasodilate the extremities, patients can learn, for example, to control tension-type and migraine headaches. Patients may be presented with one or another particular strategy for practice, like a relaxation tape or exercise, along with the therapist's coaching, and then they can proceed to learn how to influence in the appropriate directions the physiological feedback monitored on the computer by lowering surface electromyographic (sEMG) measures, for example, and raising skin temperature (sTemp) measured electronically through sensors placed on the body (60).

As an adjunct to the learning of meditative technique applied to the situation of chronic pain, biofeedback may also be used more passively, as a psychoeducational tool. Such an indirect approach can have two beneficial consequences: 1) it relieves patients who may be sensitive to the psychological burden of scrutiny or performance, especially those who would react with avoidance toward being assessed straightforwardly, and 2) it provides a suitable index, as well as a reward, for having already achieved a certain level of mastery with meditative technique. In this manner, biofeedback analysis and monitoring can prove to a patient that meditation is having a profound impact upon his physiology and reassure him that the technique is being done correctly, in effect, bypassing relaxation-induced anxiety.

When biofeedback is employed in this passive or indirect manner, the feedback loop is typically not completed during the exercise. The patient, who cannot see the physiological data being produced, may be asked to undergo one or more conditions, for example, a mildly stressed condition, during which he may be asked to recall stressful events or solve mental puzzles, followed by a period of meditation. At the end, the complete results are reviewed with the therapist, who delineates and encourages the patient's success and offers clues as to how to improve still further. Almost every patient can demonstrate success in this manner, and periodic assessment can provide an additional motivation for consistency of practice. Patients who meditate for relief of chronic pain may find that, with the addition of biofeedback analysis, their practice is easier to sustain to the point where they begin to apprehend subjective changes in their pain perception.

9. POSSIBLE ADVERSE CONSEQUENCES OF MEDITATIVE PRACTICE

The response to mind-body interventions, in general, and meditative practice, in particular, has been overwhelmingly favorable among those who have benefited from its health applications. Not only can it reduce and effectively manage a range of stress-related medical symptoms, including chronic pain, but also it is inexpensive, cost-effective, easy to learn and use for most people, and can greatly reduce medical expenses, including doctor's visits, medications, and hospital admissions (23,61). Meditation can engender optimism with regard to health and the problems of illness and can restore more of a sense of control to the patient, who may find that having direct access to an intervention providing relief from pain is a source of confidence and empowerment (23).

Meditation has been found to be generally safe, but there is evidence to suggest that intensive meditation can result in or exacerbate existing symptoms in individuals with certain psychiatric problems (7,62). Adverse effects in this population may include relaxation-induced anxiety and panic, paradoxical increases in tension, reduced motivation, pain, impaired reality testing, confusion and disorientation, dissociation, depression, and psychosis-like symptoms (7,62,63). Much of the concern about adverse effects is anecdotal (64), and the studies are generally limited to long-term meditators who devote a considerable portion of the day to meditation, but the National Center for Complementary and Alternative Medicine of the National Institutes of Health nevertheless recommends the following guidelines for the safe practice of meditation: (1) never delay seeking appropriate medical care because of reliance upon meditation or any complementary or alternative therapy, and do not rely upon meditation as the only treatment, unless in consultation with a medical provider; (2) discuss all complementary and alternative therapies with a provider, before beginning, to develop a safe, comprehensive treatment plan; (3) inquire about the training and experience of the instructor, when seeking to learn meditation; and (4) investigate what has been published by way of research on the relationship between meditation and the symptoms or condition to be addressed (17).

Despite the potential for direct harm occurring as a result of using any mind-body therapy being quite small (5), it is possible that some patients may develop excessive expectations regarding the benefits of such applications, delaying or foregoing medical treatment until the situation becomes needlessly more serious *(65)*. Some patients may also develop persistent guilt, when their results are not as successful as anticipated, holding themselves responsible for their inadequacy at mastering the technique *(66)*. Although the National Center for Complementary and Alternative Medicine has developed some helpful resources to aid prospective meditators in the selection of an instructor *(17)*, there is, to date, no widely available database for choosing a teacher who can insure that patients are not affected by these potential complications.

Many medical and mental health professionals, as well as many lay or paraprofessionals, receive training through Dr. Benson's Mind/Body Institute or Dr. Kabat-Zinn's Center for Mindfulness and combine the best of interdisciplinary skills and interests as teachers. Recognized clinical centers specializing in mind-body applications may prove to be the best training ground for teachers and providers of meditative practice and other complementary approaches to care. Licensure alone may not insure competence, since many licensed mental health providers may not be sufficiently trained in meditative technique or have enough personal experience with practice. Spiritual leaders may have practiced and taught meditation for years but may not have sufficient acquaintance with symptoms and medicine to make competent judgments with regard to the application of meditation to medical conditions. Making inquiries about the background and training of the teacher or provider and researching what has been published in the medical and popular literature about meditation and its impact on the symptoms to be treated requires motivation on the part of the patient and a collaborative temperament on the part of the provider, but may, in the end, represent the best and safest avenue of pursuing treatment.

REFERENCES

1. Benson H. 1996. Timeless Healing: The Power and Biology of Belief. New York: Scribner.
2. Taylor E. 1999–2004. Introduction. In: The Physical and Psychological Effects of Meditation. Murphy M, Donovan S, Eds. Petaluma, CA: Institute of the Noetic Sciences. Available at: http://www.noetic.org/research/medbiblio/. Accessed February 2, 2006.
3. Walsh R, Shapiro SL. The meeting of meditative disciplines and western psychology: a mutually enriching dialogue. Am Psychol 2006;61:227–239.
4. Barnes PM, Powell-Griner E, McFann K, Nahin RL. 2002. Complementary and Alternative Medicine Use Among Adults: United Sates. Advance Data from Vital and Health Statistics; No 343. Hyattsville, MD: National Center for Health Statistics, 2004.
5. Wolsko PM, Eisenberg DM, Davis RB, Phillips RS. Use of mind-body medical therapies: results of a national survey. J Gen Intern Med 2004;19:43–50.
6. Orme-Johnson DW, Alexander CN, Hawkins MA. Critique of the national research council's report on meditation. J Soc Behav Personal 2005;17:383–414.
7. Perez-de-Albenez A, Holmes J. Meditation: concepts, effects, and uses in therapy. Int J Psychother 2000:5;49–58.
8. Shapiro DH. Overview: clinical and physiological comparison of meditation with other self-control strategies. Am J Psychiatry 1982;139(3):267–274.
9. Caspi O, Burleson KO. Methodological challenges in meditation research. Adv Mind–Body Med 2005;21:4–11.
10. Murata T, Takahashi T, Hamada T, Omori M, Kosaka H, Yoshida H, Wada Y. Individual trait anxiety levels characterizing the properties of Zen meditation. Neuropsychobiology 2004;50:189–194.
11. Chandler HM, Alexander CN, Heaton DP. The transcendental meditation program and postconventional self-development: a 10-year longitudinal study. J Soc Behav Personal 2005;17:93–121.
12. Alexander CN, Rainforth MV, Gelderloos P. Transcendental meditation, self-actualization, and psychological health: a conceptual overview and statistical meta-analysis. J Soc Behav Personal 1991;6:189–247.

13. Cardoso R, de Souza E, Camano L, Leite JR. Meditation in health: an operational definition. Brain Res Protoc 2004;14:58–60.

14. Murphy M, Donovan S. 1999–2004. Physiological effects. In: The Physical and Psychological Effects of Meditation. Murphy M, Donovan S, Eds. Petaluma, CA: Institute of the Noetic Sciences, Available at: http://www.noetic.org/research/medbiblio/. Accessed February 2, 2006.

15. Bogart G. Meditation and psychotherapy. Am J Psychother 1991;45:383–412.

16. Wenk-Sormaz H. Meditation can reduce habitual responding. Adv Mind–Body Med 2005;21:33–49.

17. NIH/NCCAM (National Institutes of Health/National Center for Complementary and Alternative Medicine). Meditation for health purposes. Available at http://nccam.nih.gov/health/meditation/. Accessed March 10, 2006.

18. Travis F, Wallace RK. Autonomic patterns during respiration suspensions: possible markers of transcendental consciousness. Psychophysiology 1997;34:39–46.

19. Jevning R, Wallace RK, Biedebach M. The physiology of meditation: a review: a wakeful hypometabolic integrated response. Neurosci Biobehav Rev 1992;16:415–424.

20. Dillbeck MC, Orme-Johnson DW. Physiological differences between transcendental meditation and rest. Am Psychol 1987;42:879–881.

21. Benson H. 1975. The Relaxation Response. New York: William Morrow.

22. M/BMI (Mind/Body Medical Institute). Mind/Body Medical Institute: Treating the Total You. Available at http://www.mbmi.org/. Accessed March 23, 2006.

23. Jacobs GD. Clinical applications of the relaxation response and mind–body interventions. J Altern Complement Med 2001;7(S1):S93–S101.

24. Baer RA. Mindfulness training as a clinical intervention: a conceptual and empirical review. Clin Psychol Sci Pract 2003;10:125–143.

25. Newberg AB, Iversen J. The neural basis of the complex mental task of meditation: neurotransmitter and neurochemical considerations. Med Hypotheses 2003;61:282–291.

26. Marlatt GA, Kristeller JL. 1999. Mindfulness and meditation. In: Integrating Spirituality Into Treatment. Miller WR, Ed. Washington, DC: American Psychological Association, pp. 67–84.

27. Kabat-Zinn J. 1994. Wherever You Go, There You Are: Mindfulness Meditation in Everyday Life. New York: Hyperion.

28. SRP/CFM/UMMS (Stress Reduction Program/Center for Mindfulness/University of Massachusetts Medical School). Center for Mindfulness in Medicine, Healthcare, and Society (CFM). Available at http://www.umassmed.edu/cfm/srp/. Accessed March 23, 2006.

29. Kabat-Zinn J. 1990. Full Catastrophe Living: Using the Wisdom of Your Body and Mind to Face Stress, Pain, and Illness. New York: Delacorte.

30. Proulx K. Integrating mindfulness-based stress reduction. Holist Nurs Practice 2003:17:201–208.

31. Salmon PG, Santorelli SF, Kabat-Zinn J. 1998. Intervention elements promoting adherence to mindfulness-based stress reduction programs in the clinical behavioral medicine setting. In: Handbook of Health Behavior Change, Second edition. Shumaker SA, Shron EB, Ockene JK, Bee WL, Eds. New York: Springer, pp. 239–268.

32. Schaffer SD, Yucha CB. Relaxation and pain management: the relaxation response can play a role in managing chronic and acute pain. Am J Nurs 2004;104:75–82.

33. Randolph PD, Caldera YM, Tacone AM, Greak ML. The long-term combined effects of medical treatment and a mindfulness-based behavioral program for the multidisciplinary management of chronic pain in west Texas. Pain Dig 1999;9:103–112.

34. Hermann C, Kim M, Blanchard EB. Behavioral and prophylactic pharmacological intervention studies for pediatric migraine: an exploratory meta-analysis. Pain 1995;50:239–255.

35. Caudill M, Schnable R, Zuttermeister P, Benson H, Friedman R. Decreased clinic use by chronic pain patients: response to behavioral medicine intervention. Clin J Pain 1991;7:305–310.

36. Kabat-Zinn J, Lipworth L, Burney R, Sellers W. Four-year follow-up of a meditation-based program for the self-regulation of chronic pain: treatment outcomes and compliance. Clin J Pain 1987;2:159–173.

37. Kabat-Zinn J, Lipworth L, Burney R. The clinical use of mindfulness meditation for the self-regulation of chronic pain. J Behav Med 1985;8:163–190.

38. Kutz I, Caudill M, Benson H. The role of relaxation fin behavioral therapies for chronic pain. Int Anesthesiol Clin 1983;21:193–200.

39. Kabat-Zinn J. An outpatient program in behavioral medicine for chronic pain patients based on the practice of mindfulness meditation: theoretical considerations and preliminary results. Gen Hosp Psychiatry 1982;4:33–47.

40. Smith JC. 2005. Relaxation, Meditation, and Mindfulness: A Mental Health Practitioner's Guide to New and Traditional Approaches. New York: Springer.

41. McCaffrey R, Frock TL, Garguilo H. Understanding chronic pain and the mind–body connection. Holist Nurs Pract 2003;17:281–287.

42. Lutz A, Greischar LL, Rawlings NB, Ricard M, Davidson RJ. Long-term meditators self-induce high amplitude gamma synchrony during mental practice. Proc Natl Acad Sci 2004;101:16369–16373. Available at http://www.pnas.org/cgi/doi/10.1073/pnas.0407401101. Accessed March 29, 2006

43. Davidson RJ, Kabat-Zinn J, Schumacher J, Rosenkranz M, Muller D, Santorelli SF, Urbanowski F, Harrington A, Bonus K, Sheridan JF. Alterations in brain and immune function produced by mindfulness meditation. Psychosom Med 2003;65:564–570.

44. Cahn BR, Polich J. Meditation states and traits: EEG, ERP, and neuroimaging studies. Psychol Bull 2006;132:180–211.

45. Carlson LE, Speca M, Patel KD, Goodey E. Mindfulness-based stress reduction in relation to quality of life, mood, symptoms of stress, and immune parameters in breast and prostate cancer outpatients. Psychosom Med 2003;65:571–581.

46. Lazar SW, Bush G, Gollub RL, Fricchione GL, Khalsa G, Benson H. Functional brain mapping of the relaxation response and meditation. Neuroreport 2000;11:1581–1585.

47. Knight J. Buddhism on the brain. Nature 2004;432:670.

48. Khalsa DS, Stauth C. 2002. Meditation As Medicine: Activate the Power of Your Natural Healing Force. New York: Fireside.

49. Eimer BN, Freeman A. 1998. Pain Management Psychotherapy: A Practical Guide. New York: John Wiley & Sons.

50. Schneider JP. 2004. Living with Chronic Pain: The Complete Health Guide to the Causes and Treatment of Chronic Pain. New York: Healthy Living Books.

51. Travis F. Autonomic and EEG patterns distinguish transcending from other experiences during transcendental meditation practice. Int J Psychophysiol 2001;42:1–9.

52. Peng CK, Mietus JE, Liu Y, Khalsa G, Douglas PS, Benson H, Goldberger AL. Exaggerated heart rate oscillations during two meditation techniques. Int J Cardiol 1999;70:101–107.

53. Hugdahl K. Cognitive influences on human autonomic nervous system function. Curr Opin Neurobiol 1996;6:252–258.

54. NIH/USDHHS (National Institutes of Health/US Department of Health and Human Services). An update of NIH pain research and related program initiatives. Statement for the Record. Subcommittee on Health. Committee on Energy and Commerce. United States House of Representatives, December 8, 2005. Available at: http://www.hhs.gov/asl/testify/t051208a.html. Accessed March 29, 2006.

55. NIH/NCCAM (National Institutes of Health/National Center for Complementary and Alternative Medicine). Expanding horizons of healthcare: Strategic plan 2005–2009. Available at: http://nccam.nih.gov/about/plans/2005/. Accessed March 29, 2006.

56. Deng G, Cassileth B, Yeung KS. Complementary therapies for cancer-related symptoms. J Support Oncol 2004;2:419–429.

57. Mamtani R, Cimino A. A primer of complementary and alternative medicine and its relevance in the treatment of mental health problems. Psychiatr Q 2002;73:367–381.

58. Kabat-Zinn J. Mindfulness-based interventions in context: past, present, and future. Clin Psychol Sci Pract 2003;10:144–158.

59. Arena JG, Blanchard EB. 2002. Biofeedback training for chronic pain disorders: a primer. In: Psychological Approaches to Pain Management: A Practitioner's Guide, Second edition. Turk DC, Gatchel RJ, Eds. New York: Guilford, pp. 159–186.

60. Andrasik F. 2004. The essence of biofeedback, relaxation, and hypnosis. In: Psychosocial Aspects of Pain: A Handbook for Healthcare Providers. Progress in Pain Research and Management. Dworkin RH, Breitbart WS, Eds. Volume 27. Seattle: IASP, pp. 285–305.

61. Friedman R, Sobel D, Myers P, Caudill M, Benson H. Behavioral medicine, clinical health psychology, and cost offset. Health Psychol 1995;14:509–518.

62. Shapiro DH. Adverse effects of meditation: a preliminary investigation of long-term meditators. Int J Psychosom 1992;39:62–67.

63. Murphy M, Donovan S. 1999–2004. Subjective reports. In: The Physical and Psychological Effects of Meditation. Murphy M, Donovan S, Eds. Petaluma, CA: Institute of the Noetic Sciences. Available at: http://www.noetic.org/research/medbiblio/. Accessed February 2, 2006.

64. Yorston GA. Mania precipitated by meditation: a case report and literature review. Ment Health Religion Cult 2001;4:209–213.
65. Shine KI. A critique on complementary and alternative medicine. J Altern Complement Med 2001;7:S145–S52.
66. Davidoff F. Weighing the alternatives: lessons from the paradoxes of alternative medicine. Ann Intern Med 1998;129:1068–1070.

10 Adjunctive Hypnotic Management of Acute Pain in Invasive Medical Interventions

Gloria Maria Martinez Salazar,
Salomao Faintuch, and Elvira V. Lang

CONTENTS

Summary

Acute pain management remains a challenge to clinicians. Despite the advances in procedural techniques and pharmacologic treatment for patients, the use of narcotics and sedatives for clinical pain has considerable health system implications. An approach that safely provides comfort to patients while remaining cost-effective is highly desirable. Hypnosis as an alternative or adjunct to pharmacological management of acute pain has the potential to fulfill these requirements. This chapter presents the evidence for, and explores mechanisms of the benefits of, clinical hypnosis in acute pain management and presents a model of implementation in the modern medical environment.

Key Words: hypnosis, acute pain, medical procedures, surgery, pain management, hypnotic analgesia, anesthesia, conscious sedation

1. DEFINITION AND BACKGROUND

Hypnosis is commonly but erroneously viewed as something that is done to a person involving loss of control on the part of the subject. This, however, is not the case. Hypnosis is simply a form of focused concentration or total absorption, similar to what happens when a person becomes completely absorbed in a book or movie. Therefore, all hypnosis is essentially self-hypnosis, which permits individuals to achieve a variety of

From: *Contemporary Pain Medicine: Integrative Pain Medicine: The Science and Practice of Complementary and Alternative Medicine in Pain Management*
Edited by: J. F. Audette and A. Bailey © Humana Press, Totowa, NJ

objectives. Hypnosis in itself is not a therapy *(1)* but can be used as a powerful adjunct to treatment for both medical and psychological disorders *(2)*. As such, it is becoming an attractive treatment option in the current medical setting where recognition of the effect of the mind–body connection on pain and other medical conditions is increasing.

Within the surgical field, open surgery is being replaced more and more by less invasive alternatives. Advances in technology have permitted rapid growth of minimally invasive surgery, particularly in the interventional radiology setting *(3)*. Often such procedures no longer require general anesthesia. In 2003, approximately 43 million invasive procedures were performed, including 1.2 million cardiac catheterizations, 1.9 million arteriograms, and 1.6 million endoscopic procedures *(3)*. Interventional procedures are usually performed on awake patients and can be perceived as very painful and distressing depending on the patient *(4,5)*. Despite the evolving refinement of procedural and anesthetic techniques, pain and its pharmacologic management arise as factors limiting procedural safety *(6)*. Intravenous analgesics and sedatives are important tools in managing perioperative distress, but have limited effectiveness and serious side effects *(5)*. Therefore, a nonpharmacologic approach that reduces pain and anxiety while avoiding adverse drug effects is highly desirable. Clinical Practice Guidelines for Acute Pain Management, published by the US Public Health Service, mention relaxation exercises and cognitive approaches but do not give specifics or outcome data *(7)*. Hypnosis is increasingly emerging as an effective and practical adjunct in the management of acute pain during invasive medical interventions *(8–12)* and does not only benefit patients with considerable hypnotic talent, but also broad groups of unselected individuals. Hypnosis is a safe approach with little likelihood of causing negative side effects, *(13–15)*, but it is still underused for pain management *(16)*.

2. MECHANISM OF ACTION

The IASP (International Association for the Study of Pain) defines pain as "an unpleasant sensory and emotional experience associated with actual or potential tissue damage, or described in terms of such damage" *(17)*. The distinction between the sensory and affective experience of pain forms the basis for the understanding of hypnotic analgesia *(18,19)*. The same stimulus can elicit widely varying experiences from different people, or even from the same individual, depending on the meaning of the stimulus and the framing of the situation. Kiernan et al. investigated the multifactorial nature of hypnotic analgesia by examining changes in R-III, a nociceptive spinal reflex, in response to hypnotic suggestion aimed at reduction of pain sensation and its unpleasantness *(20)*. The authors suggested that at least three mechanisms may be involved in hypnotic analgesia: (1) sensory attenuation of the pain experience at the level of spinal cord, (2) reduction of the awareness of nociceptive input at higher centers, and (3) reduction in the experience of unpleasantness over and beyond reductions in pain sensation. Modern neuroimaging techniques provide additional experimental evidence in the processing of the pain components selectively altered by hypnotic suggestions *(19)*. Rainville et al. used positron emission tomography (PET) to differentiate cortical areas involved in pain affect. Hypnotic suggestions for increased or decreased unpleasantness of noxious stimuli were applied selectively. In this setting, PET revealed pain-related changes in regional cerebral blood flow (rCBF) in the anterior cingulate cortex, but not in the somatosensory cortex, providing direct experimental evidence in humans linking frontal-lobe limbic activity with pain affect (see Chapter 4). In subsequent experiments the same investigator group *(18)* produced the following additional observations: hypnotic suggestions for decreased pain effectively reduced the unpleasantness of pain, particularly in highly hypnotizable individuals. Suggestions for increased pain affect influenced unpleasantness more than intensity, and this effect increased with repetition of the suggestions. Moreover, there was a significant relationship between elevated heart rate and unpleasantness ratings. Suggestions to change the sensory aspects of noxious stimuli modulated pain intensity, which were paralleled by changes in unpleasantness ratings. Therefore, a successive-stage model of pain processing that distinguishes between sensory and affective dimensions, alluding to an interaction between pain affect and autonomic response was proposed *(21)*.

Specific patterns of cerebral activation associated with the hypnotic state and with the processing of hypnotic suggestions were provided by PET measurements of rCBF, electroencephalographic (EEG) determination of brain electrical activity, and self ratings of subjective feelings of mental relaxation *(22,23)*. Hypnotic states were associated with activation of the anterior cingulate cortex, the thalamus, and the ponto-mesencephalic brainstem, brain structures essential for the basic regulation of states of consciousness, self-monitoring and self-regulation.

Modulation of the primary sensory cortex activity through hypnotic suggestions has also been supported by a study that assessed perception of color by means of PET and rCBF *(24)*. The authors found that rCBF increased in the lingual and fusiform gyri when color was hypnotically added to a black-and-white image (as it would if a colored image were shown to a non-hypnotized person), and it decreased when a color image was hypnotically drained of color.

Recently, the pursuit of the neuroanatomical basis for hypnotic analgesia led researchers to postulate a relationship between the size of the corpus callosum rostrum and competence to modulate unwanted stimuli through attentional/inhibitory mechanisms in healthy individuals *(25)*. This investigation was the first to compare the corpus callosum of selected subjects with low and high levels of hypnotizability and demonstrated that highly hypnotizable individuals have a significantly larger rostrum than do those with low levels of hypnotizability. This supports the theory that highly hypnotizable individuals have more effective frontal attentional systems for implementing control, monitoring performance and inhibiting unwanted stimuli from conscious awareness.

While research progresses in further elucidating the underlying mechanisms of hypnosis, there is sufficient evidence by neuroimaging and clinical experience to demonstrate the usefulness of hypnosis as an adjunct to pain management.

3. RATIONALE FOR USE IN SPECIFIC ACUTE PAIN CONDITIONS

Given the hypnotic analgesia model discussed above, one of the most valuable applications of hypnosis is its capacity to modulate the experience of pain. Hypnosis can provide substantial aid during medical procedures, such as acute pain management *(8,12)* and post operative recovery *(26)*. We favor its use as a powerful adjunct for treatment of procedural pain. This is founded in our practice where many hypnosis-naïve patients are first presented with the concept of hypnosis at the time of their procedures when their level of hypnotizability is unknown. The majority of patients appreciate having a "safety net" of medications available, if needed, and this, in our experience, has made them more willing to engage in hypnosis in this setting. Nevertheless, hypnosis has been found to be effective as the sole means of analgesia during open surgery in selected patients *(27–39)*. Hypnosis and suggestion as adjuncts of pharmacologic analgesia are becoming attractive options. The effectiveness of hypnosis as a pain management adjunct is relatively independent of the patients' degree of hypnotizability *(8,28,40–44)*.

The literature has shown that patients offered hypnosis for various medical purposes experienced significant benefits, despite substantial variation in hypnotic techniques, *(45)* indicating an expanded role for its use. In the largest prospective randomized trial of its kind, adjunct hypnosis significantly reduced pain, anxiety, drug use and complications during invasive procedures in the vasculature and the kidneys *(8)*. Interestingly, patients assigned to the hypnosis intervention had greater hemodynamic stability, which could not be explained by decreased use of procedural drugs alone.

The physiologic responses to the use of hypnosis are also being investigated for percutaneous transluminal coronary angioplasty (PTCA). The influence of hypnosis on cardiac vegetative tone is well known *(46)*. Likewise, the regulation of the sympathetic drive during PTCA through the selective influence of hypnosis was demonstrated in 2004 *(47)*. These regulation mechanisms provided by hypnotic suggestion illustrate the safety of its use during medical procedures.

Provision of safety and efficacy in acute pain management is still a challenge for doctors, especially in the pediatric population *(6)*. The observation that children have an increased susceptibility for hypnosis *(48)* makes its use attractive for this population. As such, the benefits of hypnosis were assessed in a randomized study of 44 children undergoing voiding cystourethrography *(12)*. Children assigned to the hypnosis group demonstrated significantly lower distress levels during the procedure compared to the control group, and also parents of the children reported that the procedure was significantly less traumatic for their children compared to their previous procedures. Moreover, the medical staff reported less difficulty in performing the procedure in the hypnosis group, as well as shorter procedure times compared to the control condition.

Use of adjunctive hypnosis in more invasive procedures was also evaluated during elective plastic surgery under local anesthesia and intravenous sedation *(49)*. In this study, 60 patients were randomly assigned to stress-reducing strategies (control) or hypnosis. The results showed that peri- and postoperative anxiety and pain were significantly lower in the hypnosis group, even though this group used fewer medications as compared to the control group. The hypnosis group also presented with more stable vital signs, had better surgical conditions and higher patient satisfaction compared to the stress-reducing strategies group.

Safety and patient comfort provided by hypnosis was also highlighted in a review of more than 1,650 surgical cases that used hypnosis as an adjunct to conscious sedation *(9)*. This form of anesthesia (i.e., hypnosis with conscious sedation) was applied as an alternative to general anesthesia for a wide range of surgical procedures, including neck lift, thyroidectomy, cervicotomy for hyperparathyroidism, correction of mammary ptosis, breast augmentation, tubal ligation, nasal septorhinoplasty, debridement with skin grafting and calvarian bone graft (maxillofacial reconstruction), as well as some minor surgical procedures (e.g., turbinoplasty, wisdom teeth removal). The authors proposed the use of this technique as a safe alternative to standard anesthesia protocols, indicating that the major benefit for its use is the capability of patients' participation during their procedure, ensuing a faster recovery and shorter hospital stay. However, this evidence requires some modification of the environment in a standard surgical setting, considering the conscious state of the patient during all steps of the procedures.

The beneficial impact of the use of adjunct hypnosis in surgical patients was presented in a meta-analysis conducted by Montgomery *(44)*. After standardized methods were applied, the authors calculated 22 effect sizes of 20 controlled published studies. They categorized clinical outcomes and performed a secondary analysis of differences in the following categories: (1) negative affect (e.g., anxiety and depression), which was measured by both self-report and observations by others (e.g., nurse); (2) pain (both self-report and observations by others); (3) amount of pain medication (e.g., analgesics and anesthetics); (4) physiological indicators (e.g., blood pressure, heart rate, and catecholamine levels); (5) recovery (e.g., return of muscular strength, postoperative vomiting, and fatigue); and (6) treatment time (e.g., length of procedure and inpatient stay).

The results of these studies indicated that, on average, 89% of surgical patients benefited from adjunctive hypnosis techniques, as compared to patients in control conditions. Likewise, the beneficial effects were apparent in each of the six clinical outcome categories selected for the study. The impact of brief hypnosis has also been documented to be valuable for excisional breast biopsies in a study of 20 patients randomly assigned to a hypnosis or control group *(11)*. In this setting, hypnosis significantly reduced post-surgical pain and distress.

The benefits of using hypnosis for acute pain management was also seen in the burn care unit, where daily dressing changes and wound debridement produce significant nociception *(50)*. Numerous case reports show the benefit of hypnosis, *(51)* and the first study to investigate this in a controlled fashion was published by Patterson in 1992 *(10)*. In this investigation, 30 patients undergoing dressing changes in a major regional burn unit were randomly assigned to one of the three following conditions: hypnosis, attention and information control condition, and no-treatment control condition. The hypnosis condition was based on a rapid induction analgesia model modified for burn wound debridement *(52)*. The attention and information control condition included interaction with psychologists, leaving patients and attending nurses with the belief that subjects were being hypnotized. Subjects in the no-treatment control condition received only opioid medication. The authors compared the patients' self-ratings of pain in the first and second days of wound care for each group, and the results showed that hypnotized patients had superior pain relief compared to the no-treatment control condition, and also lower pain scores relative to the group that was led to believe they had received a hypnosis intervention.

An analysis of the literature provides evidence recognizing the safety and beneficial effects of hypnosis as an adjunct to the pharmacological approach in the acute management of pain. Hence, training in hypnosis skills for clinicians working in this medical setting has been proposed in a recent literature review, as well as considerations on how to incorporate it into their practice *(16)*.

3.1. Hypnosis in Chronic Pain Conditions

The use of hypnosis for chronic pain conditions is growing. In the chronic pain arena, the primary goal is not to just alter pain for a brief period during the hypnotic trance, but to make hypnotic suggestions and teach skills that will alter pain intensity and its impact throughout the patient's daily life. Typical suggestions made during hypnosis include direct diminution of pain, relaxation, imagined analgesia, decreased pain unpleasantness, and replacement of pain with other non-painful sensations or pain displacement (i.e., moving the pain to other non-painful areas of the body).

In a recent review of the use of hypnosis in chronic pain, the authors concluded that hypnotic analgesia produces significantly greater decreases in pain relative to no-treatment and to some non-hypnotic interventions such as medication management, physical therapy, and education/advice. The most common chronic pain condition in the review was headache, with only one or two studies included in the review on low back pain, fibromyalgia, osteoarthritis, cancer related pain, temporomandibular pain disorder, and mixed pain conditions. Interestingly, when hypnosis was compared to other mind-body interventions such as progressive muscle relaxation and autogenic training (both of which often include hypnotic-like suggestions), the positive effects of self-hypnosis training on chronic pain was similar. Patient expectancy about the positive benefits of hypnosis appeared to play a significant role in some of the studies in the review, and because a credible placebo treatment has not been developed, conclusions cannot yet be made about whether hypnotic analgesia treatment is specifically effective over and above its effects on expectancy. Finally, the review found that global hypnotic responsiveness and ability to experience vivid images are associated with positive treatment outcome in hypnosis, progressive relaxation, and autogenic training treatments *(16).*

3.2. Use in Specific Chronic Pain Conditions

In a controlled study comparing hypnosis to physical therapy, 40 subjects were randomly assigned to either eight 1-hour sessions of hypnotherapy (supplemented by a self-hypnosis home practice tape) over a 3-month period, or 12–24 hours of physical therapy (that included massage and muscle relaxation training) over a 3-month period. Outcome was assessed pre-treatment, post-treatment, and at 3-month follow-up. The hypnosis intervention began with an arm levitation induction and included standard ego-strengthening suggestions as well as suggestions for general relaxation, improved sleep, and "control of muscle pain." Larger improvements were found in the patients who received hypnosis than those who received physical therapy on measures of muscle pain, fatigue, sleep disturbance, distress, and patient overall assessment of outcome and these differences were maintained at 3-month follow-up. The average percent decrease in pain among patients who received hypnosis was 35% compared to a 2% decrease in the patients who received physical therapy *(53).*

In a study of chronic osteoarthritis pain, hypnosis was compared to a progressive muscle relaxation treatment condition and to a no-treatment control condition in 36 patients with osteoarthritis. The hypnosis treatment involved relaxation suggestions for the induction and then suggestions for pleasant memories involving the use of the joint when it was not painful. The relaxation condition was eight sessions of standard progressive muscle relaxation training. In this study, both interventions were more effective than no treatment, and there were no significant differences in outcome between the two active interventions overall. However, hypnosis did show a trend to be more effective than relaxation (56% average pre- to post-treatment improvement versus 31% improvement), and the difference in improvement between the two treatments was statistically significant at the mid-point (4 weeks after treatment began) of treatment. Patients in both treatment conditions also reported similar decreases in medication use over the course of treatment that was not observed in the no-treatment condition *(54).*

In a study, of 66 patients with chronic migraine headaches, subjects were randomly assigned to one of five different experimental conditions: Two hypnotic analgesia interventions, a hand temperature biofeedback condition, a relaxation training condition, and a 3-month standard care control condition. Participants in one of the hypnosis conditions were "instructed in self-hypnosis." Those in the second hypnosis condition were given the same instructions as those in the first condition, but also given a hypnotic suggestion to visualize putting their hands in bowls of warm water. The hand temperature biofeedback condition included standard hypnotic-like autogenic suggestions. The relaxation response intervention involved "step-by-step" instruction in obtaining a relaxation response through mental repetition of a single word following Benson's model (see Chapter 9). All treatment subjects received three sessions of weekly treatment, and outcome was assessed pre- and post treatment, as well as at 6-, 9-, and 12-month follow-up. The three outcome measures were peak headache pain intensity, number of headaches, and medication use, computed from data taken from 3-week periods of headache diaries completed just before each assessment point; standard care patients completed diaries for 3 months prior to being assigned to a treatment condition. Their results indicated that patients in both hypnosis groups showed greater decreases in all three outcome measures than these patients did during their 3 month period of standard care. The two hypnosis treatment interventions were no more effective, on average, than either relaxation response or the hand temperature biofeedback training conditions on any of the outcome measures (55).

In their review, Jensen and Patterson conclude with suggestions for future research: (1) Can the effects of hypnotic analgesia treatment be accounted for by the effects of treatment on outcome expectancy. (2) Do the relative rates of responsiveness to hypnosis treatment differ as a function of pain type. (3) How should the problem of variability in hypnosis treatments between studies be dealt with when comparing study results. (4) What are the primary components of hypnotic analgesia interventions that contribute to their efficacy? (16).

4. SAFETY BASED ON LITERATURE REVIEW AND EXPERIENCE

4.1. Contraindications for the Use of Hypnosis

There is theoretically a minor risk that psychotic patients could become worse when told to interact with their imagery during the self-hypnotic process. However, psychotic patients are typically not very hypnotizable, and thus may not respond to hypnotic suggestion as well as others (56). Very rarely, some patients might experience transitory negative effects either during or after hypnosis, (13–15,57) including: drowsiness, confusion, headaches, and less frequently, anxiety or panic described in case reports (13).

In our clinical and research practice, we always review the patients' medical records prior to the use of adjunct hypnosis. If there is any clinical evidence or suspicion of psychosis or other major psychiatric disorder, hypnosis is not provided and a mental health care specialist is consulted.

4.2. Precautions

In a 2004 review of mind-body therapies for the management of pain, the authors recommend that hypnosis and imagery should be considered as "adjunctive therapies to help ameliorate pain during invasive medical procedures" (58). However, inadequate training in hypnosis has been suggested to be associated with a greater likelihood of occurrence of negative effects *(57)*. Thus, it is important that the hypnotherapist should be sufficiently capable and prepared to recognize the potential for adverse events and intervene accordingly.

Patients tend to take suggestions literally; it is therefore important to be specific in the clinical domain. For example, when suggesting adaptation of blood pressure, exact target values must be provided. While hypnosis can be helpful in maintaining patients' hemodynamic stability *(8,49)*, one should never rely on this mechanism alone in the procedure room but be fully equipped to deal with all potential procedural complications. Hypnosis should never be used in medical settings as the sole mode of complication management. Particularly, practitioners who wish to use hypnosis to reduce bleeding have to be aware that the capillary constriction that can be elicited to reduce surface oozes has no effect in preventing exsanguination from larger vessels.

5. MODELS OF INTEGRATION

5.1. Examples of Treatment Pathways and Their Rationale

Despite technical refinements in the management of acute pain during medical interventions, patients may experience distress that exceeds their coping mechanisms *(59)* and may require a patient-oriented intervention *(60)*. To address this issue, hypnosis can be used in two basic approaches: preparation of patients in the clinic for an upcoming procedure and providing hypnosis directly on the procedure table with or without prior patient preparation.

When preparing a patient for an upcoming procedure, one must consider time, cost and also the involvement of members of the patient's family, especially in the pediatric population *(12,26)*. Individualized interventions that require repeated encounters with the hypnotherapist are less likely to be adopted in the healthcare model and may not even be necessary for most patients.

Video and audiotapes can be employed as preparatory and procedural methods that do not demand excessive amounts of staff time, and have been reported to be useful in promoting relaxation and reducing drug use during dental surgery *(61,62)*, gastrointestinal endoscopy *(63)*, and femoral angiography *(64)*. However, a 13% rejection rate was also described *(65)*, and because of the lack of a therapist-patient relationship, videos and audiotapes may not be as powerful in preventing adverse effects such as vomiting *(62)*. In general, the presence of a live therapist is felt to be preferable *(28)*. Very anxious patients may also require a process that addresses their worries specifically before they will be able to relax and engage in hypnosis. This opportunity would be lost if only a standard electronic medium were used.

Furthermore, given the patient's awareness during medical procedures *(28)* and the fact that patients who come for a doctor's visit or a medical procedure are highly suggestible *(66)*, the medical staff should be careful in their choice of words when interacting with a patient *(67)*. Unfortunately, there is a strong belief in the medical community that announcing upcoming stimuli and events as painful and then expressing sympathy is a more honest approach and therefore beneficial to their patients. Therapists who prepare patients prior to procedures and are not in the procedure room with them may want to be particularly conscious of these negative suggestions and include measures of immunization against such comments. On the other hand, it is important to recognize the emotional investment of the procedure team in the patient's pain management, and it is crucial to acknowledge their experience and enlist their contribution and collaboration when designing hypnosis programs in medical settings.

When providing hypnosis during medical procedures, the authors prefer an approach validated in the interventional radiology setting, which was proven safe for both patient and therapist in prior studies *(8,68,69)*. Typically, all hypnotic treatment is performed in the procedure room, while the patient is lying on the procedure table. In the authors' clinical practice, this is often the first time patients are exposed to the idea of having medical hypnosis during their procedure. The main reason for this setup is the lack of time and structure for a preparatory visit in the very busy clinical interventional radiology setting. Patient hypnotizability is not assessed prior to hypnosis. Emphasis is placed on rapid rapport techniques in the form of structured attentive behavior to establish a patient-provider relationship. Detailed descriptions of these standardized interventions have been published (see Table 1) *(70)*.

For guidance to self-hypnotic relaxation the authors typically use scripts, in part because much of this work occurs in a research context. Scripts assure reproducibility and also help the hypnosis providers, many of whom are trained de novo, to internalize hypnotic language. Seeing a hypnosis provider sit down, put on glasses, and start reading a script provides some comforting aspects in the procedure suite for patients and personnel. In particular, it removes notions of mind-control as asserted in stage hypnosis and movie presentations. It also demonstrates to the procedure team that with the safety blanket of the script, hypnosis is something they could learn and do, and that language matters.

5.2. Cost Structure and Financial Considerations

The clinical benefits of hypnosis can be extended to cost savings *(71,72)*. In interventional radiology, US \$338 could be saved per case if every patient were offered hypnosis as compared to standard sedation *(71)*. This is largely due to a shortening

Table 1
Components of Structured Attentive Behavior Used During Medical Hypnosis

Components	*Examples*
Match the patients' verbal communication pattern	
Match the patients' nonverbal	Cross arms during interview, if subject crosses arms
Attentive listening	
Provision of the perception of control	"Let us know at any time what we can do for you."
Swift response to patients' requests	
Encouragement	
Use of emotionally neutral descriptors when painful stimuli are imminent	"What are you experiencing?" "Focus on a sensation of fullness, numbness, coolness or warmth."
Avoidance of negatively loaded suggestions	"How bad is your pain?" "You will feel a sting and burn now." "I know that you are sore."

of the procedure (an average reduction of 17 minutes) and the saving of expensive operating-room time as well as less need for recovery. Costs for sedation are mainly driven by oversedation; therefore, any reduction in oversedation will result in shorter post-surgical observation times and admissions. Cost is less affected by undersedation, so even a "poorly performing hypnotherapist who can produce some reduction in drug use will still reduce cost. Even if the hypnotherapist were to take a long time to induce hypnosis, and keep the patient for 58.2 minutes in the suite before the procedure starts, hypnosis would still remain cost-neutral. The cost advantage of adjunct hypnosis persists in a sensitivity analysis when a healthcare provider dedicated only to performing hypnosis is added to the team, unless this person's hourly wage exceeds US $330/hour.

5.3. Training Standards

The national societies of hypnosis, The American Society of Clinical Hypnosis (ASCH), The Society of Clinical & Experimental Hypnosis (SCEH), and the associated state societies have established training guidelines for registered healthcare professionals interested in becoming hypnosis providers.

In order to be eligible for training, healthcare professionals with a D.D.S., D.M.D., M.D., or a Ph.D., Psy.D., or an M.A., M.S. must have a professional license in the state where they practice. Students of these professions can be trained but practice only under supervision of a fully credentialed specialist. The individuals providing self-hypnosis in our institution are required to have a background in the healthcare profession in accordance with requirements by the national societies set for hypnosis training.

5.4. Licensing and Credentialing Standards

According to the ASCH, there are two levels of certification in hypnosis after appropriate training: entry and advanced level. Entry level is simply called "Certification." The advanced level, called "Approved Consultant," recognizes individuals who have obtained advanced training in clinical hypnosis and who have extensive experience in utilizing hypnosis within their professional practices. Approved Consultants are qualified to provide individualized training and consultation for those seeking Certification.

Certification in hypnosis by the ASCH requires 40 workshop hours (20 basic and 20 intermediate), 20 hours of individualized consultation on clinical work and 2 years of independent practice using hypnosis. In order to become an "approved consultant" an additional 60 workshop hours, 5 years of independent practice using hypnosis and an ASCH or SCEH membership is required.

ASCH Certification in Clinical Hypnosis is distinct from other certification programs in that it ensures that the certified individual is a bona fide healthcare professional who is licensed in his or her state or province to provide medical, dental, or psychotherapeutic services. ASCH believes that persons trained only in hypnosis lack the diagnostic and therapeutic skills as well as the licensure required to safely and responsibly treat medical, psychological, or dental problems with hypnosis. ASCH Certification distinguishes the professional practitioner from the lay hypnotist.

Certified professionals are encouraged to work toward attaining the highest level of advanced specialty certification in hypnosis by obtaining Diplomate status from the

American Board of Medical Hypnosis, the American Board of Psychological Hypnosis, the American Board of Hypnosis in Dentistry, or the American Hypnosis Board for Clinical Social Work.

5.5. *Liability and Risk Management*

In general, to reduce liability and decrease risk, an individual practitioner should use hypnosis as an adjunct only for a procedure or treatment that he or she is licensed to perform.

6. RESOURCES

6.1. *Journals*

American Journal of Clinical Hypnosis (ASCH)
http://www.asch.net/ajch.htm
International Journal of Clinical and Experimental Hypnosis (SCEH)
http://ijceh.educ.wsu.edu/

6.2. *Books*

Spiegel H, Spiegel D. Trance and treatment: Clinical uses of hypnosis. New York: Basic Books, 1978.

Barabasz AF, Watkins JG. Hypnotherapeutic Techniques. 2 ed. New York, NY: Brunner-Routledge, 2005.

Hammond DC. Hypnotic induction & suggestion. Chicago , IL: American Society of Clinical Hypnosis,1998.

Hammond DC. Handbook of Hypnotic Suggestions and Metaphors. 1st ed. New York, NY: W. W. Norton & Company, 1990.

6.3. *Websites*

American Society of Clinical Hypnosis (ASCH)
http://www.asch.net/
Society for Clinical and Experimental Hypnosis (SCEH)
www.sceh.us.
The Canadian Society of Clinical Hypnosis
http://www.csch.org.
The Milton Erickson Foundation
www.erickson-foundation.org.
The American Board of Medical Hypnosis
www.abmedhyp.org.

6.4. *Acknowledgements*

This work was supported by the National Institutes of Health, National Center for Complementary and Alternative Medicine 1K24 AT 01074-01, and RO1-AT-0002-07. The content is solely the responsibility of the authors and does not necessarily reflect the official views of the funding agencies.

REFERENCES

1. Spiegel H, Spiegel D. 1978. Trance and Treatment: Clinical Uses of Hypnosis. New York: Basic Books.
2. Barabasz AF, Watkins JG. 2005. Hypnotherapeutic Techniques, 2nd edition. New York, NY: Brunner-Routledge.
3. De Frances CJ, Margaret JH, Podgornik MN. 2003. National Hospital Discharge Survey. Advanced data from Vital and Health Statistics 2005;359.
4. Mueller PR, Biswal S, Halpern EF, Kaufman JA, Lee MJ. Interventional radiologic procedures: patient anxiety, perception of pain, understanding of procedure, and satisfaction with medication—a prospective study. Radiology 2000;215:684–688.
5. Martin ML, Lennox PH. 2003. Sedation and analgesia in the interventional radiology department. J Vasc Interv Radiol 2003;14:1119–1128.
6. Yaster M, Cravero JP. The continuing conundrum of sedation for painful and nonpainful procedures. J Pediatr 2004;145:10–12.
7. Acute Pain Management Guideline Panel. Acute Pain Management: Operative or Medical Procedures and Trauma. Clinical Practice Guideline. AHCPR Pub. No.92–0032. Rockville, MD: Agency for Health Care Policy and Research, Public Health Service, U.S. Department of Health and Human Services; 1992.
8. Lang EV, Benotsch EG, Fick LJ, Lutgendorf S, Berbaun ML, Berbaun KS, Logan H, Spiegel D. Adjunctive non-pharmacologic analgesia for invasive medical procedures: a randomized trial. Lancet 2000;355:1486–1490.
9. Faymonville ME, Meurisse M, Fissette J. Hypnosedation: a valuable alternative to traditional anaesthetic technidques. Acta Chir Belg 1999;99:141–146.
10. Patterson DR, Everett JJ, Burns GL, Marvin JA. Hypnosis for the treatment of burn pain. J Consult Clin Psychol 1992;5:713–717.
11. Montgomery GH, Weltz CR, Seltz M, Bovbjerg DH. Brief presurgery hypnosis reduces stress and pain in excisional breast biopsy patients. Int J Clin Exp Hypn 2002;50:17–32.
12. Butler LD, Symons BK, Henderson SL, Shortliffe LD, Spiegel D. Hypnosis reduces distress and duration of an invasive medical procedure for children. Pediatrics 2005;115:77–85.
13. MacHovec F. Hypnosis, complications, risk factors and prevention. Am J Clin Hypn 1988;31:40–49.
14. Page RA, Handley GW. In search of predictors of hypnotic sequelae. Am J Clin Hypn 1996;39:93–96.
15. Barber J. When hypnosis causes trouble. Int J Clin Exp Hypn 1998;46:157–170.
16. Jensen M, Patterson DR. Hypnotic treatment of chronic pain. J Behav Med 2006;11:1–30.
17. Lindblom U, Merskey H, Mumford J, Nathan PW, Noordenbos W, Sunderland S. Pain terms—a current list of definitions and notes on usage. Pain 1986;24(1):S215–S221.
18. Rainville P, Carrier B, Hofbauer RK, Bushnell MC, Duncan GH. Dissociation of sensory and affective dimensions of pain using hypnotic modulation. Pain 1999;82:159–171.
19. Rainville P, Duncan GH, Price DD, Carrier B, Bushnell MC. Pain affect encoded in human anterior cingulate but not somatosensory cortex. Science 1997;277:968–971.
20. Kiernan BD, Dane JR, Philips LH, Price DD. Hypnotic analgesia reduces R-III nociceptive reflex: further evidence concerning the multifactorial nature of hypnotic analgesia. Pain 1995;60:39–47.
21. Rainville P, Bao QVH, Chretien P. Pain-related emotions modulate experimental pain perception and autonomic responses. Pain 2005;118(3):306–318.
22. Rainville P, Hofbauer RK, Bushnell MC, Duncan GH, Price DD. Hypnosis modulates activity in brain structures involved in the regulation of conciousness. J Cogn Neurosci 2002;14:887–901.
23. Rainville P, Hofbauer RK, Paus T, Duncan GH, Bushnell MC, Price DD. Cerebral mechanisms of hypnotic induction and suggestion. J Cogn Neurosci 1999;11:110–125.
24. Kosslyn SM, Thompson WL, Constantini-Ferrando MF, Alpert NM, Spiegel D. Hypnotic visual illusion alters color processing in the brain. Am J Psychiatry 2000;157:1279–1284.
25. Horton JE, Crawford HJ, Harrington GS, Downs JHI. Increased anterior corpus callosum size associated positively with hypnotizability and the ability to control pain. Brain 2004;127:1741–1747.
26. Huth MM, Broome ME, Good M. Imagery reduces children's postoperative pain. Pain 2004;110:439–448.
27. Levitan AA, Harbaugh TE. Hypnotizability and hypnoanalgesia: hypnotizability of patients using hypnoanalgesia during surgery. Am J Clin Hypn 1992;34:223–226.
28. Blankfield RP. Suggestion, relaxation, and hypnosis as adjuncts in the care of surgery patients: a review of the literature. Am J Clin Hypn 1991;33:172–186.

29. Esdaile J. 1957. Mesmerism in India and its practical application in surgery and medicine. London. Reiussued as Hypnosis in medicine and surgery. New York: Julian Press, 1846.
30. Schwarcz BE. Hypnoanalgesia and hypnoanesthesia in urology. Surg Clin N Am 1965;45:1547–1555.
31. Tinterow MT. Hypnotic anesthesia for major surgical procedures. Am Surg 1960;26:732–737.
32. Ruiz ORG, Fernandez A. Hypnosis as an anesthetic in ophthalmology. Am J Opthalm 1960;50:163.
33. Mason AA. Surgery under hypnosis. Anaesthesia 1955;10:295–299.
34. Marmer MJ. Hypnoanalgesia and hypnoanesthesia for cardiac surgery. JAMA 1959;171:512–517.
35. Levitan AA, Harbaugh tL. Hypnoanalgesia and hypnotizability. Hypnosis 1989;16:140–148.
36. Kroger WS, DeLee ST. Hypnoanesthesia for Cesarean section and hysterectomy. JAMA 1957;163:442–444.
37. Crasilneck HB, McCranie EJ, Jenkins MT. Special indications for hypnosis as method of anesthesia. JAMA 1956;126:1606–1608.
38. Bernstein MR. Significant value of hypnoanaesthesia: Three clinical examples. Am J Clin Hypn 1965;7:259–260.
39. Bowen DE. Transurethral resection under self-hypnosis. Am J Clin Hypn 1973;16:132–134.
40. Fredericks LE. Teaching of hypnosis in the overall approach to the surgical patient. Am J Clin Hypn 1978;22:175–183.
41. Rodger BP. The art of preparing the patient for anesthesia. Anesthesiology 1961;22:548–554.
42. Bonilla KB, Quigley WF, Bowers WF. Experiences with hypnosis on a surgical service. Military Medicine 1961;126:364–370.
43. Lang EV, Joyce JS, Spiegel D, Hamilton D, Lee K. Self-hypnotic relaxation during interventional radiological procedures. Effects on pain perception and intravenous drug use. Int J Exp Clin Hyp 1996;44:106–119.
44. Montgomery GH, David D, Winkel G, Silverstein JH, Bovberg DH. The effectiveness of adjunctive hypnosis with surgical patients: A meta-analysis. Anesth Analg 2002;94:1639–1645.
45. Stewart JH. Hypnosis in contemporary medicine. Mayo Clin Proc 2005;80:511–524.
46. Hippel CV, Hole G, Kaschka WP. Autonomic profile under hypnosis as assessed by heart rate variability and spectral analysis. 2001;34:11–113.
47. Baglini R, Sesana M, Capuano C, Gnecchi-Ruscone T, Ugo L, Danzi G. Effect of hypnotic sedation during percutaneous transluminal coronary angioplasty on myocardial ischemia and cardiac sympathetic drive. Am J Cardiol 2004;93:1035–1038.
48. Morgan AH, Hilgard ER. Age differences in susceptibility to hypnosis. Int J Clin Exp Hypn 1972;21:78–85.
49. Faymonville ME, Mambourg PH, Joris J, et al. Psychological approaches during conscious sedation. Hypnosis versus stress reducing strategies: a prospective randomized study. Pain 1997;73:361–367.
50. Patterson DR, Everett JJ, Bombardier CH, Questad KA, Lee VK, Marvin JA. Psychological effects of severe burn injuries. Psychological Bulletin 1993;113:362–378.
51. Patterson DR, Questad KA, Boltwood MD. Hypnotherapy as a treatment for pain in patients with burns: research and clinical considerations. Journal of Burn Care and Rehabilitation 1987;8:263–268.
52. Patterson DR, Questad KA, deLateour BJ. Hypnotherapy as an adjunct to narcotic analgesia for the treatment of pain for burn debridement. American Journal of Clinical Hypnosis 1989;31:156–163.
53. Haanen HC, Hoenderdos HT, van Romunde LK, et al. Controlled trial of hypnotherapy in the treatment of refractory fibromyalgia. J Rheumatol. 1991 Jan;18(1):72–75.
54. Gay MC, Philippot P, Luminet O. Differential effectiveness of psychological interventions for reducing osteoarthritis pain: a comparison of Erikson [correction of Erickson] hypnosis and Jacobson relaxation. Eur J Pain. 2002;6(1):1–16.
55. Friedman H, Taub HA. Brief psychological training procedures in migraine treatment. Am J Clin Hypn. 1984 Jan;26(3):187–200.
56. Spiegel D, Detrick D, Fricholz E. Hypnotizability and psychopathology. AJ Psychiatry 1982;139:431–437.
57. Lynn SJ, Martin DJ, Frauman DC. Does hypnosis pose special risks for negative effects? A master class commentary. Int J Clin Exp Hypn 1996;44:7–19.
58. Astin JA. Mind-body therapies for the management of pain. Clin J Pain 2004;20:27–32.
59. Horne DJ, Vatmanidis P, Careri A. Preparing patients for invasive medical procedures and surgical procedures. 1: Adding behavioral and cognitive interventions. Behav Med 1994;20:5–13.
60. Schupp C, Berbaum K, Berbaum M, Lang EV. Pain and anxiety during interventional radiological procedures. Effect of patients' state anxiety at baseline and modulation by nonpharmacologic analgesia adjuncts. J Vasc Intervent Radiol 2005;16.

61. Corah NL, Gale EN, Illig SJ. The use of relaxation and distraction during dental procedures. J Am Dent Assoc 1979;98:390–394.
62. Ghoneim MM, Block RI, Sarasin DS, Davis CS, Marchman JN. Tape-recorded hypnosis instructions as adjuvant in the care of patients scheduled for third molar surgery. Anesth Analg 2000;90:64–68.
63. Wilson JF, Moore RW, Randolph S, Hanson BJ. Behavioral preparation of patients for gastrointestinal endoscopy: information, relaxation and coping style. J Hum Stress 1982;8:13–23.
64. Mandle CL, Domar AD, Harrington DP, et al. Relaxation response in femoral angiography. Radiology 1990;174:737–739.
65. Smith JT, Barabasz A, Barabasz M. Comparison of hypnosis and distraction in severely ill children undergoing painful medical procedures. J Counseling Psychol 1996;43:187–195.
66. Spiegel H. Nocebo: the power of suggestibility. Prevent Med 1997;26:616.
67. Lang EV, Hatsiopoulou O, Koch T, et al. Can words hurt? Patient–provider interactions during invasive medical procedures. Pain 2005;114( ):303–309.
68. Lang EV, Berbaum KS. Educating interventional radiology personnel in nonpharmacologic analgesia: effect on patients' pain perception. Acad Radiol 1997;4:753–757.
69. Lang EV, Spiegel D, Lutgendorf S, Logan H. 1996. Empathic attention and self-hypnotic relaxation for interventional radiological procedures. Iowa City, IA: The University of Iowa.
70. Lang EV, Lutgendorf S, Logan H, Benotsch E, Laser E, Spiegel D. Nonpharmacologic analgesia and anxiolysis for interventional radiological procedures. Sem Intervent Radiol 1999;16:113–123.
71. Lang EV, Rosen M. Cost analysis of adjunct hypnosis for sedation during outpatient interventional procedures. Radiology 2002;222:375–382.
72. Faintuch S, Lang EV, Rosen MP. Cost-effectiveness of self-hypnosis during outpatient interventional radiologic procedures: update and impact. In: Sociedad Iberoamericana de Informacion Cientifica. http://www.siicsalud.com/des/des040/04no3005.htm

11 Energy-Based Therapies for Chronic Pain

Eric Leskowitz

CONTENTS

Horatio: O day and night, but this is wondrous strange!
Hamlet: And therefore as a stranger give it welcome.
There are more things in heaven and earth, Horatio,
Than are dreamt of in your philosophy.
William Shakespeare (Hamlet, I,v, 165–168)

Summary

A multidimensional model of chronic pain includes not only physiologic and psychological/emotional factors, but also the dimension of subtle energy. In this chapter, the subtle energy dynamics of chronic pain are explored by first outlining the subtle anatomy and energy physiology described in many healing traditions around the world. Then, specific pain conditions (myofascial pain, fibromyalgia, phantom pain, and complex regional pain syndrome) are reconceptualized as energy imbalances, and suggested interventions and clinical vignettes are described. A range of energy therapies is also described, including acupuncture, Reiki, Therapeutic Touch, and meridian-based psychotherapy.

Key Words: subtle energy, chakra, meridian, energy psychology, chronic pain, phantom pain, qi, aura

From: *Contemporary Pain Medicine: Integrative Pain Medicine: The Science and Practice of Complementary and Alternative Medicine in Pain Management*
Edited by: J. F. Audette and A. Bailey © Humana Press, Totowa, NJ

1. INTRODUCTION

Hamlet's friend Horatio is mystified by his encounter with a ghost because he doesn't believe in ghosts, and so Hamlet counsels his friend that life is too complex to be fully understood within a single philosophical framework. This wise advice also applies to the world of pain management. Medical theories are, after all, reflections of the prevailing scientific model; they change as philosophies change. Over the past 30 years, the field of pain management has undergone a major shift from what could be called a mechanistic model that focused exclusively on nociception, to a more interactive mind–body model that ushered in the era of multidisciplinary pain clinics and the reconceptualization of chronic pain as a behavioral syndrome. Despite the acknowledged successes of this model, however (lowered costs, improved function, and higher rates of return to work *(1)*), there is still "more to heaven and earth than is dreamed of" by even this expanded mind–body model. In this chapter, a multidimensional model of chronic pain will be proposed, in which the role of energy medicine is highlighted. This aspect of health, though unacknowledged by Western medicine, plays a central role in numerous other systems of healthcare, particularly in the East, and has been called by many names, including "subtle energy," "vital force," "qi" (in traditional Chinese medicine), and "prana" (in yoga theory).

Despite this lack of recognition by mainstream medicine, a substantial body of evidence has been compiled in recent years that appears to validate ancient mystical theories of life energy. This chapter will outline some of the evidence for the existence of this subtle energy circulation system in the human body and will consider the ways by which the disruption of this energy flow can result in the development of symptoms and illnesses (including chronic pain) by a mechanism that might be called energy physiology. Certain well-known pain syndromes will be examined through the lens of subtle energy anatomy and physiology, and the range of energy-oriented therapies that may be effective in treating these pain syndromes will be explored. Because data on many aspects of this model have not yet been fully developed, this chapter will at times adopt a more speculative tone than other sections of this textbook. However, there seems to be sufficiently established individual data points to form an energy physiology, a blueprint for future research and clinical developments in chronic pain.

2. ENERGY THEORY

In Western medicine, human beings are conceived of as extremely complex machines. Metaphors to this effect pervade medical writings: the heart is a pump, the eye is a camera, and the brain is a computer. There are unwritten assumptions in this model. For example, if we learn to subdivide defective body parts into ever more basic components, we will, presumably, be able to reconstruct a fully functioning and asymptomatic machine. Symptoms tell us where the breakdown lies, so we can appropriately repair the defective part, whether by surgery or redesigning the DNA blueprint. If pain stems from unwanted or unpleasant internal communications, then blocking those pathways can abolish it. This is the nociceptive model of pain. Within this model, the sense of "I," the individual awareness that we all experience, is simply an artifact or byproduct of our incredibly complex nervous system and brain; there is no independent self or Soul or consciousness.

In the energy model, however, human beings are conceived of as multidimensional organisms, not simply as composite machines. The "I-ness" of consciousness is seen as primary, operating within the tripartite system of body, mind and spirit. Mind is composed of thoughts and emotions, while spirit includes the transcendent level of soul as well as the more tangible force of subtle energy. For example, the yogis described a series of nested sheaths ranging from the densest one, the physical body, to the most ethereal, the Spirit. One of these layers, the subtle energy sheath, has been called the "breath body" and it parallels the acupuncture meridian system in traditional Chinese medicine. The yogis considered this dimension to be merely another subdivision of the physical body. In other words, energy and matter were thought of as poles of a continuous spectrum of which Western medicine considers only a very limited portion.

3. ENERGY ANATOMY

The energy system is classically organized into three major components: the containment vessel known as the energy field (popularly called the aura), the distribution pathways known as the acupuncture meridians, and a series of energy centers or transformers called "chakras." Problems within each of these components of subtle energy anatomy may contribute to the development of a particular pain syndrome to be discussed in subsequent sections of this chapter. These structures will, therefore, be described in more detail below.

3.1. The Energy Field

In everyday language we acknowledge the existence of a human energy field or aura whenever we talk of our "personal space." Just as magnets have electromagnetic fields (EMF) that are distributed in space beyond their physical boundaries, so it is with the human body; we don't end at our skins, and we feel something unpleasant when someone enters our personal space without our permission. Electronic measurements show the existence of an EMF extending far beyond the body, strongest in the region around the heart *(2)*, and strengthened during meditation or healing practices *(3)*. "Healthy boundaries" is a psychological concept that denotes the ability to separate self from other and to prevent psychological aggression and abuse. Perhaps these boundaries are not just metaphorical but are based on the tangible energetic boundaries that provide a protective layer at the outer reaches of our personal energy field. Therapeutic Touch (TT), to be discussed in detail later, is the energy intervention most directly focused on this energy field boundary.

3.1.1. EXPERIENTIAL EXERCISE

To have a personal experience of the type of energy we are discussing in this chapter, begin by placing your arms out in front of you, hands facing each other about 12 inches apart. Bring the hands close enough to feel the warmth but without making physical contact. Then begin to slowly move the hands farther apart and closer together, and notice any non-thermal sensations, especially when the hands are about a foot apart. By closing your eyes, you can increase your sensitivity to these subtle sensations. Many people describe a tingling or bouncing feeling, almost magnetic in quality. This is the sensation that TT practitioners use to assess the status of the energy field of their patients.

3.2. The Energy Pathways

Perhaps the best-validated components of the subtle anatomy system are the acupuncture points and meridians that were brought to Western attention by Chinese medical theory. These points were discovered and mapped in the pre-technological era of imperial China, but modern electronic detection systems have validated the existence of acupoints and meridians even though there appears to be no physical structure that underlies their presence. For example, electrical conductivity is lower at acupoints than in surrounding tissues *(4)*, and thermography reveals the presence of meridian pathways when selected points are activated by moxa heat stimulation *(5)*. Acupuncture, acupressure, and energy psychology using acupuncture meridians are the treatment modalities most directly focused on the energy pathways.

3.3. The Energy Centers

Despite a religious prohibition against anatomical dissection, Hindu scientists developed a map of the body that contained seven internal energy centers along the vertical axis of the spinal column. These centers function as energy transformers, regulating the "voltage" of universal life energy ("prana") as it flows through the human system. The functions of these energy centers range from survival and sexuality at the base of the spine, to compassion at the level of the anatomic heart, to intuition at the brow center (third eye), and enlightenment located at the crown of the head. Intriguingly, these subtle centers correspond in location and function to the seven endocrine glands of allopathic medicine, though yoga anatomists used only intro-spection during meditation to locate these psychospiritual centers. Even non-meditators have experienced their energy centers, as some common everyday sensations represent our perception of highly energized chakras. For example, butterflies in the stomach occur when our 3rd center is active (fear of public speaking), warmth in the heart when we feel love, tingling in the scalp when we're in awe *(6)*. Table 1 shows these parallels. Chelation and energy work *(7,8)* as taught by Rev. Rosalyn Bruyere and in the Barbara Brennan School of Healing, are the treatment modalities that are most directly focused on the energy centers.

Table 1
Energy/Endocrine Correspondence

Energy Center (Chakra)	Endocrine Gland	Emotional Function	Energy sensation
Crown	Pineal	Bliss	scalp tingling
Brown	Pituitary	Intuition	inner 'lightbulb'
Throat	Thyroid	Truth	choking up
Heart	Thymus	Compassion	broken heart
Solar Plexus	Pancreas	Personal power	'butterflies'
Genital	Gonads	Sexuality	sexual arousal
Root	Adrenal	survival	'adrenaline rush'

- Endocrine/energy center correspondences were discovered in introspective traditions that did not allow dissection.
- Psycho-endocrinology: the emotional functions of each energy center relates to physio-logical functions of each corresponding endocrine gland.
- Everyday experiences of intensified life energy flow represents the palpable interface of subtle energy with gross physiology.

3.4. Energy Physiology: Layers/Sheaths/Dimensions

Just as gross anatomy provides the substrate for understanding physiology in allopathic medical schools, energy anatomy provides the substrate for understanding energy physiology within the field of energy medicine. The dynamics of energy flow, and its interaction with the body, are the focus here. As the Chinese said, "The mind directs the qi (energy) and the qi directs the blood (the body)." The nature of the link between mind and body has been the oldest philosophical and neurobiological mystery facing modern Western medicine. However, this mind–body connection is a given in energy paradigms; energy is the intervening variable that connects the two, thereby resolving Cartesian dualism and the separation of mind and body. Energy physiology also has an explanation for the symptom of pain. The traditional Chinese medicine (TCM) formulation was *bu tong, ze tong; tong ze, bu tong,* which can be translated as "free flow, no pain; blocked flow, pain." In other words, any blockage to energy flow creates friction, which will be perceived as uncomfortable to variable degrees, depending on the severity of the blockage and the overall energy status of the organism. Interestingly, in TCM, someone with an overall high level of energy, such as a young athlete, may experience more significant pain than someone weakened by age or chronic illness with a sudden energy blockage. However, because of the higher level of energy in the body of the athlete, the treatment will be easier than in someone that is energy deficient, where the stagnation of the free flow of energy cannot be as easily overcome.

Another important principle of energy physiology was alluded to earlier, in the discussion of the energy/matter spectrum. It's helpful to think of consciousness as analogous to H_2O—a gas at high temperatures, a liquid at medium temperature, and a solid at low temperatures. Similarly, consciousness at its highest vibrational level is pure spirit, at a lower level is emotion and thought, and in its most condensed state is biologic matter. This condensation analogy may help to better understand acupuncture. This energy model is often dismissed as the indigenous, pre-scientific explanation of acupuncture. Acupuncture, as the most intensively studied of the energy modalities, has received the most theoretical attention as to possible mechanisms of action. Elsewhere in this text, a fascial mechanism, as well as a neuromodulation theory, for acupuncture are proposed; neither model requires nor negates the independent existence of subtle energy.

I will briefly describe a highly speculative mechanism of action for acupuncture that proposes a direct interaction between qi and neurons. The key component to this model is the relatively neglected direct current, perineural system described by neurosurgeon Robert Becker *(9)*. In contrast to the familiar digital, on-off, synaptically based neurological communication system, this analog system involves slower inter-cellular interactions that occur via ion fluxes within the extracellular matrix of the glial cells in the central nervous system (CNS) and along nerve sheaths in the peripheral nervous system (PNS). Many physiologic processes, including wound healing and possibly oncogenesis, are regulated by this system. Some healers believe this network in the CNS and along the axon sheaths in the PNS is the physical carrier of healing energy *(10)*. It is possible that the electrically charged and highly ionized solution in this matrix can be influenced by qi flow itself to induce action potentials, much like fluxes in magnetic fields can induce electrical currents in a nearby conducting medium.

Thus, the interface between qi and physiology, between electromagnetic charge and perineural conduction, may be where the neurological mechanism of acupuncture lies.

4. HYPOTHESIS OF ACTION: ENERGETIC RECONCEPTUALIZATION OF SPECIFIC PAIN SYNDROMES

Recent advances in the neuroanatomical model of pain include advanced imaging technology and an improved understanding of neuroplasicity, including the molecular biology (e.g., C-fos gene expression), and neurotransmitter-receptor activity (e.g., NMDA receptor linked wind-up of wide dynamic range neurons). However, a different model of pain etiology emerges when the energy perspective is adopted. This section will focus on the specific energy dynamics of four common pain diagnoses; myofascial pain syndrome (MPS), fibromyalgia syndrome (FMS), complex regional pain syndrome (CRPS), and phantom limb pain (PLP). The first two are characterized by specific point disturbances in local tissue, which will be related to acupuncture point (acupoint) imbalances, CRPS will be conceptualized as an imbalance with a particular deficiency of emotional energy, and PLP will be described as a disturbance in the underlying energetic matrix.

4.1. Myofascial Pain Syndrome

The key clinical finding in MPS is localized pain in a taut band of muscle called a myofascial trigger point (MTrP) (see Chapter 5). MTrPs appear to be randomly dispersed, according to the map of Western medicine, because they are found in anatomically heterogeneous tissues and locations. However, from an energy medicine or TCM perspective, they function as key acupoints. They were first linked to acupuncture points 30 years ago by Ronald Melzack, the pioneering pain psychologist (11), who found >70% correlation of MTrPs with acupuncture points. In addition, the Western medicine treatment of MPS via trigger point injections is remarkably similar to acupuncture. The trigger points are inactivated, through injection of a range of substances (whether steroids, anesthetics, or saline). A standard MPS treatment guide (12) shows just such an injection into a MTrP in the brachii triceps tendon (see Figure 1). However, if the practitioner were using a dry needling technique (without any injected liquid), the procedure would in fact be remarkably similar to acupuncture needling of the Large Intestine-10 (acupuncture point Shou San Li on the hand Yangming meridian).

The electromagnetic activity in acupoints and in MTrPs has been investigated (13, 14). The emerging consensus is that MTrPs are characterized by heightened sympathetic activity. Therefore, the energetics of MTrPs are described as having an excess of qi requiring dispersion, in contrast to the tender points of fibromyalgia which, as we'll see are deficient in qi and require tonification. From this point of view, MTrPs are generated when a physical injury results in a local or regional energy blockage that is frequently accompanied by underlying emotional factors. Unless these emotional components are addressed the block may not be released despite treatment of the physical MTrP (6). An upcoming patient vignette illustrates how the emotional root of MPS can be treated via energy therapy.

4.2. Fibromyalgia Syndrome

Two key components of FMS are primarily energetic in nature: the profound fatigue and the pathognomonic tender points. As with MTrPs, the location of FMS tender

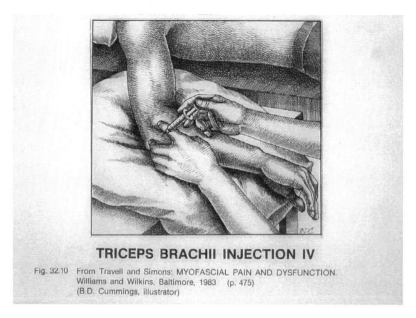

TRICEPS BRACHII INJECTION IV

Fig. 32.10 From Travell and Simons: MYOFASCIAL PAIN AND DYSFUNCTION.
Williams and Wilkins, Baltimore, 1983 (p. 475)
(B.D. Cummings, illustrator)

Fig. 1. Trigger point injection and similarity to acupuncture needling of acupuncture point Large Intestine 10 *(12)*.

points is somewhat mystifying from the anatomical perspective. The map of tender points put forward by the American College of Rheumatology (ACR) correlates exactly with key acupuncture points, including Bladder 10, Large Intestine 11, and Bladder 25 (see Figure 2).

The life history that precedes the diagnosis of FMS is often striking in the degree of cumulative stress and attendant symptomatology that occurs before medical attention is sought. From an energetic perspective, it seems likely that this accumulated physical and emotional stress has totally depleted the FMS patient's energy system. Western medicine refers to adrenal exhaustion *(15)* as an indicator of a breakdown in the "Fight or Flight" response to stress. The parallel energetic process would be a breakdown in the root center, the chakra center that regulates survival issues. One well-known experimental finding suggests that the energy drain of insomnia may create the early symptoms of FMS. Healthy volunteers who are deprived of the restorative phase of sleep known as slow wave sleep will reliably develop tender points, which then disappear when normal sleep cycles are restored *(16)*. In effect, this energetic exhaustion leads to a breakdown of the root center (the foundation of the chakra system's house of cards), which snowballs into complete energetic and endocrine collapse.

Comprehensive treatment of FMS must address all these issues. Classical homeopathy sometimes succeeds in finding the unique silver bullet known as the constitutional remedy that will specifically and directly resolve the underlying imbalance *(17)*. Dr. Jacob Teitelbaum's comprehensive FMS treatment protocol addresses endocrine dysfunction at all levels. It is one of the few FMS treatments that have shown statistically significant benefit in double blind, controlled experiments *(18)*. His protocol involves supplementation or replacement of each endocrine gland's hormonal product: DHEA supplementation restores adrenal/root chakra function, thyroxine restores

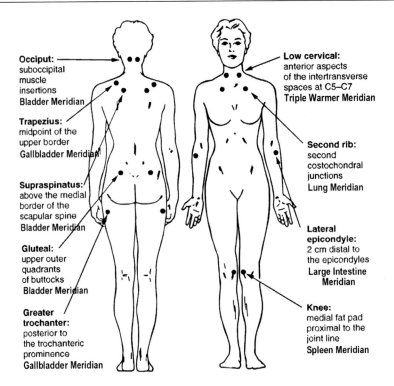

Occiput:
suboccipital
muscle
insertions
Bladder Meridian

Trapezius:
midpoint of the
upper border
Gallbladder Meridian

Supraspinatus:
above the medial
border of the
scapular spine
Bladder Meridian

Gluteal:
upper outer
quadrants
of buttocks
Bladder Meridian

**Greater
trochanter:**
posterior to
the trochanteric
prominence
Gallbladder Meridian

Low cervical:
anterior aspects
of the intertransverse
spaces at C5–C7
Triple Warmer Meridian

Second rib:
second
costochondral
junctions
Lung Meridian

**Lateral
epicondyle:**
2 cm distal to
the epicondyles
**Large Intestine
Meridian**

Knee:
medial fat pad
proximal to the
joint line
Spleen Meridian

Fig. 2. American College of Rheumatology (ACR) fibromyalgia tender point map with acupuncture point correlates (from Google Images).

thryoid/throat center function, melatonin restores crown/pineal function, and so on, as the chakra/endocrine axis is reconstructed. While his model does not use subtle energy terminology, it calls to mind the chakra/endocrine parallels outlined in Table 1.

4.3. Complex Regional Pain Syndrome

Complex regional pain syndrome (CRPS) is a pain syndrome occurring most often in an extremity that is associated with abnormal autonomic nervous system activity and trophic changes. The disorder has both nociceptive and neuropathic features and is characterized by persistent pain, allodynia or hyperalgesia, edema, alterations in skin blood flow, and sudomotor dysfunction *(19)*. The underlying pathophysiology of CRPS remains incompletely understood at this time. Until recently, the pain medicine literature has suggested that CRPS involves a significant psychosomatic component. Many now advocate that the psychological distress seen in CRPS is a late consequence of unrelenting severe pain that makes concomitant anxiety and depression a nearly universal finding in chronic CRPS. However, Ochoa and others have noted *(20)* the strong placebo responsiveness in CRPS as evidence for the psychophysiological reactivity of these patients. As of yet, the mind-body link in CRPS has been explored only via survey instruments (i.e., the incidence of childhood trauma is 30%) *(21)*. The role of physically insignificant trauma as a precipitant for the syndrome has been widely noted but not fully explored. In the course of in-depth psychodynamic interviews, these physically insignificant initial traumas (sprained ankle, stubbed toe, injection of medication) are, however, often revealed to be emotionally significant, and at times even devastating, to the patient. By adopting a specific psychodynamically cued interview technique with CRPS patients, a significant degree of unaddressed emotional pain is frequently uncovered (unreported findings by author). The intensity of these psychological symptoms does not approach that seen in post-traumatic stress disorder (PTSD) and the process can best be described as suppressed dysphoric emotion, typically anger.

The energy model of CRPS proposes that the mildly injured body part becomes so identified (often consciously) with emotional conflict that the patient chooses to ignore or at least withdraw attention from that part of the body. In other words, the qi is withdrawn from a specific region as a psychological defense against experiencing the associated unpleasant emotions that are somatically embedded in that area of the body. In time, the familiar sequence of CRPS symptoms develops—initially manifested as disturbances of the autonomic nervous system (allodynia, vasomotor instability), but ultimately progressing to frank tissue damage (loss of hair, cornification of nails, and osteoporosis). Interestingly, these latter symptoms are all characterized by loss of tissue vitality and can be readily reconceptualized as signs of chronic energy depletion. This "qi withdrawal" model may explain why energizing therapies like exercise can be so effective, particularly in younger/adolescent patients (22)—the vigorous aerobic exercise re-establishes circulation into the affected area, not only of blood, but also presumably of qi. Similarly, new work in graded motor imagery suggests that thinking about the limb can also desensitize the pain, perhaps via qi release (as the Chinese said, "the mind directs the qi") (23). When patients are again emotionally balanced enough to "reinhabit" the affected body part, symptoms will resolve.

4.3.1. CASE EXAMPLE

Micaela presented as a 20-year-old college student who had maintained a high level of function despite unremitting CRPS pain since an ankle sprain during basketball practice at age 11. At the time of her accident, she was taken to the local emergency department where she was treated aggressively for her injury. This treatment included an intramuscular injection by a physician whose manner clearly communicated to Micaela disbelief in the legitimacy of her pain. Within minutes of that intervention, pain began at the injection site and spread in characteristic CRPS fashion to the entire lower extremity over the following months. Being a "good girl," Micaela never expressed her rage and hurt at the offending doctor, yet it came to the surface readily during her initial evaluation. This case illustrates that the subjective meaning of the physical injury to the patient may be more important than the degree of tissue damage incurred.

4.4. Phantom Limb Pain

PLP provides a challenge to the neuroanatomical model, if only because of its poor response to nociceptively oriented treatments. The perceived phantom limb is generally theorized to be a cortically induced perception (in other words, a hallucination), but PLP's responsiveness to certain energy therapies (24) suggests that an energy mechanism is worth considering. Unfortunately, there is no well-established and widely accepted method to visualize energy fields, so that field anomalies could be correlated with symptoms. However, using a technique known as Kirlian photography to image electrostatic fields around living organisms, some images appear to show that an EMF exists around a leaf even after its tip has been cut off; this so-called phantom leaf effect (25) has been compared to PLP. The energy field seems to be a pre-existing matrix around which the leaf (or limb) is structured, rather than an artifact of the electrical activity that can be measured in living tissue. Analogously, iron filings arrange themselves in alignment with invisible magnetic lines of force; the force does not arise from the filings but is separate and independent. It has been hypothesized (26) that phantom pain sensations may be generated by imbalances in this invisible energy matrix that arise from the emotional trauma of the amputation. The energetic rebalancing that comes with healing the pre-existing psychological trauma should relieve the pain.

4.4.1. CASE EXAMPLE

Jeri was a 65-year-old administrative assistant with a 7-year history of PLP when she was seen in clinic. She described the onset of phantom pain following a left below-knee amputation surgery to save a limb whose circulation had been severely compromised after a fall down a flight of stairs. Pain was manageable, averaging 6/10 on a numeric pain scale with a regimen of short-acting opioid analgesics. The original treatment plan to apply Emotional Freedom Technique (EFT) desensitization (described in the next section) to her memories of the fall were changed when Jeri shared that the feeling of falling had recapitulated what she had experienced in a swimming accident at age nine when she fell into a pit of water at the beach. Instead, EFT was directed at the swimming memory. After completion of the EFT treatment course, Jeri found that she no longer had the swooning internal feeling that used to accompany this memory and her leg pain had markedly decreased. She went on to experience her first pain-free period in the 7 years since the surgery.

5. ENERGY THERAPIES: RATIONALE FOR USE

The following examples each focus on a specific energy therapy that has been effective in treating chronic pain. Of course, many other energy therapies are not represented in this section, due to space limitations. Case vignettes and research citations accompany the brief descriptive overviews.

5.1. Therapeutic Touch

Therapeutic Touch (TT) was developed by the partnership of a clinical nurse and an energy healer more than 35 years ago, in an attempt to develop a healing methodology that would be acceptable in medical settings and that would build on nursing's tradition of compassionate hands-on caring. The technique involves no physical contact but rather an assessment of the state of the energy field surrounding the patient by using energy sensitivity of the practitioner's hands. At the core of the practice is the assumption by the practitioner of an attitude of centered compassion toward the patient and adoption this state of mind is the key first step of the healing process (27). The assessment phase is then followed by an unruffling/balancing process to clear any perceived blockages in the field. There is a large body of experimental evidence validating TT for a range of conditions, from pre-surgical anxiety to osteoarthritis. Unfortunately, the two best-known TT studies are marred by controversy. Briefly, a study published in JAMA in 1998 that claimed to show no benefit for TT (28) has been shown to be methodologically flawed (29), while a 1990 study purporting to show that TT accelerated wound healing in healthy human subjects (30) has recently been shown to be fraudulent (31). Caveats aside, TT has been taught to more than 100,000 nurses in North America and is available in many major medical centers.

5.1.1. Case: TT and Phantom Limb Pain

Joe was a 35-year-old cargo loader whose leg had been crushed in a work injury, necessitating an above-knee amputation five years before he presented to our clinic. His chronic phantom limb pain was only marginally responsive to a regimen of antidepressants and opiates. He did not benefit from cognitive-behavioral retraining and was offered a trial of TT, about which he knew nothing. During the assessment phase, there was a similar energy presence sensed by the practitioner in the region of his missing leg that was also felt around the remainder of his intact body (much like the sensation from the Experiential Exercise in Section 3.1.1). At that moment, the patient reported sensing his phantom limb being touched. As the treatment continued, Joe reported that the pain sensations seemed to be draining out the bottom of his phantom foot. Surprisingly, he asked for the treatment to be stopped before the pain could be completely alleviated, saying that he feared becoming pain-free because this would be proof to him that his leg was in fact missing. In other words, his pain served the psychological function of defending him against the shock that would come with full acceptance of his loss (for a more detailed discussion of this case, see reference 32).

5.2. Energy Psychology

The Emotional Freedom Technique (EFT) is the most widely taught and widely used protocol *(33)* among the array of new techniques that fall under the umbrella of energy psychology (EP). This relatively new discipline *(34)* derives from early observations that acupuncture treatment can cause strong emotional reactions and that certain meridians seemed to correlate strongly with specific emotions. Building on a lineage that includes acupuncture, chiropractic, psychiatry, and martial arts, EP has evolved a series of "tapping" protocols in which the major acupuncture meridians are self-activated by finger tapping or pressure at the same time that psychologically problematic material is being discussed or thought about by the patient. In a sort of "flushing out" process, the EFT activations are thought to clear or balance negative emotions. Anecdotal evidence is prolific, but well designed studies are few and far between. The following vignette is illustrative of EFT's potential in myofascial pain syndrome. Figure 3 shows a common EFT protocol.

5.2.1. Case Example: EFT and Post Traumatic Stress Disorder

Maria was a 35-year-old woman who received mild concussion and cervical hyperextension injuries in a boating accident. Her neck and shoulder pain syndrome was largely myofascial in nature and responded only minimally to standard stress management training and stretching/strengthening exercises in physical therapy. During a course of EFT, she was able to access memories of the event (she was able to remember her subjective experience of the time when she was outwardly appeared to be unconscious) in a way that triggered a dramatic healing response. She described this recovery of memory as being psychologically crucial to restoring her sense of wholeness. Within minutes of completing the EFT process, she was able to demonstrate full range of motion in her neck and shoulder, and her pain level almost completely disappeared (for a more detailed discussion of the case, see reference 35).

5.3. Reiki

Reiki has become the most widely known of the hands-on energy therapies, in part due to the apparent ease of training—typically attendance at a weekend workshop grants

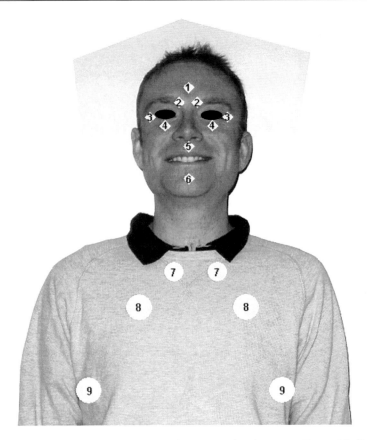

Fig. 3. Acupressure points used in EFT protocol *(from E. Leskowitz: www.EnergyMedicine101.com).*

the practitioner Level 1 mastery. No graduate-level training or clinical experience is required, as it is not intended to be restricted to healthcare professionals; an estimated 80,000 Americans have been trained in the past year *(36)*. A recent research review *(37)* highlights the current challenges of working within a medical model. As with TT, the most tightly controlled studies demonstrated subjective improvements rather than organic changes. The method itself was introduced to America about 70 years ago from Japan, and involves direct hand contact to transmit a healing energy that the practitioner has been attuned to receive and transmit. No specific diagnostic steps are taken, nor does the practitioner intentionally modify the healing energy in any way. Distant healing is also felt to occur in certain forms of Reiki.

5.4. Homeopathy

Homeopathy is the energy modality that is most amenable to randomized controlled trials (RCTs) with blinded methodology because the protocols can be adapted from pharmaceutical testing. An extensive supportive literature exists, showing that in many conditions—asthma, infant diarrhea, otitis, etc.—the benefits of homeopathy are clear and not explicable by placebo or expectancy factors *(38,39)*. However, the literature on homeopathy for pain illustrates another common pitfall of assessing energy modalities. In classic homeopathic prescribing, the clinician arrives at a designated individualized remedy after detailed history taking; three patients with allopathically similar diagnoses (fever and productive cough, for example) might receive three different homeopathic remedies. However, research protocols are often set up to offer only a limited number of treatment options—in an extreme example with a widely reported negative finding, 500 marathon runners were all treated with the same remedy at identical dosages. They did not respond positively to a statistically significant degree *(39)*. However, lack of individualized prescribing, and suboptimal dosing render these study results meaningless.

By contrast, a more appropriately designed trial of homeopathy for fibromyalgia *(18)* included fully individualized dosing and generated positive results in treating this notoriously refractory condition. A subgroup of excellent responders was identified, not only by clinical response, but also by using a novel form of EEG screening (alpha concordance measurement) to identify likely positive responders to homeopathy.

5.5. Acupuncture

For a discussion of the wide range of clinical uses of acupuncture in pain management, refer to Chapter 17.

6. SAFETY

Practitioners of energy medicine typically stress the safety of energy interventions relative to allopathic medicine. The incidence of clinically significant side effects is miniscule in such modalities as Reiki and TT, while homeopathy does acknowledge the phenomenon of the "healing crisis" during which symptoms initially increase after a treatment until the body's innate vigor can overcome the symptom and return to a state of greater balance. A similar process of initial symptom exacerbation is described in the acupuncture and energy healing literature. However, emergent symptoms are usually mild enough (headache, jitteriness, muscle soreness) that simple supportive measures like fluid and bed rest are sufficient to resolve the problem. Hence, contraindications are practically nonexistent for energy therapies.

There is, however, a distinct possibility of energy "overdose" in certain situations. Patients must become familiar and comfortable with energy sensations in order to work optimally with the healing process, and overzealous use of "high voltage" interventions early on can backfire, with patient drop out a possible result. In addition, some patients may become so enraptured with the internal energy states cultivated using techniques like tai chi or qi gong that intensive practice regimens can lead to fairly violent purgings, typically manifested in such psychological symptoms as anxiety and agitation. Obviously, some patients will be more sensitive than others to these effects, and a teacher, mentor or clinician should be available to attend to these dynamics.

There is another important caveat to be made in patient selection for some of the hands-on forms of energy therapy. Specifically, patients with a prior history of abuse (physical, emotional, or sexual) should be offered hands-on treatment only after careful psychological screening. Manual treatments may sometimes be experienced, either consciously or unconsciously, as boundary violations that re-traumatize the patient and lead to a flare-up of PTSD symptoms or borderline personality behaviors.

Hence, psychological training should be a core component of any training program for the energy practitioner. The growing subgroup of energy workers who hold advanced degrees in mental health is at the forefront of this issue. In the absence of such expert dually trained providers, a conventional clinician referring to an energy therapist should enquire about back-up psychological support. This may be available in the form of psychologists or psychiatrists with whom the energy practitioner has an ongoing collegial referral relationship.

6.1. Contraindications

As mentioned previously, hands-on therapies must be used with care in the presence of co-morbid psychiatric conditions. One important psychiatric contraindication would be a diagnosis of borderline personality disorder or history of abuse or PTSD (these three often co-exist). A good outline of how to pursue psychotherapy of these patients while remaining sensitive to their energetic boundary issues is available *(40)*. Psychotic states can sometimes be calmed by energy interventions, but their use depends on the existence of a prior relationship of trust with the provider, and in general should be approached very cautiously.

6.2. Precautions

In common with other passive therapies like massage or craniosacral treatment, hands-on energy techniques like TT and Reiki can foster dependence in patients—not in the sense of drug dependence or tolerance, but in the sense of reliance on others for treatment. Given that most pain management programs stress the development of self-management skills, this dependency potential can become an obstacle in patients who gain secondary benefits from being in the passive patient role (i.e., increased attention, decreased responsibility, etc.). Fortunately, most energy therapies can be adapted to become self-administered, such as self-acupressure, self-Reiki, and qi gong training. Their use, therefore, need not be in opposition to the overarching treatment philosophy of patient independence.

Adverse interactions between energy therapies and traditional medical treatments are rare. Prescription pharmaceuticals, however, are believed by many energy practitioners to create their own disruptions of energy fields, and the treatment goal of energy therapy is often to taper and ultimately discontinue prescription medications. Obviously, an integrative and collaborative approach best serves the majority of patients. For example, tapering off of opiate medications can sometimes proceed safely when the patient's innate energy flows are reconstituted by appropriate energy interventions. In general, central nervous system depressants like opioids, tranquilizers, and hypnotic agents impair the efficacy of energy therapies, with practitioners reporting a sense that energy movement is more sluggish in these patients. Research on this issue has not developed beyond the level of individual case reports.

7. MODELS OF INTEGRATION

One possible model of integration of energy therapies into a pain medicine practice is to train the clinician members of an interdisciplinary pain treatment team in various energy healing modalities. By developing and monitoring the plan of care for all patients in regular Patient Care Conferences (PCCs), the interdisciplinary team, which includes physicians, psychologists, nurses, and physical and occupational therapists, functions as a forum where all aspects of healing can be addressed. When issues arise that are outside an individual provider's scope of expertise, a colleague's assistance is easily sought. For example, if emotional issues surface during the course of manual therapy with PT, a referral to the team psychologist can be made to help deal with the underlying issues, whether trauma, depression, or secondary gain.

In such settings, a "cross-training" model of integration is frequently employed. Staff energy medicine practitioners would all have expertise, credentials, and licensure as conventional medical practitioners. For example, the team could consist of a Registered Nurse with Barbara Brennan Energy Healer training, an Energy Psychology therapist who is a psychiatrist, a physician acupuncturist, and physical and occupational therapists who practice Tai Chi, acupressure, and Reiki therapies.

8. SCOPE OF PRACTICE

In the above model, energy clinicians are dually trained, while operating under their primary conventional license. They follow the scope of practice restrictions of their conventional discipline, and use consultations with colleagues to address potential boundary issues.

9. COST STRUCTURE

Billing issues can be problematic, given that energy therapies are not covered by most health insurance plans as of yet. However, in inpatients settings, these services can often be bundled into the day rates for hospital services so that the patients do not accrue an additional charge. For example, the salaried RN can do TT without needing to bill for it as a separate procedure. In the outpatient setting, patients may either be charged out-of-pocket for an energy intervention (particularly acupuncture or Reiki), or at other times energy treatments may be integrated into a procedure that is already covered by insurance (i.e., EFT desensitization as part of psychotherapy). Within the Worker's Compensation system, it is sometimes possible to negotiate for coverage of a course of energy therapy, especially acupuncture.

Other funding options include the use of a sliding scale to set self-pay rates and obtaining foundation funding to either subsidize treatment costs or to pay directly for a therapist's salary. There is also the time-honored option of practitioners performing their services pro bono. It should be remembered that after the initial consultation with a homeopathic provider, the remedies themselves are often quite inexpensive, costing only a few dollars per month.

10. TRAINING STANDARDS

- Reiki: Level 1 after two weekend workshops (12 hours); Level 2 (distant healing) requires an additional workshop. Different traditions within Reiki use the term "Master" to refer to varying levels of training.
- Barbara Brennan School of Healing: 4-year program with quarterly residential trainings (5 days), including lectures and supervised practice; students are also required to undergo a course of individual psychotherapy during their training. No state certification or licensure is currently required or available.
- Therapeutic Touch: 3 levels of certification, as practitioner, teacher and mentor.
- Association of Comprehensive Energy Psychology (ACEP): Annual conference with workshops: a program is being developed by ACEP for formal certification that requires a minimum number of approved workshop attendance and clinical supervision hours.

- Healing Touch (HT): Five stages of training are required to become a fully certified HT practitioner, totaling 100 hours; further training is required to be certified as an instructor.

11. LICENSING AND LIABILITY

As of this writing, acupuncture and homeopathy practitioners are the only energy therapists required by most state boards to obtain licensure. There is great variability among the states in the development of licensure and liability standards for the range of energy therapies. Several references provide specific information on the ethics, malpractice issues and licensing process of various energy practices *(41,42)*.

12. RESOURCES FOR TRAINING AND PRACTITIONER AVAILABILITY

- Reiki: No nationally recognized central organization or clearinghouse exists; www.reikialliance.com is a useful starting point.
- Therapeutic Touch: www.therapeutic-touch.org
- Barbara Brennan School of Healing: www.barbarabrennan.com
- Energy Psychology (Association of Comprehensive Energy Psychology): www.energypsych.org
- Healing Touch: www.healingtouchinternational.org

REFERENCES

1. Flor H, Fydrich T, Turk, DC. Efficacy of multidisciplinary pain treatment cetners: a meta-analytic review. Pain 1992;49(2):221–230.
2. McCraty R, Childre D. The appreciative heart: the psychophysiology of positive emotions and optimal functioning, 2003. Available at: http://www.heartmath.org/.
3. Green E, Parks P, Buher P, Fahrion S, Coyne L. Anomalous electrostatic phenomena in exceptional subjects. Subtle Energies 1992;2(3):69–94.
4. Kwok G, Cohen M, Cosic I. Mapping acupuncture points using multi-channel device. Austalas Phys Eng Sci Med 1998;21(2):68–72.
5. Schlebusch K-P, Maric-Oehler W, Popp F-A. Biophotonics in the infrared spectral range reveal acupuncture meridian structure. J Alt Comp Med 2005;11(1):171–174.
6. Myss C, Norman S. The Creation of Health, Walpole NH:Stillpoint Press.
7. Brennan B. 1990. Hands of Light. NY: Bantam New Age.
8. Bruyere, R. 1994. Wheels of Light:Chakras, Auras, and the Healing Energy of the Body. NY: Fireside/Harper Collins.
9. Becker R. 1990. CrossCurrents: The Perils of Electropollution, the Promise of Electromedicine. Bear and Co.
10. Kepner J. Energy and the nervous system in embodied experience. Available at http://www.pathwaysforhealing.com/resources.html.
11. Melzack R, Stillwell D, Fox S. Trigger points and acupuncture points for pain:correlations and implications. Pain 1977;3:3–23.
12. Travell J, Simons D. 1983. Myofascial Pain and Dysfunction: The Trigger Point Manual, Baltimore MD: Williams and Wilkins.
13. Colbert A, Hammerschlag R, Aickin M, Mcnames J. Reliability of the Prognos electrodermal device for measurements of electrical skin resistance at acupuncture points. J Alt Comp Med 2004;10(4): 610–616.
14. Borg-Stein J, Stein J. Trigger points and tender points: One and the same? Does injection treatment help? Rheum Dis Clin North Am 1996;22(2):305–322.
15. Fries E, Hesse J, Helhammer J, Helhammer D. A new view on hypocortisolism, Psychoneuroendocrinology 2005;30(10):1010–1016.
16. Moldofsky H. Sleep and musculoskeletal pain. Am J Med 1986;81(3A):85–89.

17. Bell I, Lewis D, Schwartz G, Lewis S, Caspi O, Scott A, Brooks A, Baldwin C. Electroencephalographic concordance patterns distinguish exceptional clinical responders with fibromyalgia to individualized homeopathic medicines. J Alt Comp Med 2004;10(2):285–300.

18. Teitlebaum J. Effective treatment of chronic fatigue syndrome and fibromyalgia—a randomized, double-blind, placebo-controlled, intent to treat study. J Chr Fatigue Synd 2001;8(2).

19. Bailey A, Audette J. 2007 Complex Regional Pain Syndrome. In: Essentails of Physical Medicine and Rehabilitation. Elsevier, St. Louis MO. 2nd edition. Frontera W, Silver J, Robinson L, Eds. (In press).

20. Ochoa JL, Verdugo MJ. Reflex sympathetic dystrophy: a common clinical avenue for somatoform expression. Neurol Clin 1995;13(2):351–363.

21. Goldberg RT, Pachas WN, Keith D. Relationship between traumatic events in childhood and chronic pain. Disabil Rehabil 1999;21(1):23–30.

22. Sherry DD, et al. Short- and long-term outcomes of children with CRPS type I treated with exercise therapy. Clin J Pain 1999;15(3):218–223.

23. Moseley, GL. Graded motor imagery for pathologic pain: a randomized controlled study. Neurology 2006;67:2129–2134.

24. Bradbrook, D. Acupuncture treatment of phantom limb pain and phantom limb sensation in amputees. Acupunct Med (UK) 2004;22(2): 93–97.

25. Worsley J. 1973. In The Kirlian Aura: Photographing the Galaxies of Life. Krippner S, Rubin D, Eds. NY: Doubleday Anchor, p. 165.

26. Leskowitz, E. Phantom limb pain: subtle energy perspectives. Subtle Energy Energy Med 2001;8(2):125–152.

27. Mulloney S, Wells-Federman C. Therapeutic TOUCH: a healing modality. J Cardiovasc Nurs 1996;18(3):v-x.

28. Rosa L, Rosa E, Sarner L, Barrett S. A close look at Therapeutic Touch, JAMA 1998;279:1005–1101.

29. Leskowitz E. Un-Debunking Therapeutic Touch, Alt Ther Health Med 1998;4(4):101–102.

30. Wirth D. The effect of non-contact therapeutic touch on the rate of healing of full thickness dermal wounds. Subtle Energies 1990;1(1):1–20.

31. Solfvin J, Benor DJ, Leskowitz E. Concerning the work of Daniel P. Wirth (letter). J Altern Complem Med 2006;11(6):949–950.

32. Leskowitz E. Phantom limb pain treated with therapeutic touch: a case report. Arch Phys Med Rehabil 2000;81:522–524.

33. Emotional Freedom Technique: http://www.emofree.com/

34. Feinstein D. The promise of energy psychology, Tarcher, 2005.

35. Leskowitz E. Nonlocal and subtle energetic aspects of chronic pain, Altern Ther Health Med 2001;7(5):144–145.

36. Reiki: http://www.reiki.com/

37. Miles P, True G. Reiki: a review of a biofield therapy history, theory, practice and research. Alt Ther Health Med 2003;9(2):62–72.

38. Walach H, Jonas W, Ives J, Wijk K, Weingartner O. Research on homeopathy: state of the art. J Alt Comp Med 2005; 11(5):813–829.

39. Vickers AJ, Fisher P, Smith L, Wylie S, Rees R. Homeopathic arnica 30x is ineffective for muscle soreness after long-distance running: a randomized, double-blind, placebo controlled trial. Clin J Pain 1998;14:227–231.

40. Kepner J. 1993. Body Process: Body-Centered Psychotherapy. Jossey-Bass, San Francisco, CA.

41. Cohen M. http://www.camlawblog.com/

42. Cohen M. 2003. Future Medicine: Ethical Dilemmas, Regulatory Challenges, and Therapeutic Pathways to Health Care and Healing in Human Transformation. Ann Arbor, MI: University of Michigan Press.

12 Tai Chi in Pain Medicine

Joseph F. Audette

CONTENTS

INTRODUCTION
HISTORY AND PHILOSOPHY
TRAINING
MECHANISM OF ACTION
TAI CHI FOR PAIN MANAGEMENT
FUTURE RESEARCH
PRACTICAL CONSIDERATIONS
CONCLUSION

Summary

Tai Chi Chuan (TCC) was developed many centuries ago as one of many different styles of Chinese martial arts and continues to be enjoyed in a form true to its beginnings throughout the world. The name is derived from the Chinese characters that mean "The Great Ultimate," indicating the high historic regard that exists for this physical art. On a philosophical level, the principles of TCC are founded on the teachings of Taoism and the writings of Lao Tzu (770–221 B.C.E.). The central method of achieving tranquility was to align oneself with the *Tao*, a term which has been translated as "the way" or "the path." These philosophical roots point to the fact that Tai Chi practice places great emphasis on training both the mind and the body to reach spiritual unity. In this chapter, TCC will be introduced as a therapeutic exercise rather than a martial art. Information about the history and philosophy of TCC will also be provided with a detailed review of the scientific literature, particularly for pain management. Finally, two case examples of the practical application of TCC for painful conditions will be given.

Key Words: Tai Chi, Qi Gong, pain, arthritis, elderly, balance, heart rate variability

1. INTRODUCTION

There is growing understanding both among patients and healthcare practitioners that the modern biomedical healthcare model is not equally effective for all types and stages of illness. The tremendous advancements in medical technology over the last 60 years have not been as helpful as we would like in treating individuals with chronic disease, especially those with persistently painful conditions. As a result, many in the healthcare community have looked to the medical wisdom of our historic past to find alternative solutions to modern problems, especially in the area of health promotion, disease prevention, and pain management. A particularly rich area of ancient knowledge

From: *Contemporary Pain Medicine: Integrative Pain Medicine: The Science and Practice of Complementary and Alternative Medicine in Pain Management*
Edited by: J. F. Audette and A. Bailey © Humana Press, Totowa, NJ

can be found by exploring the health value of movement therapies. These exercises offer great potential for informing new therapies in the rehabilitation and pain arena for the treatment of a variety of chronic conditions.

There are a number of Eastern movement practices that have gained popularity in the West. These include Tai Chi, Qigong, and Yoga. Although each of these practices has a distinct origin, the current focus of research and general use is to apply these movements to the development of physical, mental, emotional, and spiritual well being, as well as disease prevention and treatment. Unique among these, Tai Chi Chuan (TCC) had clear martial beginnings and was considered an effective means of self-defense. In the last 50 to 70 years, however, the primary application of this ancient art has been directed at health promotion.

2. HISTORY AND PHILOSOPHY

Tai Chi Chuan (TCC) (also written as Tai Chi, Tai Chi Quan, Taijiquan, or T'ai Chi) developed many centuries ago as one of many different styles of Chinese martial arts and continues to be enjoyed in a form true to its beginnings throughout the world. The name is derived from the Chinese characters that mean "The Great Ultimate" (Figure 1). This refers to the dynamic and fundamental balance between opposites in the universe (Yin or unity balanced with Yang or change).

Taoist theories of health and longevity are based in part on the theory that exercise practices such as TCC that can enhance the flow and balance of Qi or vital energy. Disease is believed to occur when the Qi is out of balance or blocked, and TCC is one of a number of techniques used to help restore this dynamic, energetic equilibrium in the body. Even today, the practice of TCC is an important feature of the Chinese approach to health maintenance and disease prevention and the practice continues to be taught to students in traditional Chinese medical schools. As anyone who has visited

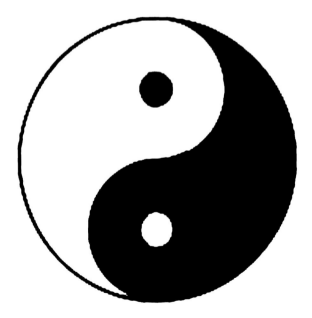

Fig. 1. The Great Ultimate.

China knows, TCC has also become popular among Chinese elders who practice in large numbers in the streets and parks of China for primarily the health benefits.

The historical origins of TCC are controversial and steeped in legend. Douglas Wile has sorted the various historical accounts into different categories to help with the scholarly endeavor of tracing back the true beginnings of this unusual form of exercise. Conceptually, TCC can be traced back to its philosophical origins, the origins of various training techniques and combat strategies, and the origins of the modern postures and forms *(1)*.

On a philosophical level, the principles of TCC are founded on the teachings of Taoism and the writings of Lao Tzu (770–221 B.C.E.). The central method of achieving tranquility was to align oneself with the *Tao*, a term which has been translated as "the way" or "the path." The Tao is the central mystical underpinning of Lao Tzu's philosophy and is characterized as the formless, unfathomable source of all things. Historically, at the very least, the writings of Lao Tzu have provided ample inspiration for the movements and theory of Tai Chi. Lao Tzu writes, "Yield and overcome. Bend and be straight." "Returning is the motion of the Tao. Yielding is the way of the Tao." "Stiff and unbending is the principle of death. Gentle and yielding is the principle of life" *(2)*.

Legend has it that the synthesis between Taoist thought and TCC movements occurred some eight centuries ago with Chang San-feng. The available historical data suggests that Chang San-feng may have lived as long ago as the Sung period (960–1279) or as late as the Ming (1368–1644). A legendary Taoist priest, it is told that he developed Tai Chi-like movements based on the inspiration of observing a fight between a crane and a snake. In this skirmish, he saw how the soft and yielding could overcome the hard and inflexible. The fundamental wisdom of self-defense lay in the knowledge of softness in the face of strength. The principles of yielding, softness, slowness, balance, suppleness, and remaining rooted and centered are essential tenets of Taoist philosophy that Tai Chi has drawn upon in its understanding of movement, both in relation to health and also in its martial applications.

The legend of Chang Sang-feng is tied to the present with the publication of Huang Tsung-hi's (1610–95) *Epitaph for Wang Cheng-nan*, and his son Pai-chia's work; *Methods of the Internal School of Pugilism (3)*. These writings organize various systems of martial arts into internal (soft) and external (hard) styles. The underlying principle of an internal school is illustrated by the aphorism "stillness overcoming movement." Internal styles of martial arts reversed the principles of the older Shao-lin Temple styles where only superior force could win. Pai-chia traces the transmission of this philosophy of pugilism back to Chang Sang-feng. TCC was subsequently labeled as an internal style and as a result, identified with the Chang San-feng legend, without there being direct evidence of more than a philosophical connection to modern styles.

3. TRAINING

In subsequent years foreign invasions of China and domestic peasant uprisings stimulated the diffusion of martial arts among the people. With the destruction of the Shao-lin temple, a new form of boxing evolved and developed with the Chen family that closely resembles styles of TCC practiced today (Chen family boxing 1771–1853). The Yang family then inherited and transformed the Chen Tai Chi movements (Yang Lu-ch'an 1799–1872), and then later the Wu family (Wu Chien-ch'üan 1870–1942), and the Sun family (Sun Lu-t'ang 1861–1932) created distinct styles *(1)*.

Based on these early family traditions, there are several styles of Tai Chi currently practiced (five main schools, and numerous subdivisions under each school): Chen (quick and slow, large movements), Yang (slow, large movement), Wu (mid-paced, compact), Sun (quick, compact), and Hao style (related to the Wu style). Among these styles, Chen is the oldest, and Yang is the most commonly practiced (see Table 1).

There are 108 movements in the traditional long form of the Yang style. Yang Ch'eng-fu (1883–1936, grandson of Yang Lu-ch'an) is credited with establishing the Yang style of TCC as the dominant internal martial art system in China. His period of greatest influence was in the 1920s and 1930s. Perhaps Yang Ch'eng-fu's most famous student in the United States was Professor Cheng Man-ch'ing (1900–1975), who taught in New York for many years and has published a number of books on Tai Chi (4). He created a shortened version of the Yang style that is 37 movements long and has many adherents in the United States, including the late T.T. Liang. Another accomplished student of Yang Ch'eng-fu's was Han Ch'in-tang. Han Ch'in-tang also studied with Yang Ch'eng-fu's older brother, Yang Shao-hou, whose style was more compact than his younger brother. Currently, Han Ch'in-tang's son-in-law, Leung Kai-chi, and daughter, Han Lin, teach in the United States and continue the tradition of teaching the long form of the Yang style.

In the 1950s, a National Physical Fitness Program incorporating TCC was first instituted in China. A simplified set of TCC exercise based on the most popular sequences of the Yang school was issued in 1956 by the Chinese National Athletic Committee. This form consists of 24 movements which progress logically from the

Table 1
Tai Chi Styles

Style	Historical background	Comments
Chen	Chen family boxing (1771–1853)	Quick and slow, large movements, more martial and powerful in appearance
Yang	Yang Lu-ch'an (1799–1872) and later his grandson Yang Ch'eng-fu (1883–1936)	Slow, large movement
Wu (Jianchuan)	Wu Chien-ch'üan (1870–1942), who learned from his father a student of Yang	Mid-paced, compact
Hao (Sometimes also referred to Wu style)	Wu Yu-hs'iang (1812–1880), who learned the style from Yang and another Chen family member who then passed the style on to Hao Weizheng (1849–1920)	Slow and loose movements which are close-knit that combine elements of Yang and Chen style
Sun	Sun Lu-t'ang (1861–1932), who learned from Hao who had prior training	Quick, compact

easy to the difficult and which takes five minutes to complete. Finally, TCC was first included in the martial arts division of the 11th Asian games in 1990.

4. MECHANISM OF ACTION

TCC is now predominantly used as a therapeutic exercise, both in China and in the West. There is evidence that TCC can have a significant positive effect on reducing frailty and improving strength, balance and fitness, especially in the elderly (5). In addition to the health benefits associated with TCC practice gained from improved cardiovascular fitness (see Chapter 8), TCC also incorporates a form of cognitive, mindfulness training (see Chapter 9). Much like Qi Gong, TCC has been shown to have a positive effect on mood and measures of general well being that may be related to this cognitive component of TCC training (6,7).

Our knowledge about the influence of cognitive states and the relaxation response on health and disease has greatly increased in the last 10 years. Little attention, however, has been given to the physiological relationship between exercise and the relaxation response nor has work been done to compare their relative health benefits. Clearly, the potential health benefits of cognitive and physical practices are not the same, as has been illustrated in a recent study, where a 4-month stress management intervention was found to be superior to an exercise intervention in reducing ischemic events in patients with coronary artery disease (8). In addition, there has not been a great deal of research looking at whether there is an additive effect on physiologic outcomes when combining the relaxation response with exercise.

In an attempt to better understand this relationship, low and moderate intensity walking was compared to a mindfulness exercise group performing TCC to determine if the cognitive effect of TCC provided a therapeutic benefit over and above its exercise effect. Subjects were sedentary adults (69 woman and 66 men) randomized to light to moderate walking exercise without a mindfulness component versus TCC. Outcome measures included self-assessment questionnaires measuring different domains of mood and general health. The most significant finding was that woman in the TCC group experienced significant improvements in depression scores and other measures of mood disturbance when compared to the walking interventions (9). The men did not show the same response to TCC. This difference between the male and female response to TCC may reflect interesting differences in the willingness to learn the cognitive aspects of TCC.

A study by Jin compared 33 experienced TCC practitioners with 33 beginners (total group age range, 16–75) (10). The experienced practitioners exhibited increased heart rate, increased noradrenaline excretion in urine, but decreased salivary cortisol concentration following practice when compared to the beginners. It was noted in the study that the more experienced group had lower, more strenuous postures during the movements, thus practice inducing a higher heart rate response and stronger catecholamine activation. However, the greater physical stress of the practice was not accompanied by an increase in cortisol levels, as would normally be expected. These data are compatible with the notion that experienced TCC practitioners are less stress reactive due to the induction of the relaxation response during exercise.

Chen has reviewed the effects of Tai Chi when used as a technique to reduce stress–elated illnesses, such as pain, mood disorders, and nightmares. In one study reviewed, the effectiveness of mind–body interventions in reducing chronic low back pain was assessed. The mind–body interventions including education, relaxation response training, and movement therapy (Tai Chi or Qigong) were taught in combination. All groups were matched relative to gender, age, and pain scores on visual analog scales. Findings confirmed that this combination of mind–body interventions produced an improvement in affective mood state, pain perception, and functional state *(11)*. However, because of the combined therapies, the specific outcome effect of TCC is not known.

Jin reported that mood states became more positive during TCC, and they remained positive even one hour following the exercise. Relative to base line levels subjects reported less tension, depression, anger, fatigue, confusion, and state anxiety, felt more vigorous and, in general, had less total mood disturbance during and after Tai Chi *(12)*. Similar findings have been found in a population of patients with Multiple Sclerosis following TCC practice *(13)*.

Finally, there may be some influence on healing that comes from slow stretch on the fascia given the slow repetitive movements of TCC based on the theory outline by Langevin (see Chapter 6).

5. TAI CHI FOR PAIN MANAGEMENT

Tai Chi is a CAM movement therapy that is especially popular among the elderly because of the gentle nature of the exercise, safety, and low cost *(14)*. By the year 2030, people older than 65 will comprise 20% of the total population in the United States *(15)*. In a recent large survey, the most common explanation for disability reported by older persons is musculoskeletal pain *(16)*. Whether due to arthritic or non-arthritic causes, pain is a major factor in disability in this age group even when other impairments and symptoms are taken into account *(17,18)*. Although pain, in and of itself, is a primary concern to elderly, it is the associated impairments that have the most devastating impact on quality of life and morbidity and mortality *(19)*. For example, musculoskeletal pain has been found to be a substantial risk factor for falls in older women with disabilities *(20)*.

There are no standards for the treatment of pain in the elderly and, as has been seen in younger populations, given the lack of guidance, the elderly are increasingly seeking complementary and alternative medical (CAM) treatments for the treatment of chronic pain *(21)*. In a survey of elderly with chronic pain by Lansbury, it was found that the least preferred treatment by elderly are conventional treatments that involve use of medications, exercise or physical therapy while they are turning more to CAM modalities *(22)*. Others have found a poor tolerability of pharmacological interventions in the elder population with greater risks for falls and complications from the adverse cognitive side effects *(23)*. Eisenberg has reported low back pain and arthritis as two of the top five conditions for which people over 65 years of age seek CAM treatment *(24)*. In addition, a recent survey of 3 ethnically diverse, elderly populations has shown a high proportion of CAM use in these groups as well *(25)*.

5.1. Significance of a Sedentary Lifestyle in Chronic Pain

A Sedentary lifestyle across all age groups, but particularly with the elderly, has serious adverse health consequences, including diminished quality of life, reduced functional capacity, increased risk for cardiovascular morbidity and mortality, and increased medical costs *(26–28)*. Poor exercise capacity has been found to be a powerful predictor of subsequent cardiovascular related mortality and all-cause mortality in both men and woman *(29–38)*. In fact, poor cardiovascular fitness is a more important risk factor for all-cause mortality than is obesity *(39)*. Regular physical activity and general aerobic fitness has been found to be protective against mortality risks with some evidence that the response to exercise follows a normal dose-response curve *(40–42)*. In particular, in the elderly, adherence to a regular exercise program or increased leisure time physical activity has been found to be protective from all-cause mortality *(43–46)*. The implications of these findings for the chronic pain population are significant, as persistent pain has been found to be an independent risk factor for a sedentary lifestyle in an elderly Canadian population with arthritis *(47)*.

5.2. Autonomic Nervous System Response to Exercise and Its Clinical Implications

A number of physiologic mechanisms have been proposed to explain how physical activity might decrease the risk of cardiovascular morbidity and mortality in normal elderly subjects and in elderly with heart disease and these same factors may apply to sedentary elderly with chronic pain. The primary and common denominator among all of these mechanisms appears to be a shift in autonomic balance, specifically the augmentation of parasympathetic activity with increased activity or fitness. Exercise in the elderly is known to cause positive changes in autonomic regulation of blood pressure and circulation, which may also influence pain modulation *(48,49)*. Cardiac parasympathetic tone can be determined in an individual with ECG monitoring to provide measures of heart rate variability (HRV) where increased variability is found with more parasympathetic input. There is a steady decline in HRV with age, and low HRV has been shown to predict risk of coronary heart disease and mortality in the elderly *(50,51)*.

There is a significant relationship between exercise and improved autonomic control of the heart, and this improvement has been shown to take place in people of all ages *(52–55)*. For example, in patients with moderate to severe congestive heart failure, exercise training lead to increased parasympathetic cardiovascular control *(56)*. These autonomic effects of regular physical activity are seen in healthy individuals as well as patients with CAD, in young and aged subjects *(30,57–60)*. Given the variety of treatments possible for elders who have pain, it would be of considerable value to recommend an intervention that can influence both pain, function, mobility and fitness especially with reference to the changes in the autonomic nervous system, and the evidence presented below suggests that TCC is unique in being able to effect these outcomes.

5.3. Effect of Tai Chi Chuan on Pain in the Elderly

We hypothesize, as have others, that because the literature suggests that TCC has significant impact on measures of fitness, function, and psychosocial quality of life, that there may also be a positive influence on chronic pain *(61)*. TCC has been shown to be well tolerated in the elderly, even in subjects with rheumatoid arthritis *(62,63)*. A recent study specifically looked at the effect of TCC on elderly with osteoarthritic (OA) knee pain and showed significant improvements in pain, stiffness and perceived difficulty in physical functioning *(64)*. An abbreviated Sun style of TCC (12 movements) was used because it was hypothesized that the higher stance used with this style would put less stress on the subjects arthritic joints. In this study, 72 subjects with knee OA mean age 63 were randomized to either a 12 week course of TCC versus a sedentary control group. Diagnosis of OA was made using the American College of Rheumatology classification and plain films with degenerative changes based on the Kellgren-Lawrence scale grading of ≥2. Outcomes included the Korean Western Ontario and McMaster Osteoarthritis Index (K-WOMAC), and measures of balance, strength, flexibility, and cardiovascular conditioning. At conclusion of the study intervention there was a significant reduction in the joint pain, and stiffness, as well as an improvement in physical function subscores on the K-WOMAC when compared to the sedentary controls. This change was found without there being a significant change in the cardiovascular conditioning of the participants as measured by a standard sub-maximal exercise bike test, suggesting that the beneficial pain response was not due to the possible aerobic conditioning effect of TCC.

5.4. Effect of TCC on Function in Elderly

TCC has also been shown to have a significant effect on reducing frailty in the elderly with positive benefits on improving measures of psychosocial well-being, lower extremity strength, balance and, importantly, falls reduction *(6,65–67)*. A recent review of the effect of TCC on postural control provides a detailed summary on the positive effect of TCC on lower extremity strength, increased joint flexibility, improved single leg stance times, and other measures of balance *(68)*. Other randomized controlled studies have shown significant improvements in measures of function and ADL's with Tai Chi interventions of 8 to 24 weeks in older adults using a subset of questions focused on the physical functioning domain of the Medical Outcomes Study Questionnaire (SF-36) when compared to sedentary control groups *(7,69)*.

5.5. Effect of TCC on Cardiovascular Fitness

There is a growing literature that suggests that TCC has a measurable effect on cardiovascular and physical fitness in the elderly *(70–76)*. The metabolic demand of Tai Chi has been shown in a number of studies to be equivalent to light to moderate aerobic activity, depending on the TCC form practiced and the age group studied. In one study of men and woman from age 58 to 70 years old using the 108 movement Yang style of TCC, the exercise intensity was 52–63% of the predicted target heart rate *(71)*. In a comparison of the metabolic energy equivalents (MET's) of the TCC short-form (24 movements) with that of the long-form (108 movements), the short form was estimated to cost about 2.9 MET's, compared to 4.1 MET's for the long form *(77)*. In another study of a modified short form of TCC called T'ai Chi Ch'ih, the MET's were estimated to be 1.5 when doing the movements in a sitting position, 2.3 MET's for slow standing movements, and 2.6 for the same form but with a faster pace. In this group, mean maximum heart rates ranged from 43% to 49% of the predicted maximum heart rate for age. An 8% increase in mean systolic and diastolic blood pressures was observed during TCC. There was no difference in response to the movements by gender or experience with Tai Chi exercise *(78)*. Table 2 summarizes the current research on the metabolic demand of different TCC styles relative to brisk walking.

These studies confirm that a gentle style of TCC requires energy expenditure comparable a moderate walking pace and would be safe for persons with low exercise

Table 2
Comparison of the Metabolic Demands and Changes in Heart Rate Seen in TCC

Author	Tai Chi style	METs	HR (% of max)	Equivalent activity
Zhuo	Yang long form	4.1		Brisk walking (3.5 mph)
	Yang short form	2.9		Walking (3 mph)
Fontana	TC Ch'ih sitting	1.5		Sewing or eating
	TC Ch'ih slowly	2.3	43%	Slow walking (2–2.5 mph)
	TC Ch'ih fast	2.6	49%	Walking (2.5 mph)
Lan	Yang long form		52–63%	
Lai	Yang long form		70%	
Jin	Yang long form		58%	Brisk walking (4 mph)
Schneider	Yang long form	4.6	59.8%	Brisk walking (4 mph)

tolerance. TCC has been shown in one study to have a positive effect on increasing HRV (79). In a recent study, 27 community-dwelling, sedentary women (average age 71.4 ± 4.5 years) were randomly assigned to Tai Chi Chuan (TCC; n = 11) or brisk-walking group (BWG; n = 8), with those that could not exercise 3 days a week assigned to a sedentary control group (SCG; n = 8) (80). The exercise groups met for 1 hour, 3 days per week for 12 weeks. Outcomes measured before and after training included estimated VO$_2$max and the spectral analysis of heart rate variability (high frequency, HFnu, and low frequency power, LFnu, in normalized units) as a measure of autonomic control of the heart. Significant improvement was seen in estimated VO$_2$max in the TCC group (TCC vs. SCG, p = 0.003; TCC vs. BWG, p = 0.08; BWG vs. SCG, p = 0.085). The mean within-person change for HFnu increased (8.2 [0.14 to16.3]), representing increased parasympathetic activity, and LFnu decreased (−8.7 [−16.8 to –0.5]), representing decrease sympathetic activity, in the TCC group only. Significant gains were also seen in the non-dominant knee extensor strength and single leg stance time (TCC vs. BWG, p < 0.05).

6. FUTURE RESEARCH

Most of the Tai Chi trials reviewed had a relatively small sample size. These factors limit our ability to generalize from the results of these studies. Another factor that must be considered when reviewing the effects of TCC is the influence of the practice parameters and style on the outcome. This is a problem that is found in other complementary and alternative interventions, where the skill of the practitioner has a great deal to do with the treatment effect.

Because TCC has many different styles, diverse movement protocols, and various teaching methods, researchers should have a solid understanding of the key elements of a particular TCC technique before implementing it in a study. When learning Tai Chi, a novice should be periodically evaluated on the progress and program adherence, such as cognitive response, muscular tension, balance, and flexibility to ensure optimal results.

Furthermore, longitudinal studies are essential to substantiate the long-term training effects of Tai Chi. This is particularly important with a practice like TCC that requires learning to integrate a state of deep cognitive relaxation with specific breathing and movement techniques and can not be learned quickly. Since this mind and body integration is essential for optimal benefit from the practice of TCC, the physiological effects are likely to be more pronounced with sustained practice.

7. PRACTICAL CONSIDERATIONS

TCC takes between 5 and 25 minutes to perform. When practicing Tai Chi, the lower body moves within a square, based on the four cardinal directions and their diagonals, while the upper body moves in multi-planed circles. The original intent of the circular movement was to allow the interception of aggression in a fluid motion and deflect it away. Today, the circular movements of the hips and waist promote flexibility and central balance. TCC training also teaches one to have an open, quiet mind. Training must emphasize complete relaxation, and effortless movement to achieve the intended results. A sense of grounded buoyancy must be achieved that Cheng Man-ch'ing related to the sensation of swimming or floating in air. From a martial point of view, this was felt to improve reaction time and enhance sensitivity to the actions of the opponent. Today with the focus on the health benefits of TCC, the importance of this sense of floating is still primary, as it allows integration of mindfulness and the relaxation response with conscious movement.

Despite the fact that the individual styles of TCC appear distinct, they share common properties. From a Taoist point of view, all TCC styles seek to balance and strengthen Qi (vital energy) in the body's meridians, consequently reducing the potential for developing serious illness. The *correct* practice of the styles then was motivated to enhance this balance. From a more pragmatic point of view, there are still certain essential elements to the modern practice of TCC that enhance the health benefits.

The first thing a beginner of TCC has to learn is to completely relax. This can be surprisingly difficult for many beginners. TCC practice encourages a state of cognitive relaxation that is similar to that found with meditation-based stress reduction techniques. Qigong breathing exercises, which are often incorporated in TCC practice, have been recognized to have a similar physiologic effect as mind-body relaxation techniques (81–83). This state of mindfulness meditation has been shown to have a regulating effect on the autonomic nervous system (84,85). Randomized studies of TCC in healthy subjects have had mixed results on measures of mood when compared to control groups. Shaller found no improvement in mood with a 10-week TCC intervention, but Ross found significant improvement in mood in a healthy elderly population (86,87). Finally, Li has found that TCC can improve self-efficacy, which may have an effect on improving exercise adherence (88), When commencing Tai Chi, progressive muscle relaxation techniques can be utlized to first relax the facial muscles, then the neck and shoulder muscles, and so on down the body to facilitate the relaxation response. Second, the pattern of movements must be accompanied by a sense of lightness or a floating sensation. To accomplish this, the body should be extended and relaxed, the elbows should always hang to the floor and not point out to the sides, and the body should be kept erect, as if there is a string pulling lightly on the crown of the head. Movements should not be exaggerated or forced, but flow from the center of mass below the umbilicus. Third, all movements require the well-coordinated sequencing of body segments. Awareness of this sequencing originates with the center of mass and involves rotation at the waist and upper hips. The movement then flows outward from this center balance point to propel the arms in circular movements. The movements progress in the semi-squat position and utilize the principle of single weighting, where the weight of the body continuously shifts from one leg to the next and back again without jerky or bobbing movements of the head and shoulders. Finally, breathing should be deep and regular. By using the diaphragm, each breath should expand the lower abdomen. With practice, the breath frequency should match the pace of the movements with each weight shift accompanied by the alternation of inhalation and expiration. Wolf has published a sequence of 10 TCC movements that he believes distills out these essential elements for practice in the elderly without being overly complex or physically demanding (Figure 2).

7.1. Case 1: Cerebral Palsy with Painful Spasticity

Eve is a 31-year-old woman with spastic paraparesis secondary to cerebral palsy. Although functional and independent in ambulation with bilateral loft-strand crutches, movement can often be seriously impaired by periods of excessive spasticity in her lower extremities that is accompanied by hip pain. Eve is generally intolerant of oral anti-spasticity agents due to cognitive clouding and fatigue. Standard physical therapy techniques such as stretching, proprioceptive neuromuscular facilitation (PNF), and progressive muscle relaxation techniques were only partially beneficial for relieving the episodes of excessive lower extremity tone. Eventually, Eve had the opportunity to attempt practice of a simplified form of TCC. The form had to be even further modified due to Eve's inability to stand without use of her crutches. This was accomplished by having Eve perform the practice sitting, but still motivated her arm movement

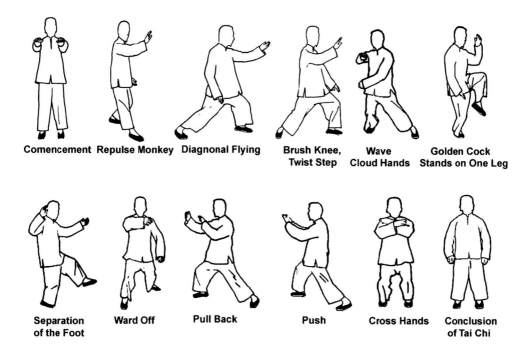

| Comencement | Repulse Monkey | Diagnonal Flying | Brush Knee, Twist Step | Wave Cloud Hands | Golden Cock Stands on One Leg |

| Separation of the Foot | Ward Off | Pull Back | Push | Cross Hands | Conclusion of Tai Chi |

Fig. 2. Standard movements used in Tai Chi Chuan practice.

from the area of her center of mass below the umbilicus. Her breathing pattern was diaphragmatic and timed with her movements. Practice two to three times per week had a profound effect on her normal ambulation and movements, dramatically reducing the episodes of incapacitating spasticity.

7.2. Case 2: Peripheral Neuropathy

Aida is a 53-year-old woman with a painful 5-year history of an ideopathic peripheral sensory polyneuropathy affecting her hands and feet. She experienced balance problems and pain related to the abnormal sensations in her extremities. She had become increasingly isolated and depressed as a result of the discomfort and was unable to exercise because use of her arms or legs would increase her pain. Tai Chi was started, initially focusing on gentle movements of her upper extremities in a standing position without moving her feet. Initially, this actually made her hand pain worse with increased stinging sensation in her hands and she wanted to stop after the first few sessions. However, with individual counseling, having her focus her mind onto her center of mass, below the umbilicus, she was able completely to eliminate the stinging sensations. Eventually, her exercise tolerance increased and she regained normal function for most activities.

8. CONCLUSION

TCC is known as a slow, smooth, and graceful form of Chinese exercise that includes a form of mindfulness meditation that is renowned for its health benefits. TCC practice has been shown to improve balance, strength, and coordination of body movements and can reduce the risk of falls in the elderly. In addition, TCC has been shown to be a safe method of exercise for the elderly from a cardiovascular point of view and to reduce pain and stiffness from OA of the knee.

TCC requires a state of mind that is similar to that found with meditation-based stress reduction techniques. Qigong breathing exercises, which are often incorporated in TCC practice, have been recognized to have a similar physiologic effect as mind–body relaxation techniques. This state of mindfulness has been shown to have a regulating effect on the autonomic nervous system and immune function.

Tai chi, qigong, and yoga represent a class of exercise that differs from the routine strengthening and stretching programs currently employed in physical medicine. Practicing Tai Chi appropriately has various physiological effects beyond pain control (e.g., balance improvement, fall prevention, cardiovascular enhancement, stress reduction, etc.), and therefore may provide more health benefits than standard exercise routines in certain populations.

These techniques incorporate a "mind–body" approach to the rehabilitation of disorders commonly seen by clinicians. Methods such as TCC and Qigong serve to add valuable options to the continuity of care of ambulatory and non-ambulatory patients with various chronic illnesses. In the interim, there is a clear challenge to practitioners of Western medicine to continue to explore the basis of the beneficial effects seen from the practice of this time-honored exercise.

REFERENCES

1. Wile D. 1996. Lost Tai Chi Classics from the Late Ch'ing Dynasty. New York: SUNY Press.
2. Liang TT. 1977. T'ai Chi Ch'uan for Health and Self-Defense: Philosophy and Practice. New York: Vintage Books.

3. Goodrich LC. 1966. The Literary Inquisition of Ch'ien Lnug. New York: Paragon Books (Reprint), p 65, 247.

4. Cheng M-ci. 1981. Tai Chi Ch'uan: A Simplified Method of Calisthenics For Health and Self Defense. Berkely, CA: North Atlantic Books.

5. Gallagher B. Tai Chi Chuan and Qigong—Physical and mental practice for functional mobility. Top Geriatric Rehabil. 2003;19(3):172–182.

6. Wolf SL, Barnhart HX, Kutner NG, et al. Reducing frailty and falls in older persons: an investigation of Tai Chi and computerized balance training. J Am Geriatr Soc. 1996;44(5):489–497.

7. Hartman CA, Manos TM, Winter C, Hartman DM, Li B, Smith JC. Effects of T'ai Chi training on function and quality of life indicators in older adults with osteoarthritis. J Am Geriatr Soc. 2000;48(12):1553–1559.

8. Blumenthal JA, Jiang W, Babyak MA, et al. Stress management and exercise training in cardiac patients with myocardial ischemia—Effects on prognosis and evaluation of mechanisms. Arch Int Med. 1997;157(19):2213–2223.

9. Brown DR, Wang YD, Ward A, et al. Chronic psychological effects of exercise and exercise plus cognitive strategies. Med Sci Sports Exerc. 1995;27(5):765–775.

10. Jin PT. Efficacy of Tai Chi, Brisk walking, meditation, and reading in reducing mental and emotional-stress. J Psychosom Res. 1992;36(4):361–370.

11. Chen K, Snyder M. A research-based use of Tai Chi/movement therapy as a nursing. J Holistic Nurs. 1999;17(3):267–79 (Sep. (33 ref)).

12. Jin P. Changes in heart-rate, noradrenaline, cortisol and mood during Tai Chi. J Psychosom Res. 1989;33(2):197–206.

13. Mills N, Allen J. Mindfulness of movement as a coping strategy in multiple sclerosis—a pilot study. Gen Hosp Psychiatry. 2000;22(6):425–431.

14. Yan JH, Downing JH. Tai Chi: an alternative exercise form for seniors. J Aging Phys Activity. 1998;6(4):350–362.

15. Kane RL, Ouslander JG, Abrass IB. 1994 Essentials of Clinical Geriatrics, 3rd edition. New York, NY: McGraw Hill.

16. Leveille SG, Fried L, Guralnik JM. Disabling symptoms—what do older women report? J Gen Int Med 2002;17(10):766–773.

17. Scudds RJ, Robertson JM. Pain factors associated with physical disability in a sample of community-dwelling senior citizens. J Gerontol Ser A: Biol Sci Med Sci 2000;55(7):M393–M399.

18. Scudds RJ, Robertson JM. Empirical evidence of the association between the presence of musculoskeletal pain and physical disability in community-dwelling senior citizens. Pain 1998;75(2–3): 229–235.

19. Woolf AD, Pfleger B. Burden of major musculoskeletal conditions. Bull World Health Organ 2003;81(9):646–656.

20. Leveille SG, Bean J, Bandeen-Roche K, Jones R, Hochberg M, Guralnik JM. Musculoskeletal pain and risk for falls in older disabled women living in the community. J Am Geriatr Soc 2002;50(4):671–678.

21. Ehrlich GE. Low back pain. Bull World Health Organ 2003;81(9):671–676.

22. Lansbury G. 2000. Chronic pain management: a qualitative study of elderly people's preferred coping strategies and barriers to management. DisabilRehabil 10–20;22(1–2):2–14.

23. Weiner DK, Hanlon JT, Studenski SA. Effects of central nervous system polypharmacy on falls liability in community-dwelling elderly. Gerontology 1998;44(4):217–221.

24. Eisenberg DM, Davis RB, Ettner SL, et al. Trends in alternative medicine use in the United States, 1990–1997: results of a follow-up national survey (comment). J Am Med Assoc 1998;280(18): 1569–1575.

25. Najm W, Reinsch S, Hoehler F, Tobis J. Use of complementary and alternative medicine among the ethnic elderly. Alt Ther Health Med. 2003;9(3):50–57.

26. Wang G, Helmick CG, Macera C, Zhang P, Pratt M. Inactivity-associated medical costs among US adults with arthritis. Arthritis & Rheum 2001;45(5):439–445.

27. Penninx BW, Messier SP, Rejeski WJ, et al. Physical exercise and the prevention of disability in activities of daily living in older persons with osteoarthritis. Arch Int Med 2001;161(19): 2309–2316.

28. Schroll M. Physical activity in an ageing population. Scand J MedSci Sports 2003;13(1):63–69.

29. Myers J, Prakash M, Froelicher V, Do D, Partington S, Atwood JE. Exercise capacity and mortality among men referred for exercise testing (comment). N Eng J Med 2002;346(11):793–801.

30. Billman GE, Schwartz PJ, Stone HL. The effects of daily exercise on susceptibility to sudden cardiac death. Circulation 1984;69(6):1182–1189.

31. Blair SN, Kohl HW III, Paffenbarger RS, Jr., Clark DG, Cooper KH, Gibbons LW. Physical fitness and all-cause mortality. A prospective study of healthy men and women (comment). J Am Med Assoc 1989;262(17):2395–2401.

32. Erikssen G, Liestol K, Bjornholt J, Thaulow E, Sandvik L, Erikssen J. Changes in physical fitness and changes in mortality. Lancet 1998;352(9130):759–762.

33. Era P, Schroll M, Hagerup L, Jurgensen KSL. Changes in bicycle ergometer test performance and survival in men and women from 50 to 60 and from 70 to 80 years of age: two longitudinal studies in the Glostrup (Denmark) population. Gerontology. 2001;47(3):136–144.

34. Gulati M, Pandey DK, Arnsdorf MF, et al. Exercise capacity and the risk of death in women: the St James Women Take Heart Project (comment). Circulation. 2003;108(13):1554–1559.

35. Laukkanen JA, Lakka TA, Rauramaa R, et al. Cardiovascular fitness as a predictor of mortality in men. Arch Int Med 2001;161(6):825–831.

36. Mora S, Redberg RF, Cui Y, et al. Ability of exercise testing to predict cardiovascular and all-cause death in asymptomatic women: a 20–year follow-up of the lipid research clinics prevalence study. J Am Med Assoc 2003;290(12):1600–1607.

37. Prakash M, Myers J, Froelicher VF, et al. Clinical and exercise test predictors of all-cause mortality—results from >6,000 consecutive referred male patients. Chest. 2001;120(3):1003–1013.

38. Lissner L, Bengtsson C, Bjorkelund C, Wedel H. Physical activity levels and changes in relation to longevity—a prospective study of Swedish women. Am J Epidemiol 1996;143(1):54–62.

39. Farrell SW, Braun L, Barlow CE, Cheng YJ, Blair SN. The relation of body mass index, cardiorespiratory fitness, and all-cause mortality in women. Obes Res 2002;10(6):417–423.

40. Blair SN, Cheng Y, Holder JS. Is physical activity or physical fitness more important in defining health benefits? Med Sci Sports Exerc 2001;33(6 Suppl):S379–399 (discussion S419–320).

41. Lee AP, Ice R, Blessey R, Sanmarco ME. Long-term effects of physical training on coronary patients with impaired ventricular function. Circulation. 1979;60(7):1519–1526.

42. LaMonte MJ, Durstine JL, Addy CL, Irwin ML, Ainsworth BE. Physical activity, physical fitness, and Framingham 10-year risk score: the cross-cultural activity participation study (comment). J Cardiopulm Rehabil 2001;21(2):63–70.

43. Morey MC, Pieper CF, Crowley GM, Sullivan RJ, Puglisi CM. Exercise adherence and 10-year mortality in chronically ill older adults (comment). J Am Geriatr Soc 2002;50(12):1929–1933.

44. Talbot LA, Morrell CH, Metter EJ, Fleg JL. Comparison of cardiorespiratory fitness versus leisure time physical activity as predictors of coronary events in men aged < or = 65 years and > 65 years. Am J Cardiol 2002;89(10):1187–1192.

45. Sandvik L, Erikssen J, Thaulow E, Erikssen G, Mundal R, Rodahl K. Physical-fitness as a predictor of mortality among healthy, middle-aged Norwegian men. N Engl J Med 1993;328(8):533–537.

46. Kushi LH, Fee RM, Folsom AR, Mink PJ, Anderson KE, Sellers TA. Physical activity and mortality in postmenopausal women (comment). J Am Med Assoc 1997;277(16):1287–1292.

47. Kaplan MS, Huguet N, Newsom JT, McFarland BH. Characteristics of physically inactive older adults with arthritis: results of a population-based study. Prev Med 2003;37(1):61–67.

48. Seals DR, Monahan KD, Bell C, Tanaka H, Jones PP. The aging cardiovascular system: changes in autonomic function at rest and in response to exercise. Int J Sport Nutr Exerc Metabol 2001;11:S189–S195.

49. Schuit AJ, van Amelsvoort L, Verheij TC, et al. Exercise training and heart rate variability in older people. Med Sci Sports Exerc 1999;31(6):816–821.

50. Dekker JM, Crow RS, Folsom AR, et al. Low heart rate variability in a 2-minute rhythm strip predicts risk of coronary heart disease and mortality from several causes—the ARIC study. Circulation 2000;102(11):1239–1244.

51. Lauer MS, Francis GS, Okin PM, Pashkow FJ, Snader CE, Marwick TH. Impaired chronotropic response to exercise stress testing as a predictor of mortality (comment). J Am Med Assoc 1999;281(6):524–529.

52. Heath GW, Hagberg JM, Ehsani AA, Holloszy JO. A physiological comparison of young and older endurance athletes. J Appl Physiol 1981;51(3):634–640.

53. Denis C, Chatard JC, Dormois D, Linossier MT, Geyssant A, Lacour JR. Effects of endurance training on capillary supply of human skeletal–muscle on 2 age-groups (20 and 60 Years). J Physiol 1986;81(5):379–383.

54. De Meersman RE. Respiratory sinus arrhythmia alteration following training in endurance athletes. Eur J Appl Physiol Occup Physiol 1992;64(5):434–436.

55. De Meersman RE. Aging as a modulator of respiratory sinus arrhythmia. J Gerontol 1993;48(2): B74–78.

56. Powell KE, Thompson PD, Caspersen CJ, Kendrick JS. Physical activity and the incidence of coronary heart disease. Ann Rev Public Health 1987;8:253–287.

57. Wyatt HL, Mitchell J. Influences of physical conditioning and deconditioning on coronary vasculature of dogs. J Appl Physiol: Respir, Environ Exerc Physiol 1978;45(4):619–625.

58. Leon AS, Bloor CM. Effects of exercise and its cessation on the heart and its blood supply. J Appl Physiol 1968;24(4):485–490.

59. Coats AJS, Adamopoulos S, Radaelli A, et al. Controlled trial of physical-training in chronic heart-failure—exercise performance, hemodynamics, ventilation, and autonomic function. Circulation 1992;85(6):2119–2131.

60. Gregoire J, Tuck S, Yamamoto Y, Hughson RL. Heart rate variability at rest and exercise: influence of age, gender, and physical training. Can J Appl Physiol 1996;21(6):455–470.

61. Yocum DE, Castro WL, Cornett M. Exercise, education, and behavioral modification as alternative therapy for pain and stress in rheumatic disease. Rheum Dis Clin North Am 2000;26(1):145 and more pages.

62. Lam P. Tai Chi for older adults and for arthritis. J Aging Phys Activity 1999;7(3):302–304.

63. Kirsteins AE, Dietz F, Hwang SM. Evaluating the safety and potential use of a weight-bearing exercise, Tai-Chi Chuan, for rheumatoid-arthritis patients. Am Jof Phys Med Rehabil 1991;70(3):136–141.

64. Song R, Lee EO, Lam P, Bae SC. Effects of tai chi exercise on pain, balance, muscle strength, and perceived difficulties in physical functioning in older women with osteoarthritis: a randomized clinical trial. J Rheumatol 2003;30(9):2039–2044.

65. Wolf SL, Coogler C, Xu TS. Exploring the basis for Tai Chi Chuan as a therapeutic exercise approach. Arch Phys Med Rehabil 1997;78(8):886–892.

66. Wolf SL, Sattin RW, O'Grady M, et al. A study design to investigate the effect of intense Tai Chi in reducing falls among older adults transitioning to frailty. Control Clin Trials 2001;22(6):689–704.

67. Wu G. Evaluation of the effectiveness of Tai Chi for improving balance and preventing falls in the older population—a review. J Am Geriatr Soc 2002;50(4):746–754.

68. Wayne PM, Krebs DE, Wolf SL, et al. Can Tai Chi improve vestibulopathic postural control? Arch Phys Med Rehabil 2004;85(1):142–152.

69. Li JX, Hong Y, Chan KM. Tai chi: physiological characteristics and beneficial effects on health. Br J Sports Med 2001;35(3):148–156.

70. Lan C, Lai JS, Wong MK, Yu ML. Cardiorespiratory function, flexibility, and body composition among geriatric Tai Chi Chuan practitioners. Arch Phys Med Rehabil 1996;77(6):612–616.

71. Lan C, Lai JS, Chen SY, Wong MK. 12-month Tai Chi training in the elderly: its effect on health fitness. Med Sci Sports Exerc 1998;30(3):345–351.

72. Lan C, Chen SY, Lai JS, Wong MK. The effect of Tai Chi on cardiorespiratory function in patients with coronary artery bypass surgery. Med Sci Sports Exerc 1999;31(5):634–638.

73. Lan C, Lai JS, Chen SY, Wong MK. Tai Chi Chuan to improve muscular strength and endurance in elderly individuals: a pilot study. Arch Phys Med Rehabil 2000;81(5):604–607.

74. Lan C, Chen SY, Lai JS, Wong MK. Heart rate responses and oxygen consumption during Tai Chi Chuan practice. Am J Chin Med 2001;29(3–4):403–410.

75. Young DR, Appel LJ, Jee SH. The effects of aerobic exercise and Tai Chi on blood pressure in the elderly. Circulation 1998;97(8):828.

76. Lai JS, Lan C, Wong MK, Teng SH. 2-year trends in cardiorespiratory function among older Tai-Chi-Chuan practitioners and sedentary subjects. J Am Geriatr Soc 1995;43(11):1222–1227.

77. Zhuo D, Shephard RJ, Plyley MJ, Davis GM. Cardiorespiratory and metabolic responses during Tai Chi Chuan exercise. Can J Appl Sport Sci (J Can Sci Appl Sport) 1984;9(1):7–10.

78. Fontana JA, Colella C, Wilson BR, Baas L. The energy costs of a modified form of T'ai Chi exercise. Nurs Res 2000;49(2):91–96.

79. Lee MS, Huh HJ, Kim BG, et al. Effects of Qi-training on heart rate variability. Am J Chin Med 2002;30(4):463–470.

80. Audette JF, Jin YS, Newcome R, Stein L, Duncan G, Frontera WF. Tai Chi versus brisk walking in elderly women. Age Ageing 2006;35(4):388–393.

81. Astin JA, Shapiro SL, Eisenberg DM, Forys KL. Mind-body medicine: state of the science, implications for practice. J Am Board Fam Pract 2003;16(2):131–147.

82. Tsang HWH, Cheung L, Lak DCC. Qigong as a psychosocial intervention for depressed elderly with chronic physical illnesses. Int J Geriatr Psychiatry 2002;17(12):1146–1154.

83. Luskin FM, Newell KA, Griffith M, et al. A review of mind/body therapies in the treatment of musculoskeletal disorders with implications for the elderly. Alt Ther Health Med 2000;6(2):46 and more pages.
84. Sakakibara M, Takeuchi S, Hayano J. Effect of relaxation training on cardiac parasympathetic tone. Psychophysiology 1994;31(3):223–228.
85. Vempati RP, Telles S. Yoga-based guided relaxation reduces sympathetic activity judged from baseline levels. Psychol Rep 2002;90(2):487–494.
86. Schaller KJ. Tai Chi Chih: an exercise option for older adults. J Gerontol Nurs 1996;22(10):12–17.
87. Ross MC, Bohannon AS, Davis DC, Gurchiek L. The effects of a short-term exercise program on movement, pain, and mood in the elderly. Results of a pilot study. J Holistic Nurs 1999;17(2):139–147.
88. Li FZ, McAuley E, Harmer P, Duncan TE, Chaumeton NR. Tai Chi enhances self-efficacy and exercise behavior in older adults. J Aging Phys Activity 2001;9(2):161–171.

13 Yoga in Pain Management

Loren Fishman and Ellen Saltonstall

CONTENTS

HISTORY OF YOGA
MECHANISMS OF ACTION
THE BODY AND THE MIND
THE YOGA ROAD REACHES AS FAR AS THE TRAVELER
CONDITIONS RESPONDING WELL TO YOGA THERAPY
SAFETY
MODELS OF CARE
GENERAL RULES FOR SPECIFIC SITUATIONS
YOGA AS THERAPY
RESOURCES

Summary

Yoga is a practice that has evolved and survived over thousands of years, its teachings adapting to many cultures and eras of history. Until recently, yoga was known in the West mostly for the extraordinary feats of its adepts: voluntarily stopping and then restarting of the heart, holding the breath for extended periods, or contortionist positions of the body. Now, with more cross-fertilization in all aspects of physical fitness, yoga has become mainstream. What may be lost in this process is the greater picture of where yoga came from, what it is, and its many uses, including medical pain relief. This chapter is meant to acquaint the reader more fully with the practice of yoga and its potential roles within an integrative pain medicine practice.

Key Words: health, mind–body, exercise, hatha yoga, yoga therapy, therapeutic yoga, pain medicine, neurophysiology in yoga, Iyengar yoga, anusara yoga

1. HISTORY OF YOGA

The word *yoga* means "to yoke" or "to join." Classically this means that the individual consciousness links itself to a universal or supreme consciousness, and in doing so attains greater freedom and joy. Even though this definition identifies yoga as a spiritual practice, anyone can practice yoga along with his or her chosen religious affiliation, or with none. Yoga is theistic but non-sectarian. It has no clergy.

Yoga itself is not a religion. It is undenominational, relying not on faith but on a number of techniques that gradually lead the individual to the direct experience of those truths on which religion rests. "We can call it the inner spirit of religion *(1)*."

From: *Contemporary Pain Medicine: Integrative Pain Medicine: The Science and Practice of Complementary and Alternative Medicine in Pain Management*
Edited by: J. F. Audette and A. Bailey © Humana Press, Totowa, NJ

As will be discussed further in this chapter, some schools of yoga focus more on philosophy, while others focus more on physical and mental practices. But yoga has an imperishably spiritual character.

Yoga is often compared to a tree, with roots that are buried deep in history, a strong trunk composed of practices and philosophical teachings, and many branches. The branch that addresses bodily health is called "Hatha Yoga;" the word 'hatha' refers to a balancing of opposing forces.

The practice of the postures or *asanas* is common to yoga classes all over the world today. Yet this is just one of many yoga practices. Others include philosophical study, known as *Jnana* yoga; worship of deities, known as *Bhakti* yoga; and *Karma* yoga, which involves devoting one's worldly activities to helping others. *Asana* is Sanskrit for "seat," and in spite of their variety, these postures hearken back to the origins of yoga, which were inextricably bound to meditation.

The roots of the yoga tree originate before the Vedic Age, thousands of years before the Common Era. The Vedas, which date from the fourth and fifth centuries BCE, are among the oldest living scriptures, yet they include references to yoga practices that have been carried through to the present day. Originally, knowledge was passed on orally from teacher to student, making this history difficult to trace. However, scholars have found evidence of yoga practices in a sophisticated civilization that existed in India as far back as 2600 BCE.

In approximately the fifth or sixth century CE, the trunk of the tree split into three main branches that became known as Hinduism, Buddhism, and Jainism. The practice of Hatha yoga is intertwined with these spiritual traditions to this day. A radical idea appears here—that tending to the human body and keeping it strong and fit is part of a way of life that honors the inherent connectedness of body, mind, and spirit.

From pre-Socratic, Platonic, Manichaean, and Christian times, mind and spirit have often been opposed to the material, animal, bodily, or physical "world." This has yielded the extremely difficult situation Descartes encountered: a ghost in a machine, with no possible connection between the mind and the body.

In contrast, contemporary integrative medicine has more affinity with the non-dualistic Advaita Vedanta tradition of Shankara (circa 800 CE), possibly reborn with Sigmund Freud. It seeks to understand the relationship between the mind and the body. For all its otherworldliness, Hatha yoga focuses less on worship and more on spirituality of the self; its orientation is far more to psychology than theology.

The next important development in yoga's history came through the work of Patanjali, a physician and grammarian who compiled the prevalent teachings of yoga into a work called the *Yoga Sutra* circa the second century of the Common Era. This is a collection of nearly 200 aphorisms, which state much of the philosophy and practice of yoga in condensed form. What arose from this pivotal time in yoga's history is called Classical yoga, which followed the teachings laid out in the *Yoga Sutra*. These are available in several excellent translations, such as those of Taimni, Feuerstein, and Shearer *(1–3)*.

In 1893, yoga was first introduced in the West by the missionary work of Swami Vivekananda who represented Hinduism at the Parliament of Religions in Chicago. After that event, many seekers traveled to India and found teachers from various branches of the tree, leading to the spread of yoga throughout the Western world. Throughout the end of the 19th and beginning of the 20th centuries, other teachers, such as Paramahansa Yogananda, Swami Satchidananda, Swami Sivananda Saraswati,

Table 1

The Four Major Schools of Yoga Originating from the Lineage of Krishnamacharya, the 20th Century Luminary Who Vastly Widened the Scope of Modern Yoga, Teaching such Contemporary Figures as B.K.S. Iyengar, and Pattabhi Jois (Ashtanga Yoga), and T.K.V. Desikachar (Krishnamacharya Yoga Mandiram).

Name	Developer	Primary focus/ characteristics	Training	Intensity	Additional features
Iyengar yoga	B.K.S. Iyengar	Precision of alignment, details on how to perform each pose	3–5 years, etc.	Strenuous	Extensive use of props, anatomically sophisticated, therapeutically oriented
Viniyoga	T.K.V. Desikachar	Individually prescribed sequences of poses		Varies	Attention to the health needs of the students
Ashtanga yoga	Pattabhi Jois	Poses performed in continuous series, coordinated with the breath		Strenuous	Few instructions given, Intense cardiovascular and strengthening exercise
Anusara yoga	John Friend	Precision of alignment, connection to inward source of spiritual support	3–5 years, etc.	Varies from gentle to strenuous	Props used to adapt poses, attention to individual needs, anatomically sophisticated, therapeutically oriented

and Swami Muktananda, were promoting yoga. Their influence pervades many of the styles practiced in the West today, leading to the yoga systems of the Self-Realization Fellowship and Kriya Yoga centers, and Integral Yoga, Sivananda and Vedanta Yoga Centers, and the Siddha Meditation Centers of Swami Chidvilasananda, respectively, for the teachers mentioned.

Each teacher drew on the yogic traditions, then restated and recombined them, resulting in an array of smaller branches of the tree. All modern-day yoga classes have lineages dating back to one of these or perhaps ten other major teachers. The schools that have emerged are the same in their ultimate goal: to convey the understanding "that the human being is more than the physical body and that, through a course of discipline, it is possible to discover what this 'more' is" (4). The schools differ, however, in the intensity of the physical exertion, in their balancing of active and meditative practices, and in the specific instructions given.

Western culture and traditions also had important influences on the development of yoga. European gymnastics caught the eye and imagination of the Maharaja of Mysore's court and others, leading to the rich and anatomically refined Hatha yoga styles that we see today (5,6).

Because of this diversity in approach and practice, yoga has something for everyone and anyone can do it. Many beginners say, "I can't do yoga. I'm too stiff...." But that stiffness is, in itself, a very good reason to practice yoga. A properly trained and experienced yoga instructor can usually identify a student's needs and capabilities. Starting with one-on-one instruction, yoga reliably proceeds in a safe, enjoyable manner that usually succeeds in relieving pain. Individual instruction may continue for a few sessions or a few years. Reasonably quickly the student/patient can practice at home, and soon has progressed enough to fit into regular classes.

2. MECHANISMS OF ACTION

2.1. Simple Stretching and Balancing

The practice of Hatha yoga increases body awareness, and depending on how it is performed, can build muscle strength as well as flexibility. Improvements in these areas may reduce musculoskeletal pain. A well-designed yoga regimen takes the body through a full range of movements to a greater extent than most sports or mechanical workouts.

The styles of yoga that provide detailed instruction about body alignment give a model for musculoskeletal health that will help to relieve and prevent much musculoskeletal pain. When an individual is misaligned, such as in the case of a chronically kyphotic thoracic spine or torticollis, the muscles, tendons, and ligaments are under constant strain. These weak and contracted muscles may initiate a vicious cycle of increasingly asymmetrical strain that can lead to and perpetuate myofascial pain. Conversely, good alignment supports symmetrical functioning, which in many cases will relieve the pain.

It is a relatively simple matter to improve alignment through yoga. However, in the context of pain, individual instruction with a well-trained teacher is often required. Working with an experienced yoga therapist can provide patients with a series of postures that address the deficits in strength, flexibility and balance that perpetuate their specific patterns of strain.

2.2. Golgi Tendon Organs Versus Intrafusal Fibres: The Tortoise and the Hare

Small spindle-like receptors in muscles themselves (the intrafusal receptors) are activated every time any muscle is stretched. They *excite* or *facilitate* contraction of that muscle to protect it and the joint from over-stretching. Yet each muscle also has at least one tendon, and in each tendon are Golgi tendon organs that are activated whenever they are stretched. Being part of the tendon, they are stretched whenever the muscle is stretched and also each and every time it contracts. When they are stretched, these Golgi tendon organs send out signals that *inhibit* the muscle from contracting, again protecting the muscle, the joint, and the muscle-bone connection. Intrafusal receptors and Golgi tendon organs promote and restrain every muscle-driven movement, balancing strength and enhancing control (7). The antagonistic influences of intrafusal end organs (facilitating) and Golgi tendon organs (inhibiting) integrate information about the speed and intensity of every muscle contraction and the amount of resistance it encounters (8–10). This information is processed and modulated at spinal motor centers and several coordinative loci in the medulla, cerebellum and possibly higher locations in the brain (7–10). See figure 1.

Table 2
Other Styles of Yoga Widespread in the United States

Name	Developer	Primary focus/characteristics	Training	Intensity	Additional features	References
Bikram yoga	Bikram Choudhury	Performed in hot room to encourage release of tension and detoxification	500 hours over 9 weeks in Los Angeles	26 poses repeated in each session	Same series of poses repeated, unsuited to therapeutic work	Bikram's Yoga College of India, World Headquarters La Cienaga Blvd., Los Angeles, CA
Integral yoga	Satchidananda	Integrate spiritual teachings into daily life	250 hours for basic course	Gentle	Provides no-impact, general fitness benefits; special asanas for children with Down's syndrome, cerebral palsy, attention deficit disorder and learning disabilities	Satchidananda Ashram, Yogaville, VA
Integrative yoga therapy	Joseph Le Page	Eclectic method specifically developed for mainstream medical settings	200 hours	Gentle	Uses assisted postures, guided imagery and breathing techniques; therapeutically oriented	IYTyogatherapy.com Many articles by Joseph Le Page
Jivamukti yoga	Sharon Gannon and David Life	Fast-paced style that includes intellectual	200 hour residential program: 5	Vigorous	Performed to new age and traditional Indian music in a	Jivamukti.com

(Continued)

Table 2
(*Continued*)

Name	Developer	Primary focus/characteristics	Training	Intensity	Additional features	References
		considerations of yoga philosophy	book-reports for admission		large group with chanting	
Kundalini yoga	Yogi Bhajan	Emphasizes the breath to induce deeper body awareness	Various programs	Rapid repetitive "cleansing" movements	Basic attention to "energy flow" within and between chakras	International Kundalini Yoga Teachers Association
Kripalu yoga	Amrit Desai	Developing awareness of movement and concurrent psychological state	200 hours	Gentle at first, poses then held longer	A number of teachers with varied approaches.	Kripalu.org
Phoenix Rising yoga therapy	Michael Lee	Classical yoga postures combined with mind body psychology	200 hours for certification	Holistic	Practitioner physically assists the student and has dialogue. One-on-one and couples	Donna Raskin "Profound Presence." *Fit Yoga*, November, 2005
Sivananda yoga	Swami Sivananda; Swami Vishnu-Devananda	Uses breathing, postures, meditation	1 month residential program	Gentle	Indian culture, chanting, meditation and lectures	International Sivananda Yoga Vedanta Center
Svaroopa yoga	Rama Berch	Development of consciousness using the body as a tool	5 days to learn 16 basic asanas, hierarchical progress thereafter	Gentle	Special needs yoga	Masteryoga.org

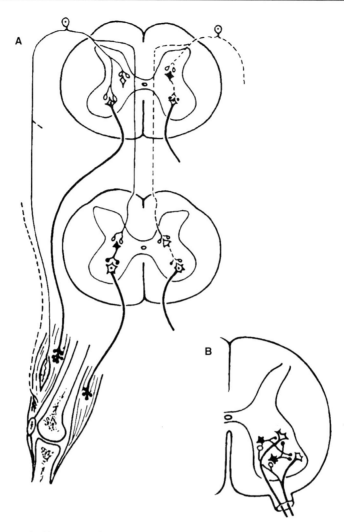

Fig. 1. Facilitatory spindles are modulated by internal muscle fibres that alter their arousal thresholds. Inhibitory Golgi tendon organs respond to tension in a linear fashion. Dotted lines and clear cells are inhibitory. (**A**) One model of a possible inhibitory central circuit (**B**), after Eccles.

These nuclei are sensitive to hormonal, metabolic, and psychological factors. Awake or asleep, they coordinate and regulate the strength and contour of each muscle's every contraction at any given time.

2.2.1. How Do These Reflexes Work in Pain Medicine?

Many yoga postures utilize the biological fact that the intrafusal fibers respond to the speed of motion, and generally have their greatest influence in facilitating contraction *early* in muscle stretch *(9)*, while Golgi tendon organs *continue* to exert their inhibitory influence at their original strength *throughout* contractions of any duration *(10)* (see Figure 2). Electrophysiological studies of corticospinal tract activation support the concept that muscle stretch (eccentric contraction) involves inhibition not present in concentric contraction *(11)*. In general, any sustained muscle stretch will then, over time, tend toward a relaxation response in that muscle *(10)*. Naturally, any painful

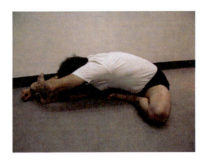 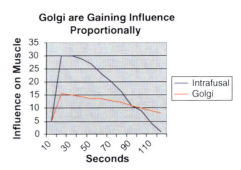

Fig. 2. At first, intrafusal fibers react to activate contraction, overwhelming Golgi tendon organs' inhibition. In less than two minutes, intrafusal fibers reduce their influence, and Golgi tendon organs induce relaxation.

stimuli that are activated during that same time period will have a contrary, unsettling, and excitatory effect. The yoga poses that have endured over the centuries succeed in accomplishing sustained stretch and relaxation, without undue antagonistic, painful or arousing side effects.

2.3. The Agonist—Antagonist Reflex

A second reflex of great utility in yoga is the agonist–antagonist reflex. When the biceps contracts to flex the elbow, the triceps must relax enough to permit the movement. These reflexes often operate over large groups of muscles. When extensors arch the back, abdominal musculature has to relent. Whether hard-wired or picked up early in life, these complex reflexes are mediated at the spinal cord level. They are used in yoga to help stretch muscles and increase the range of motion of joints and to quiet the painful spasms that are the greatest single cause of back pain.

Paschimottanasana is a good example of both of these principles. At first it is painful; the spindles stimulate contraction of the hamstring muscles precisely because they are elongated. But within two minutes the Golgi tendon organs' inhibitory input overtakes the flagging spindles' influence and calms down the muscles, causing them to evenly and pleasantly stretch. In musculoskeletal back pain, in which there is no neurological involvement, stretching the hamstrings and the extensor muscles of the dorsal spine and legs can be facilitated by contracting the quadriceps and the abdominal flexor groups. This natural reflex helps calm spastic back muscles within a few minutes (see Figure 3).

Further, contracting the quadriceps to keep the legs straight in *Paschimottanasana* is hard-wired to relax the hamstring muscles, their antagonists. These are the two powerful reflexes that yoga has harnessed here which help one's overly tight hamstrings to relent, making them much more accessible and much less painful to stretch.

One characteristic of yoga practice that is common to all yoga styles is the development of awareness. A more refined awareness of the body may allow one to make small adjustments in posture and habitual movement patterns that will help to relieve pain, particularly that of habitual, postural, or myofascial origin. Yoga allows one to learn and change the habits that may perpetuate myofascial pain and in the process become more sensitive to how these movements influence sensation.

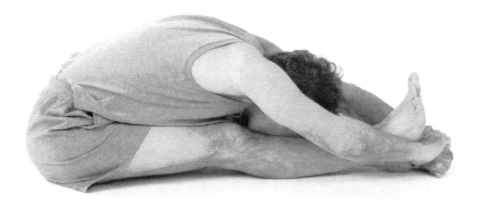

Fig. 3. Paschimottanasana.

When the means are available, we learn how to avoid pain or reduce disability with very little training. This skill of adaptation is not the same in all of us and rarely maximized. Yoga has been shown to increase adaptation in the young and in the old. Telles et al. have shown significantly increased motor learning in a group of children taught yoga for one month versus a control group matched for age and grade level *(12)*. DiBenedetto et al. report gait improvement in elderly patients begun on a program of gentle Iyengar yoga *(13)*. Further work with hemispheric electroencephalogram (EEG) recordings and electrophysiological markers of autonomic activity suggests that cortical circuitry is quite readily affected by yogic breathing techniques and useful in reducing anxiety and stress *(14–16)*. A number of studies report such effects as increased cortical thickening with meditation, enhanced adaptability of motor control systems, and changes in signaling molecules with yoga, suggesting that yoga may enhance central nervous system plasticity *(7,12,17,18)*.

3. THE BODY AND THE MIND

One of the greatest challenges for the pain medicine practitioner is management of the anxiety and depression that accompany chronic pain syndromes. These emotional and cognitive effects of pain frequently are quite devastating and have an impact on the recovery process itself *(19)*. Meditation and the practice of Hatha yoga have been documented to relieve these symptoms and simultaneously give the patient additional resources for managing the pain itself *(15,19)*.

It is often said that most people start a yoga practice in order to relieve musculoskeletal pain or reduce stress. One British study found that Complementary and Alternative Medicine (CAM) techniques, including yoga, were most often sought to relieve anxiety and stress *(20)*. Making allowances for inherent limitations due to illness or age, a careful practice of yoga appears to enhance parasympathetic function, soothing the practitioner and quieting the nervous system *(3,4)*. Recent studies at Yale and Harvard suggest that yoga works to reduce "mental strain" *(4,19,20)*.

The actual neurobiology of this effect has been sought and analyzed in some detail *(16)*. Herbert Benson's laboratory has suggested endocannabinoids' coupling to nitric oxide as part of the explanation of the relaxation response *(17)*. Historically, the practice of Hatha yoga was intended to prepare a person to meditate. We have reviewed how deliberate, vigorous stretching activates reflexes that improve the ability to sit quietly for meditation. Although there are many different styles of meditation, with varying techniques, they all aim to focus one's attention and to uncover a reservoir of subtle understanding and peace that is within us. Most styles of yoga include meditation in their classes.

A key premise of yoga is that the mind and body are inextricably linked. In fact, in the *Bhagavad Gita*, another fundamental source of yoga teachings from the fifth century BCE, yoga is defined as "evenness of mind." Steadiness and clarity in the body brings steadiness and clarity in the mind, and the reverse is also true. Calming and regulating the nervous system reduces pain and the fear of pain. *Pranayama*, the practice of expanding the breath, is yoga's most powerful link between mind and body. Working with the breath, either along with *asana* or as a practice in itself, is a fruitful route to healing, and one that is utilized specifically for reduction of stress and pain *(20)*. We have found one simple exercise in *Pranayama, Viloma,* extremely useful with insomnia. After a little practice, many people fall asleep before they finish the exercise. Research shows that parasympathetic function is altered with deep breathing, even in beginners without prior yoga skills *(3,4,17)*.

4. THE YOGA ROAD REACHES AS FAR AS THE TRAVELER

As a spiritual self-improvement program, yoga distinguishes itself from many other types of therapies. Physical therapy, occupational therapy, Alexander technique, Feldenkrais, Pilates, Taibo, Jazzercize, and the myriad health club and outdoor fitness regimens also encourage specific activities. However, when the client or patient has reached a state of normalcy, these disciplines have done their work, and apart from "upkeep," pursue no further goals. This is unlike yoga, which takes practitioners from painful, weak, and disabled conditions back to good health and attempts to carry them on toward more and more liberation, and toward spiritual lives.

This spiritual aspect of yoga may be of additional importance within a pain medicine practice. By re-framing the philosophical and psychological constructs by which patients interpret their pain, yoga may act as cognitive-behavioral therapy, enabling patients to adopt more constructive attitudes about their chronically painful conditions. Some key concepts from two ancient texts on yoga, the *Bhagavad Gita* and the *Yoga Sutra*, can help to illuminate this yoga of the mind. These concepts form the basis of a "yogic way of life." *Viveka*, or discrimination, is the ability to distinguish the true from the false, what is necessary from what is not, that which can change from that which cannot change. In dealing with physical pain, we want to be able to determine clearly whether there are any causative lifestyle factors that can be altered to relieve it. *Ahimsa*, or non-violence, is practiced both in relation to others and to oneself. Another definition of *ahimsa* is compassion or respect for life. Often physical pain is perpetuated or increased by some sort of violence to oneself, and by practicing *ahimsa* (preceded by *viveka*) through a well-designed yoga regimen, pain can be diminished.

In Western culture there is a high value placed on speedy results and bottom-line benefits. We want to see improvements right away, and we want to know exactly what those improvements are going to be. Two fundamental teachings of yoga, *abhyasa* and *vairagya*, exemplify the Eastern attitude of patience and detachment. *Abhyasa*, or constant practice over a long period of time, has been a yogic virtue for thousands of years. The complex nature of the human organism requires perseverance over time for change. *Abhyasa* implies a willingness to see the process through, to commit to the long haul, and to accept that changes may be gradual. *Vairagya* means not being attached to one particular outcome but being open to whatever results come: flexibility or adaptability.

Perhaps the most difficult yogic attitude or virtue for Westerners is *santosha*, or contentment. Here is a system of ethics with a *commandment* "Be Content!" How could anyone who is in pain practice contentment? Yoga teachings always come back to the idea of seeing the bigger picture in any situation and seeing the good wherever possible. Cultivating and appreciating whatever gives comfort and solace can reduce the intensity of suffering. We have found in our clinical practice that simple pleasures such as the company of a pet or reading humorous stories can change our patients' experiences of pain. Being aware of the variability of one's own responses to pain gives an authentic degree of control, an antidote to the "helpless victim" attitude that generally intensifies suffering.

Another spiritual aspect of yoga is the renunciation of desire. While the majority of Americans who attend Hatha yoga classes may have other goals, yoga itself has been, for thousands of years, a practice stressing equanimity in the presence of either pleasure or pain. This is particularly important for those instances in which pain cannot be eliminated. Yoga then attempts to minimize the pain's impact on the life and soul of the sufferer. In this way, the goals of the pain medicine physician and the yoga therapist coincide at the threshold between the mind and the body. A translation of the *Bhagavad Gita* states "Yoga is the severing of the union with pain" *(4)*.

5. CONDITIONS RESPONDING WELL TO YOGA THERAPY

The substantiated claims that yoga therapists make include many critical areas of medicine that are not covered here in any detail, such as asthma and depression *(15,20,21)*. Each is best treated as part of an integrated program. Physical therapy, oral or injected medication, and other modalities frequently combine to the patients' advantage. The ones we'll consider are—

- Low back pain
- Sciatica and piriformis syndrome
- Carpal tunnel syndrome
- Multiple sclerosis
- Osteoarthritis
- Rotator cuff tears

5.1. Low Back Pain

Low back pain is one of the most common conditions seen in pain medicine practices and is one of the most common reasons patients seek CAM *(20)*. Muscle spasm is the most common cause of lower back pain, and yoga, with its emphases on stretching and relaxation, is particularly well suited to counter it. The McKenzie technique, involving lower spinal extension, also employs a number of movements and positions that are familiar to yoga practitioners. Spondylolisthesis, hyperlordosis, spinal stenosis and sacroiliac joint derangement are often ameliorated or cured through postural work, another of yoga's mainstays *(19,21–28)*.

There is now substantial data to support the use of yoga in the treatment of chronic low back pain. Williams et al. used Iyengar yoga in a 16-week controlled trial of patients with more than 10 years of chronic low back pain *(26)*. Univariate analyses of medical and functional outcomes recorded at 3 months' follow-up found significant reductions in pain intensity (64%), functional disability (77%), and pain medication usage (88%) in the yoga group *(26)*. Sherman et al. randomized 101 patients into three groups, giving one group yoga, a second physical therapy, and assigning the third control group a self-help book. Yoga outperformed the self-help book group on the Roland 24 scale at 12 and 26 weeks (p < .001 in each case), and outperformed physical therapy on a "bothersomeness scale" at 12 weeks (p <0.001) *(28)*.

There are, of course, different causes and therefore different treatments for back pain. For example, although extension may be helpful in herniated disc conditions *(22)*, it will significantly reduce the intraspinal space in spinal stenosis *(23,25)*. Recent literature has begun examining particular approaches to yoga for particular types of lower back pain. Clinicians have analyzed the kinesiological characteristics of the different conditions that cause low back pain, and then found yoga poses that remediate them. In this case, the use of specific yoga postures is, of course, dependent on the diagnosis. This may mean using magnetic resonance imaging (MRI), electromyogram (EMG), CT myelograms, and sometimes trials of diagnostic injections to establish as specific a diagnosis as possible. Epidural steroid injections and non-steroidal anti-inflammatory medications may prepare appropriate patients for the definitive yoga treatment that will help ameliorate the majority of their pain and prevent future episodes. One recent book provides pictures of these diagnosis-specific poses for sacroiliac joint derangement, musculoskeletal causes, herniated nucleus pulposus, spinal stenosis, piriformis syndrome, segmental rigidity, back pain associated with pregnancy, arthritis and obesity, and post-surgical pain *(27)*.

Physical therapy and physiatric texts rightly promote dorsolumbar extension as a means of reducing the severity of herniated lumbar discs *(26)*, and the value of flexion postures for spinal stenosis *(27)*. Lumbar extension may reduce the intramedullary space by up to 63% *(25)*, while forward flexion will often extend a herniated nucleus pulposus further *(27)*. Therefore backbends such as the Cobra, the Camel or *Urdhva Dhanurasana* are reserved for herniated discs, and forward bends such as *Janusirsasana* and P*aschimottanasana* work well for spinal stenosis. Piriformis syndrome, a common spasm-related cause of sciatica, is best treated by an integrative combination of injection, physical therapy and a "home exercise" yoga program *(27,29,30)*. This will include *Parivrtta Trikonasana*, the twisted triangle, a pose well suited for stretching the piriformis muscle, utilizing the reflex mechanisms cited earlier but inappropriate for either of the other main causes of sciatica, radiculopathy and spinal stenosis *(27,30)*.

5.2. Sciatica and Piriformis Syndrome

This is the one condition we treat in depth.

Definition: Pain along the course of the sciatic nerve, originating from irritation of or trauma to its fibers above the knee.

It is a symptom-with-a-range-of-causes: In the literature of 15th century Florence, the term sciatica described pain at the ischial tuberosity. Tuberculosis and arthritis were cited as suspected causes. Historically, a broad and varying definition suggested unclear pathogenesis. Distal pedal pain due to intermittent claudication and nerve entrapment at the fibular head are now termed "pseudo-sciatica" and "peroneal palsy," respectively, but they have often been mistaken for sciatica. More recently, similar symptoms deriving from thalamic cerebrovascular accident, multiple sclerosis, thoracic spinal fracture, and "phantom limb" phenomena have been called sciatica because they share a similar distribution of pain. Symptoms from these causes differ from our core concept in that they involve only the upper motor and sensory neuron. While a patient may accurately describe the pain as "sciatic," the word would describe only the symptom and not the common pathophysiology. We suggest that a cerebrovascular accident infarction in the conus medullaris might be a limiting example of true sciatica if it involved the lower motor and sensory neurons, but question whether anything more rostral could be true sciatica. Another borderline case would be a (rare) mononeuropathy multiplex involving the proximal sciatic nerve.

A study of 700 surgical cases performed under local anesthesia confirmed the utility of our definition, finding symptoms were reproduced only when the sciatic nerve or its involved roots were stimulated, stretched, or compressed. Regardless of other tissue involvement or injury, the closer the stimulus to the site of nerve compression or tension, the greater the pain suffered by the patient. This pain could always be eliminated by injection of Xylocaine beneath the nerve sleeve proximal to the site of compression *(31)*.

Due to variance in definition, studies putting the lifetime prevalence of "generic sciatica" at 35% must be interpreted cautiously *(32–34)*. Two independent studies with more precise definitions similar to ours yield lifetime prevalence of true nerve-related sciatica at 5% in men and 4% in women *(32,35)*. It is thought that back pain affects approximately 14% of adults annually; about 1–2% also have sciatica *(36)*. This amounts to 13% of 40,000,000 back pain cases per year.

Three pathogenic groups contain the common causes of sciatica. They are intraspinal, neuroforaminal and extraspinal. There are also a number of infrequent causes as well as a short list of habitual impostors.

1. Neuroforaminal

   - One level

     - Laterally herniated nucleus pulposus (HNP)/bulging disc
     - Spondylolisthesis

   - Multiple levels

     - Arthritis

2. Intraspinal

   - One level

     - Medially HNP/bulging disc
     - Spondylosisthesis

   - Multiple levels
   - Boney/Ligamentum flavum

3. Extraspinal

   - Piriformis syndrome

     - Overuse/sitting

  - Traumatic
  - Anatomical

- Ischial tunnel

  - Overuse
  - Traumatic

Uncommon causes

- Infectious: e.g., tuberculosis
- Autoimmune: e.g., lupus erythematosus,
- Lumbosacral plexus
- Neuropathy: e.g., mononeuropathy monoplex
- Neoplastic
- Trauma

  - Fracture
  - Gunshot

Impostors

- Sacroiliac joint derangement
- Intermittent claudication
- Thalamic CVA
- Peroneal palsy
- Morton's neuroma

Differential diagnosis begins with the location of the pain and the accompanying symptoms and signs.

1. Diagnosis from muscle weakness

  - Flexing the thigh (with knee bent)—Dx: Radiculopathy at L1–2
  - Extending the knee—Dx: Radiculopathy at L3–4
  - Walking on the heels—Dx: Radiculopathy L4–5
  - Walking on the toes—Dx: Radiculopathy L5–S1
  - Difficulty controlling the bowel or bladder—Dx: S1–2–3

Note: Physical therapists often treat each of these conditions with McKenzie exercises appropriate for the level and severity of injury.

2. Diagnosis from numbness and/or paresthesias

  - Inguinal region, including side of testicle, labia majoris: L1
  - Upper front and side of thigh: L2
  - Main region of front of thigh down to or including knee: L3
  - Inside of calf, top of foot: L4–5
  - First web space, very outside of foot, outside of calf: S1
  - Middle back of thigh: S2
  - Middle portion of testicles, penis, labia majora, anus: S3
  - Glans penis, clitoris: S4

*Adapted from Fishman LM, Ardman CA. 2006. Sciatica Solutions: Diagnosis, Treatment and Cure of Spinal and Piriformis problems. New York: W.W. Norton.

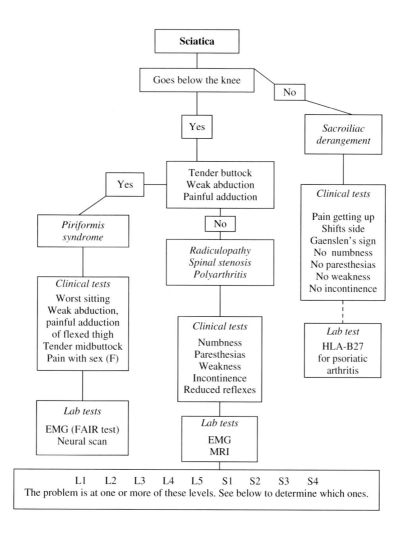

5.2.1. PRE-DIAGNOSTIC TREATMENT FOR SCIATICA

Given the painful nature of sciatica, analgesia often precedes diagnostic workup. Many patients present already having started a pain control regimen with ibuprofen or another over-the-counter non-steroidal anti-inflammatory. Non-steroidal analgesia can be used in ascending order of potency: tramadol (g of Ultram), acetaminophen (g), meloxicam (g of Mobic), celecoxib (g of Celebrex), ketorolac (g of Toradol), diclofenac (g of Voltaren), indomethacin (g). If ineffective, propoxyphene HCI (g of Darvon), acetaminophen/hydrocodone (g of Vicodin), meperidine (g of Demerol), codeine, acetaminophen/codeine (g of Tylenol #3), acetaminophen/oxycodone (g of Percocet), hydromorphone (g of Dilaudid), and oxymorphone (g of Opana) can be utilized. It should be noted that some common synthetic and semi-synthetic opiates include enough acetaminophen to approach hepatotoxicity at prolonged higher dosages.

5.2.2. PRACTICAL DIAGNOSIS

The diverse etiology of sciatica makes it necessary to be comprehensive and precise when evaluating a patient. Many clinicians rely on imaging early on in a patient's treatment. Plain radiographs are rarely useful in the initial evaluation of non-geriatric acute back pain. They do not reveal herniated intervertebral discs nor spinal stenosis, and the findings on plain films are often unrelated to symptoms. For example, spondylolisthesis can be seen in up to 5% of the normal subjects (37). Immediate X-ray of the lumbar spine should be reserved for patients with alarm symptoms suggestive of infection, cancer, or fracture; however, a normal plain film itself does not rule out these conditions. In general, MRI or CT and EMG are required for definitive diagnosis of many spinal conditions. Nonetheless, these studies are not acutely necessary in patients with sciatica unless major neurological deficits or severe pain are present. Imaging studies can usually be deferred until after 4–6 weeks of failed conservative therapy.

Once obtained, there can still be an issue of misdiagnosis. One well-known study found that more than 30% of a group of pain-free subjects had serious spinal abnormalities on their MRIs (38). If spinal pathology can be painless, it can also co-exist with sciatica that has a different cause. This prompts the clinician to use EMG as an extension of the history and physical exam to confirm the diagnosis.

5.2.3. TREATMENT FOR RADICULOPATHY AND SPINAL STENOSIS BY CAUSE

Herniated Nucleus Pulposus. Whether central or lateral, usual treatment begins with McKenzie and manual medical techniques, extension exercises, paraspinal myofascial work, modalities, Alexander work, and/or yoga. Tapering oral steroids (starting dose often dexamethasone 8–16 mg) over a 6-day to 3-week period may dramatically lower a patient's pain, enabling him or her to tolerate an effective therapy program. Translaminar or transforaminal epidural injections are sometimes beneficial, though studies demonstrating the efficacy of these common practices are lacking.

True disc-related sciatica has a very high morbidity. This makes surgery an appealing alternative to conservative treatment for some patients. Many studies support surgery as the most efficient treatment. One analysis of medication use, ability to return to work, leisure activity, and pain score found that after the first year of treatment, 30% of conservatively treated patients were satisfied with their outcome, while 60% of surgically treated patients reported satisfaction with their outcome (39). Surgery continued to lead until differences became insignificant at 10 years and beyond. Another study found 99.99% identical outcomes in surgical and non-surgical patients after 10 years (40). It should be noted that in most studies, the more severely involved patients tended toward the surgical group.

One study followed patients hospitalized for disc-related sciatica for 5 years, comparing the one-third that refused surgery with the two-thirds that did not. At 5 years, 82% of the non-surgically treated patients still had pain in a sciatic distribution, versus 68% of the surgically treated patients. More than 13% of the surgical group required an additional operation for recurrent disc herniation. Outcome studies of these patients found 84% in the WHO "Severe handicap" group (41).

Surgery may be an appealing option for many patients given the generally more favorable outcome. However, a recent study found little risk of serious or permanent injury when surgery for simple sciatica was delayed more than 7 months (42). Given this information, a reasonable approach to treating sciatica clearly caused by a herniated disc is to attempt conservative treatment for 4–6 weeks. If intractable pain persists, a microdiscectomy or similar procedure can reasonably proceed.

Anterior Spondylolisthesis. Anterior spondylolisthesis is the most common form of spondylolisthesis, in which the upper vertebra is moved forward relative to the one below, may cause radiculopathy if it truncates neuroforamina, and/or spinal stenosis if the intraspinal space is narrowed. It is graded I through IV by the quartiles of vertebral body displacement. It is often successfully treated with an abdominal binder or lumbosacral corset, abdominal strengthening, and postural training (the latter by a physical therapist or Alexander therapist). Yoga and Feldenkreis are also helpful. Beyond grade II, be it antero-, retro-, or lateral listhesis, surgical procedures that re-establish the proper alignment often utilize hardware such as titanium cages, and usually meet with considerable, but sub-total improvement that may not last more than 4–5 years. Studies of conservative or surgical treatment of spondylolisthesis are few.

Arthritis. Arthritis may narrow neuroforamina to cause radiculopathy unilaterally or bilaterally at one or more levels. Often, periodic episodes of increasing severity, frequency, and duration occur after the age of 65–70 years. Pain as well as motor and sensory complaints will be gradual in onset, and at least early on, are often positional. Conservative strategy reduces the attendant inflammation, lowers peripheral and central sensitization, and increases range of motion at neighboring joints to reduce compromise at the affected level(s) *(43)*. Non-steroidal and/or steroidal anti-inflammatories, yoga, and physical therapy often accomplish these three goals Training in yoga allows patients to maintain the beneficial effects of stretching with home practice *(44–46)*. Although quite effective, steroids must be used with caution in osteoporotic patients. More advanced or complicated cases of arthritis may require surgery to remove deteriorated bone and disc material, osteophytes, or other matter impinging on the nerves. In these refractory patients, an EMG is helpful in identifying and characterizing the levels warranting treatment. If yoga does anything, it stretches.

Boney Growth and/or Swelling of the Ligamentum Flavum. Boney growth and/or swelling of the ligamentum flavum may narrow the lumbar intraspinal canal, causing single or multiple level spinal stenosis and resultant sciatica. The former may have genetic or arthritic pathogenesis, the latter inflammatory or traumatic. Conservative treatment aims to reduce the girth of the canal's contents: tapered oral or epidural steroids, traction, and postural work by physical therapists, yoga therapists, Alexander therapists, and osteopathic physicians have had success.

While ligamentous swelling may subside naturally, boney narrowing will not. Surgical intervention, sometimes requiring stabilization procedures as well, should be considered when a progressive boney thickening is documented, but before emergent intervention is required. Cauda equina syndrome, a rare complication of spinal stenosis in which ascending numbness or weakness and bladder or bowel incontinence, results from extreme pressure on descending rootlets within the intraspinal space, is one such surgical emergency.

In a recent study of non-emergent spinal stenosis surgery, outcome comparison of control and intervention groups at 1 and 4 years favored surgical treatment. After 8–10 years, a similar percentage reported low back pain that was improved but sciatica relief continued to favor the surgical group *(47)*. Because it is generally progressive, surgery for spinal stenosis may wisely occur before it is utterly mandatory, since its necessity may arise after the patient is too frail for it *(48)*.

Piriformis syndrome. Piriformis syndrome is an under-recognized cause of sciatica. This was validated when 239 patients who failed conservative or surgical treatment for the above causes underwent MR neurography. Piriformis involvement was found in more than two-thirds of them *(49)*. Symptoms arise from compression of the sciatic nerve as it exits the buttock in relation to the piriformis muscle, due to spasm or tightness in the muscle. The chief environmental causes are overuse at health clubs, from running, outdoor activities, excessive sitting, trauma from auto accidents, and falls. Anomalous relationships between the sciatic nerve and the inferior gluteal artery or vein at the greater sciatic foramen are uncommon but demonstrated anatomic bases for pain.

Diagnosis is made by EMG through delay of H-reflexes in flexion, adduction, and internal rotation (the FAIR test). Comparing affected with unaffected limbs helps rule out radiculopathy or spinal stenosis, and may be used in the 90% of cases that are unilateral *(50)*. Neural scan imaging (NMR) will show asymmetrical development of the affected piriformis muscle, and evidence of inflammation or focal narrowing of the sciatic nerve. EMG and NMR will only be positive if sciatic compression in the buttock is present, not with sacroiliac derangement alone. However, these conditions occur together with some frequency. Since the piriformis muscle arises in part from the sacroiliac joint, it is possible that sacroiliac joint derangement causes piriformis muscle spasm in these cases.

Conservative treatment begins with EMG-guided or fluoroscopically guided steroid and lidocaine/Marcaine injection of the piriformis muscle near its lateral musculo-tendinous junction, as well as stretching and relaxing the muscle, using ultrasound, myofascial release, and spray/stretch techniques. Appropriate home yoga therapy is often successful over time *(51)*. Yoga poses in which the hip is adducted and flexed will stretch the restricting gluteal and lateral thigh muscles. This can be done with standing or seated poses; *Parivrtta trikonasana* (standing revolved triangle pose). *Parivrtta ardhachandrasana* (standing revolved half moon pose) and *Ardha Matsyendrasana* (Seated twist named after a sage) are poses that we have used with success. *(51)*. Botulinum neurotoxin A or B, 300 or 12,500 units, respectively, in four locations throughout the muscle, are reported to significantly relieve 60–90% of the resistant cases *(52)*. Neurovascular anomalies and ventral piriformis muscle scars require surgery, which appears to benefit 60–80% of cases *(53)*.

5.2.4. CONFUSION RESOLVED

While the rare vascular and neurological abnormalites have been shown to cause piriformis syndrome, the common variations in anatomy do not. Piriformis syndrome is often attributed to the sciatic nerve passing through the piriformis muscle, an anatomic "anomaly." Cadaveric studies show that approximately 15% of the population has at least one branch of the sciatic nerve that travels such a course. Interestingly, in these people, the anatomy is bilateral more than 90% of the time. The "anomaly" theory comes into question in that complaints consistent with piriformis syndrome are bilateral in less than 10% of patients. Further, at surgery only 15% of patients have had anatomy consistent with the "anomaly" theory, the same percentage that is seen in the general population *(54)*.

5.2.5. ISCHIAL TUNNEL SYNDROME

The FAIR test is occasionally positive when entrapment is at a site other than the piriformis muscle. Four percent of sciatic nerve entrapment in the buttock is due to entrapment as the nerve passes close to the ischium *(55)*. The pudendal nerve may be separately involved. Neural scan is the definitive diagnostic tool for ischial tunnel syndrome. In these cases, treatment begins with myofascial release, modalities, and postural re-training. Surgery is reported but outcome studies lack sufficient numbers to be persuasive. Again, yoga poses in which the thigh is adducted and flexed will stretch the restricting soft tissue in the gluteal area and lateral thigh. One particular pose that is applicable here is *Gomukhasana*, a seated pose in which both femurs are adducted maximally. This pose can be learned in a gentle way while sitting in a chair, then progressing to sitting on a folded blanket on the floor.

There are many other causes of sciatica, ranging from tumor and fracture to gunshot wound. In all, the pathogenetic mechanism and the diagnosis can be understood on the anatomical bases that we have attempted to provide. Multiple conditions can co-exist in which the analytical "either–or" approach is not recommended: proper initial treatment for a herniated disc is extension exercises, which is contraindicated in spondylolisthesis and non-disc forms of spinal stenosis. For these last conditions, flexion is standard, which is contraindicated for most herniated discs. In the occurrence of both conditions, lateral strengthening and spinal work such as the yoga pose *vasisthasana* have proven useful in alleviating pain, with Fonar evidence of anatomical improvement *(56)*.

5.3. Carpal Tunnel Syndrome

One of yoga's first incursions into mainstream medicine was the result of Garfinkel's study *(18)* indicating reduced levels of discomfort in patients with moderately severe carpal tunnel syndrome after a short course of yoga. Here again, diagnosis usually requires EMG or musculoskeletal ultrasound. Oral non-steroidals and steroidal injections with night splints are compatible with yoga. If this fails, a simple and effective surgery may be followed by a different set of asanas that often hasten recovery and sustain full hand use *(26)*. In milder cases, and those for which a non-repetitive incident is the cause, yoga may be combined with wrist splints for recovery. Most of the better studies and the best treatment use EMG to monitor progress.

5.4. Multiple Sclerosis

One of the most disabling and frustrating parts of chronic relapsing or chronic progressive multiple sclerosis (MS) is fatigue. Oken et al. have shown *(57)* the efficacy of yoga in diminishing, if not eliminating, fatigue in patients with MS. Here, too, the practice of yoga might enable the patient to participate in physical therapy and other active treatments. Yoga and medications do not interfere with one another; on the contrary, they are mutually beneficial. In our clinical experience, the generous use of props in Iyengar and Anusara yoga are greatly appreciated by our MS patients. A book on this subject intended for patients with MS was published in May 2007 *(58)*.

5.5. Osteoarthritis

The neurological advantages of stretch apply forcibly to osteoarthritis, since reducing the tendency to maintain agonist-antagonist tension may slow progress of the "wear-and-tear" disease. Stretching has obvious implications for increasing joint range and other measures of improved joint function *(59)* and thereby reducing discomfort *(60)*. In addition, the slow, no-impact movement of joints to their extremes also promotes circulation of joint fluid. Since the inner adjacent surfaces of joint cartilage lack perichondrium *(61)*, chondrocytes depend on this circulation for their nutrition and for carrying away the products of metabolism. Work in France documents that mast cell and nitrite concentration is higher in osteoarthritic synovial fluid than in rheumatoid synovial fluid, implying that these elements are active in osteoarthritis. This too suggests a beneficial role to improving synovial circulation *(62)*.

As well as improving functional movement in the joints, yoga safely develops the arthritic practitioner's awareness of all the coordinating structures (muscles, tendons, capsules, ligaments) that influence the joints and are affected by their welfare *(12)*. Joints act in concert, and each must adapt to the limitations of the other joints near it. Increasing range of motion is a major goal. Yoga is a natural ally here. Combined with non-steroidal anti-inflammatory medications, periodic focal physical therapy for particular problems, and judiciously placed injections, yoga can be a great boon to patients as well as healthcare payers and providers. Inherent in yoga is a self-checking and very low-injury means of prolonging the functional life of joints while stretching and coordinating the muscles, ligaments and capsules that cross them. Yoga delays joint restrictions that make movement painful.

Activating the agonist–antagonist mechanism has implications for strengthening as well. One example is reversing painful and unsafe weakness in the quadriceps through the forward bend (Figure 3). This manner of "dynamic tension" is a clear isometric strengthening technique with benefits for both muscle groups involved. Yoga strengthens muscles in other ways, including important muscles that have no physiological antagonists. Sometimes it is wise to begin with non-steroidals and withdraw them gradually as the yoga enables activity in normal ranges of motion.

Our book *Yoga for Arthritis,* published by WWNorton 2008, outlines a full program of yoga for osteoarthritis. This text can offer clinicians and patients a useful guide for yoga techniques, arranged by joint, with detailed instructions.

5.6. Rotator Cuff Tear

Rotator cuff tears are a major cause of shoulder pain and can be treated non-surgically by teaching patients the Iyengar-method headstand. It generally trains patients to replace supraspinatus contraction with subscapularis-plus-deltoid activity *(63–65)* in the 80–120 degree range of abduction and flexion. This enables painless full active range, and rests the supraspinatus, possibly allowing it to heal.

Rotator cuff tears are more frequently seen in the aging population *(66)*. Some are irreparable. For others, MRI, arthrogram or ultrasound confirms a serious rupture suggesting surgery *(66)*. The yoga method that trains use of the subscapularis-plus-deltoid to relieve the pain and reduce the disability was successful in a pilot study *(63–65)*. A controlled study is in progress. The yoga work is typically integrated with physical therapy and short-term analgesics. In fourteen patients thus far, this integrated treatment has nearly quadrupled range of motion for abduction and flexion to 168 and 170 degrees, respectively, and decreased the mean pain score from 4.8 to 1.2 on the ten-point visual analogue scale *(65)*. These gains are comparable to those reported in the most successful surgical studies, and superior to most *(67)*. Physical therapy for strengthening, a short-term sling, and repeat MRI after six months are also included in this treatment plan.

5.7. Piriformis Syndrome

A group of neurosurgeons, radiologists, anaesthesiologists, and physiatrists at UCLA used neural scans to identify the cause of sciatica in 238 patients with normal lumbosacral MRIs or unsuccessfully operated lumbar spines. Piriformis syndrome was found to be the cause in more than 66% of them *(29)*. This group projects that piriformis syndrome may be as common a cause of sciatica as herniated nucleus pulposis. Modern diagnosis for the condition is by H-reflex delay and neural scan. Conservative treatment by EMG- or image-guided steroid/lidocaine or botulinum neurotoxin injection, and physical therapy *(29,30,68–70)* improves more than 80% of the patients diagnosed and treated this way at least 50% within 2–3 months. This is reduced to 2–3 weeks after botulinum injection. Post-treatment patients *continue* to do much better with home exercise programs *(68–70)*. Yoga exercises significantly prolong these results *(27,71)*, and are available with pictures in a text *(27)*. Some examples of poses that may be useful in piriformis syndrome are *Ardha Matsyendrasana, Jathara Parivarthasana,* and the already mentioned *Parivrtta Trikonasana (27)*. These poses flex and adduct the thigh, stretching the soft tissue of the lateral thigh and hip.

6. SAFETY

Although yoga is no-impact, low-speed, and introspective, injuries do occur. These fall chiefly into two categories:

1. beginners taught in undersupervised or overcrowded conditions, and
2. advanced practitioners who have surpassed their anatomical or fitness-related limits.

Injured beginners often have placed themselves in positions that either strain the patello-femoral joint in V*irasana* (see Figure 2), their lumbar spine (back bends or *Paschimottanasana* (see Figure 3), or mildly derange their sacroiliac joints (standing poses or twists). In clinical settings, hiring competent and experienced yoga teachers or therapists and making them aware of the patient's relevant medical history minimizes these injuries. Of course, one-to-one teaching insures a measure of safety that large classes cannot provide. More advanced and adventurous practitioners can help themselves more and hurt themselves less by learning anatomy and physiology, and by practicing carefully with an understanding of their own limitations.

7. MODELS OF CARE

These examples may have already persuaded the reader that yoga fits very well into the rubric of integrative medicine. It is a practice that can be done at home, with virtually no equipment, generating no noise or medical waste, is utterly transportable, and reasonably easily learned in a safe and low-cost context and is eminently adaptable to other modalities of treatment. We very frequently use injections, oral medications, physical therapy, Alexander technique, massage, acupuncture, and kinetic awareness methods in conjunction with Hatha yoga and simple meditation and breathing techniques. When these fail, we may use yoga, physical therapy, and modalities in rehabilitation post-surgically.

8. GENERAL RULES FOR SPECIFIC SITUATIONS

Specifically, trigger point, nerve block, and chemodenervation injections are useful to prepare muscles for the obedient stretching that reduces piriformis syndrome. Muscle relaxants and analgesics are rarely needed. For sacroiliac joint derangement,

Table 3
Useful Yoga Terms and Definitions

Term	Definition
Hatha yoga	Identifies the practice as physical exercise; does not imply a particular school of training
Vinyasa	Postures are practiced as a continuous flow from one to another; Vinyasa classes usually move fairly quickly
Power yoga	Physically demanding style of yoga similar to Ashtanga with a Western spin
Open class	Indicates that people of any experience level, including beginners, are welcome

non-steroidal anti-inflammatory medications accompany muscle energy and strain-counterstrain techniques and a number of yoga and non-yoga home exercises. Versions of the Peacock, *Gomukhasana,* and *Garudasana* are particularly successful. Herniated discs require the extensions mentioned earlier and sometimes *Salabhasana,* the Locust, and *Adho Mukha Svanasana,* the Downward Dog, as well as many modified and improvised maneuvers. Here we might use anything from epidural steroids to medications, acupuncture for pain relief, and meditation as well as McKenzie exercises in physical therapy. For musculoskeletal pain, massage, Feldenkrais, kinetic awareness and Alexander technique, alone or in combination with yoga, usually require only very short-term medicinal adjuncts.

9. YOGA AS THERAPY

The cost of yoga *therapists* may be $50—$200 per hour, but usually only a few therapeutic sessions are needed. After that, most stable patients may attend regular yoga classes once weekly for $10–$20 and/or practice daily at home.

Liability is reduced by keeping up communication among the primary referring clinician and the yoga practitioner, and, of course, the patient.

10. RESOURCES

Because the tree of yoga has so many branches and its current popularity has led to the creation of hundreds of teacher training programs around the world, interested people may be challenged to know where to turn. Many of the types of yoga listed maintain certification programs that set professional standards in the Western sense. These styles of yoga, as mentioned, differ in emphasis. However, the personality and degree of training of the teacher can matter as much as the style or technique. The best way, therefore, to find a yoga class is probably to try a few and see what fits the individual. Try diligently, but don't be afraid to say, "I don't want to try that one." Yoga Alliance has a registry of their approved schools and approved teachers but not therapists.

A number of teachers are therapists, but specifically for *therapeutics*, examine a teacher's *curriculum vitae*, or ask directly about training and experience using yoga therapeutically. We believe that a yoga therapist should have practiced yoga for a minimum of ten years. At the time of this writing many schools have their own standards of training. The *Journal of the International Association of Yoga Therapists* is an invaluable source of information about therapists who belong.

Websites of each style of yoga can easily be found on the Internet.

http://www.iayt.org/: International Association of Yoga Therapists.

http://www.iyta.org/: Integral Yoga Teachers Association.

http://www.yogaalliance.org/: Yoga Alliance.

http://www.yogajournal.com/: Yoga Journal magazine.

http://www.anusarayoga.com/: Listings of Anusara trained teachers.

http://www.iynaus.org/: Listings of Iyengar trained teachers.

www.yrec.org: Yoga Research and Education Center.

A few of the many books and tapes currently available: *Light on Yoga*. B.K.S. Iyengar. Schocken Books, New York, many editions. The classic modern text with more than 600 pictures.

Relief is in the Stretch. Loren Fishman and Carol Ardman. W.W. Norton, New York, 2005. Yoga for back pain by diagnosis.

Yoga for Multiple Sclerosis. Loren Fishman and Eric Small. Demos Medical Publishing May, 2007. Pictures and instructions for every level of ability.

Yoga for Arthritis. Loren Fishman and Ellen Saltonstall. W.W. Norton, March, 2008. Detailed help for most common arthritic conditions.

Yoga Rx. Larry Payne and Richard Usatine. Broadway Books, New York, 2002. Sensible overview.

The Woman's Book of Yoga and Health: a Lifelong Guide to Wellness. Linda Sparrowe and Patricia Walden. Shambhala, Boston, 2002. Compendious and safe.

Back Care Basics: A Doctor's Gentle Yoga Program for Back and Neck Pain Relief. Mary Pullig Schatz. Rodmell Press, Berkeley, California, 1995. Somewhat difficult but smart, anatomically-designed and beneficial program.

The Heart of Meditation: Pathways to a Deeper Experience. Swami Durgananda (Sally Kempton). SYDA foundation, South Fallsburg, NY. 2002.

Excellent introduction to meditation that goes quite deep.

The Yoga Sutra of Patanjali, Translated and Introduced by Alistair Shearer, Bell Tower, New York, 1982. Definitive earliest work.

The Bhagavad Gita, translated and introduced by Juan Mascaro, Penguin Books, 1962. Central Hindu text that has bearing on the spirit of yoga.

The Yoga Tradition. Georg Feuerstein, Hohm Press, 1998.

Scholarly work with breadth and insight similar to Jakob Burckhardt.

The Science of Yoga. I.K. Taimni. Quest Books, Theosophical Publishing House, Wheaton, Illinois. 1972. The Yoga sutra in Sanskrit with transliteration, translation, and excellent explanatory commentary.

Light on the Yoga sutra of Patanjali. B.K.S. Iyengar. Thorsons, an Imprint of Harper Collins Publishers, 1996. Another well-received version of the work.

Relax and Renew: Restful Yoga for Stressful Times. Judith Lasater. Rodmell Press, Berkeley California, 1995. Practical and spiritual application of yoga by a Ph.D. and profound and sensitive world-wide teacher.

Stress-reduction programs incorporating yoga, books, tapes. Jon Kabat Zinn Stress Reduction Clinic, University of Massachusetts Medical Center.

Yoga Unveiled. DVD that gives history and overview of yoga.

REFERENCES

1. The Yoga Sutra of Patanjali. 1982. Translated and Introduced by Alistair Shearer. New York: Bell Tower, p. 26.
2. Feuerstein G. The Yoga Sutra of Patanjali: A New Translation and Commentary. Inner Tradit Int 1991.
3. Taimni IK. 1994. The Science of Yoga. Theosophical Publishing House.
4. Feuerstein G. 2003. The Deeper Dimensions of Yoga, Shambhala Books, p. 10.
5. Cushman A. New light on Yoga. Yoga J 1999;44–49.
6. Norman S. 1996. The Yoga Tradition of the Mysore Palace. South Asia Books (Referred to in Cushman).
7. Lazar SW, Kerr CE, Wasserman RH, Gray JR, Greve DN, Treadway MT, McGarvey M, Quinn BT, Dusek JA, Benson H, Rauch SL, Moore CI, Fischl B. Meditation experience is associated with increased cortical thickness. Neuroreport 2005;16(17):1893–1897.
8. Peng, C, Henry, IC, Mietus, JE, Hausdorff, JM, Khalsa, G, Benson, H, Gokdberger, AL. Heart rate dynamics during three forms of meditation Int J Cardiol 2004;95(1):19–27.
9. Granit, R., Holmgren, B. Two pathways from brain stem to gamma ventral horn cells. Acta Physiol Scand 1955;35: 9–108.
10. Sekiguchi H, Nakazawa K, Suzuki S. Differences in recruitment properties of the corticospinal pathway between lengthening and shortening contractions in human soleus muscle. Brain Res 2003;977(2):169–179.
11. Granit R. 1955. Receptors and Sensory Perception. New Haven, CT: Yale University Press:
12. Telles S, Hanumanthaiah BH, Nagarathna R, Nagendra HR. Plasticity of motor control systems demonstrated by yoga training. Indian J Physiol Pharmacol 1994;38(2):143–144.
13. DiBenedetto M, Innes KE, Taylor AG, Rodeheaver PF, Boxer JA, Wright HJ, Kerrigan DC. Effect of a gentle Iyengar yoga program on gait in the elderly: an exploratory study. Arch Phys Med Rehabil 2005; 86:1830–1837.
14. Raghuraj P, Telles S. Effect of yoga-based and forced uninostril breathing on the autonomic nervous system. Percept Mot Skills 2003;96(1):79–80.
15. Brown RP, Gerbarg PL. Sudarshan Kriya yogic breathing in the treatment of stress, anxiety, and depression: part I—neurophysiologic model. J Altern Complement Med 2005;11(1):189–201 (Erratum in: J Altern Complement Med. 2005;11(2):383–384).
16. Deckro GR, Ballinger KM, Hoyt M, Wilcher M, Dusek J, Myers P, Greenberg B, Rosenthal DS, Benson H. The evaluation of a mind/body intervention to reduce psychological distress and perceived stress in college students. J Am Coll Health 2002;50(6):281–287
17. Stefano GB, Esch T, Cadet P, Zhu W, Mantione K, Benson H. Endocannabinoids as autoregulatory signaling molecules: coupling to nitric oxide and a possible association with the relaxation response. Med Sci Monit 2003;9(4)RA:63–75.
18. Garfinkel JS, Singhal A, Katz WA, Allan DA, Reshetar R, Schumacher HR. Yoga-based intervention for carpal tunnel syndrome: a randomized trial. J Am Med Assoc 1998;280(18):1601–1603.
19. Koleck M, Mazaux JM, Rascle N, Bruchon-Schweitzer M. Psycho-social factors and coping strategies as predictors of chronic evolution and quality of life in patients with low back pain: a prospective study. Eur J Pain 2006;10(1):1–11.
20. Long L, Huntley A, Ernst E. Which complementary and alternative therapies benefit which conditions? A survey of the opinions of 223 professional organizations. Complement Ther Med 2001;9(3): 178–185.
21. Williams AL, Selwyn PA, Liberti L, Molde S, Njike VY, McCorkle R, Zelterman D, Katz DL. A randomized controlled trial of meditation and massage effects on quality of life in people with late-stage disease: a pilot study. J Palliative Med 2005;5:939–52.
22. Lyle MA, Manes S, McGuinness M, Ziaei S, Iversen MD. Relationship of physical examination findings and self-reported symptom severity and physical function in patients with degenerative lumbar conditions. Physical Ther 2005;85(20):120–133.
23. Swami Muktibudhananda. 1998. Hatha Yoga Pradipika. Bihar School of Yoga, 4th Rep. edition.

24. McKenzie, Robin. 1997. Robin Treat your own Back. Orthopedic Physical Therapy Products, 7th edition.
25. Vo AN, Kamen LB, Shih VC, Bitar AA, Stitik TP, Kaplan RJ. Rehabilitation of orthopedic and rheumatologic disorders. Lumbar spinal stenosis. Arch Phys Med Rehabil 2005;86(3Suppl 1): S69–S76.
26. Williams KA, Petronis J, Smith D, Goodrich D, Wu J, Ravi N, Doyle EJ, Jr., Gregory Juckett R, Munoz Kolar M, Gross R, Steinberg L. Effect of Iyengar yoga therapy for chronic low back pain. Pain 2005;115(1–2):107–117.
27. Fishman LM, Ardman CA. 2005. Relief is in the Stretch: End Back Pain Through Yoga. New York: W.W. Norton and Co.
28. Sherman KJ, Cherkin DC, Erro J, et al. Comparing yoga, exercise, and a self-care book for chronic low back pain: a randomized trial. Ann Int Med 2005;143:849–856.
29. Filler AG, Haynes J, Jordan SE, Prager J, Villablanca JP, Farahani K, McBride DQ, Tsurudu JS, Morisoli B, Batzdorf U, Johnson JP, Sciatica of nondisc origin and piriformis syndrome: diagnosis by magnetic resonance neurography and interventional magnetic resonance imaging with outcome study of resulting treatment. J Neurosurg Spine 2:99–115.
30. Fishman LM, Dombi GW, Michaelsen C, Ringel SV, Rosbruch J, Rosner B, Weber C. Piriformis syndrome: diagnosis, treatment and outcome—a ten year study. Arch Phys Rehabil 2002;83:(3) 295–302.
31. Kuslich SD, et al. The tissue origin of low back pain and sciatica: a report of pain response to tissue stimulation during operations on the lumbar spine using local anesthesia. Orthop Clinic North Am 1991;22:181–187.
32. Heliovaara M, et al. Lumbar disc syndrome in Finland. J Epidemiol Community Health 1987;41: 251–258.
33. Svensson HO, Andersson GBL. A retrospective study of low back pain in 38- to 64 year old women: frequency and occurrence and impact on medical services. Spine 1988;13:548–522.
34. Svensson HO, Andersson GBL. Low back pain in forty to forty-seven year old men: work history and work environment factors. Spine 1983;8:272–276.
35. Manninen P, et al. Incidence and risk factors of low-back pain in middle-aged farmers. Occup Med 1995;45:141–146
36. Deyo, RA, Tsui-Wu, YJ. Descriptive epidemiology of low back pain and its related medical care in the United States. Spine 1987;12:264.
37. Rothman RH, Simeone FA. Spondylolisthesis. The Spine, Vol 1, 1992. pp. 913–969.
38. Jensen MC, Brant RC, Obuchowski N, Modic MT, Malkasian D, Ross JS. Magnetic resonance imaging of the lumbar spine in people without back pain. N Engl J Med 1994;69–73.
39. Weber H. 1982 Volvo Award in Clinical Science. Lumbar disc herniation: a controlled, prospective study with ten years of observation. Spine 1983; 8(2):131–140.
40. Agency for Health Care Policy and Research. Acute Low Back Problems in Adults. Clinical Practice Guidelines No. 14, Publication 95-0642, 1994 Rockville, MD.
41. Nykvist F, et al. A prospective 5-year follow-up study of 276 patients hospitalized because of suspected lumbar disc herniation. Int Disabil Stud 1989;11(2):61–67.
42. Carragee E. Surgical treatment of lumbar disk disorders. JAMA 2006;296:2485–2487.
43. Wolff CJ, Salter MW. Neuronal plasticity: increasing the gain in pain. Science 2000;288:1765–1768.
44. Raghuraj P, Telles S. Effect of yoga-based and forced uninostril breathing on the autonomic nervous system. Percept Mot Skills 2003; 96(1):79–80.
45. Telles S, Hanumanthaiah BH, Nagarathna R, Nagendra HR. Plasticity of motor control systems demonstrated by yoga training. Indian J Physiol Pharmacol 1994;38(2):143–144.
46. Williams KA, Petronis J, Smith D, Goodrich D, Wu J, Ravi N, Doyle EJ Jr., Gregory Juckett R, Munoz G, Kolar M, Gross R, Steinberg L. Effect of Iyengar yoga therapy for chronic low back pain. Pain 2005;115(1–2):107–117.
47. Atlas SJ, Keller RB, Wu YA, Deyo RA, Singer DE. Long-term outcomes of surgical and nonsurgical management of lumbar spinal stenosis: 8 to 10 year results from the maine lumbar spine study. Spine 2005;April 15;30(8):936–43.
48. Agency for Health Care Policy and Research. Acute Low Back Problems in Adults. Clinical Practice Guidelines No. 14, Publication 95-0642, 1994 Rockville, MD.
49. Papadopoulos, EC, Khan, SN. Piriformis syndrome and low back pain: a new classification and review of the literature. Orthop Clin North Am 2004;35:65.

50. Fishman LM, Zybert PA. Electrophysiologic evidence of piriformis syndrome. Arch Phys Med Rehabil 1992;73(4):359–364.
51. Fishman L, Ardman C. 2005. Relief is in the Stretch. New York: W.W. Norton.
52. Fishman LM, Konnoth C, Rozner B. Botulinum neurotoxin type B and physical therapy in the treatment of piriformis syndrome: a dose-finding study. Am J Phys Med Rehabil 2004;83(1):42–50.
53. Mizuguchi T. Division of the piriformis muscle for the treatment of sciatica. Postlaminectomy syndrome and osteoarthritis of the spine. Arch Surg 1976;111(6):719–722.
54. Broadhurst NA, Simmons DN, Bond MJ. Piriformis syndrome: Correlation of muscle morphology with symptoms and signs. Arch Phys Med Rehabil 2004;85(12):2036–2039.
55. Filler AG, Haynes J, Jordan SE, et al. Sciatica of nondisc origin and piriformis syndrome: diagnosis by magnetic resonance neurography and interventional magnetic resonance imaging with outcome study of resulting treatment. J Neurosurg Spine 2005;2(2):99–115.
56. Fishman LM and Saltonstall E. 2008. Yoga for Osteoarthritis. New York: W.W. Norton. Scheduled for publication in Spring.
57. Oken BS, Kishiyama S, Zajdel D, Bourdette D, Carlsen J, Haas M, Hugos C, Kraemer DF, Lawrence J, Mass M. Randomized controlled trial of yoga and exercise in multiple sclerosis. Neurology 2004;62(11):2058–2064.
58. Fishman LM, Small E. Yoga for Multiple Sclerosis 2007 Demos Medical Publishing, New York (Scheduled for publication March, 2008)
59. Kolasinski SL, Garfinkel M, Tsai AG, Matz W, Van Dyke A, Schumacher HR. Iyengar yoga for treating symptoms of osteoarthritis of the knees: a pilot study. J Altern Complement Med 2005;11(4):689–693.
60. Garfinkel MS, Schumacher HR, Jr., Husain A, Levy M, Reshetar RA. Evaluation of a yoga based regimen for treatment of osteoarthritis of the hands. J Rheumatol. 1994;21(12):2341–2343.
61. Junqueira LC, Carneiro J. Basic Histology, 10th edition. McGraw-Hill, p.136.
62. Renoux M, Hilliquin P, Galoppin L, Florentin J, Menkes CJ. Cellular activation products in osteoarthritis synovial fluid. Int J Clin Pharmacol Res 1995;15(4):135–138.
63. Fishman LM, Polesin A, Konnoth C. Headstand in the treatment of rotator cuff syndrome – *Sirsasana* or surgery. J Assoc Yoga Ther (16):2006,137–45.
64. Fishman LM, Konnoth C. Role of headstand in the management of rotator cuff syndrome. Am J Phys Med Rehabil 2004: 83(3):228 (abstract).
65. Fishman LM, Polesin A, Konnoth C. Headstand in the treatment of rotator cuff syndrome – *Sirsasana* or Surgery. J Int Assoc Yoga Ther (16):2006,137–45.
66. Laudicina L, D'Ambrosia R. Management of irreparable rotator cuff tears and glenohumeral arthritis. Orthopedics 2005;28(4):382–388.
67. Van Linthoudt D, Deforge J, Malterre L, Huber H. Rotator cuff repair. Long-term results. Joint Bone Spine 2003;70(4):271–275.
68. Fishman LM, Konnoth C, Rosner B. Botulinum neurotoxin type B and physical therapy in the treatment of piriformis syndrome: a dose-finding study. Am J Phys Med Rehabil 2004;83:42–50.
69. Childers MK, Wilson DJ, Gnatz SM, Conway RR, Sherman AK. Botulinum toxin in piriformis muscle syndrome. Am J Phys Med Rehabil 2002; 81(10):751–759.
70. Fishman LM, Konnoth C, Rozner B. Botulinum neurotoxin type B and physical therapy in the treatment of piriformis syndrome: a dose-finding study. Am J Phys Med Rehabil 2004;83:42–50.
71. Fishman LM, Saltonstall E. Yoga for Arthritis. W.W. Norton, New York, 2008.

14 Contemporary Aquatic Therapy and Pain Management

Douglas W. Kinnaird and Bruce E. Becker

CONTENTS

CONTEMPORARY AQUATIC THERAPY AND PAIN
    REHABILITATION: OLD WINE IN NEW BOTTLES
WHY WATER?
AQUATIC THERAPY AND PAIN REHABILITATION
AQUATIC THERAPY TECHNIQUES—APPLYING THE PRINCIPLES
CONTRAINDICATIONS AND PRECAUTIONS
INTEGRATING AQUATIC THERAPY INTO A PAIN PRACTICE
THERAPISTS LEAD ADVANCES IN PRACTICAL APPLICATIONS

Summary

Though the therapeutic use of water is an ancient practice, American interest waned after the end of the polio epidemic in the 1950s. NASA studies and research into the physiological effects of immersion, however, revived interest in the 1990s. Meanwhile, physicians and therapists in other countries continued to research and to develop techniques that now compose the primary approaches to aquatic therapy and rehabilitation in the United States. Aquatic therapy and rehabilitation is considered a multi-disciplinary specialty with some technique certifications and overall certification offered by the National Commission for the Credentialing of Aquatic Rehabilitation Disciplines (NCCARD).

The essential properties of water—density, buoyancy, viscosity and specific heat—act on essentially every homeostatic system of the body, reducing edema, enhancing circulation, measurably reducing weight-bearing stress, and relieving pain.

Turbulence, caused by moving water around the body, or by moving the body through water, provides further therapeutic benefits: thermal conductivity is enhanced; drag forces challenge movement and balance to strengthen muscles and improve proprioception; viscosity helps prevent the risk of falling; resistance to movement can be balanced between agonists and antagonists; painful movements can be stopped instantly to prevent damage; and combined with hydrostatic pressure, turbulence acts to further reduce pain.

The multiple effects of immersion and movement in water provide a rich field for research. While research is not lacking internationally, much that has been done with aquatic therapy and rehabilitation is based on anecdotal or experiential evidence. With modern tools for measurement and quantification, scientific evidence for the value of the therapeutic use of water could lead to its greater acceptance and utilization, reducing healthcare costs and improving outcomes for millions of Americans.

From: *Contemporary Pain Medicine: Integrative Pain Medicine: The Science and Practice
of Complementary and Alternative Medicine in Pain Management*
Edited by: J. F. Audette and A. Bailey © Humana Press, Totowa, NJ

Key Words: aquatic therapy, water therapy, Watsu®, Bad Ragaz Ring Method, Halliwick Concept, Burdenko Method, and Ai Chi

1. CONTEMPORARY AQUATIC THERAPY AND PAIN REHABILITATION: OLD WINE IN NEW BOTTLES

A frail, elderly woman, obviously in pain, pushes her walker to the stairway. Grasping the handrail, she sidesteps carefully down. As she settles into the warm therapy pool, a blissful smile spreads over her face and she walks easily toward deeper water.

The last decade of the 20th century, up to the present, has seen an American renaissance of one of mankind's oldest approaches to health and healing. Using water for therapy and rehabilitation predates recorded history and has been practiced by almost every known civilization.

Art, texts, and ruins from Mesopotamia, Egypt, India, and China attest to the use of baths and pools for the healing of body, mind, and spirit. Spas of ancient Greece and Rome were integral to those civilizations. The word *spa* derives from the Latin: *spargere*—"to pour forth" *(1)*.

Most modern nations have maintained, and even built on, traditional water therapies. Polio influenced modern use of aquatic therapy, with the addition of active movement to the more traditional method of passive immersion, which had prevailed since the Middle Ages *(2)*. In health spas throughout the world, patients lay on submerged plinths for passive and assisted range-of-motion exercises or sometimes even walked in the buoyant environment of deeper water.

Therapists in Wildbad, Bavaria, began using flotation rings during the 1930s to support patients for two-dimensional water movements. In 1957, therapists in Bad Ragaz, Switzerland, adopted ring flotation for use with a wider range of active exercises, including proprioceptive neuromuscular facilitation (PNF) *(3)*.

Hydraulics engineer James McMillan stirred a revolution in 1950, maintaining that buoyant equipment was both unnecessary and inhibiting to neuromuscular training. Using fluid dynamics, he developed adaptive swimming techniques for children with cerebral palsy. McMillan taught his Halliwick Concept in England, moving later to Bad Ragaz, where he continued researching and teaching until 1994.

Advances in medical specialization and pharmaceutical research, such as the development of the new polio vaccines, overshadowed American interest in aquatic therapy for years. Two areas of research, neither directly related to therapy or rehabilitation, eventually brought a renewal of interest. First was recognition that immersion is ideal for studying the physiological effects of sudden changes in blood volume, in the cardiac, pulmonary and renal systems. The second involved space travel, as NASA scientists used water's buoyancy as a simulation to study the human response to weightlessness. They found effects, both immediate and delayed, on every homeostatic system of the human body, many of which were therapeutically significant. Data also suggested that therapeutic effects could be obtained with a wider margin of safety than almost any other treatment approach *(4)*.

These studies in what has become known as *medical hydrology* laid the scientific groundwork for a closer look at the growing popular interest in therapeutic aquatics during the last two decades of the 20th century. Popular interest, stemming from such influences as athletic injury treatment, new-age relaxation techniques like Watsu®, and aquatic exercise, grew as an aging population sought more natural approaches to health and healing.

Current American aquatic therapy and rehabilitation is a multi-disciplinary specialty within various licensed disciplines such as physical therapy, occupational therapy, therapeutic recreation, kinesiotherapy, massage therapy, etc., practiced in hospital pools, private clinics, athletic clubs, and community aquatic facilities.

2. WHY WATER?

Three essential physical properties of water, *density*, *viscosity*, and *specific heat*, make it uniquely suitable for therapy, rehabilitation, and pain management. Practical use integrates these three properties, but understanding how each contributes requires separate consideration of the physical properties involved.

2.1. Hydrostatic Pressure

Mass, the measure of the fundamental amount of matter in a substance or object, is a constant, essentially unchanged by pressure or temperature. *Density*, which describes how closely the molecules of a substance are arranged, is a variable. Molecules become more active with increased temperatures and move farther apart, so density decreases but mass remains constant. As temperatures decrease, molecules move more slowly and density increases.

Density gives water *weight*, the result of gravitational pull on the substance or object. Weight produces pressure, which in water is referred to as *hydrostatic pressure*. Water's density is the standard against which the density of all other substances is measured. Its density of 1 gram per cubic centimeter gives it a value of 1 in density-comparison ratios.

A solid object exerts pressure only between its resting surfaces and its area of contact. But fluid molecules move freely, so water confined in a vessel exerts pressure equally on all sides of an immersed point, proportional to the immersion depth (Pascal's law).

Water exerts pressure equal to that of 22.4 mm of mercury (Hg) for each foot of depth (22.4mm Hg/ft) *(4)*. Standing in 48 inches of water subjects the feet and ankles to 89.6 mm Hg (4' × 22.4) of hydrostatic pressure, well above average diastolic blood pressure of 80 mm Hg, helping to resolve edema and assist venous return of blood to the central volume (see Figure 1). Concentrating blood in the central volume affects the heart, the lungs, and the kidneys. The heart's right atrium expands, causing more forceful contractions (Starling's law), which increases ejection fractions, stroke volume, and cardiac output (see Figure 2) *(4)*.

Increased cardiac output forces more blood into the pulmonary vessels *(5,6)*. Higher internal pressure, combined with hydrostatic pressure on the thorax, reduces tidal volume, expiratory reserve volume (ERV), and inspiratory reserve volume (IRV) *(7)*. The work of breathing one liter of air increases by 60% with immersion to the neck *(7–10)*. Experience with athletes indicates that this can have a conditioning effect on respiratory musculature *(4)*. Higher vascular pressure in the central volume increases renal output and excretion of solutes such as sodium, potassium and creatinine, which can help to regulate blood pressure *(11–13)*. All of these physiological effects may contribute to pain reduction and management, but hydrostatic pressure also seems to work directly on the nervous system *(14)*.

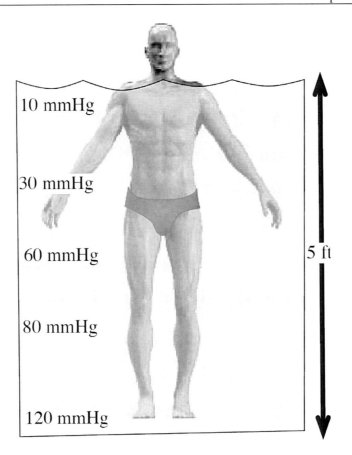

10 mmHg

30 mmHg

60 mmHg

80 mmHg

120 mmHg

5 ft

Fig. 1. Pressure gradients during immersion.

According to the gate control theory, stimulation of type Aβ sensory afferents (large myelinated nerve fibers that mediate touch and proprioception) *(15)* inhibit synaptic transmission from C (unmyelinated nerve fibers that mediate nociception) and Aδ (thinly myelinated nerve fibers that mediate nociception) sensory fibers to second-order neurons of the spinothalamic tract, blocking pain impulses. Stimulating type Aβ fibers can also trigger the release of enkephalins, the body's endogenous opioids, for pain relief. This helps to explain the tendency to rub a sore spot, and is one explanation for the analgesic effects of massage (see Chapter 17), acupuncture (see Chapter 18) and transcutaneous electrical nerve stimulation (TENS).

Hydrostatic pressure appears to have a similar effect. This may explain why fibromyalgia (FMS) patients experience significant pain relief with immersion *(16)*. Proper training permits pain-free exercise with little or no exercise-induced pain *(17)*. Similar results are reported by arthritis exercise participants and by others with chronic pain conditions *(18,19)*.

Gate control theory, however, is an incomplete explanation of the pain modulatory system, and Melzack has recently proposed the neuromatrix theory better to capture the multidimensional nature of the human experience of pain (see Chapter 3) *(20–22)*. Briefly, the neuromatrix theory posits that a combination of cognitive-evaluative, sensory-discriminative, and motivational-affective inputs over a period of time produce individualized output patterns of pain experience. Therefore, an individual patient's

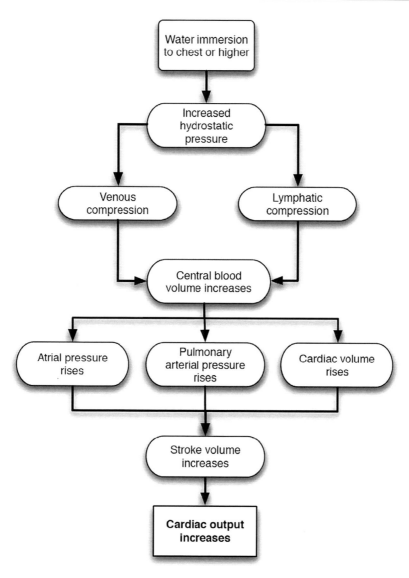

Fig. 2. The cardiovascular effects of immersion, which ultimately influence all the body's homeostatic mechanisms, suggest a number of ways that water therapies are effective in relieving pain.

pain presentation will depend upon the unique collection of sensory and affective stimuli he has experienced over his or her life (see chapter 2).

McEwen, building on Selye's work, *(23–25)* demonstrates how stress, a normal initial response to challenge, excitement, or danger, contributes to a wide range of pathologies when it becomes a chronic condition *(22)*. Individual responses to any given stressor, however, appear related to attitude and knowledge, so one person may be strongly affected while another experiences little or no distress, which seems to correlate with Melzack's Neuromatrix concept. Therefore, techniques that decrease stress responses in patients with chronic pain are integral in altering pain perceptions. This is another likely mechanism by which hydrostatic pressure exerts its pain-modulatory effects. There is evidence as shown by the work of Mano and others in space research programs that immersion suppresses sympathetic nervous system activity, the so-called "fight or flight" response *(26,27)*. Other studies show that water-based exercise has stress-reduction effects that are equal to, if not greater than, similar effects seen with land-based exercise *(28,29)*. We have postulated elsewhere that this effect is likely to be multifactorial and could also involve modulation of the reticular-activating system *(4)*.

Buoyancy results as an immersed object displaces water equal in mass to its own submerged mass (Archimedes' Law), and upward-thrusting hydrostatic pressure forces counteract gravity-induced downward forces *(4)*. Variations in substance density are expressed as specific gravity (SG), the ratio of the density of a given substance to that of water, with its SG of 1. Substances with SG <1 float; those with SG > 1 sink. With an average SG of 0.974, the human body floats, though differences in mass (i.e.: obesity vs loan muscle) cause individuals to reach neutral buoyancy at different levels. Buoyant off-loading from standing in water reduces compressive forces in joints, reducing pain and freeing movement (see Figure 3). Tight muscles relax and the body feels lighter.

Off-loading, which is directly proportional to immersion depth, is clinically significant. Effective body weight reduces to approximately 10% of total with neck-

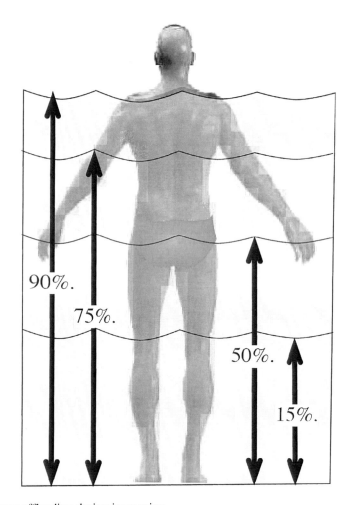

Fig. 3. Buoyancy offloading during immersion.

deep immersion, with the effective body weight becoming progressively greater with movement to shallower water *(4)*. This permits exercise within weight-bearing parameters such as those prescribed for joint replacement or injury recovery. It also enables persons with arthritic conditions to move more freely and strengthen joint-supporting musculature without the pain of walking on land.

Buoyancy is a versatile tool for aquatic therapy. In addition to vertical off-loading, some of its many uses include assisting or resisting movement, positioning a person for manual therapies or exercise in horizontal or diagonal planes, and training exercises for posture, gait, and balance. Technological advances in the design and manufacture of buoyant equipment have greatly expanded the possibilities for using water in rehabilitation, offering support for further off-loading and comfort, as well as variable resistance for exercise. Buoyancy, however, is only one benefit of immersion. Effective as passive immersion may be, movement enhances everything.

2.2. Viscosity and Turbulence

Viscosity is the measure of friction between the molecules of a fluid, which creates resistance to movement. Higher-viscosity fluids flow more slowly than do those of lower viscosity. Friction also impedes the movement of objects through the fluid, and of the fluid through a channel or pipe, as contact between fluid molecules and other surface areas slows their velocity. Theoretically, unimpeded water can be thought of as flowing in laminar sheets. Friction against the sides of the channel disrupts this *streamline flow*, as do objects within the stream. The result is called *turbulent flow* or *turbulence*.

For example, moving, especially walking, through water creates pressure in front of the body. Water moves upward, toward the area of lower atmospheric pressure, and toward the sides of the body, creating a *bow wave*. Surface friction against the sides of the body creates turbulence in the form of *eddy currents*, as water molecules move toward areas of lower pressure. As the body moves forward, the considerably lower pressure of the water behind it creates a *wake*, which tends to pull the body backward. As eddy currents from the sides of the body meet the wake, pressure differentials form an asymmetric pattern, presenting a challenge to proprioception and balance that can be used therapeutically to enhance both.

These *drag forces* also are responsible for most of the work required to move through water. Only 10% of the total effort of forward walking goes into overcoming *frontal resistance*. Most of the remaining work is created by the *tail suction* of the wake, with a small portion derived from surface friction and eddy currents. Both frontal resistance and drag forces increase with speed. This permits exercise for progressive strengthening, with direct control of the level of resistance, while maintaining smoothly coordinated movement patterns. Pain occurring within the range of motion may often be avoided through decreasing the force of movement, allowing joint motion through a complete range *(30)*.

Streamlining a shape permits freer movement but generates its own effects. "Slicing" a hand through a horizontal plane, for example, creates the same kind of lift as an airplane wing. The movement causes turbulence above the hand, reducing pressure relative to the upthrust of pressure below. These effects of turbulence are invaluable in aquatic therapy, rehabilitation, and pain treatment. For example, turbulence can be used to challenge or assist balance, to assist or resist movement, to stretch or strengthen musculature, to enhance proprioception, and to reduce pain directly through stimulation of cutaneous Aβ nerve receptors.

2.3. Specific Heat and Thermal Energy Transfer

All forms of water, liquid, solid, and gas have therapeutic applications due to the physics of thermodynamics. Aquatic therapy relies primarily on water in liquid form, using temperature differentials to meet varying needs. Every substance possesses energy stored in the form of heat, referred to as its *specific heat*. The unit of measurement for this heat is the *calorie (cal)*, defined as the heat required to raise the temperature of 1 gram of water by 1°C. Water's specific heat at 15°C is 1.00 cal. In comparison, the average human body has a specific heat of 0.83 cal.

The human body converts food energy into forms of energy that sustain life. Only about 20% of this energy is expressed as kinetic energy, and roughly 80% is used to produce heat. Without regulating homeostatic mechanisms, the body's core temperature would rise 3°C per hour with light exertion. The vascular system circulates heat from the core to the skin, which dissipates it as necessary into the external environment.

The law of conservation of energy states that energy can neither be created nor destroyed. The first law of thermodynamics states that change in the internal energy of a system is equal to the heat added to the system minus the work done by the system. Immersing a body in water creates an interactive energy system. If the body is warmer than the water, energy transfer cools the body and warms the water until equilibrium is attained. If the water is warmer, the reverse occurs. This makes the choice of water temperature a critical factor in therapy and rehabilitation.

Energy can be transferred by way of *conduction, convection,* and/or *radiation.* Conduction is the transfer of energy across an imaginary membrane between two masses in contact with one another. Convection is similar, but moving molecules of a liquid or gas speed the transfer, as immediately adjacent molecules are not allowed to form a thermal envelope around an immersed body. Radiation transmits heat by way of electromagnetic waves.

Free nerve endings transmit both pain (*nociception*) and sensations of heat and cold (*thermoreception*). Information on pain and temperature is necessary for survival and activation of these receptors triggers immediate homeostatic responses. Cold water, for example, causes restriction of blood flow to the skin to reduce the speed of thermal energy transfer and maintain core temperature *(31)*. Exercising in warm water, on the other hand, causes dilatation of capillary beds in the skin to dissipate heat and protect vital organs from overheating *(32–34)*.

Ideally, water temperature is determined by the therapeutic need. The choice of water temperature for therapeutic uses depends on such factors as activity level, individual physiological responses to temperature, pathologies exacerbated by heat or cold, and desired results. Acute injuries respond best to cold water, reducing blood flow to the trauma site, slowing subcutaneous bleeding, and blocking pain by decreasing sensory nerve conduction velocities *(35)*. Neurological conditions like multiple sclerosis that affect temperature regulation can lead to overheating, so water in the 84–87°F range is preferable for exercise, although some authors have used higher temperatures without clinically ill effects *(36)*. The same temperature range, slightly higher than that for a recreational swimming pool, also is generally preferred for inflammatory arthritis, as it permits active exercise without overheating *(19)*.

Warmer water of 90–94°F, approximately the same as skin temperature, is considered *thermoneutral*. This temperature range is considered the most appropriate for a therapy pool, providing maximum comfort for both therapist and patient while permitting light to medium levels of exercise without overheating. Individuals with conditions ranging from FMS to stroke or spinal cord injury, or other conditions where there could be temperature-regulating deficiencies may find that water temperatures below 92°F can cause discomfort, inappropriate muscle spasms, or both. Immersion in thermoneutral or warmer water often provides immediate subjective pain relief. Again, the reasons probably are multifactorial, with neural effects as described above *(28)*. But evidence also points to metabolic and circulatory effects of warm water on muscle tissue as a significant factor *(37)*. Warmer water, on the other hand, may not provide adequate cooling during strenuous exercise for those with hypertension who must moderate their activity to avoid overheating.

Studies suggest that increased cardiac output resulting from hydrostatic pressure redistributes blood to skin and muscle rather than to splanchnic beds *(32)*. Sympathetic vasoconstriction of resistance vessels in skeletal muscle prevents blood pooling in gravity-dominant conditions, but with immersion this biologic need is fulfilled by hydrostatic pressure, and vessels relax, allowing greater flow *(32)*. Thermal influences might be expected to further promote vasodilatation, as temperature-regulating mechanisms redistribute heat away from the core. Pre-immersion baseline blood flow of 1.8 mL/min/100g in muscle tissue has been shown to increase to 4.1 mL/min/100g with neck-deep immersion, an increase of more than 125% *(37)*. Such increases are significant in the effort to counter hypoxic conditions and may contribute to the clearance of pain-inducing lactates and other metabolic end products.

3. AQUATIC THERAPY AND PAIN REHABILITATION

The combination of buoyancy-produced joint offloading plus the thermal gain effects of warm water make the aquatic environment an ideal place for rehabilitation of low back injuries and pain. A number of studies have shown benefit, including several randomized prospective studies, although methodological issues permeate this literature *(38–42)*. There does seem to be support for an increased return-to-work rate in the low back pain population following an aquatic therapy program *(43)*.

A Turkish study published in 2004 compared pool exercise to balneotherapy, which is simply immersion in thermal or mineral-rich water. Two groups of 25 women diagnosed with FMS participated. Group 1 exercised in a warm pool for 35 minutes, 3 times a week for 12 weeks. Group 2 followed the same schedule, bathing in warm water without exercise. Evaluations were made pre-treatment, at the end of week 12, and at 24 weeks. Researchers concluded that both approaches brought significant relief from most FMS symptoms but found no statistically significant difference between the exercise and non-exercise groups, except for longer-term relief in the exercise group *(44)*.

In a recent review of fibromyalgia, Nampiaparampil and Shmerling cite studies supporting a hypothesis that local tissue hypoxia in muscles plays a role in causing FMS pain symptoms *(45)*. Related histological changes, however, cannot yet be identified as a cause or effect of FMS. The physiological effects of immersion, coupled with the hypoxia hypothesis, might help explain how warm water relieves pain, whether or not exercise is incorporated with immersion. Clearly, the psychological, stress-relieving benefits of immersion must also play a role.

4. AQUATIC THERAPY TECHNIQUES—APPLYING THE PRINCIPLES

Five primary approaches, each with innumerable modifications by individual therapists, currently comprise the state of the art in aquatic therapy in the United States: Watsu®, the Bad Ragaz ring method (BRRM), the Halliwick Concept, the Burdenko Method, and Ai Chi. This list is not exclusive; other techniques exist, but this is a representative list of the most widely used approaches (see Table 1).

4.1. Watsu®

Harold Dull began developing Watsu® (WAter + shiaTSU) in 1980, at Northern California's Harbin Hot Springs. As a student of Eastern philosophies of healing and meditation, he linked meditation practice with a style of Japanese massage and flowing movements in a warm water pool. The first publication of his technique was in his 1987 book, *Bodywork Tantra on Land and in Water*.

Watsu is a passive form of therapy. It was originally practiced to relax and energize the body, but its calming effects, passive joint ranging, and muscular relaxation proved valuable for a wide scope of therapeutic interventions, in both neurological and orthopedic conditions.

As the technique evolved and became more widely utilized, it has been modified by a number of practitioners. Brazilian Mario Jahara introduced "third arm" flotation to ease handling and increase range of motion possibilities. Peggy Schoedinger, PT, pioneered clinical applications for rehabilitation *(46)*. In Germany, Arjana Brunschwiler and Aman Schroter added underwater movements, in what they called *Wassertanzen*, or Waterdance.

Watsu, as well as all of its modifications, is performed in warm water, with the patient cradled in the therapist's arms. All variations revolve around gentle passive stretching, ranging joints of the spine and extremities, and relaxing musculature; but the effects go beyond musculoskeletal considerations. A profound parasympathetic response occurs with this approach; heart and respiration rates slow, blood circulation improves, and the relaxation response ensues. Patients experience deep relaxation, often accompanied by emotional releases.

Schoedinger states that therapists are impressed by the benefits for patients with traumatic brain injury, spinal cord injury, stroke, Parkinson's Disease, arthritis, cerebral palsy, chronic pain, fibromyalgia, ankylosing spondylitis, post-mastectomy, post-thoracic surgery, post- traumatic stress disorder, and those with functional limitations secondary to pain, stiffness, muscle spasm, or spasticity *(46)*. Mary Essert, a pioneer in use of the technique for post-mastectomy patients, has taught her methods to therapists throughout the world *(47)*. Because hydrostatic pressure easily exceeds lymphatic pressures even with edema, there is often a reduction of lymphedema following a period of immersion. The Worldwide Aquatic Bodywork Association (WABA) requires extensive training and practice for certification of Watsu practitioners and providers, who practice the modality within their respective disciplines.

Table 1
Five Primary Approaches to Aquatic Therapy in the United States

Technique	Passive/active	Support	Position	Pain treatment values
Watsu®	Passive	Therapist	Supine	Reduce stress, reduce muscle tension, improve joint mobility, enhance mental-emotional state, balance *chi* flow (similar to acupressure or shiatsu)
Bad Ragaz Ring Method	Both - therapist-dependent	Buoyant Equipment, minimally at neck and S2 segment	Supine	Passive, active-assisted, active, and active-resisted range of motion for relaxation, joint mobility, and strengthening
Halliwick Concept	Both - initially therapist-dependent, but moving to independence	Therapist, initially, but moving to none	All positions - floating, standing, sitting	Neurodevelopmental aspects of Water- Specific Training enhance balance, coordination, and movement
Burdenko Method	Active - Integrated Water/Land Program	No therapist support - extensive use of buoyant equipment	Primarily Vertical, but all positions	Works to maintain and enhance performance; athletic-injury based rehabilitation training applies widely to functional improvement, minimizing movement-induced pain
Ai Chi	Active	None - stand on pool floor	Vertical, Standing	Breath control, stress reduction, reduce muscle tension, increase strength, improve joint mobility, enhance mental-emotional state, balance *chi* flow

4.2. Bad Ragaz Ring Method

The Bad Ragaz Ring Method (BRRM), as previously noted, was adopted in 1957 from the earlier work of Knupfer and Suden in Bavaria. The original, non-weight-bearing (NWB) exercises were performed from a supine position in warm water with buoyant support at the neck, pelvis and extremities. Egger and McMillan, at Bad Ragaz, eventually modified the technique with 23 patterns of closed kinetic chain exercises, from a supine position, including bilateral-symmetrical and bilateral-reciprocal lower extremity patterns, trunk patterns, and upper extremity patterns *(3)*.

Hydrodynamic principles of frontal resistance and drag forces provide viscous resistance in BRRM. A therapist can use these principles to stretch, to challenge and strengthen isometric muscle contractions, to assist active movement, or to resist active movement. In one open-chain exercise for lateral trunk stability the therapist stabilizes the patient's hips. On cue, the patient isometrically holds a stable trunk position as the therapist moves, using frontal resistance, drag forces, and velocity, to challenge core strength (see Figure 4).

In a closed-chain exercise, the therapist's hand position provides a fixed point as the patient is cued to move in relation to that point. For example, stabilized at the hip and knee, a patient might be instructed to abduct and adduct the contralateral extremity. The effect is to engage hip-stabilization musculature on the fixed side and hip-mobilization musculature on the other. Even minimal effort produces motion, so muscle strength can be developed from trace levels to significant power by increasing the speed and, thereby, resistance to the movement (see Figures 5 and 6). While certification programs are available in Europe, most American therapists train in workshops to learn BRRM, utilizing the technique without certification, as a modality within their discipline's scope of practice.

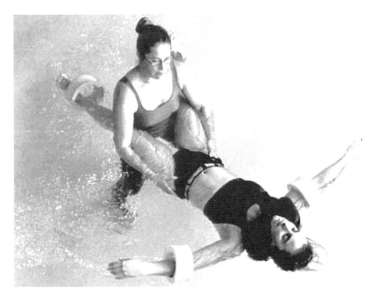

Fig. 4. Bad Ragaz Ring Method—pelvic hold/isometric trunk stabilization. Stabilizing the pelvic girdle at the trochanters and ilia, therapist cues patient to "hold" during lateral movement (here, patient is being moved to her right). This exercise is designed to strengthen muscles that support the spine laterally. (Illustration courtesy of Julia Meno Fettig, Florence McCall, photographer)

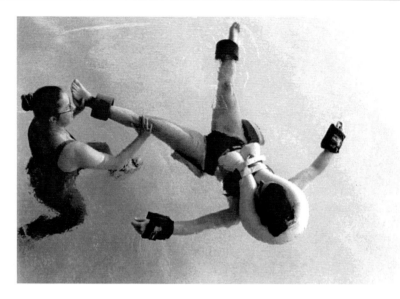

Fig. 5. Bad Ragaz Ring Method—open kinetic-chain lower extremity abduction. Therapist, engaging at knee and ankle, cues the patient to abduct ("feet apart"), while providing resistance against the movement of the left lower extremity. This movement promotes mobility of the free limb and strengthening of the other. (Illustration courtesy of Julia Meno Fettig, Florence McCall, photographer.)

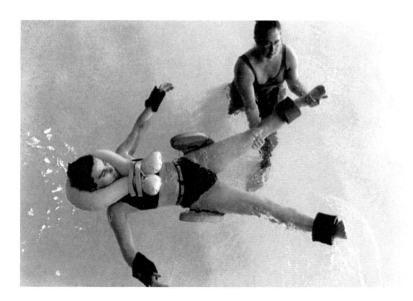

Fig. 6. Bad Ragaz ring method—open kinetic-chain lower extremity adduction. Therapist, engaging at knee and ankle, cues the patient to adduct ("feet together"), while providing resistance against the movement of the left lower extremity. As in Figure 5, this movement promotes mobility of the free limb and strengthening of the other. (Illustration courtesy of Julia Meno Fettig, Florence McCall, photographer.)

4.3. Halliwick Concept

Though James McMillan was not a therapist and had no medical training, as an hydraulics engineer, his knowledge of fluid mechanics informed his work as a swimming teacher. At the Halliwick School for Girls in Bath, England, he saw children with cerebral palsy wearing buoyant equipment in the pool. Insisting that flotation devices were unnecessary and inhibiting to skill development, he developed the Halliwick Concept of adapted swimming.

McMillan's "Ten-Point Program" is divided into three phases, to meet three goals (see Table 2):

- to encourage participation in water activities
- to encourage independent movement
- to teach swimming

The program provides a logical progression from initial immersion, through breath control, to balance control and, finally, to basic swimming skill. Though one phase evolves into the next, overlapping occurs, and each earlier skill is practiced repeatedly throughout the training until the student becomes a fully competent swimmer *(48)*. Evidence showed that students not only learned to swim, but also made significant neurodevelopmental advances, enhancing their activities of daily life. Breath control, head balance, trunk stability, limb control and movement, and self-esteem all improved. This became the focus of McMillan's life's work, which he called Water Specific Training. Research continues today, and as Europe's dominant modality of aquatic therapy, the Halliwick concept is used to treat congenital conditions like cerebral palsy, for rehabilitation following stroke or spinal cord injury, and for neurological conditions

Table 2
The Ten-Point Program and the Three Phases
of the Halliwick Concept *(49)*

Ten Points	Phases
1. Mental Adjustment and disengagement	Mental adaptation (adjustment)
2. Sagittal rotation (control)	
3. Transversal rotation (control)	Balance control
4. Longitudinal rotation (control)	
5. Combined rotation (control)	
6. Upthrust / mental inversion	
7. Balance in stillness	
8. Turbulent gliding	
9. Simple progression	
10. Basic Halliwick Movement	Movement

like multiple sclerosis and Parkinsonism. While certification training is available, it is not required in the United States. McMillan, however, believed that basic and advanced training was necessary to be truly effective.

4.4. Burdenko Method

Igor Burdenko, PhD, emigrated in 1981 from the Soviet Union, where he was a professor of Sports Medicine at Moscow Pedagogical Institute and author of a standard text for athletic conditioning. Today, he works primarily with Olympic and professional athletes, elite amateurs, and professional dancers. His Burdenko method is an integrated land-and-water approach to therapy and rehabilitation, designed to develop balance, coordination, flexibility, endurance, speed, and strength in the same way athletes build these qualities.

Burdenko makes extensive use of buoyant equipment in aquatic work, and simple props such as rubber tubing, PVC pipes and exercise benches in land exercises. He describes the main characteristics of his method as:

- a combination of land and water exercises that challenge the center of buoyancy and center of gravity
- exercising only in basically vertical positions in the water
- developing the six essential qualities: balance, coordination, flexibility, endurance, speed and strength
- exercising the body in multiple directions
- performing all exercises at different speeds: slow, medium, and fast(50)

Though the Burdenko method does not focus specifically on pain treatment or management, its emphasis on overall physical fitness is valuable in reducing the pain-inducing effects of poor posture, low endurance, and deconditioning, in general.

4.5. Ai Chi

Jun Konno, a decorated Japanese swimming coach and aquatic fitness authority, says he observed that Asian people prefer low-intensity, gentle movement for exercise. He also found that, though Watsu is popular as a therapeutic intervention in Japan, many find the close contact between therapist and client uncomfortable. He describes Ai Chi *(EYE-chee)*, a new form of exercise he created in the early 1990s, as his "way of creating a stepping stone to Watsu, but it now stands alone as a form of exercise" *(51)*. Working with aquatic fitness expert Ruth Sova, Konno introduced Ai Chi to the United States in the late 1990s. Since then, with its slow, gentle movements that painlessly stretch and move every part of the body, it has become a popular form of aquatic exercise for people with fibromyalgia and arthritis.

Ai Chi is performed in shoulder-depth warm water—the recommended temperature range is 88–96°F, (30°C+)—to maximize muscular relaxation, a key aspect of the exercise. The beginning stance is relaxed, with the feet placed at least shoulder-width apart. Hips and knees are slightly flexed, with toes and knees pointed slightly outward. The back is kept straight and the head erect. Breath control, using slow, steady abdominal breaths, is primary to Ai Chi, as it is to traditional martial arts. Movements are similar to those in the martial arts of Tai Chi and Qi Gong, but specifically designed to utilize the hydrodynamic principles of aquatic immersion. They are never done in a start-stop fashion, as in many calisthenics, but are rounded and

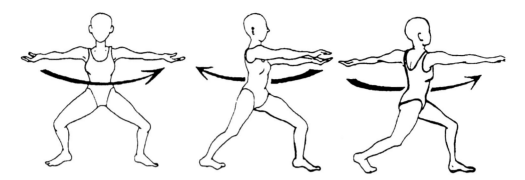

Fig. 7. "Freeing," one of 16 basic sets in Ai Chi. Movements are performed in a continuous flowing motion, circling from one direction to the next, without stops or starts. (Illustration courtesy of Ruth Sova.)

connected. And all positions are performed either bilaterally or mirrored, left and right (see Figure 7).

Basic Ai Chi has 16 different movements, divided into Breathing Movement (#1), Upper Extremity Movements (#2–5), Trunk Stability Movements (#6–10), Lower Extremity Movements (#11–13), and Total Coordinated Body Movements (#14–16). Three optional movements, known collectively as Cultivating the Chi, may also be included for advanced students. Ai Chi Ne, a partner-stretching program for two people working together, was originally intended as an extension of Ai Chi, but also has been found useful by therapists working with neuromuscular conditions or severely deconditioned patients.

While considerable subjective and anecdotal evidence supports its effectiveness, Ai Chi still is too new to have generated a major body of research. However, studies at the Universities of Tsukuba and Tokai, in Japan, found that oxygen consumption during Ai Chi rose by 4–7% and research into the effects of martial arts may provide further evidence in its support *(51)*.

Studies have shown, for example, that the traditional Chinese art of Tai Chi improves lung function in older adults, *(52)* raises heart rate during exertion, *(53)* increased noradrenaline excretion in urine, and reduces salivary cortisol concentration *(53)*. Subjects also reported lower levels of tension, depression, anger, fatigue, confusion and anxiety, in addition to feeling more vigorous and experiencing fewer mood disturbances (see Chapter 12) *(53)*. Its similarity to Tai Chi suggests that there could be similar therapeutic benefits from Ai Chi practice with the added benefits of immersion in thermoneutral water. While certification as an Ai Chi instructor is provided only upon completion of training by an approved provider, it is widely practiced and taught by non-certified therapists and fitness trainers.

5. CONTRAINDICATIONS AND PRECAUTIONS

Water's properties and its effects on the body make it a clinically safe environment for therapy and rehabilitation *(2)*. Contraindications are minimal, and observing practical precautions ensures patient health and safety. The following considerations are generally advised:

5.1. *Contraindications*

- Open or draining wounds that cannot be covered with an occlusive dressing
- Severe burns
- Fever over 100°F or sepsis
- Vomiting
- Bowel incontinence
- Unstable congestive heart failure
- Severely unstable blood pressure
- Untreated acute deep vein thrombosis
- Uncontrolled epilepsy
- Severe urinary tract infection
- Menstruation without internal protection
- Severe respiratory infection
- Severe or contagious dermatological disorders (i.e., impetigo, severe active psoriasis)
- Tracheostomy (though some physicians and therapists do permit)
- Non-tunnel catheters (PIC, Intrasil, supra-pubic catheters*)
- Compromised immune function (for patient safety)
- Intoxication

5.2. *Precautions*

- Small open wounds*
- Uncontrolled high/low blood pressure
- Cardiac conditions (unstable angina, arrhythmia - monitor closely)
- Intravenous lines (heplocks, hickman lines)*
- Heat intolerance or poor temperature regulation (precaution for water temperature)
- Excessive skin sensitivity, especially to chlorine
- Ear infections or perforated ear drums
- Cerebral hemorrhage (wait at least 3 weeks after bleeding ceases)
- Vertigo or dizziness (precaution for some movements)
- Absence of cough reflex
- High risk pregnancy
- Behavior problems
- Extreme fear of water
- Dysphasia (communication problem)
- Hyponatremia (water intoxication encountered with autistic children who drink pool water)
- Serious debilitation or deconditioning
- Autonomic dysreflexia (especially for SCI patients, T6 and higher)
- Orthopedic precautions (fractures, fresh total joint replacements, etc.)
- Atlanto/occipital instability (no diving, precaution for deep head immersion, etc.)

6. INTEGRATING AQUATIC THERAPY INTO A PAIN PRACTICE

The multiple benefits of immersion and aquatic movement make aquatic therapy a useful tool in any pain practice. In making the choice for aquatic therapy, the questions to ask are—

---

* Smaller wounds, operative sites and some tubes may be covered with a waterproof barrier membrane such as Op-Site™, DuoDERM™, or Tegaderm™.

- Can satisfactory results be obtained without putting the patient into water?
- Why use water? What benefits of immersion and/or aquatic movement apply?
- Will immersion and/or aquatic movement enhance outcomes?
- Do medical issues indicate or contraindicate immersion or aquatic movement?
- Are therapists trained, experienced, and certified in aquatic therapy?
- Are pools with appropriate temperature and depths available?
- Are the pool and facilities properly operated and maintained, and are lifeguards on duty?

Rheumatologists refer arthritis or fibromyalgia patients to warm water pools, for both immediate and long-term effects. Movement is easier and less painful, and the cumulative effects of exercise reduce pain, so patients are compliant, and usually enthusiastic, about maintaining a regular regimen. This also can be a cost-effective way to treat pain, as many communities offer aquatic exercise classes at affordable rates in public pools, YMCAs, YWCAs, and Jewish Community Centers (JCCs). Arthritis Foundation-approved classes, taught by trained instructors, are preferable, when offered.

Orthopedists find aquatic therapy valuable for pre-surgery strengthening prior to joint replacement procedures and again for post-surgery rehabilitation. The authors have extensive experience with patients who report faster, and more satisfactory, post-surgical outcomes, with less pain, when rehabilitation included aquatic therapy. Occlusive dressings such as Tegaderm®, DuoDERM™, or Op-Site™, make immersion possible as soon as a patient is medically stable, and buoyancy permits exercise of supporting musculature at any prescribed level of weightbearing, including NWB.

Successful rehabilitation of elite athletes (e.g., Burdenko's work) provides evidence for the effectiveness of aquatic therapy in reducing the time and cost of rehabilitation from work-related injuries. Employing aquatic movement immediately can minimize post-trauma atrophy of unaffected musculature as injury sites heal. Then, as healing progresses, the water permits gradual, low-stress, work hardening toward full recovery *(54)*.

An increasing number of neurologists find the aquatic environment ideal for treating neurological impairments. Balance and gait training for progressive disorders such as Parkinsonism, multiple sclerosis, muscular dystrophy, ALS, peripheral neuropathy, etc., is easier and safer for both patient and therapist. Buoyancy and turbulence provide challenges to proprioception, enhancing body awareness and control while reducing or eliminating the pain associated with movement.

For non-progressive neurological disorders such as cerebral palsy, stroke (CVA), spinal cord injury, traumatic brain injury, etc., water provides a safe, supportive environment to maintain fitness, and to enhance posture and function. Pool temperature is a factor when a patient's condition impairs homeostatic temperature regulation, but when a warm pool is not available, neoprene clothing (similar to wet suits for divers) can prevent chilling.

Mary Essert, BA, ATRIC, a breast cancer survivor herself, has developed Breast Cancer Waterwork, a program for cancer patients to rehabilitate from surgery, safely regain range of motion, and maintain fitness through cross-training with land exercise. Since the early 1980s, she has trained hundreds of therapists internationally for working with cancer patients in medical settings as well as community programs. Essert's whole-person approach emphasizes that intervention in the pain cycle is vital, prioritizing treatment goals as—

- Pain reduction
- Increased range of motion
- Increased strength
- Increased cardio-respiratory conditioning
- Increased relaxation and stress management
- Provision of support, social and outreach opportunities *(47)*

7. THERAPISTS LEAD ADVANCES IN PRACTICAL APPLICATIONS

Three organizations, the Aquatic Therapy and Rehab Institute (ATRI), the Aquatic Resource Network (ARN), and the Aquatic PT Section of the American Physical Therapy Association (APTA), have been active in spreading the growth of therapeutic aquatics in this country (see Table 3 for summary of training resources).

ATRI, an outgrowth of the Aquatic Exercise Association, is largely credited with the American revival of practical therapeutic applications of medical hydrology. The non-profit institute has presented multi-disciplinary educational programs since 1990, publishes the *Aquatic Therapy Journal*, maintains a web site (www.atri.org), and established the country's first industry-wide certification for aquatic therapy specialists.

ARN collects and disseminates research findings on aquatic therapy and offers a number of educational programs. The organization publishes a magazine, *The Aquatic Therapist*, maintains an extensive library of academic publications in the field that is

Table 3
Aquatic Therapy Resources in the United States

Organiation	*Contact Information*	*Publications*
Aquatic Therapy and Rehab Institute (ATRI)	13297 Temple Blvd West Palm Beach Fl, 33412 Phone 866.462.2874 E-mail: atri@atri.org Web: www.atri.org	*Aquatic Therapy Journal* (quarterly/ subscription) Free e-list: register at website
Aquatic PT Section of the American Physical Therapy Association (APTA)	7400 East Arapahoe Road, Suite 211 Centennial, Colorado 80112 Phone 303.694.4728, ext. 35 E-mail: aquaticpt@assnoffice.com Web: aquaticpt.org	Journal of Aquatic Physical Therapy
Aquatic Resource Network (ARN)	3500 Vicksburg Ln. N, #250 Plymouth MN 55447 Phone: 715.248.7258 E-mail: info@aquaticnet.com Web: www.aquaticnet.com	*The Aquatic Therapist* Books and Manuals Free e-list: register at website
National Commission for the Credentialing of Aquatic Therapy Disciplines	12400 Hwy 71 West, Ste 350-150, Austin TX 78378 Phone: 512.263.8890 Web: www.thenccard	No Publications

a major source of such material, and has a web site (www.aquaticnet.com) that offers free articles.

APTA's Aquatic PT Section is concerned with research, education, and practice standards in aquatics, specifically as it applies to physical therapy. The group publishes the *Journal of Aquatic Physical Therapy* and a newsletter, and maintains a web site (www.apta.org).

Certification of aquatic therapy and rehabilitation in the United States is relatively new, as most modern development has occurred since 1990. The Aquatic Therapy and Rehab Institute (ATRI) created the first industry-wide certification in 1989. The International Council for Aquatic Therapy (ICATRIC) and Rehabilitation was formed in 2001 and took responsibility for certification as an independent, not-for-profit organization.

ICATRIC, in turn, has since been dissolved, and replaced by a new, independent body, the National Commission for the Credentialing of Aquatic Rehabilitation Disciplines (NCCARD). The first NCCARD examinations, to be held in 2008, will be offered for applicants seeking certification, according to professional discipline, as either Aquatic Physical Therapist or Aquatic Therapy Practitioner. Further information is available on the organization's web site (www.thenccard.org).

REFERENCES

1. deVierville J. 1997. A History of aquatic rehabilitation. In: Comprehensive Aquatic Rehabilitation. First edition. Becker BE, CA, Ed. Newton MA: Butterworth-Heinemann.
2. De Vierville JP. 2004. Aquatic Rehabilitation: A Historical Perspective. In: Comprehensive Aquatic Therapy. Second edition. Cole AJ BB, ed. Philadelphia, PA: Butterworth Heineman, pp 1–18.
3. Lambeck J GU. History of Bad Ragaz Ring Method. http://www.multimediasupport.nl/badragaz/index_E.html. (online)
4. Becker BE. 2004. Biophysiologic aspects of hydrotherapy. In: Comprehensive Aquatic Therapy. Cole AJ BB, Ed. Philadelphia PA: Elsevier, Inc, pp 19–56.
5. Arborelius M, Jr., Balldin UI, Lilja B, Lundgren CE. Regional lung function in man during immersion with the head above water. Aerosp Med. 1972;43(7):701–707.
6. Arborelius M, Jr., Balldin UI, Lilja B, Lundgren CE. Hemodynamic changes in man during immersion with the head above water. Aerosp Med. 1972;43(6):592–598.
7. Hong SK, Cerretelli P, Cruz JC, Rahn H. Mechanics of respiration during submersion in water. J Appl Physiol. 1969;27(4):535–538.
8. Taylor NA, Morrison JB. Pulmonary flow-resistive work during hydrostatic loading. Acta Physiol Scand. 1991;142(3):307–312.
9. Taylor NA, Morrison JB. Static and dynamic pulmonary compliance during upright immersion. Acta Physiol Scand. 1993;149(4):413–417.
10. Taylor NA, Morrison JB. Static respiratory muscle work during immersion with positive and negative respiratory loading. J Appl Physiol. 1999;87(4):1397–1403.
11. Epstein M. Cardiovascular and renal effects of head-out water immersion in man: application of the model in the assessment of volume homeostasis. Circ Res. 1976;39(5):619–628.
12. Epstein M. Renal effects of head-out water immersion in humans: a 15-year update. Physiol Rev. 1992;72(3):563–621.
13. Epstein M, Levinson R, Loutzenhiser R. Effects of water immersion on renal hemodynamics in normal man. J Appl Physiol. 1976;41(2):230–233.
14. Mano T, Iwase S, Yamazaki Y, Saito M. Sympathetic nervous adjustments in man to simulated weightlessness induced by water immersion. J Uoeh. 1985;7(Suppl):215–227.
15. Melzack R, Wall PD. Pain mechanisms: a new theory. Science. 1965;150(699):971–979.
16. Mannerkorpi K, Nyberg B, Ahlmen M, Ekdahl C. Pool exercise combined with an education program for patients with fibromyalgia syndrome. A prospective, randomized study. J Rheumatol 2000;27(10):2473–2481.

17. Jentoft ES, Kvalvik AG, Mengshoel AM. Effects of pool-based and land-based aerobic exercise on women with fibromyalgia/chronic widespread muscle pain. Arthritis Rheum Feb 2001;45(1):42–47.

18. Hall J, Skevington SM, Maddison PJ, Chapman K. A randomized and controlled trial of hydrotherapy in rheumatoid arthritis. Arthritis Care Res 1996;9(3):206–215.

19. Danneskiold-Samsoe B, Lyngberg K, Risum T, Telling M. The effect of water exercise therapy given to patients with rheumatoid arthritis. Scand J Rehabil Med 1987;19(1):31–35.

20. Melzack R. From the gate to the neuromatrix. Pain Aug 1999;(Suppl 6):S121–126.

21. Melzack R. Pain—an overview. Acta Anaesthesiol Scand 1999;43(9):880–884.

22. Melzack R. Phantom limbs and the concept of a neuromatrix. Trends Neurosci 1990;13(3):88–92.

23. Selye H. The evolution of the stress concept. Am Sci 1973;61(6):692–699.

24. Selye H. Forty years of stress research: principal remaining problems and misconceptions. Can Med Assoc J. 1976;115(1):53–56.

25. Selye H. Stress and the reduction of distress. JSC Med Assoc 1979;75(11):562–566.

26. Mano T, Iwase S, Yamazaki Y, Saito M. Sympathetic nervous adjustments in man to simulated weightlessness induced by water immersion. J Uoeh 1985;7(Suppl):215–227.

27. Miwa C, Sugiyama Y, Mano T, Iwase S, Matsukawa T. Spectral characteristics of heart rate and blood pressure variabilities during head-out water immersion. Environ Med 1996;40(1):91–94.

28. Robiner WN. Psychological and physical reactions to whirlpool baths. J Behav Med 1990;13(2):157–173.

29. Watanabe E, Takeshima N, Okada A, Inomata K. Comparison of water- and land-based exercise in the reduction of state anxiety among older adults. Percept Mot Skills 2000;91(1):97–104.

30. Kottke F. 1971. Therapeutic exercise. In: Handbook of Physical Medicine and Rehabilitation. Krusen K, Ellwood, Ed. Philadelphia, PA: W. B. Saunders 424–426.

31. Mathew L, Purkayastha SS, Selvamurthy W, Malhotra MS. Cold-induced vasodilatation and peripheral blood flow under local cold stress in man at altitude. Aviat Space Environ Med 1977;48(6):497–500.

32. Bonde-Petersen F, Schultz-Pedersen L, Dragsted N. Peripheral and central blood flow in man during cold, thermoneutral, and hot water immersion. Aviat Space Environ Med 1992;63(5):346–350.

33. Koga S. The regional difference of thermal response to immersion during rest and exercise. Ann Physiol Anthropol 1985;4(2):191–192.

34. Craig AB, Jr., Dvorak M. Thermal regulation of man exercising during water immersion. J Appl Physiol 1968;25(1):28–35.

35. Swenson C, Sward L, Karlsson J. Cryotherapy in sports medicine. Scand J Med Sci Sports 1996;6(4):193–200.

36. Peterson C. Exercise in 94 degrees F water for a patient with multiple sclerosis. Phys Ther 2001;81(4):1049–1058.

37. Balldin UI, Lundgren CE, Lundvall J, Mellander S. Changes in the elimination of 133 xenon from the anterior tibial muscle in man induced by immersion in water and by shifts in body position. Aerosp Med 1971;42(5):489–493.

38. Ariyoshi M, Sonoda K, Nagata K, et al. Efficacy of aquatic exercises for patients with low-back pain. Kurume Med J 1999;46(2):91–96.

39. Sjogren T, Long N, Storay I, Smith J. Group hydrotherapy versus group land-based treatment for chronic low back pain. Physiother Res Int 1997;2(4):212–222.

40. Constant F, Collin JF, Guillemin F, Boulange M. Effectiveness of spa therapy in chronic low back pain: a randomized clinical trial. J Rheumatol 1995;22(7):1315–1320.

41. Queneau P, Francon A, Graber-Duvernay B. Methodological reflections on 20 randomized clinical hydrotherapy trials in rheumatology. Therapie 2001;56(6):675–684.

42. Balogh Z, Ordogh J, Gasz A, Nemet L, Bender T. Effectiveness of balneotherapy in chronic low back pain—a randomized single-blind controlled follow-up study. Forsch Komplementarmed Klass Naturheilkd. 2005;12(4):196–201.

43. LeFort SM, Hannah TE. Return to work following an aquafitness and muscle strengthening program for the low back injured. Arch Phys Med Rehabil 1994;75(11):1247–1255.

44. Altan L, Bingol U, Aykac M, Koc Z, Yurtkuran M. Investigation of the effects of pool-based exercise on fibromyalgia syndrome. Rheumatol Int 2004;24(5):272–277.

45. Nampiaparampil DE, Shmerling RH. A review of fibromyalgia. Am J Manag Care 2004;10 (11 Pt 1):794–800.

46. Schoedinger P. Benefits of Watsu for People with Orthopedic, Neurologic and Rheumatologic Special Needs. (online reference) http://www.waba.edu/watsu/Watsu%20with%20Special%20Needs.htm.

47. Essert M. Breast Cancer Water Work Management Through Aquatic Exercise and Rehab Techniques. Conway AR: Essert Associates; 2004.
48. Gresswell A MJ. Principles of Halliwick and Its Application for Children and Adults with Neurological Conditions. Paper presented at: HACP Study Day, 2000.
49. Lambeck J SF, Kinnaird DW. 2004. The Halliwick concept. In: Comprehensive Aquatic Therapy. Second edition. Cole AJ BB, Ed. Philadelphia PA: Butterworth Heinemann, pp 73–98.
50. Burdenko I. 2000. Functional Rehab—The Burdenko Method. Paper presented at: Aquatic Therapy and Rehab Symposium, Orlando FL.
51. Sova R KJ. 1999. Ai Chi—Balance, Harmony & Healing. Port Washington WI: DSL Ltd.
52. Lai JS WN, Lan C, Chong CK, Lien IN. Cardiorespiratory responses of t'ai chi Ch'uan practitioners and sedentary subjects during cycle ergometry. J Formosan Med Assoc 1993;92:894–899.
53. Jin P. Changes in heart rate, noradrenaline, cortisol and mood during Tai Chi. J Psychosom Res 1989;33(2):197–206.
54. Thein JM, Brody LT. Aquatic-based rehabilitation and training for the elite athlete. J Orthop Sports Phys Ther 1998;27(1):32–41.

15 Osteopathic Medicine in Chronic Pain

James H. Gronemeyer
and Alexios G. Carayannopoulos

CONTENTS

Summary

Osteopathic medicine traditionally emphasizes the unison of all body systems including the musculoskeletal system. This recognition includes a reciprocal relationship between structure and organic function. The musculoskeletal system, including the bones, muscles, soft tissues, nerves, and spinal column can exhibit primary disorders, usually secondary to injury and degenerative changes, but it can also reflect many internal illnesses and may influence the process of disease through the circulatory, lymphatic, nervous, or other body systems.

In this review, the authors make no attempt to include all aspects of the Osteopathic philosophy and how it may influence medical care. However, in the treatment of chronic pain, as well as other fields of medicine, osteopathic approaches have long included the assessment of nociceptive and proprioceptive mechanisms in diagnosis and treatment. In this review, key anatomic, physiologic and homeostatic mechanisms, their scientific basis, and the influence they have on pain under pathological conditions are highlighted. A review of Osteopathic treatment techniques and examples of how they may enhance treatment strategies will follow.

Key Words: osteopathy, osteopathic medicine, manual medicine, spinal manipulation, craniosacral therapy, somatic dysfunction

From: *Contemporary Pain Medicine: Integrative Pain Medicine: The Science and Practice of Complementary and Alternative Medicine in Pain Management*
Edited by: J. F. Audette and A. Bailey © Humana Press, Totowa, NJ

1. INTRODUCTION

Osteopathic medicine traditionally emphasizes the unison of all body systems including the musculoskeletal system. This recognition includes a reciprocal relationship between structure and organic function. The musculoskeletal system including the bones, muscles, soft tissues, nerves and spinal column represents about 60 percent of the body composition. This system can exhibit primary disorders, usually secondary to injury and degenerative changes, but it can also reflect many internal illnesses and may influence the process of disease thru the circulatory, lymphatic, nervous or other body systems.

The early osteopaths stressed a detailed understanding of anatomy and physiology as the foundation for developing a rational medical treatment protocol. The manual techniques that developed from this philosophy were utilized in addition to all of the recognized medical procedures and technologies for the prevention, diagnosis and treatment of disease. This included drugs, botanicals, surgery, and radiation.

In this review, the authors make no attempt to include all aspects of the osteopathic philosophy and how it may influence medical care. However, in the treatment of chronic pain, as well as other fields of medicine, osteopathic approaches have long included the assessment of nociceptive and proprioceptive mechanisms in diagnosis and treatment. In this review, we plan to highlight key anatomic, physiologic and homeostatic mechanisms, their scientific basis, and the influence they have on pain under pathological conditions. A review of osteopathic treatment techniques and examples of how they may enhance treatment strategies will follow.

2. HISTORY

Following the Civil War, multiple approaches to medicine were popular and competing. Manual medicine had thousands of years of history in multiple cultures. In Europe "bone-setters" practiced manual medicine and kept their techniques in families as a secret trade. The Sweet family of Rhode Island was known for skilled bone setting in America during this period. A principle thinker and visionary in manual medicine at that time was Andrew Taylor Still, M.D. He was trained in the apprentice method, which was common in those days. It is unclear if there was a direct influence of Dr. Still by a descendant of the European bonesetters, but these were transcendental times with influences from around the world stimulating contemporary thinking.

American medicine in the 1860s was not very sophisticated and included purgatives, laxatives, blood letting, and the administration of narcotics, mercury, and arsenic compounds for various therapeutic purposes. Dr. Still's disenchantment with these primitive methods was strengthened when neither he nor any of his medical associates could save the lives of three of his children from an epidemic of meningitis. The system of medicine developing at the time was called "allopathy" which is currently defined as "that system of therapeutics in which diseases are treated by producing a condition incompatible with or antagonistic to the condition to be cured or alleviated" *(1)*. In contrast, homeopathy was also popular in the mid 19th century and was founded on the principle that a disease could be treated by the administration of highly dilute concentrations of substances that would normally produce like symptoms of the disease in healthy persons. Botanicals, nutritional, Native American healing, magnetic healing, hypnotism, and spiritualism, among others, were also popular healing traditions at the time.

Dr. Still developed a philosophy recognizing the importance of the neuromusculoskeletal system and developed a system of manual medicine to assist the natural immune system and the self-regulatory mechanisms of the body. He espoused the unity of the body and applied the principle of the interrelationship of structure and function as part of the reciprocal integration of the total body. Recognizing the body's ability to heal, he stressed prevention, proper diet, and fitness. These concepts, while popular today, were revolutionary in the medical culture of the mid 19th century.

Initially, Dr. Still avoided teaching specific techniques for treating various diseases and stressed a thorough understanding of the anatomic and physiologic principles associated with diseases to enable an astute practitioner to apply various osteopathic techniques in an advantageous manner. As enrollment in osteopathic colleges increased many of his students continued the research and development of osteopathic concepts. One of Dr. Still's students who is relevant today is William G. Sutherland, DO. He completed the understanding of the cranial concept first pointed to by Dr. Still. Called Osteopathy in the Cranial Field, it added the integration of the cranial and spinal dura structurally with the inherent self-correcting mechanism of the central nervous system. The Sutherland Cranial Teaching Foundation was formed to promote graduate education of his understanding. Several of his principle teaching associates have become well known to the current generation of physicians practicing manual medicine because of a resurgence of interest in alternative and complimentary medicine. One notable associate was Anne L Wales, DO who continued to teach and write about Dr Sutherland's work into her late 90's, influencing multiple generations. Another early colleague was Robert Fulford, DO who became well known for his work with children and inspired many notable alternative practitioners. These and many others provided a continuity of understanding and practice of Dr. Still's teachings and its extension as scientific understanding progressed.

3. OSTEOPATHIC PRINCIPLES

A distinguishing concept in the principles and practice of osteopathic medicine is that of somatic dysfunction. Historically termed the "osteopathic lesion", functional musculoskeletal restrictions that are associated with pain and autonomic arousal are believed to be a source or result of visceral dysfunction and disease. Somatic and visceral dysfunctions are characterized by the following:

1. Changes in texture or tone of soft tissues,
2. Mechanical hyperalgesia or increased sensitivity to touch,
3. Altered range and ease of motion,
4. Anatomic asymmetry of the affected region *(2)*.

These changes are usually identified by subtle palpation as part of an osteopathic structural examination of a patient.

Somatic dysfunctions may be caused by musculoskeletal restrictions in a single joint. More frequently they include widespread changes in posture, mobility, and regional function as compensatory changes that develop in response to an initial restriction or injury. These somatic dysfunctions have been demonstrated to involve edema, inflammation, and thickening of connective tissue *(2)* rather than gross muscle or ligament tears, fractures or avulsions. Gross injuries, once healed, may also develop into a somatic dysfunction as the body adapts to the secondary consequences of that injury including loss of joint range of motion and soft tissue restrictions.

Typically, the restrictions associated with somatic dysfunction and its related autonomic arousal and visceral dysfunction are anatomically related. They tend to follow 'segmental' patterns based on the embryologic innervation of the developing tissues. However, autonomic dysfunction may be more widespread. These dysfunctions may develop from somatic or visceral disease or trauma, peripheral nerve or central nervous system trauma, and even as a consequence of more subtle musculoskeletal restrictions or postural habits that may develop over time. Osteopathic approaches in the treatment of disease or chronic pain include those directed at removing physical or irritative processes that may potentiate or facilitate disease or perpetuate pain.

4. PATHOPHYSIOLOGY OF SOMATIC DYSFUNCTION

Several models may be employed to understand the concept of somatic dysfunction and rational approaches to treatment utilizing osteopathic methods in manual medicine. Beginning with the effects of tissue injury and the subsequent inflammatory response, multiple chemical mediators are released from various types of cells in the fascia to stimulate repair and tissue growth. Simultaneously, these mediators stimulate nociceptive nerve endings in the injured tissue and signal the spinal cord through the primary afferent fibers (see Chapter 2). Primary afferent fibers are divided into two major categories based on structure and function. The large caliber fibers are well myelinated and rapidly conducting. They project from the periphery to the somatosensory cortex through the spinal cord in a discrete and precisely mapped manner. They carry discriminate touch and proprioception from specialized, encapsulated endings such as Pacinian corpuscles, Merkel discs, or Ruffini endings responding to light touch, vibration or tissue movements.

4.1. Neuroanatomy of Pain

The small caliber primary afferent fibers are unmyelinated or lightly myelinated nerves that terminate with naked nerve endings in the peripheral tissue. A large percentage of the small fibers carry information about actual or potential injury to the surrounding tissue to multiple areas of the brainstem, thalamus, limbus, and somatosensory cortex with less precise somatotopic mapping. Intensity of stimulation to small fiber afferent nerves produces a variable response. While low-level stimulation produces a sensation of crude touch or contact, high intensity stimulation produces the sensation of pain and may activate the arousal system triggering endocrine and immune response. An important characteristic of this system is its ability to become sensitized to repetitive stimuli and lower the threshold of activation.

The small afferent fibers innervate all the tissues of the body except the center of the vertebral disc, hyaline cartilage and the parenchyma of the central nervous system (CNS). These include the connective tissue of the dermis and deep epidermis, fascias of blood vessels and nerves, as well as muscles, tendons, ligaments, joint capsules and synovial linings including the outer third of the intervertebral discs. The viscera and their support structures contain similar small fiber components. The central nervous system contains small caliber fibers extending from the meningeal blood vessels. The activation of these fibers by chemical, mechanical or thermal stimuli is called nociception and they are often termed primary afferent nociceptors.

The inflammatory changes associated with somatic dysfunction can affect the nociceptive nerve endings in an adverse manner thru the release of prostaglandins, histamine, bradykinin, and changes in pH. As the nociceptive fibers become more active, the C fibers (or group IV fibers in muscle) can exhibit a secretory response as well as the afferent response, with the release of neuropeptides from their peripheral terminals. These neuropeptides can increase vasodilation and stimulate mast cell degranulation there by further irritating the peripheral nociceptors. As this condition progresses, hyperalgesia develops as previously low-level noxious stimulus begins to produce increased pain. When tissues become so sensitive that normally non-painful stimuli produce pain, the resultant condition is called allodynia. This process of altered thresholds of nociceptors is termed peripheral sensitization.

As the primary afferent nociceptors enter the dorsal horn of the spinal cord, they terminate on interneurons that map to the lateral columns (leading to an autonomic efferent response), the ventral horn (providing guarding response to the motor system), and multiple segments of the spinal cord of the propriospinal system. The related segmental interneuronal pool also receives input from the descending pain modulatory system emanating from the midbrain and can provide either inhibitory or, under certain conditions, excitatory input to the dorsal horn. Damage to the soma can, through the small caliber fibers, modify the response of the related segmental large fiber afferent system in and motor system out. This facilitated segment can lead to changes in visceral function, somatic muscle tone, tone of the vaso vasorum and tissue fluid balance from increased motor facilitation modifying adaptive responses in the peripheral tissues.

4.2. Models of Spinal Facilitation

The processes described above have given rise to several models that encompass the osteopathic concept in restoring function or assisting regulation of altered physiology in pain conditions. The model of nociception and spinal facilitation, best described by Willard (3), might be summarized as follows. Tissue injury may modify pain related sensory neurons resulting in changes of joint mobility, and changes in related autonomic, visceral and immunologic systems. Normally, the effect of activation of primary afferent nociceptors on the dorsal horn of the spinal cord is modulated via inhibition, either locally or from descending pathways from the cerebral cortex or brainstem. However, under sustained afferent drive pathologic changes can occur in the spinal cord, which may include inhibitory neuron cell death, as well as wind up and sensitization of the 2nd order neuron in the dorsal horn. Concurrently, the autonomic response to sustained nociception can evoke changes in assorted visceral, inflammatory, and immunological functions. Once established, spinal facilitation may persist even if peripheral afferent drive is eliminated. This model of a chronically facilitated segment can also account for the more global CNS activity including the patterns of altered behavior, sleep patterns, depression, hyper or hypo-asthenia, as well as other manifestations, seen in chronic pain syndromes.

Van Buskirk (4) presented a model of somatic dysfunction that built on the early research and neural models of somatic dysfunction by Denslow and Korr. This model describes restriction in mobility and autonomic, visceral, and immunological changes that are produced by pain-related sensory neurons and their reflexes. Activation of nociceptors is known to produce guarding reactions, as well as autonomic activation, following stress or damage to musculoskeletal tissue. Musculoskeletal guarding results in abnormal position and range of motion in the related tissue. Local inflammatory responses and autonomic reflexes enhance nociceptive activity, facilitating further restriction. The resulting maintenance of muscles, joints, and related tissues in an abnormal guarding pattern produces changes in connective tissues reinforcing the abnormal postural patterns. Attempting to stretch these modified tissues into a normal range of motion can further stimulate the nociceptive response, reflexively reinforcing the abnormal musculoskeletal response.

Another older model is based on muscle spasm leading to muscle spindle dysfunction. Muscle length is determined by afferent stimulus from the Golgi tendon apparatus and muscle spindle fibers, followed by efferent stimulation of alpha and gamma efferents to elicit appropriate contraction or relaxation. Joint motion will become altered and dysfunctional in the face of a related tonically over tightened muscle. For example, a tightened paraspinal muscle may cause spinal facet dysfunction, which in turn lead to further tightening of the involved muscles and a vicious cycle develops. A normal stretching routine may not return the muscle to its normal resting length because of altered spindle activity driven by the somatic dysfunction. Efforts to reset the muscle spindle activity level to baseline by post isometric contraction stretching is the basis for some osteopathic treatment techniques.

5. OSTEOPATHIC PRACTICE IN PAIN MEDICINE

Contemporary multi-disciplinary pain programs are frequently related to rehabilitation programs or anesthesia departments and are often directed by Anesthesiologists, Physiatrists, or Neurologists. They have the benefits of integrating physical medicine, pain medicine, physical therapy, occupational therapy, pain psychology, and other behavioral approaches for improved treatment of difficult pain cases. Unfortunately, some cases of chronic pain persist. Osteopathic evaluation and treatment can prove valuable in many situations. A representative example will be reviewed to encourage a careful full body examination locating distant postural causes for difficult pain syndromes.

5.1. Low Back Pain

Low back pain may be the most common patient complaint and sometimes, even with the best medical or surgical care, results in a failed back syndrome. Employing the more subtle soft tissue palpation techniques often used in osteopathic evaluation often reveals structural or myofascial changes referred to as somatic dysfunctions as described above. These can maintain a pain pattern or chronically facilitated segment long after successful surgical or epidural injection techniques have improved the acute symptoms.

A common example is an acute psoas spasm following a lifting, sports, fall or other acute injury. The sensation that 'I can't stand up straight' or 'I walk leaning to the side' usually improves in several days or weeks with usual treatment. However, persistent restriction in the lumbar facet joints or sacroiliac joint may create late effects in local or distant tissues as the result of postural compensation or splinting. In the lumbar region hyper-tonicity in the piriformis, paraspinal muscles or quadratus lumborum develops and becomes a risk factor for reinjury from otherwise benign activities. A pelvic obliquity and short leg syndrome may follow, leading to altered tone in the postural muscles and a shift to the opposite side when standing to maintain balance and stability (see Figure 1). The pelvic bone, which is restricted in the swing phase of the gait, tends to externally rotate the leg at the hip. However, foot mechanics require the lower leg to turn in for good heel-toe weight transfer. This process stretches an already hypertonic piriformis muscle and may lead to leg pain and its other manifestations. The same altered postural dynamics can simultaneously affect the tensor fascia lata, iliotibial band (ITB), and biceps femoris with late pain effects on the knee, ankle and foot. Conditions such as ITB syndrome, heel pain, or plantar fasciitis frequently follow.

5.2. Neck Pain

Other late effects of persistent somatic dysfunctions from the example above can affect thoracic, cervical or cranial regions. A compensatory scoliosis develops in

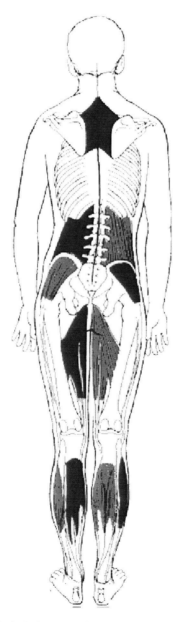

Fig. 1. Illustration of the muscle imbalances and compensation scoliosis that develops in response to a pelvic obliquity.

response to short leg syndrome, with alternating lateral curves made necessary for postural stability and to maintain the center of mass over midline. As a result of this compensation pattern, a compression syndrome may develop at the apex of the spinal curve or at transition points where the curvature shifts from one direction to the other. Facet syndrome or chronic rib pain may develop with local myofascial changes including the development of trigger points. In the thorax, joint dysfunction of the spine may cause secondary facilitated segments that can affect the function of the shoulder girdle and upper extremity. Facilitation or inhibition of the lower trapezius, serratus muscles, pectoralis, and rhomboids can lead to rotator cuff dysfunction and related pain syndromes.

Cervical facet syndromes are known to cause sclerotomal referral patterns with pain symptoms frequently traveling to the upper extremity and thorax, as well as associations with cervcogenic head pain. Current attention to uncinate or chronic zygapophyseal joint pain and diagnosis with medial branch blocks does not account for all the possible causes of inflammation in that region. While degenerative joint disease and prior cervical trauma may account for some of the cases, some patients with cervical facet syndrome may have had no known trauma to the neck but rather a history of a low back or lower extremity injury, or even a difficult labor and delivery, again suggesting that the cervical pain is a late secondary effect that has developed in response to a compensation pattern from the remote trauma.

Other common pain syndromes in the region of the cranio-cervical junction including myofascial pain, headache, cranio-facial pain, cervicogenic vertigo, and tempo-mandibular joint dysfunction, among others, can share injury to remote structures as an etiology. Accessing and including the treatment of distant postural or late effects of prior injury may add an important and missing treatment modality in the treatment of chronic pain, especially pain that has not responded to local treatment. The example used here is not exhaustive or definitive, but is presented to encourage an expanded view of causality sometimes associated with chronic pain syndromes. These approaches have been successful in improving outcomes of patients who had failed previous chronic pain treatment programs.

5.3. Integrative Approach

It is important to note that often gentle, indirect osteopathic treatment modalities are better tolerated in chronic pain patients and provide longer lasting results by engaging the patients' postural or motor reflexes rather than a quick high velocity joint manipulation. This indirect approach promotes retraining of altered motor firing patterns, improvement of inhibited or facilitated postural patterns and, ultimately, reduction in the afferent drive fueling a facilitated pain pathway. Frequently, physical therapies or trigger point treatments, which were not effective before osteopathic treatment was initiated, become successful and stabilizing for the patient following osteopathic care.

Concurrent medical treatment is recommended to address the multiple components or pathways associated with chronic pain. The use of non-steroidal anti-inflammatory drugs (NSAIDs) can be useful to reduce inflammation and peripheral sensitization. Tricyclics may be helpful in decreasing central facilitation and loss of inhibitory circuits also associated with chronic pain. Other supplements sometimes used in multidisciplinary treatment programs include the omega 3 and 6 fatty acids as found in borage oil, fish oil or flax seed oil. Vitamin E, glucosamine and possibly chondroitin in combination with glucosamine are popular with many practitioners. Adequate sleep is important with multiple choices of medications. The use of low dose muscle relaxants such as cyclobenzaprine or tizanidine may improve sleep and reduce myofascial symptoms. Of course medications for neuropathic pain, opioids or their devativies, topicals such as lidocaine patches, botox and current pain ablation techniques may be indicated. It is important to remember the substantial benefits of heat or cold applications and the use of daily gentle exercise program.

6. OSTEOPATHIC PROFESSION

In the United States, Doctors of Osteopathic Medicine (DOs) are fully licensed physicians and surgeons, able to practice medicine alongside their Medical Doctor (MD) colleagues in every state. They hold the same unlimited rights as MDs and are recognized by the AMA as full-practice physicians admitting and treating patients in both osteopathic and allopathic hospitals and clinics. DOs undergo osteopathic and/or allopathic post-graduate training and are governed by the same state licensing and credentialing boards as MDs. At this time post-graduate training is predominantly in mixed staff hospitals. Osteopathic physicians utilize all of the recognized procedures and modern techniques for prevention, diagnosis, and treatment of disease, which include drugs, injections, radiation, and surgery, but are encouraged to use their hands to diagnose and treat somatic dysfunction and its clinical manifestations. DOs can be found in clinical, academic, as well as industrial settings, including the public, private, as well as national defense sector.

Although osteopathic physicians represent only 5% of the national medical work force, it continues to be a fast growing segment of the medical field, with the number of trainees and training institutions growing tremendously in the last 30 years. Like its allopathic counterpart, the AMA, the American Osteopathic Association (AOA), governs the osteopathic profession, and retains substantial influence over the training, certification, and continuing medical education of osteopathic medical students, residents, and board eligible/qualified physicians. It has maintained its independence from the AMA and has been instrumental in promoting its unique perspective for over 100 years.

Although the holistic tradition of osteopathic medicine is reflected in the fact that a large percentage work as primary care practitioners, DOs are fully qualified to pursue every specialty from the medical to the surgical arena. Even when a DO becomes a specialist, however, they may retain the unique philosophy taught in osteopathic medical schools to regard each patient as a whole person, to understand the inter-relatedness of all body systems, and to stress that illness can have its origin in another part of the body.

7. SAFETY

In general, osteopathic manipulative medicine is very safe and efficacious when used by trained, experienced hands. However, despite being used safely for many years, there is little in the literature to support the low morbidity and mortality rate. Most early reports were in the form of case studies. More recently, carefully designed studies have reported complications mostly related to techniques employing the use of thrusts or force. The growing interest in Complementary and Alternative Medicine (CAM) as well as tighter regulations by the medical insurance sector has forced the profession to attempt to better quantify and qualify not only their efficacy, but also the potential complications arising from osteopathic treatment or spinal manipulation.

When looking at complications, it is important to consider a few issues. First, statistics for rates of complications are generated from case reports, surveys, and medico-legal statistics. These statistics may be influenced by reporting bias of the practitioners involved since it is not always advantageous to advertise their adverse outcomes producing statistics that may underreport true risks involved. Second, it is important to distinguish between true adverse side effects and transient symptom exacerbations, which may occur following manual treatments. For example, some patients experience a transient increase in pain or soreness after manipulation, possibly from increased range of motion and function. True complications are those that result in the development of new injury or dysfunction and are the direct result of the manipulative treatment. Third, since case reports often only describe the most serious complications, the medical literature may not be reporting on the less severe side effects, such as mild or transient neurological symptoms, which often herald more sinister pathology.

7.1. Risk of Major Complications

From the literature, most studies quantify the risk of major or serious complications in the range of 1 in 400,000 to 1 in 1 million *(5)*. The true risk per patient is highly dependent on the skills of the practitioner, the particular treatments used, and the comorbidities of the patient. Most attention to rates of complications has been given to cervical manipulations, but evidence does exist for other aspects of osteopathic and spinal manipulative medicine. Currently the literature does not adequately distinguish between the type of provider (i.e. MD, DO, DC, PT) or the type of treatment (manipulation vs. mobilization). Most reported cases of adverse outcome have been associated with "Thrust" or "High Velocity/Low Amplitude" methods of treatment. One of the most comprehensive assessments of the complications of spinal manipulation was conducted by Assendelft et al in 1996, who identified relevant case reports, surveys, and review articles using a comprehensive search of online databases. Based on case reports and surveys, estimation was made of the risk for the most frequently reported complications, which included vertebrobasilar accidents (VBAs) and cauda equina syndrome (CES). They found that VBAs occurred mainly after a cervical manipulation with a rotatory component with an estimated occurrence of 1 per 20,000 patients to 1 per 1 million cervical manipulations. They reported the risk of CES to be 1 in a million.

Dvorak and Orelli reported a serious complication incidence to be 1 in 400,000 procedures when they surveyed the Swiss Manual Medicine Society in 1981. Most of these, including loss of consciousness or neurologic events, were related to high velocity cervical manipulation. These were reported much less frequently in the lumbar than cervical spine *(6)*. Minor sequelae reported included transient vertigo or temporary exacerbation of pain. Although this study did not include US trained osteopathic physicians, this carefully designed study was one of the first to show the relative safety of manipulative medicine. As a follow-up, Dvorak reported a zero incidence of manipulation related complications in his own practice at a lecture ten years later at an osteopathic college.

Patijin reviewed several papers in 1991 for cases of manipulation-related complications. He notes that the majority (67%, 85 cases) involved chiropractors; none were specific to osteopathic physicians. He found that the most significant complication (65%) involved injury to the vertebral artery and all appeared to be related to high velocity, thrusting applications. On average, these incidences occurred highest in the relatively young age group of 35-40 years, but were still less than the rate of spontaneous dissection and embolus *(7)*. Interestingly, Koss reported a higher incidence of side effects from medications vs. manipulative treatments with a rate of hospital admissions secondary to drug side effects to be 5% *(8)*.

Kleynhans divides causes of manipulation complications into two categories: physician related, and patient related. The former are secondary to diagnostic errors, poor technical skill, and poor interdisciplinary communication and consultation. The latter are secondary to medical co-morbidities, subjective pain response, psychobehavioral issues, congenital abnormalities, previous negative manipulative experiences, and discordant expectations between patient and practitioner *(9)*. Furthermore, this study pointed out the importance of appropriate physician assessment before each and every encounter.

Oliphant et al performed a qualitative systematic review of the risk of chiropractic spinal manipulation in the treatment of lumbar disc herniations (LDH) to estimate the risk of spinal manipulation causing a severe adverse reaction, such as clinically worsened disc herniation or cauda equina syndrome, in a patient presenting with LDH. He found the risk to be less than 1 in 3.7 million, thereby concluding that it is relatively safe, especially when compared to other common treatments for LDH, such as NSAIDS and surgery. Moreover, he posited that spinal manipulation may be no more dangerous than activities of daily living, in their relation to causing LDH *(10)*.

Finally, Vick et al looked at the safety of manipulative treatment from 1925 to 1993 to determine how commonly injuries occur from osteopathic manipulative medicine (OMM), as well as other types of manipulative treatment. A total of 128 articles were examined, of which 98 reported a total of 185 specific cases of major complications in the cervical, thoracic, and lumbar spine from manipulation as well as spontaneous trauma or insult. They concluded that manipulative treatment remains an extremely safe, therapeutic modality, when performed by a knowledgeable and skilled practitioner after a thorough history and physical examination is performed to ensure the health and safety of the patient *(11)*.

In summary, most studies have shown that the most frequent and serious complications are related to techniques that use high velocity, low amplitude (HVLA) thrusting, with the cervical region surpassing the thoracic and lumbosacral, especially when combined with movements of extension and rotation. The most frequent of these complications, which range from 1 in 20,000 to 1 in 1 million, is neurovascular compromise, including stroke, vertebral thrombosis, and arterial dissection. As noted in Grant's atlas, "The cervical spine is, without doubt, quite resistant, and the atheromatous vertebral arteries quite tolerant" *(12)*. However, patients with rheumatoid arthritis and Down's syndrome are at an increased risk during cervical manipulation secondary to potential weakening and increased susceptibility to rupture of the odontoid ligament with resultant pithing of the cord. Other complications of HVLA have included fractures in predisposed patients and cauda equina syndrome. It has been shown that there is a lower chance of injury when the neck is maintained in midline if cervical flexion and side-bending maneuvers are used.

7.2. *Other Complications*

Other manipulative procedures, including muscle energy, counterstrain, and craniosacral treatments have also been examined. The most frequent complication from muscle energy is a temporary increase in pain. Poor efficacy of treatment and muscle soreness can occur if concomitant soft tissue procedures are not performed prior to treatment. Contraindications include fractures and neurologic compromise. Complications from counterstrain also include temporary flare-up of pain, especially in antagonist muscles. Precautions include positions that fail to relieve pain and discomfort as well as positions that produce dizziness or radicular pain. Patients with poor bone mineralization should not be placed in extremes of spinal flexion. Complications of craniosacral treatment are more frequently encountered by unskilled practitioners, and these include temporary nausea, vertigo, lightheadedness, headache, loss of appetite, and sleep difficulties. Most are transient and respond to rest *(5)*.

Although complications from OMM are relatively benign and infrequent, there are steps the osteopathic physician can take to prevent their occurrence. Foremost on this list is a thorough understanding and training in osteopathic principles and practice, including excellent manipulative skills. In addition, a thorough history and physical examination with a carefully selected treatment paradigm based on structural examination, functional anatomy, and biomechanics is essential. Absolute contraindications for manipulative medicine may include acute arthropathies, acute fractures and dislocations, signs of ligamentous rupture or instability, bone malignancies and metastases, infections of bone and joint, acute myelopathy, and cauda equina syndrome. Relative contraindications are spondylolisthesis with progressive slippage, articular hypermobility, post-surgical joints, acute soft tissue injuries, demineralization of bone (eg. osteoporosis), benign bone tumors, and clinical manifestations of vertebrobasilar insufficiency, aneurysm, anticoagulant therapy, and blood dyscrasias *(13)*. Precautions should be taken by referring physicians for patients with any of the following: age greater than 50, history of significant trauma, fever greater than 100 degrees F, history of prolonged corticosteroid use, unexplained weight loss, history of cancer, adenopathy, history of serious systemic inflammatory arthritides or vasculitidies, endocrinopathies that affect calcium metabolism, and presence of neurological deficit *(14,15)*.

8. OSTEOPATHIC TECHNIQUES

There are a wide variety of techniques used by US trained osteopathic physicians. These treatments are founded on the belief that the body's structure and function are interdependent and that all systems are interrelated through the common fascia (see Figure 2). Each of the techniques requires a hands-on approach. Most treatment paradigms used are a combination of several techniques, which are individually tailored based on findings of the structural exam. Techniques may be active in which the patient assists the physician contracting various muscles or passive were the patient is relaxed. These techniques employ several physiologic principles including the stretch reflex, the muscle spindle reflex, the Golgi tendon organ reflex, reciprocal inhibition and the crossed extensor reflex.

8.1. *Soft-Tissue Technique*

These techniques are usually applied to the paraspinal muscles and consist of three basic mechanisms; traction, or stretching, in which the origin and insertion of

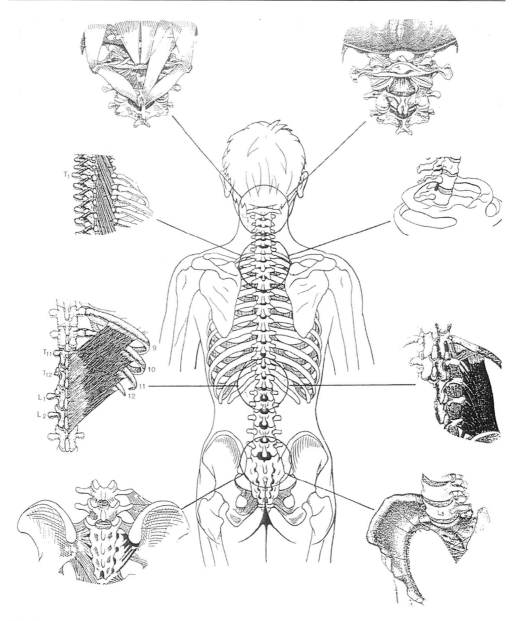

Fig. 2. Interconnected areas of treatment focus in Osteopathic Manipulative Medicine (OMM). A: Cranio-cervical junction; B: Cervico-thoracal junction; C: Thoraco-lumbar junction; D: Lumbo-sacral junction.

myofascial tissues are longitudinally separated, inhibition using sustained deep pressure over a hypertonic structure, and kneading, a rhythmic, lateral stretching of myofascial structures. The focus is on the movement of tissue fluids, such as edema, and the relaxation of tightened muscles and fibrous bands, which are often associated with somatic dysfunction.

8.2. Myofascial Release

This technique is used to treat the myofascial system. It can be divided into direct and indirect approaches. In the direct approach, a restrictive barrier is engaged and the tissue is subsequently loaded with a constant force until the barrier is released. In the indirect approach, the restricted tissues are guided along a path of least resistance until the barrier is indirectly released and unrestricted movement is achieved.

8.3. Muscle Energy Technique

This technique involves active participation of the patient whereby he/she is instructed to contract a muscle in a specific direction and position against a counter force applied by the practitioner. The goal is to restore motion, decrease muscle hyper-activity and tissue restriction, and ultimately restore symmetry.

8.4. Counterstrain

Originally referred to as 'spontaneous release by positioning' by its' discoverer it was given a shorter term to describe the method of technique. This technique entails passive movement of the patient's body away from a restriction into the position of greatest comfort. At that point, an asymptomatic strain is created in order to relieve somatic dysfunctions that are usually too acute or too sensitive to treat with the other techniques.

8.5. Thrust Techniques

These techniques involve the targeted application of controlled high velocity/low amplitude thrusts to restore specific joint motion. The goal is to restore normal range of motion and to re-set neural reflexes. In turn, this will treat somatic dysfunction, resulting in relaxation of tissues, restoration of symmetry, relief of tenderness, and resumption of movement.

8.6. Lymphatic Techniques

This technique is designed to encourage the circulation of the lymphatic system and the removal of toxic metabolic wastes. It is used to relieve edema and has been helpful in upper and lower respiratory infections. It is mostly used on inpatients with systemic disease, post-operative patients, and cancer patients as it uses gentle alternating pressure to assist the bodies' respiratory system.

8.7. Cranial Osteopathy

Osteopathy in the Cranial Field (often called Cranial Osteopathy) is a systematic approach to diagnosis and treatment utilizing the body's self-regulatory mechanism inherent in the central nervous system. The cranium is accommodative to the function of the central nervous system, cerebrospinal fluid and dural membranes that function as a unit. The regulatory forces emanating from the head region function through out the body facilitating diagnosis and treatment of the whole person. For example, if the cranial structures are brought into a state of imbalance from trauma, changes in postural balance will cause compensatory changes throughout the neuromusculoskeletal system in an effort to maintain equilibrium.

8.8. Balanced Ligamentous Tension

This technique is a component of Osteopathy in the Cranial Field used in treating strains throughout the body. When joints are strained, it is primarily the ligaments that are involved in maintaining the restriction of function termed "ligamentous articular strain" by Dr. Sutherland. Treatment entails gently exaggerating the position of the ligaments to a point of balance where splinting or other dysfunction can be released promoting improved function.

9. OSTEOPATHY IN A HOSPITAL BASED PRACTICE

Although most applications of osteopathic medicine occur in the outpatient setting, the same principles and practice can be applied to an inpatient population experiencing pain. The goals might include a decrease in pain score, shorter hospital stay, fewer medications, concomitant decrease in medication side effects, and lower utilization of costly hospital resources. Most pain services in acute care hospitals see pain patients in consultation. The inpatient pain consult includes an in-depth, focused history whenever possible, physical examination including palpatory diagnosis, clinical correlation with assessment and diagnosis, and finally, a pertinent OMM treatment plan when appropriate. The addition of osteopathic manipulative medicine can complement medical and surgical treatment.

9.1. Reduced Hospital Length of Stay

Several studies have attempted to look at inpatient osteopathic manipulative treatment (OMT). Fitzgerald and Stiles reported reduction in hospital length of stay when osteopathic manipulative medicine was used for patients with asthma (14%), pneumonia (10%), cholecystectomy (7%), and hysterectomy (12%). They also found a concomitant reduction in shock, dysrhythmias, and mortality when osteopathically oriented manipulative care was integrated into the care of patients with myocardial disease *(16)*. More recently, Klock and Cantieri performed a retrospective chart review of four hundred and eighty-four patients admitted to a hospital who had received PTCA (Percutaneous Transluminal Coronary Angioplasty) with or without stent placement, one hundred thirty-four of whom received adjunctive care in the form of a structural examination and OMT. This was in an effort to determine if structural abnormalities were a reliable predictor of coronary artery disease and if the two patient populations differed significantly in terms of mortality rates, length of stay, and readmission within 31 days of discharge. He found a statistically significant difference between patients who received manipulative care during their hospitalization and those who did not. The most significant finding was a reduction in length of stay for the patients who also had chronic obstructive pulmonary disease *(17)*. Finally, Cantieri reports on a survey of the use of OMT in 18 osteopathic hospitals. In those diagnostic groups with documentation of more than 10 patients receiving OMT, a decreased length of stay of one day or more was noted, including GI-related, psychiatric, neurological, and cardiovascular diseases *(18)*.

9.2. Acute Pain Management

Extrapolation of these results to the general inpatient acute pain patient lies in the application of the osteopathic structural examination. Osteopathic physicians have used the presence of somatic dysfunction as in indicator of visceral pathology or autonomic dysfunction. Because most pain syndromes can involve a disturbance of the somatic, visceral, or autonomic systems, a keen understanding of the structural findings and their relation to the concept of central facilitation allows the osteopathic physician to identify alterations in normal body homeostasis, which may contribute to pain. Structural abnormalities, such as muscular imbalance, tissue texture abnormalities, temperature change, and restricted spinal segments help to provide an overall understanding of the interplay of related systems and provide direction for a treatment plan. By including OMM treatment to reverse the restrictions found on structural examination, the physician may enhance treatment of the pain syndrome by reducing functional limitations and analgesic requirements.

Hospital patients experience some element of acute or acute-on-chronic pain. Pain may be secondary to the principal diagnosis, such as tumor-related pain, mechanics of a surgical procedure such as incisional pain, or to the post-operative reaction of the body, such as edema and localized inflammation. Each of these requires a slightly different approach. OMM on inpatients experiencing pain is designed to hasten the patient's discharge and to facilitate return-to-normal function of the cardiovascular, neurologic, renal, pulmonary, gastrointestinal and musculoskeletal systems. Pain in these areas includes, but is not limited to alterations in: neurologic tone, vascular or lymphatic flow, fascial or myofascial tension, axoplasmic transport, and overall efficiency. This can lead to vasospasm, venous stasis, lymphatic pooling, ileus, urinary retention, and DVT. Each can be addressed with a variety of gentle, non-thrusting techniques. The basis of some of the more popular techniques is described below. For more detailed information, consultation with a comprehensive source such as Kuchera or Graham is advised *(19,20)*.

9.3. Common In-Patient Osteopathic Techniques

1. Occipito-atlantal/Cranial Base (O/A/CB) Decompression and Release: This technique addresses somatic dysfunction, muscle spasm, fascial and myofascial tension caused by generalized edema or muscle spasm in the cervical area, which can lead to direct muscular pressure on the vagus nerve and jugular vein as they exit through the jugular foramen, with resultant compromise of the normal function of the vagus nerve. Resultant adverse effects include: bronchoconstriction with excessive mucus production causing pleuritic pain; excessive input to the vomiting center with nausea and vomiting causing headache and generalized malaise; adverse alteration of heart rate, conduction, and cardiac output causing chest pain and palpitations; disruption of GI peristalsis and sphincter tone causing ileus and abdominal discomfort and restriction of the vagus nerve. This technique aims to reverse this pathological process.

2. Rib raising/walking: This technique addresses pleuritic and chest wall pain. Its focus is to decrease pulmonary congestion, enhance and encourage pulmonary expectorant function, facilitate venous and lymphatic circulation, increase ribcage mobility, increase pulmonary excursion, and increase sympathetic tone through pumping action on the sympathetic chain ganglia located on the rib heads. This will in turn decrease pulmonary congestion, cause bronchodilation, decrease atelectasis and pneumonia, maximize O2 and CO2 ventilation and exchange, maximize natural and adaptive immunity, and improve delivery of antibiotics and other medications to the lungs and throughout the circulation. Rib raising is also pivotal to allow for other organs to recover from generalized stasis caused by acute illness, trauma, or surgery.

3. Kidney Pump: This technique is performed through a pumping action of the inferior ribs *(13–15)*, to restore normal physiologic function of the kidney. Congestion of the filtration system may cause fluid overload and systemic toxicity. This can often manifest as flank or low back pain. The pumping and milking action of this technique encourages urine flow and facilitates removal of dead cells and toxins to mechanically decrease congestion and inflammation and increase venous and lymphatic drainage of the area. Additionally, the mechanical pumping will improve arterial flow, increase oxygenation, improve delivery of medications and intrinsic healing factors, and ultimately prevent further damage and facilitate return of normal kidney function.

4. Lumbosacral/Pelvic Soft tissue articulation and release: This technique is directed at low back and pelvic pain patients, addressing the somatic dysfunction, muscle spasm, and myofascial tension of the lumbar vertebrae and sacrum. This can cause facilitation of the sympathetic and parasympathetic nervous system, which compromises normal physiologic function and tone of the pelvic viscera resulting in stasis, accumulation of excess gas, constipation, urinary retention, decreased kidney and adrenal function, decreased urine output and altered catecholamine levels. This technique has the ability to decrease myofascial tension and facilitate the normal function of the distal colon, bladder, and kidneys.

5. Pedal fascial pump: This technique is most helpful in the post-surgical patient or after prolonged bed rest. It provides a gentle ballottement of the organs in the thoracic and abdominal cavities to stimulate the internal organs to return to normal physiologic function. This is akin to early ambulation after surgery or bed rest, which helps to overcome organ stasis, increased fluid in the extra cellular space, and decreases the potential for deep vein thrombosis in the post-operative or sedentary patient.

These techniques are only a portion of the available options specific to treating somatic dysfunction and related pain disorders in the inpatient population. For a more comprehensive, the reader should refer to a standard osteopathic text (See Resources Section).

9.4. Manipulation Under Joint Anesthesia

Manipulation under joint anesthesia/analgesia (MUJA) is a technique used by some physicians to treat patients with chronic, recalcitrant spinal axis pain. It is performed using fluoroscopically-guided intraarticular synovial joint injections with a variety of corticosteroid and anesthetic agents, which are followed by targeted manipulations of the affected joint(s). This combination of procedures can be performed by one exceptionally skilled physician but is usually performed through a collaborative effort by two or more specialists.

Although MUJA has recently gained favor, the practice of combining spinal manipulation with injections is not a new idea. It was first described in 1938 by Haldeman and Soto-Hall, who used a blind injection followed by manipulation of the sacro-iliac joint *(21)*. It was researched by Bloomberg et al, who combined blinded corticosteroid injections with manipulation in a group of back pain patients, and found encouraging results *(22)*. Other reports include those of Ben-David et al *(23)*, Geraci et al *(24)*, Nelson et al *(25)*, and Aspergen et al *(26)*. To date however, there have been no randomized controlled trials or meta-analyses in the literature. Nonetheless, practitioners using this technique have reported anecdotal success with patients who are non-responsive to more conservative treatment options.

According to Michaelson, the following patients should be considered for MUJA:

(1) Patients with predominant spinal axis pain who have not progressed over sufficient time (2 months) from the delivery of prior treatments, including spinal manipulation;
(2) Patients with pain so severe that standard manipulation cannot be delivered with technical success due to an increase in pain and subsequent rigidity;
(3) Patients with complex problems, in whom the diagnosis of synovial joint-mediated spinal pain must be established before the safe delivery of manipulative therapy *(27)*. Despite these guidelines, individual practice parameters vary widely.

MUJA is closely related clinically to manipulation of the spine under general anesthesia (MUA), which is somewhat controversial. However, the benefits reported by proponents of MUA are similar to MUJA in that both can potentially facilitate spinal manipulation through the reduction of pain, guarding, and spasm. MUJA has the added benefit of providing diagnostic information to the physician as to the specific pain generating spinal segment. However, MUA has additional risks associated with general anesthesia. MUJA carries the combined risks of the individual components involved, with the risk varying according to the region of the spine being treated *(27)*.

10. OSTEOPATHIC RESEARCH

The state of osteopathic medical research is in a transition period. In the past, the art of osteopathy was taught through mentorship and sharing of anecdotal experiences by clinically oriented practitioners. With the Flexner report of the early part of the twentieth century, osteopathic medical education underwent reorganization just as the allopathic medical profession did, changing the way students were trained, and enforcing higher standards for a more scientifically based foundation. With the growth of evidence-based medicine in the latter half of the last century, the profession entered a new era. While the quality and quantity of research on osteopathic principles subsequently expanded with many case-reports and pilot studies in the osteopathic literature, it lagged behind its allopathic counterpart with only a few randomized, prospective clinical trials.

10.1. Methodological Considerations

When evaluating research, it is important to understand the semantic differences between the various terms used by other providers of manual skills, such as chiropractors, physical therapists, and massage therapists. Primarily chiropractors refer to spinal manipulation and manual medicine in treatment, while physical therapists use mobilization and massage therapists do bodywork. Osteopathic manipulative medicine does not equal allopathic medicine plus chiropractic and therefore much of the available research, which investigates the effect of chiropractic or physical/massage therapy techniques on various pain conditions, does not directly reflect the state of osteopathic medicine today.

Because osteopathic medicine involves much more than manipulation, it is a more comprehensive philosophy of care that cannot be encompassed by the results of manipulation trials. It is steeped in history and tradition. Although osteopathic and chiropractic medicine have similar roots, their paths diverged over a century ago. Massage and physical therapists may perform similar techniques, however the rigor and depth of their training is not comparable to that of osteopathic physicians. Therefore, the clinical evidence regarding chiropractic, physical, or massage therapy, which form the bulk of the literature, does not adequately assess the clinical and scientific merit of osteopathic medicine.

The gold standard of clinical research today is the randomized controlled trial, whereby the treatment of interest is compared to placebo or standard of care in a randomized, blinded fashion. Although there have been studies comparing osteopathic medicine to conservative treatment for spinal pain, it has not been compared to placebo or "sham" manipulation for obvious technical challenges. Moreover, the act of "laying hands" on a patient, even if during a sham manipulation and not as part of a formalized osteopathic treatment paradigm, may have a significant placebo effect, which cannot necessarily be distinguished from the effect of osteopathic manipulation in a small clinical trial.

Osteopathic manipulative medicine is an art as well as a science. There is not "one classic" osteopathic treatment that can be standardized and examined individually or independently from the others. The practice of OMM includes a number of different treatment options, which vary depending on the style, preference, and clinical acumen and experience of the practitioner. It is as much a philosophy of looking at the human body in terms of interrelated parts, as it is a practical application of this vantage.

Performing research on the subject of osteopathic medicine is challenging from a logistical perspective because many of the studies relevant to the subject do not come up on standard medical search engine databases such as PUBMED or MEDLINE. Many of these studies can only be found on complementary and alternative medicine websites, such as MANTIS (Manual Alternative and Natural Therapy Index System), CINAHL (Cumulative Index to Nursing and Allied Health Literature), or the Osteopathic Database. For example, Murphy et al. looked at the yield of Pub Med MEDLINE for complementary and alternative medicine (CAM) studies compared to other databases in an effort to formulate an effective search strategy to answer a sample research question on spinal palpation. They showed that commonly used databases do not provide accurate indexing or coverage of CAM publications and that subject-specific databases were more useful. They also identified that access, cost, and ease of using specialized databases were limiting factors (28).

Another difficulty with the literature is that often the duration of pain in the study population is not made clear (29). Some authors have defined the acute period from 1 to 14 days after onset, while others have described it as acute episodes of "less than 10 weeks duration". Skouen et al suggested the following time frames for spinal pain: acute (< 28 days duration), sub acute (4–12 week's duration), and chronic (> 12 weeks duration). A randomized controlled study, in addition to describing a standardized treatment protocol, should clearly define the duration of spinal pain in its study group (30).

10.2. Clinical Research

Despite these caveats, from the 1950s to latter 1990s, many studies were published pertaining to spinal manipulation. The vast majority of these were from the chiropractic perspective. The bulk of these studies suffered from multiple methodological weaknesses, including but not limited to small sample sizes, poor standardization of treatments, lack of long-term follow-up, and heterogeneous patient populations with widely different types of back pain, inconsistent definitions of disease acuity, and statistical Type 1 and Type 2 errors. Because of the inherent difficulties in deciphering these suboptimal data, several scientists attempted independent reviews of the available literature, the first of which was Koes et al, who performed a blinded review in 1991

(31). Their MEDLINE review from 1966 to 1990 produced 35 RCTs comparing spinal manipulation to other treatments. They scored each study on 17 items including study population, interventions, measurement of effect, and data presentation and analysis. With a maximum score of 100, no trial had more than 56 points, reflecting the perceived quality of the available literature. Overall, 56% of the studies showed positive results. The authors concluded that although the results were promising, more trials were needed with more attention paid to methodological consistency. They also postulated that the results might indicate that manipulation might be effective only in certain subgroups of patients with back and neck pain *(31)*.

Shekelle et al performed a second review at RAND/UCLA. They searched Index Medicus and MEDLINE from 1952 to 1992 and found 25 controlled trials examining the efficacy of spinal manipulation for low back pain. Using the same scoring system as Koes et at, each study was given a score from 1 to 100. Despite consideration of 23 of the same trials, the reviewers came up with different results in eighteen of them. They concluded that although spinal manipulation is of short-term benefit for some patients with uncomplicated acute low back pain, insufficient data are available concerning the efficacy of spinal manipulation for chronic low back pain *(32)*.

Finally, Anderson et al then reviewed many of these same studies by applying their own analytical approach *(33)*. They reviewed articles on Index Medicus with a supplement from the Chiropractic Research Archives Collection from 1980 to 1989. They scored studies with emphasis on randomization, blinding of patients and evaluators, description of interventions and quality of intervention controls, good description of treatment, and outcome measures. Scores ranged from 9 – 73 out of a total possible of 135. Interestingly, their three highest scores were not among the high scores given by Koes et al or Shekelle et al. These differences among these three reviews of the same or similar lot of trials revealed the significant variability in interpretation possible with literature review and emphasized the difficulty in generalizing conclusions from the myriad of studies published during the period of consideration that were heterogeneous in size, design, and quality of performance.

Since these reviews, many trials have been conducted several other groups. Bronfort et al looked at the relative efficacy of spinal manipulation combined with trunk exercise or NSAID therapy combined with trunk exercise for chronic low back pain. They concluded that all three therapeutic regimens were associated with similar and clinically significant improvement over time, which was considered superior to the expected natural history of chronic low back pain *(34)*. McMorland and Suter concluded that spinal manipulation was beneficial for the treatment of cervical and lumbar pain, despite the fact that their study design did not account for the natural history of such pain *(35)*. Hurwitz et al looked at the literature to assess the evidence for the efficacy of cervical manipulation for neck pain and headache. They concluded that cervical spine manipulation and mobilization probably provide at least short-term benefits for some patients with neck pain and headaches and compared favorably to medical care in terms of long-term low back and disability outcomes with greater improvement and satisfaction in those patients in those patients treated by chiropractic vs. family physicians *(36)*. Stig et al looked at a group of chiropractic patients with long lasting or recurrent low back pain and found that they improved early in the course of treatment *(37)*. Meade et al looked at what happens in day-to-day practice of patients treated by chiropractors vs. hospital therapists and found that patients in the former group derived more benefit and long-term satisfaction than the latter *(38)*. Ernst and Pittler found that expert opinion preferred the efficacy of the osteopathic and chiropractic approach for patients with uncomplicated low back pain *(39)*. Finally, Giles and Muller concluded that spinal manipulation, if not contraindicated, resulted in greater improvement than acupuncture or medicine, despite the shortcomings disclosed in the study *(40)*.

In terms of specific osteopathically oriented research, there have been two pivotal studies in the last decade, which should be mentioned. Andersson et al performed a randomized, controlled trial that involved patients who had back pain for at least 3 weeks but less than six months. The patients were randomized into a standard care MD group (72 patients), or a DO manipulation specialty group (83 patients). A variety of outcome measures were used including the Roland–Morris and Oswestry questionnaires, a visual-analogue pain scale, as well as objective measurements of range of motion and straight leg raise over a twelve-week study period. Over the course of the study, patients in both groups improved. There was no statistically significant difference between the two groups in any of the primary outcome measures. The osteopathic treatment group, however, did require fewer PT visits and significantly less medication, including analgesics, anti-inflammatory agents, and muscle relaxants *(41)*.

In another important trial, Williams et al looked at effectiveness and health care costs of a practice-based osteopathy clinic for subacute spinal pain. The study included a total of 201 patients with neck or back pain of 2–12 weeks duration, which were allocated at random between usual care given by a general practitioner and an additional three treatment sessions of osteopathic spinal manipulation. The primary outcome measure was the Extended Aberdeen Spine Pain Scale (EASPS). Secondary measures included SF-12, EuroQol, and Short-form McGill Pain Questionnaire. Health care costs were estimated from the records of referring general practitioners (GPs). Results of the study revealed that more patients improved who received the additional osteopathic treatment. At two months, this improvement was significantly greater in EASPS, but at six months, this difference was no longer significant for EASPS, but remained significant for SF-12 mental score. Mean health care costs attributed to spinal pain were significantly greater in the osteopathy group. Conclusions drawn were that a primary care osteopathy clinic improved short-term physical and longer psychological outcomes, with reasonable extra cost *(42)*.

10.3. The Future of Spinal Manipulation Research

Given the growing popularity of complementary and alternative therapeutic options, including osteopathic and spinal manipulative medicine, as well as the increasingly knowledgeable and demanding patient population seeking such services, several research forums were developed to wade through and decipher the growing amount of literature and its discordant findings. From 1975 until 2001, the National Institutes of Health sponsored the first of a series of eight international interdisciplinary conferences inquiring into the scientific basis of spinal manipulative treatment in America. Their goals included determining the state of research, identifying future areas of study, and examining various models and mechanisms to explain how manual medicine worked. Among the many conclusions drawn from these meetings was that despite their methodological flaws, the myriad of trials available during the period of consideration adequately demonstrated the efficacy for the use of manipulative medicine when dealing with acute and acute recurrent mechanical low back pain, but none of the trials adequately dealt with chronic low back pain. This eventually led to the inclusion of spinal manipulative treatment in the Agency for Health Care Policy and Research (now

AHQR – Agency for Healthcare Quality and Research) Guidelines for the Management of Acute Low Back Pain, which was published in 1994 *(43)*. Numerous studies then began to further evaluate efficacy, safety, and clinical relevance of manipulation, with the majority being on the topic of acute or chronic low back pain. This was followed by clinical practice guidelines for the use of manual techniques in cases of mechanical neck disorders *(44)*. From these later position papers, it was concluded that moderate but conflicting evidence existed to support spinal manipulation in cases of chronic non-specific or mechanical low back pain for short-term relief of symptoms to enable increased activity levels and less reliance on medications. Finally, recommendations from the National Guideline Clearinghouse were established for disorders of the neck and upper back, as well as for acute low back pain. In the neck and upper back, manual therapy was recommended on the second visit at between 1 and 4 weeks follow up if at least 50% disability remains and if no neurological findings exist. Chiropractic manipulation, not osteopathic, was specifically contraindicated in patients with a risk of stroke *(45)*. In terms of the low back, manual therapy was recommended at follow up visits 1-3 weeks after initial evaluation if indicated, but only if pre-manipulative testing peripheralized symptoms and only if used to progress an individual toward independence in exercise and self-care for a total of 4 – 6 visits. They considered the prescription of high-grade mobilization/manipulation to have Grade 1 or the strongest clinical evidence, if followed by appropriate active rehabilitation *(46)*.

Subsequently, several systematic Cochrane reviews were issued, with the latest amendments made in 2004. With respect to mechanical neck disorders (MNDs), 33 trials were reviewed to assess whether manipulation and mobilization (osteopathic treatment is not mentioned), either alone or in combination with other treatments, relieve pain or improve functional disability, patient satisfaction, and global perceived effect. They concluded that: "Multimodal care has short-term and long-term maintained benefits for sub-acute/chronic MNDs with or without headache. The common elements in this care strategy were mobilization and/or manipulation plus exercise." The evidence did not favor manipulation or mobilization alone or in combination with various other physical medicine modalities, nor when compared to each other *(47)*.

The Cochrane Review also amended spinal manipulative therapy for low-back pain in 2004. The objectives were to review randomized controlled trials that evaluated spinal manipulative therapy for patients with low back pain, with at least one day of follow up, and at least one clinically relevant outcome measure to resolve the discrepancies related to its use. Additionally, they sought to update previous estimates of effectiveness, by comparing spinal manipulative therapy to other therapies and incorporating data from recent high quality RCTs into the analysis. After reviewing 39 RCTs, the authors concluded that there was no evidence that spinal manipulative therapy was superior to other standard treatments for patients with acute or chronic low back pain *(48)*. There is no mention of osteopathic medicine in the review.

In all, the state of research in osteopathic and spinal manipulative medicine is growing. Without a doubt, it has progressed from simple case reports and anecdotal "truths" to a more scientifically based collection of studies. However, more research is needed with larger sample sizes, improved standardization of treatments, long-term follow-up, homogeneous patient populations with comparable types of back pain, consistent definitions of disease acuity, and optimized methodological study design.

11. RESOURCES

11.1. Books

Foundations for Osteopathic Medicine by Robert C. Ward (Editor), et al. 2nd Edition. Published: Philadelphia, Lippincott Williams & Wilkins, 2003. (The official textbook for the osteopathic profession. Contains information on how osteopathic theory and methods are incorporated in every aspect of medicine).

Principles of Manual Medicine by Philip E. Greenman. 3rd Edition Published: Philadelphia, Lippincott Williams & Wilkins, 2003.

An Osteopathic Approach to Diagnosis and Treatment by Eileen L. Digiovanna, Stanley Schiowitz. 2nd Edition. Published: Philadelphia, Lippincott- Raven, 1997. (A text that organizes currently taught concepts and techniques which serves as a reference for osteopathic medical students).

11.2. Website

The Philadelphia College of Osteopathic Medicine (PCOM) has an excellent website with multiple resources and numerous links to Osteopathic Professional Organizations and Training Resources.: http://www.pcom.edu/Library/Internet_Guides/IG_osteopathic_resources/osteopathic_resource.html.

12. CONCLUSION

Optimized care in the chronic pain field is always a goal. The early integration of Osteopathic Manipulative Medicine into the overall care plan has been demonstrated to improve outcomes and facilitate a multidisciplinary treatment approach. Typically, patients presenting to a tertiary care pain program have had initial evaluation with a primary care provider, neurologist, or orthopedist and treatment that may include medications, physical therapy, and/or exercise. Reassessment may be made by a pain physician or by multiple members of a team including physical therapy, occupational therapy, psychology or psychiatry. It is common that patients presenting to specialty programs have failed one or more treatment modalities. Many patients self-refer to Chiropractic, acupuncture, massage or other bodywork, or exercise programs with limited or temporal benefit only. In our experience, when well-qualified practitioners are consulted in a serial manner without integration of treatment, outcomes are often suboptimal.

Bringing multiple skills together often improves pain related outcomes. Especially if refinements in diagnosis can identify components of the patients problem not previously resolved. Osteopathic training includes more subtle assessment of joint and somatic function that may be related to prior injury, degenerative disease, or fibrosis. Additionally, direct manipulation or mobilization when inflammation or significant protective splinting is present in a patient may be aggravating. Employing gentle indirect osteopathic treatment has facilitated improved function, decreased pain, and facilitated the patient's ability to complete PT, OT, and other rehabilitation modalities *(49)*.

REFERENCES

1. Dorland. Dorland's Medical Dictionary, 30th edition.
2. Denslow JS. Soft tissues in areas of osteopathic lesion. 1947. J Am Osteopath Assoc 2001;101(7):P406–409.

3. Willard F. 2003. Nociception, the neuroendocrine immune system, and osteopathic medicine. In: Foundation for Osteopathic Medicine, 2nd edition. Ward RC, Executive Ed. Philadelphia, PA: Lippincott, Williams & Wilkins, pp 137–156.

4. Van Buskirk RL. Nociceptive reflexes and the somatic dysfunction: a model. JAOA 1990;90:792–794.

5. Kuchera ML, DiGiovanna EL, Greenman PE. Efficacy and complications. In: Foundations for Osteopathic Medicine. Ward RC, Ed. Baltimore, MD: Williams & Wilkins. 2002: 1143–1152.

6. Dvorak J, Orelli FV. How dangerous is manipulation to the cervical spine? Case report and results of a survey. Man Med 1985;2:1–4.

7. Patijin J. Complications of manual medicine: a review of the literature. Man Med 1991;6:89–92

8. Koss RW. Quality assurance monitoring of osteopathic manipulative treatment. JAOA. 1990;90(5):427–434.

9. Kleynhans AM. 1980. Complications of and contraindications to spinal manipulative therapy. In: Modern Developments in the Principles and Practice of Chiropractic. Haldeman S, Ed. New York, NY: Appleton-Century-Crofts, pp 359–384.

10. Oliphant, D. Safety of spinal manipulation in the treatment of lumbar disk herniations: a systematic review and risk assessment. J Manipulative Physiol Ther 2004;27:197–210.

11. Vick DA, McKay C, Zengerle CR. The safety of manipulative treatment: review of the literature from 1925 to 1993. JAOA 1996;96:113–115.

12. Basmajian JV. 1983. Grant's Method of Anatomy, 8th editon. Baltimore, MD: Williams & Wilkins.

13. Anonymous. 1993. Contraindications and complications. In Guidelines for Chiropractic Quality Assurance and Practice Parameters—Proceedings of the Mercy Center Consensus Conference. Haldeman S, Chapman-Smith D, Petersen DM, Eds. Gaithersburg, MD: Aspen, pp 159–77.

14. Curtis P, Bove G. Family physicians, chiropractors, and back pain. J Fam Pract 1992;35:551–555.

15. Shekelle PG, Adams AH, Chassin MR, et al. 1991. The appropriateness of spinal manipulation for low back pain-indications and ratings by a multidisciplinary expert panel. Santa Monica, Calif: Rand.

16. Fitzgerald M, Stiles E. 1984. Osteopathic hospitals' solution to DRG's may be OMT. The DO. November, pp 97–101.

17. Klock BG. The impact of osteopathic manipulative medicine on inpatient outcomes. AAO J 2002; 33–38.

18. Cantieri MS. Inpatient osteopathic manipulative treatment: impact on length of stay. Available at http://www.ohhpf.org/research96.html.

19. Kuchera ML, Kuchera WA. 1994. Osteopathic Considerations in Systemic Dysfunction. Second edition.

20. Kenneth G. 2003. Osteopathic Manipulative Medicine Guidelines for the Hospitalized Patient. Third edition.

21. Haldeman KO, Soto-Hall R. The diagnosis and treatment of sacroiliac conditions by the injection of procaine (Novocain). J Bone Joint Surg Am 1938;20-A:675–685

22. Bloomberg S, et al. Manual therapy with steroid injections: a new approach to treatment of low back pain. Spine 1994;19:569–577.

23. Ben-David B, Raboy M. Manipulation under joint anesthesia combined with epidural steroid injection. L Manipulative Physiol Ther 1994;17:605–609.

24. Geraci M, Alleva J. 1996. Prather H. Manipulation Under Anesthesia. Physical Medicine and Rehabilitation Clinics of North America. Philadelphia: WB Saunders, pp 897–913.

25. Nelson L, Aspegren D, Bova C. The use of epidural steroid injection and manipulation on patient with chronic low back pain. J Manipulative Phyiol Ther 1997;20:263–266.

26. Aspegren D, Wright R, Hemler D. Manipulation under epidural anesthesia with corticosteroid injection: two case reports. J. Manipulative Physiol Ther 1997:20:263–266.

27. Michaelson MR. Manipulation under joint anesthesia/analgesia: a proposed interdisciplinary treatment approach for recalcitrant spinal axis pain of synovial joint origin. J Manipulative Physiol Ther 2000:23;2:127–129.

28. Murphy LS, et al. Spinal palpation: the challenges of information retrieval using available databases. J Manipulative Phsiol Ther 2003;26:374–382.

29. Waddell G, Feder GM, McIntosh A, et al. 1996. Low Back Pain Evidence Review. London: Royal College of General Practitioners.

30. Giles LF, Muller R. A randomized clinical trial comparing medication, acupuncture, and spinal manipulation. Spine 2003;28(14):1490–1503.

31. Koes BW, Assendelft WJJ, van der Heijden MG, et al. Spinal manipulation and mobilization for back and neck pain: a blinded review. Br Med J 1991;303:1298–1303.

32. Shekelle PG, Adams AH, Chassin MR, et al. Spinal manipulation for low back pain. Ann Intern Med 1992;117:590–598.
33. Anderson R, Meeker WC, Wirick BE, et al. A meta-analysis of clinical trials of spinal manipulation. J Manipulative Physiol Ther 1992;15:181–194.
34. Bronfort G, Goldsmith CH, Nelson CF, et al. Trunk exercise combined with spinal manipulation or NSAID therapy for chronic low back pain: a randomized, observer-blinded clinical trial. J Manipulative Physiol Ther 1996;19:570–582.
35. McMorland G, Suter E. Chiropractic management of mechanical neck and low back pain: a retrospective, outcome-based analysis. J Manipulative Physiol Ther 2000;23:307–311.
36. Hurwitz EL, Aker PD, Adams AH, et al. Manipulation and mobilization of the cervical spine: a systematic review of the literature. Spine 1996;21:1746–1759.
37. Stig L-C, Nilsson O, Leboeuf-Yde C. Recovery pattern of patients treated with chiropractic spinal manipulative therapy for long lasting or recurrent low back pain. J Manipulative Phsyiol Ther 2001;24:288–291.
38. Meade TW, Dyer S, Browne W, et al. Low back pain of mechanical origin: randomized comparison of chiropractic and hospital outpatient treatment. Br Med J 1990;300:1431–1437.
39. Ernst E, Pittler H. Expert's opinions on complementary/alternative therapies for low back pain. L Manipulative Physiol Ther 1999;22:87–90.
40. Giles LGF, Muller R. Chronic spinal pain syndromes: a randomized clinical trail comparing medication, acupuncture, and spinal manipulation. Spine 28(14):1490–1503.
41. Andersson GBJ, Lucente T, Davis AM, et al. A comparison of osteopathic spinal manipulation with standard of care for patients with low back pain. N Engl J Med 1999;341:1426–1431.
42. Williams NH, Wilkinson C, Russell I, et al. Randomized osteopathic manipulation study (ROMANS): pragmatic trial for spinal pain in primary care. Fam Pract 2003;20:662–669.
43. Bigos SJ, bowyer OR, Braen GR, et al. 1994. Acute low back pain problems in adults. Clin Pract Guideline No. 14. AHCPR Publication No. 95–0642. Rockville, MD: Agency for Health Care Policy & Research.
44. Gross A. R. et al. Clinical practice guidelines for the use of manipulation or mobilization in the treatment of adults with mechanical neck disorders. Manual Ther 2002;7:193–205.
45. Work Loss Data Institute. 2003. Disorders of the Neck and Upper Back. Corpus Christi (TX): Work Loss Data Institute, p 109.
46. Institute for Clinical Systems Improvement (ICSI). 2002. Adult Low Back Pain. Bloomington (MN): Institute for Clinical Systems Improvement (ICSI), p 61.
47. Gross AR, Hoving JL, Haines TA, Goldsmith CH, Kay T, Aker P, Bronfort G. 2004. Manipulation and mobilisation for mechanical neck disorders (Cochrane Review). In The Cochrane Library, Issue 2, UK: John Wiley & Sons, Ltd.
48. Assendelft WJJ, Morton SC, Yu EI, Suttorp, MJ, Shekelle PG. 2004. Spinal manipulative therapy for low back pain (Cochrane review). In The Cochrane Library, Issue 2, UK: John Wiley & Sons Ltd.
49. Gronemeyer J, Audette J, Drexler J, Hough J. Retrospective outcome analysis of osteopathic manipulation in a treatment failure setting. JAOA 2006;106(*).

16 Chiropractic Pain Management

An Integrative Approach

Norman W. Kettner

CONTENTS

Summary

Chiropractic management of spinal pain is increasingly utilized as an alternative or complement to pharmaceutical treatment. This chapter presents the role of chiropractic management, particularly spinal manipulative therapy in the treatment of spinal pain. The chapter presents an overview of the the historical roots of chiropractic education and practice, and contrasts them with contemporary education, practice, and the evolution of modern chiropractic research. The role of joint dysfunction as a pain generator is reviewed. The mechanisms underlying spinal manipulative therapy (SMT) are presented in the context of biomechanical and neurophysiological models as well as mind–body integration. The clinical setting for the delivery of chiropractic care in pain management is outlined. Clinical indications and contraindications for SMT are presented. The effectiveness and safety of SMT are reviewed. Research horizons are suggested which target questions ranging from the basic sciences, such as the biological mechanisms underlying joint dysfunction and SMT, to clinical sciences and the possible role of SMT in rehabilitation and post-operative care.

Key Words: chiropractic, pain management, joint dysfunction, vertebral subluxation, spinal pain, CAM, biomechanics, joint neurophysiology, spinal manipulative therapy, adjustment.

1. DEFINITION AND BACKGROUND

The chiropractic profession has, since its inception in 1895, provided healthcare utilizing the integrative relationship between the musculoskeletal and nervous system. In addition, a foundation principle of clinical practice has been an emphasis on the whole person and the innate capacity for self-healing. Another tenet of the chiropractic profession has been the identification of a dysfunctional state of the neuromusculoskeletal system, described with various terms including subluxation, segmental joint dysfunction, or functional spinal lesion *(1)*. Contemporary chiropractic care

From: *Contemporary Pain Medicine: Integrative Pain Medicine: The Science and Practice of Complementary and Alternative Medicine in Pain Management*
Edited by: J. F. Audette and A. Bailey © Humana Press, Totowa, NJ

utilizes a number of conservative healthcare treatment techniques in addition to manual therapy (manipulation, mobilization and massage). These may include physiotherapeutic modalities such as ultrasound and electrostimulation, acupuncture, dietary counseling, rehabilitation, exercise, activity modification, and health promotion. The Association of Chiropractic Colleges in a position paper in 1996, defined the practice of chiropractic as the focus on the relationship between structure (primarily the spine) and function (as coordinated by the nervous system) and how that relationship affects the preservation and restoration of health. In addition, it advocated doctors of chiropractic working in cooperation with other healthcare practitioners when in the best interest of the patient (2) (Figure 1).

Pain management is an emerging chiropractic specialty, with a potential to contribute to the broader field of pain medicine. The objective of this chapter is to present an overview of the history, theory, and practice of the most widely utilized chiropractic intervention, spinal manipulative therapy (SMT). The scope of this chapter is not to present an overview of chiropractic patient management; its emphasis is narrowly directed towards the use of SMT in pain management. As way of an introduction to the chiropractic profession, a brief historical perspective is presented, highlighting the tumultuous cultural, political, legal, and educational origins of the profession. The definitions and mechanisms of segmental joint dysfunction will be reviewed; biomechanical and neurophysiological models of SMT are then addressed. The clinical setting for the delivery of SMT in chiropractic pain management will be surveyed along with data on its efficacy and safety. Lastly, selected basic and clinical science questions will be highlighted with the hope of stimulating further research into the biological and clinical mechanisms underlying SMT.

Chiropractic Scope of Practice (ACC)

Diagnosis

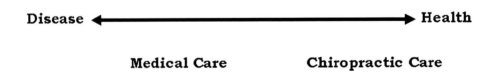

Disease ⟷ Health

Medical Care   Chiropractic Care

Collaborative Care

Palliation Advanced Sign Symptom Dysfunction Subluxation Health
            Disease   Promotion

Management

Fig. 1. Chiropractic scope of practice (ACC).

   It is useful to understand the historical context in which the founder of the chiropractic profession, Daniel David Palmer, established the principles of chiropractic
theory and practice *(3)*. The late 19th century was a period of enormous cultural,
political and scientific upheaval in the United States. The practice of orthodox medicine
at this time was poorly regulated and its clinical outcomes were often dominated by
iatrogenesis. The roots of today's alternative healthcare movement were undergoing
formation as a variety of healing methods, ranging from magnetic healing, bonesetting,
homeopathy, herbalism, and osteopathy were emerging as healing techniques. Trained
medical providers were a scarcity; in addition, family members often viewed health as
an individual responsibility and provided most of the day-to-day family healthcare.

   DD Palmer, a self-educated man, with a strong interest in vitalism, metaphysics, as
well as biology, began practicing Franz Anton Mesmer's magnetic healing technique in
the late 1880s *(4)*. By 1895, Palmer had incorporated a role for vertebral displacement
in his theory of disease and began utilizing manual thrusts along with the manual passes
of magnetic therapy. Palmer utilized the term *subluxation* to describe the vertebral
anatomic displacements that caused nerve interference and inflammation. Unfortunately, the term *subluxation* was already in clinical use to describe severely deranged
articulations, not the subtle version Palmer envisioned. This unfortunate selection of
such a critical definition has led to generations of bitter confusion, controversy, and
rejection by other medical disciplines. The term *chiropractic* was soon coined, taken
from the Greek *cheiros* and *praktikos* meaning "done by hand." In 1896, the Palmer
School of Chiropractic opened, and one of its first graduates, was B.J. Palmer, the son
of D.D. Palmer. It was B.J. Palmer who would be considered the early champion and
developer of the chiropractic profession.

   In the early 20th century, numerous proprietary chiropractic teaching institutions
were established in the United States. Without regulatory agencies or accrediting
bodies, chiropractic curricular offerings and teaching facilities were meager and training
typically limited to 18 months. Underwritten by federal vocational funding for World
War I veterans, for a short period, there was a sudden increase in the numbers of
chiropractors being graduated in the United States. This growing supply of practitioners faced the dilemma of a limited number of states with chiropractic licensure.
Without state licensure, many thousands of chiropractors were jailed for practicing
medicine and osteopathy. Chiropractors frequently offered as legal defense, an alternative medical language, even embracing vitalistic and religious views. Chiropractors
performed "analysis" not diagnosis, it was an "adjustment" not a manipulation, and
it was the innate intelligence of the body that cured, not the doctor. In one legal
case, chiropractic was distinguished from osteopathy by its "supremacy of the nervous
system" in contrast to osteopathy, which proclaimed the "supremacy of the artery."
Such legal woes began to diminish as the first state chiropractic license was granted in
1915; however, the last was not provided until 1974 *(4)*. Today there are about 70,000
chiropractic physicians licensed in the US.

   By the 1930s, educational reforms were being advanced by the National Chiropractic
Association, the forerunner of today's American Chiropractic Association. The establishment of higher standards, such as non-profit colleges with a 4-year curriculum and
the offerings of basic and clinical science training, touched off a divisive battle with
the International Chiropractors Association, organized by followers of B.J. Palmer.
Division over such issues as the extent of diagnostic responsibility, the role of vertebral
subluxation in disease pathogenesis, and even the chiropractic scope of practice has

continued to beleaguer even modern-day chiropractors (5–7). In 1962, the National Board of Chiropractic Examiners was formed to administer basic and clinical science exams for chiropractors. The Council on Chiropractic Education (CCE) was eventually established in 1971 and recognized by the US Office of Education in 1974. The CCE today serves as the accrediting body for the 18 teaching institutions in the US.

Today, the goals of chiropractic education and licensure are to produce a portal of entry healthcare practitioner who is competent in the specific principles and practice of chiropractic and who is able to work both independently and on a healthcare team with other professionals. Chiropractors are trained to assess clinically the health status in every physiological system, perform a differential diagnosis, screen patients requiring medical or other care, as well as perform a precise neuromusculoskeletal diagnosis as a basis for the delivery of chiropractic care.

Marginalized for much of the 20th century, the chiropractic profession has continuously elevated the standards of its educational system, and within the last 30 years, undertaken the development of a research infrastructure to propel its practice into the contemporary healthcare mainstream (8). This new role for scientific research, and in particular, the use of the randomized controlled trial (RCT), is a recent development in the field of chiropractic and in complementary and alternative medicine (CAM) in general. There are inherent difficulties, however, in employing the RCT, with its reliance on population-based studies. Many CAM providers have unique models of illness and healing that recognize disease only within the context of the individual. Procedural techniques such as manual therapy or acupuncture are nearly impossible to double blind as is readily performed in RCTs using medication. In addition, many CAM therapies recognize and practice the use of vitalistic and often non- quantifiable, (even though perceptible), disease models. This perspective challenges study within the framework of the RCT (9).

The earliest organized effort to evaluate spinal manipulative therapy (SMT) scientifically was convened in 1975 by the National Institute of Neurologic and Communicative Diseases and Stroke (NINCDS). It assembled chiropractors, osteopaths, manual therapists, and researchers, who presented the state of knowledge concerning SMT. Much of the evidence presented was theoretical, anecdotal, and observational. Although it concluded that claims of the value of SMT were unsubstantiated, continued research was encouraged. This NIH conference was considered a watershed event in the history of the chiropractic profession, as it catalyzed political, educational, and scientific efforts toward the development of a discipline devoted to chiropractic research. Two avenues of research were initiated, basic mechanisms of SMT and clinical outcome studies, including RCTs. In 1993, the Office of Alternative Medicine (OAM) was established within the NIH. This was a landmark development in CAM research as it provided the opportunity for federally funded research across most CAM techniques.

The NIH's National Center for Complementary and Alternative Medicine (NCCAM) the successor to the OAM and the Canadian Institutes of Health Research (CIHR) recently convened a historic second conference titled the "Conference on the Biology of Manual Therapies." It focused on the biological mechanisms underlying SMT including research findings in the fields of neuroscience, biomechanics, immunology, endocrinology and imaging (10). The 2005 conference proceedings resulted in recommendations for new funding initiatives by NCCAM and the CIHR to study the biology of manual therapies. Today more than 73 RCTs of spinal manipulative therapy have been reported in the English language, most of them evaluating spinal pain syndromes *(11)*. Scientific evaluation of chiropractic principles and practice will continue to shape and refine the profession in the future. Today, there is a growing level of professional prominence and the influence of the chiropractic profession on healthcare is increasingly visible *(12)*. In the United States, chiropractic institutions have been awarded federal funds for scientific investigations. Although still relatively limited, the scholarly output of the chiropractic profession is emerging and this work can be found both within chiropractic and non-chiropractic periodicals. The chiropractic profession is still evolving its cultural authority with respect to its clinical domain of healthcare. It is still unclear whether chiropractors practice as a spine specialty or as primary care or both, and this topic is the subject of ongoing debate *(13)*. As scientific evidence continues to support the safety and cost-effectiveness of spinal manipulation and other CAM approaches, it is likely that more chiropractic physicians will become a part of multidisciplinary or integrative medicine practices to the ultimate benefit of their patients.

2. MODELS OF SPINAL MANIPULATIVE THERAPY

Spinal manipulative therapy is one of the most frequently utilized forms of complementary and alternative medicine *(14)*. Several clinical disciplines employ SMT with the majority in the US delivered by chiropractors *(15)*. SMT is a subtype of manual therapy, which also refers to the related techniques of joint mobilization and massage. In SMT, a manually controlled, localized, high-velocity low-amplitude thrust is directed at a clinically specified spinal segment variably termed segmental joint dysfunction, functional spinal lesion or subluxation *(1,16)*. The intent of the localized thrust is to reduce the underlying pathomechanical dysfunction (load distribution) in the articular and para-articular soft tissue structures related to the segmental joint dysfunction. Herzog reported the specific forces exerted onto patients during spinal manipulative therapy of the spinal column *(17)*.

It is important to remember that segmental dysfunction, as the term implies, is functional, not an anatomic designation. Clinically, segmental joint dysfunction is typically identified as a spinal segment demonstrating altered range of motion and increased local motor tone giving rise to altered alignment, inflammation and local, as well as referred pain *(3,11)*. Another intriguing model has been hypothesized which emphasizes the interaction between joint pathomechanics and muscle dysfunction. Murphy has suggested that segmental joint dysfunction triggers nociceptive input through the spinal cord interneuron connection with the gamma motor neuron *(18)*. This barrage of abnormal input is thought to alter the efferent activity of the gamma motor neuron that regulates muscle tone through the muscle spindle. Myofascial trigger points and eventually faulty movement patterns may be initiated. This model, like others, suggests that the altered segmental biomechanics (pathomechanics) are able to propagate maladaptive segmental as well as central neural responses resulting in abnormal pain and movement behaviors.

Segmental joint dysfunction may exist as primary or secondary findings in the genesis of spinal pain and is one of several models of that await scientific and clinical validation. Recent evidence, however, raises questions regarding the need or even the capacity to clinically localize the spinal joint targets of SMT. Joint mobilization observed under kinematic MRI displayed intervertebral movements throughout the lumbar spine following contact and posteroanterior impulses at a single vertebral segment *(19)*. This lack of segmental specificity was also reported in the cervical spine *(20)*. The accuracy of site-specific SMT delivery has always been assumed, but this too, has been challenged. In a recent study using a method of cavitation localization, about one-half of the SMT in the lumbar spine was accurately targeted (average miss of one segment), however, better accuracy was seen in the thoracic spine *(21)*.

The clinical benefit of SMT is likely expressed through several physiological systems including musculoskeletal, neurological, immunological and endocrine *(22)* (Table 1). An overview will be provided addressing the putative biomechanical and neurophysiological correlates of segmental joint dysfunction and its treatment with SMT.

Most cases of chronic spinal pain do not have identifiable pathology and are termed nonspecific *(23)*. This does not mean the patient is normal, but rather that there is a limited understanding of the cause of the pain syndrome. The original model of subluxation as expressed by Palmer emphasized vertebral misalignment resulting in neuroforaminal encroachment followed by nerve compression and neural dysfunction. Palmer named the latter entity nerve interference *(4)*. To date, Palmer's model has not been validated, as modern spinal imaging techniques such as MRI have not demonstrated misalignment induced nerve compression or dysfunction. Components of the Palmer model, which are valid, but not in the context of vertebral misalignment, are neural foraminal stenosis leading to nerve dysfunction. Stenosis and nerve root compression syndromes occur, for example, in the setting of degenerative disc disease including disc herniation and spondylosis, as well as zygapophyseal joint arthritis and spinal stenosis. These degenerative joint changes are limited to patients in middle age and beyond and would not explain the clinical benefit of SMT observed in younger patients. In an investigation of the effects of spinal mobility on joint degeneration, Cramer recently identified an intriguing relationship between spinal joint fixation (hypomobility) and time-dependent degenerative changes of the zygapophyseal joints in an animal model *(24)*. Degenerative changes in these joints are a source of acute and chronic spinal pain and can give rise to neural foraminal stenosis. These findings emphasize a dynamic link between functional joint changes (segmental joint dysfunction) and the potential complication of osseous neural foraminal stenosis, rather than the anatomic model of misalignment induced neural foraminal stenosis originally advanced by Palmer.

A robust biomechanical model of segmental joint dysfunction that may explain both the biomechanical and clinical responses to SMT is spinal segmental buckling *(1,25,26)*. In this model, injurious static or dynamic loading, results in a rapid uncontrolled, nonlinear displacement of a joint's instantaneous axis of rotation, but the displacement

Table 1
Potential Mechanisms Underlying SMT

Reduced spinal buckling (joint dysfunction/subluxation)
Proprioceptor-triggered pain gating
Beneficial neuroplastic modulation
Enhanced mind–body integration
Placebo enhancement
Sympathovagal modulation
Diffuse noxious inhibitory control activation
Released entrapped meniscus/disc fragment
Reflexive motoneuron inhibition

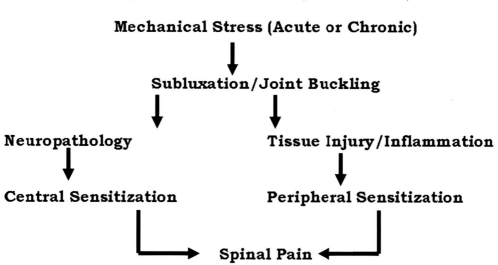

Spinal Pain and Joint Dysfunction (Triano)

Fig. 2. Spinal pain and joint dysfunction.

is maintained within the physiological range of motion. This shift in the axis of rotation results in stress load transfers into multiple local tissues of the functional spinal unit, ultimately provoking tissue injury and spinal pain (Figure 2). Segmental buckling may occur as a primary or secondary finding accompanying other spinal disorders. The predominant clinical expression of tissue injury will depend on the type of injured tissue. For example, if nerve root injury occurs, dermatomal radiation with hypoesthesia may follow, if a capsule ligament is damaged, facet joint symptoms may be detected. The resultant neurogenic and non-neurogenic inflammatory response may generate acute or in the worse case, following central sensitization, chronic pain. The use of SMT introduces force that reduces or eliminates buckling and stiffness in the functional spinal unit, increases the range of motion, and normalizes the distribution of forces in the target joint. In vitro studies of segmental and regional spinal functional units have verified the presence of buckling behavior *(25)*. Fluoroscopic imaging of a weightlifter revealed the presence of segmental buckling *(27)*. The buckling model of spinal segmental joint dysfunction is a promising and an important objective for future clinical research.

Another biomechanical mechanism of segmental joint dysfunction gaining scientific momentum is the study of abnormal spinal mobility. Recent studies have persistently verified the presence of abnormal (decreased or excessive) spinal mobility in patients with low back pain *(28–30)*. The neurophysiological consequence of joint hypomobility is poorly understood but investigation is evolving. Joint (limb) immobilization has been reported to reduce motor neuron firing, induce neuroplasticity and to trigger cortical reorganization related to the associated immobilized muscle *(31)*. Such findings are not generally appreciated outside of disciplines that use manual therapies and reinforce the need to continually validate clinical and biomechanical models of segmental joint dysfunction. An accurate clinical characterization of segmental joint dysfunction is important because of its impact on the outcomes of SMT. If a segmental lesion is incorrectly identified, the effects of SMT may be less than optimal. However, the sensitivity, specificity, and predictive value required of any diagnostic technique have not been established for segmental joint dysfunction.

Several other biomechanical models have been proposed to explain the effects of SMT. They include the release of trapped meniscoid fragments, repositioning of posterior discal fragments, and reduction of fibrosis-induced tissue stiffness. The interactive nature of spinal mechanical stability and related neurological function has evolved as an important model for studying spinal pain. Panjabi has advanced a biomechanical model of spinal pain that emphasizes the requirement of normal function in the active, passive and neural integration systems of the spine as a prerequisite for stability. The loss of spinal stability occurs when one of the components of the active (musculotendinous), passive (ligamentous), and neural integration (proprioceptors, nociceptors) becomes dysfunctional. This is necessarily followed by compensations of the other systems *(32,33)*. Such compensatory responses may trigger movement impairments such as pain avoidance or control impairments such as pain provocation. Chronic low back pain is usually mechanically induced and patients typically present with maladaptive primary physical and secondary cognitive-affective compensations that can become a mechanism for persistent pain. Patients may present then, with an excess or deficiency in spinal stability *(34)*.

In addition to biomechanical models, neurophysiological mechanisms are often used to explain the diverse clinical effects of SMT, including increased pain tolerance, reduced alpha-motor neuron activity, increased proprioceptive function, and autonomic modulation *(3,35)*. The neurophysiological mechanisms underlying SMT have yet to be clarified but are thought to include peripheral (local), and central (systemic) effects. The SMT activated proprioceptive afferents (groups I and II) serve as a reasonable model to invoke inhibitory pain gating in spinal and supraspinal circuitry *(36)*. Gating refers to the suppression of afferent information and is known to occur in the somatosensory system resulting from either inhibitory motor output or sensory afferent inputs, as afferents can gate one another *(37)*. Supraspinal pain gating mechanisms, triggered by SMT, could operate through the supraspinal pain neuromatrix and the descending inhibitory pathways, which are relayed from the forebrain to the brainstem. Such a gating mechanism could reduce noxious and possibly even innocuous subthreshold neural inputs arising from segmental joint dysfunction *(22)*. Supraspinal inhibition of the pain matrix is a reasonable hypothesis, given the reported clinical benefits of SMT in the treatment of chronic low back pain (CLBP) *(38)*. The unique interactions of biomechanical and neurophysiological factors associated with segmental joint dysfunction are emerging as an important focus of basic, clinical and neuroimaging research.

In addition to segmental joint dysfunction or subluxation, examples of spinal pain generators include disorders of musculotendinous, ligamentous, articular and neural structures. Eventually, if persistent, these initiating pain generators are surpassed in significance by genetic, electrophysiological, inflammatory, and neuroimmune responses. These factors somehow interact to increase the risk of persistent or chronic pain. Degenerative disc disease, disc herniation complicated by radiculopathy, facet syndrome, sprain, and strain and myofascial trigger points are frequent generators of spinal pain. Nociceptive activity arising from these disorders may be severe or involve neuropathic pain and, if persistent, maladaptive neuroplastic structural and functional changes occur in the central nervous system. This state leads to peripheral and central sensitization, enhanced neural excitability and, pathologic, rather than physiologic pain (39,40).

Chronic pain eventually may become independent of the degree of peripheral nociceptive activity arising from tissue inflammation and damage. Neuroplastic mechanisms such as central sensitization are eventually initiated, and maintained, playing a role more important than the activity of the specific nociceptive generator. Central pain processing is thus augmented, likely characterized by impaired inhibitory (or facilitatory) neural activity, with resultant hyperactive components of the pain neuromatrix (see Chapter 3).

Functional magnetic resonance imaging (fMRI), a brain mapping technique (see Chapter 4) has verified augmentation and hypersensitivity of elements in the pain matrix in complex regional pain syndrome, fibromyalgia, chronic low back pain and carpal tunnel syndrome (41–45).

The clinical benefits of SMT in chronic spinal pain syndromes suggest a neurophysiological mechanism interacting with pathways exhibiting pain neuroplasticity. One way to address this question is through the use of functional neuroimaging modalities such as fMRI, an imaging modality that monitors brain activation. The fMRI mapping of cortical and subcortical brain responses to SMT could illuminate the role of neuroplastic changes in the clinical response of CLBP. Following a course of SMT, hyperactivation in the pain matrix could hypothetically normalize, the result of improved inhibitory and facilitatory function in the descending pain system. This hypothesis is somewhat supported by preliminary fMRI research findings appropriated from another commonly utilized CAM technique, acupuncture. Manual and electroacupuncture were used in the treatment of chronically painful carpal tunnel syndrome (CTS) (46). Cortical processing using fMRI revealed maladaptive neuroplastic reorganization in median nerve finger somatotopy with abnormal (overlapping) somatotopic digit spacing in the sensorimotor cortex. Hyperactivated and increased extent of digit somatotopy was also seen in CTS patients compared to normal controls. Persistent and coherent afferent activity resulting from paresthesias and pain in CTS was the likely driver of the cortical maladaptive reorganization. Following a five-week course of acupuncture, there were improvements in clinical measures (including reduced neuropathic pain), reduced (improved) median nerve latencies, normalized sensorimotor cortical function (reduced hyperactivation) and improved median nerve digit somatotopy (46). The results of this study suggest a peripheral and central benefit was realized, utilizing a 5-week course of acupuncture treatment. This is an example of how conditioning sensory inputs may be employed to facilitate beneficial and adaptive neuroplastic restoration including restored neurological function and chronic pain reduction. Would a course of SMT trigger similar beneficial neuroplastic modulation in chronic low back pain (47)? This question defines another important research question waiting to be addressed. The underlying neurophysiological mechanisms of beneficial neuroplasticity are speculative but may include recruitment or uncovering of "latent" neural connections with the eventual development of dendrite and synaptic remodeling (48).

Both SMT and acupuncture treatments appear to share neurophysiological properties that are capable of benefiting chronic pain management. Both techniques are known to trigger similar populations of proprioceptive afferents (groups I and II) that can gate nociception in the dorsal horn (36). Either technique may activate the diffuse noxious inhibitory control system (DNIC) (49). This is an anti-nociceptive or analgesic pathway activated over a short time period and triggered by nociceptive conditioning stimuli. This mechanism then, uses a nociceptive input, to block pain in some other location. There are important and intriguing differences in the two techniques aside from the differences in the mechanism of sensory stimulation delivery. Acupuncture stimulation is delivered over a 20–30 minute period with intermittent periods of needle rotation and manipulation. SMT is delivered over a period of approximately 500 ms, a temporal difference of several orders of magnitude compared with acupuncture. Continued basic and clinical investigation of the biomechanical and neurophysiological mechanisms underlying SMT will benefit the understanding of other CAM interventions like acupuncture, massage and rehabilitation.

Another important aspect of SMT and CAM techniques in general, which must be emphasized, is the so-called mind/body interaction. The bi-directional linkage of the neuroendocrine and immune system is the scientific foundation of psychoneuroimmunology (50). The early observations in this field demonstrated that cognitive and affective states could modulate the immune system responses to infection and cancer. Pert described the molecular link between emotions and neurobiology (51). Mapping the neuropeptide receptors in the limbic system, endocrine glands and the immune system, she had discovered the "molecules of emotion". Her work led to the awareness of an ongoing biochemical interaction between the body and the mental state. Thus thoughts, attitudes, and emotions, form a critical neurological circuit with the autonomic nervous system. Pain is then felt, not only as a mental sensation, but also as physiological changes including increased pulse, blood pressure, respiration, muscle tone and even metabolic rate.

The perception of threat to one's well-being, no matter how ingenuine, triggers the hypothalamic-pituitary-adrenal (HPA) axis and initiates arousal of the sympathetic nervous system. Persistent HPA axis arousal, in the absence or failure of stress- coping strategies, plays a role in the pathogenesis of numerous disease states including chronic pain, hypertension, cardiac dysrrhythmia, insomnia, and viral respiratory infection (52–56). The use of SMT may activate parasympathetic responses potentially countering the presence of chronic sympathetic arousal (57,58). Can SMT reduce stress levels as a potential mechanism for improvement of the trauma or psychological stress? This answer awaits further investigation. Integrated with other "vagalizing" CAM techniques such as meditation, acupuncture, and aerobic exercise, it may be possible to reduce chronic sympathetic dominance.

Chiropractic patients consistently rate their care with high levels of satisfaction (59–61). Is it possible that chiropractic physicians empower their patients, foster an expectation of change and increase their locus of control? All of these variables are important psychosocial approaches serving to reduce anxiety and HPA axis arousal. Understanding the patient's physiological interactions in response to the nuances of the doctor-patient relationship (including placebo/nocebo) and other complex body-mind variables will serve as important scientific challenges in the advance of chiropractic research.

3. THE CLINICAL ENCOUNTER

Most patients consulting a chiropractic physician do so for a chief complaint of axial pain, especially the lumbar and cervical spine. Low back pain is a common cause of chronic pain with prevalence in North America of 6.8% (62). The etiology of chronic low back pain is initially at least multifactorial, and typically originating as mechanical injury. Risk factors are numerous and include variables of physical, psychosocial, occupational, and genetic origins. Although most cases of low back pain are considered to be nonspecific, chiropractic patients routinely undergo a history and general physical examination *(3)*. There is a clear intent of excluding underlying pathological sources of pain and dysfunction i.e. malignancy, which constitutes a contraindication to SMT and requires medical or surgical management. This clinical responsibility is required of any portal of entry provider and this aspect of diagnostic evaluation would resemble that of any other medical provider. In addition, it is important to establish the presence and level of a neurological deficit, if present; as such a finding may also constitute a sign of underlying an underlying pathological pain generator. Another major objective of the clinical encounter is the identification of a segmental joint dysfunction, the target of SMT. Segmental joint dysfunction may couple with remote spinal regions, as abnormal forces are transmitted through the articular linkage system of the pelvis and vertebral column. The finding of segmental joint dysfunction is thought to propagate adverse biomechanical and neurophysiological effects throughout the peripheral and central nervous system, which are eventually reduced or eliminated by SMT *(22)*.

The history, review of systems and general physical examination with emphasis on orthopedic and neurological examination provides a holistic assessment of the patient's functional capacity, disease risk and the presence of pathology. A manual physical examination of the chief complaint is then conducted with attention directed towards the involved articular mobility, including evidence for disc derangement (centralize/peripheralize pain), positive neural tension tests and a soft tissue evaluation for myofascial trigger points and abnormal muscle tone. Qualitative and quantitative clinical measures may be obtained depending on the clinician's preferences. For example, palpation for tenderness is qualitative (but reliable) algometry is quantitative. In addition, there are a variety of health outcome assessment tools that may be employed to gauge the level of disability in the spine as well as to monitor treatment response. Following the identification of the pain generator, a diagnosis and treatment plan is established. This includes prognosis and prevention care necessary to address comorbid conditions complicating the case. The clinical indications for SMT include many acute and chronic pain disorders involving the neuromusculoskeletal system (Table 2). Contraindications for SMT arise in conditions such as acute inflammatory

Table 2
Clinical Indications for SMT

Joint dysfunction/subluxation
Strain/sprain
Facet syndrome
Degenerative disc disease (herniation)
Costovertebral joint dysfunction
Osteoarthritis
Thoracic outlet syndrome
Temporomandibular joint dysfunction
Nonspecific spinal pain (acute or chronic)
Primary headache
Myofascial pain syndrome

Table 3
Contraindications for Local SMT

Os Odontoideum
Spinal Osteomyelitis
Abdominal Aortic Aneurysm
Malignant Vertebral Neoplasm
Acute Inflammatory Arthropathy
Acute Traumatic Joint Instability
Spinal Cord Neoplasm
Post- Traumatic Spinal Stenosis

arthropathy, neoplastic or acute traumatic instability (Table 3). Often, a trial of care is initiated as a diagnostic measure; if the patient's clinical response is not forthcoming, appropriate para-clinical testing is considered. Such testing may involve laboratory, neurophysiologic, i.e., EMG and diagnostic imaging *(3)*.

In general, the chiropractic clinical encounter emphasizes patient communication, high touch and low tech (Figure 3 photograph of SMT). This setting reinforces a strong doctor—patient relationship that in turn reinforces the psychosocial aspects of care. This is particularly important (and effective) in the management of chronic pain. Pain reduction is not the primary objective in the management of chronic pain; it is functional restoration and improved quality of life. This will require enlisting the patient's commitment to participate in rehabilitation activities. Patient participation in their own care reinforces the patient's role and responsibility in their management; it empowers them with confidence and fosters an expectation of change.

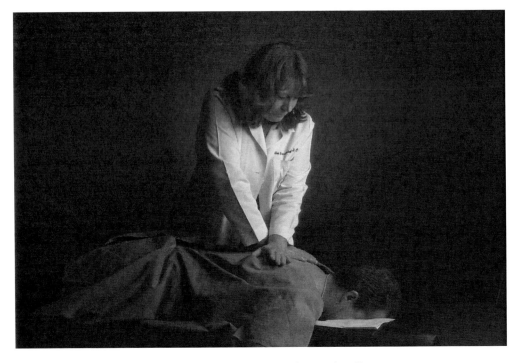

Fig. 3. The delivery of a high-velocity low-amplitude chiropractic adjustment.

4. IS SPINAL MANIPULATIVE THERAPY EFFECTIVE?

As mentioned earlier, there are more than 73 RCTs evaluating SMT, making it one of the most investigated treatments for spinal pain *(11)*. Members of the medical discipline have authored many of these trials and they were published in respected and authoritative journals. Most studies evaluated pain syndromes involving the low back, neck and headaches. The designs included controls that varied from placebo to comparisons with standard medical treatments. Meeker has reviewed a total of 43 RCTs using SMT for acute, subacute and chronic low back pain *(11)*. Thirty of these RCTs favored SMT over the comparison treatment in at least one patient subgroup. The remaining 13 reported no significant differences and none of the RCTs reported that SMT was less effective than the comparison treatment. Eight of the 11 placebo-controlled trials of low back pain favored the use of SMT. With respect to the evaluation of SMT in the treatment of cervical spine pain; the results of the RCTs were more equivocal. Eleven RCTs have been conducted, 4 with positive results and 7 which were equivocal. In the RCTs evaluating SMT for the headache treatment, 7 of the 9 RCTs for were positive. Systematic reviews and meta-analyses over the last 10 years have been somewhat positive concerning the effectiveness of SMT for low back, neck pain and headache, as methodological concerns were raised *(11)*. Recent systematic reviews have been contradictory and unable to clarify the role of SMT in spinal pain management *(63–69)*. The effect size in most of these studies was considered small but not insignificant when viewed in the light of the safety profile, availability, and cost-effectiveness of SMT.

In a more recent RCT, positive effects of SMT in spinal pain management were reported *(70)*. The assessment of short- and long-term effects of spinal manipulations on acute back pain and sciatica with disc protrusion were compared with active and simulated manipulations in 102 ambulatory patients. Inclusion required at least moderate pain on a visual analog scale for local and/or radiating pain. Outcome measures included pain-free patients at the end of treatment; treatment failure (proportion of patients stopping the assigned treatment); number of days with no, mild, moderate, or severe pain; quality of life; number of days on non-steroidal anti-inflammatory drugs; number of drug prescriptions; VAS 1(local) and VAS 2 (radiating) scores; quality of life and psychosocial findings; and reduction of disc protrusion on magnetic resonance imaging. Manipulations or simulated manipulations were done 5 days per week with a maximum of 20 treatments. Treatment was provided by experienced chiropractors.

Manipulations were more effective on the basis of the percentage of pain-free cases, number of days with pain and number of days with moderate or severe pain. Patients receiving manipulations had statistically lower mean VAS 1 and 2 scores. The authors concluded that active manipulations had more effect than simulated manipulations on pain relief for acute back pain and sciatica with disc protrusion.

5. SAFETY ISSUES AND SMT

The topic of complications arising from SMT has been a source of great controversy since the first report in 1925 *(71)*. Fortunately, most adverse responses are transient, resolving in 1–2 days, and are clinically benign. There is evidence that these responses are more common than previously recognized. Nearly a third of the patients undergoing cervical SMT in a recent RCT experienced adverse responses, with one-fourth describing increased pain or stiffness within 24 hours *(72)*. Similar short-lived and benign adverse responses consisting of headache and stiffness have been reported with upper cervical spine manipulation which was an independent predictor *(73)*. It is the more serious adverse responses to SMT that have been the greatest source of controversy. Adverse clinical events such as cauda equina syndrome and vertebral artery dissection have been difficult to evaluate, as these events are quite rare. This is especially true regarding vertebral artery dissection with subsequent cerebrovascular accident (CVA). This latter adverse event is so rarely seen that comprehensive scientific study has been difficult. None of the 73 previously mentioned RCTs or any case series reported a serious complication *(11)*. There are estimates drawn from retrospective case reports and unsubstantiated practitioner surveys for cervical SMT-induced CVA. They range from 1 in 400,000 to 3–6 per million *(74,75)*. In a Danish series, inclusive of 99% of chiropractors over a 10-year period, five cases of CVA and one death were identified *(76)*. This represented one serious complication per 1 million cervical manipulations. It is likely that vertebral artery dissections are the result of cumulative events which are non-manipulative i.e., (childbirth, overhead work, head rotation while driving, beautyparlor events) extending over a period of time rather than triggered by SMT alone *(77)*. In a retrospective review of 64 medical legal cases of CVA temporally associated with cervical SMT, it was concluded that CVA should be considered a random and unpredictable complication of any neck movement, including cervical manipulation *(78)*. The authors also concluded that evolving dissection is the likely cause of neck pain motivating the patient to seek care. Additionally, the CVA may occur at any point in the course of treatment and with any method of cervical manipulation. It must be emphasized there is risk inherent in all treatments, and that risk is relative, and although there is a slight risk of CVA following SMT, comparison with the risks of other care is important. For example, there are 225,000 deaths annually in the US resulting from iatrogenic sources; making it the third leading cause of death *(79)*. In addition, cervical SMT is hundreds of times safer as a treatment for neck pain, compared with non-steroidal anti-inflammatory drugs (NSAIDS), which are associated with gastrointestinal bleeding *(80)*.

6. RESEARCH HORIZONS

The evolution of a research community in the chiropractic profession constitutes one of its most pressing and urgent needs. In the past, legislative and legal successes marked its progress but those victories were often shallow and short-lived. Today, all strata of the healthcare industry from consumer to provider, to third-party payer, and governmental agencies, are increasingly turning to published scientific research for answers about cost-effectiveness and safety. There are many research questions begging to be answered in regards to chiropractic principles and practice in pain management. These questions could conceivably encompass and interact with disciplines including basic and clinical science, psychology, sociology, and even healthcare economics. A few examples are offered for consideration. Taking advantage of the recent advances in functional neuroimaging modalities, such as functional magnetic resonance imaging (fMRI), could increase our understanding of the CNS (brain and brainstem) correlates of SMT. Mapping the SMT inputs as they interact with the brain's pain circuitry (neuromatrix) or with the autonomic nervous system could significantly expand our understanding of the beneficial sensory, motor and autonomic clinical responses to SMT reported in acute and chronic pain.

Significant questions concerning the clinical role of SMT in pain management need to be addressed. Can SMT be utilized as the initial rung in the ladder of acute (or chronic) pain management? Can SMT reduce the risk of transformation from acute to chronic pain? Other related clinical issues are equally as pressing. Not all patients respond to SMT. Identification of the patient subtype most responsive to SMT is a critical need that would increase the cost-effectiveness and safety of SMT. Recently, effort in this direction was achieved. Rather than identify a specific biomechanical joint target as the only indication for SMT, 4 out of 5 selected criteria were employed (Table 4). These clinical prediction rules were used to identify over 90% of LBP patients who experienced a successful clinical outcome in one week of SMT treatment *(81)*. The definition of segmental joint dysfunction is controversial and requires clarification of its risk factors, pathophysiology and clinical presentation. There is little evidence of interexaminer reliability in its detection by motion palpation examination procedures *(82,83)*. The testing performance profile of segmental joint dysfunction as a diagnostic marker, i.e., sensitivity, specificity, and predictive value are unknown. Additionally, the natural history of segmental joint dysfunction needs to be understood; is it transient and self-resolving, or does it eventually erupt into symptomatic orthopedic and neurological findings? What does the SMT dose-response curve look like? What is the pharmacologic analgesic equivalent of SMT? Non-specific (placebo) effects accompany all interventions, how much of the clinical benefit of SMT is non-specific, and the result of expectancy and placebo effect? There are also abundant questions to be answered concerning the clinical benefit of chiropractic pain management at the extremes of the life spectrum i.e. pediatrics and geriatrics *(84)*.

An issue of a more social impact, fruitful for study, is the role of chiropractic physicians practicing in medical and surgical environments. Is it possible to integrate alternative and complementary practices into a traditional medical system? Such integrative practices are sporadic but appear to be increasing in number. A question that is increasingly relevant concerns the role of SMT in post-operative pain management. Will surgical outcomes be enhanced by SMT postoperatively? Could a course of SMT preoperatively benefit surgical outcomes? Then, there are sociological sources of concern that have been voiced within the chiropractic profession. For example, if integrated into the medical practice model, can the chiropractic profession maintain autonomy, or does it risk coaptation by mainstream medicine *(85)*? Will chiropractors continue to embrace a vitalistic premise in healthcare delivery or utilize an exclusively mechanistic

Table 4
LBP Clinical Prediction Rules (Flynn)

Criteria	Positive
Symptom location	no symptoms distal to the knee
Duration of Current Episode	<16 days
FABQ (Fear Avoidance Belief Questionnaire Work Subscale)	< 19
Lumbar Segmental Mobility (PA)	1 hypomobile segment
Hip Internal Rotation ROM	at least 1 hip with > 35°

approach? Are these views necessarily antagonistic and mutually exclusive, can they interact synergistically?

These are merely a handful of questions and speculations that face researchers in the chiropractic community as well as the field of healthcare at large. Many of these questions are testable hypotheses and are solvable with sufficient financial and human resources. Continued expansion of high quality chiropractic scholarship and research, will hopefully provide answers to even a few of these open questions. If successful in this effort, it is likely that the impact on patient care, especially those suffering in pain, will be significant. Pursuit of such research objectives sends a clear message that the chiropractic profession embraces the responsibility for contributions toward the advance of 21st century healthcare.

REFERENCES

1. Triano JJ. Biomechanics of spinal manipulative therapy. Spine J 2001;1(2):121–130.
2. http://www.chirocolleges.org/paradigm_scopet.html (1996) Chiropractic Scope and Practice. Volume.
3. Haldeman S. 2005. Principles and Practices of Chiropractic, Third edition. McGraw Hill.
4. Keating J, Cleveleand C, Menke M. 2004. Chiropractic History: A Primer. Davenport IA: Association for the History of Chiropractic.
5. Charlton KH. A Chiropracticness test. Chiropr Osteopat 2005;13:24.
6. Keating JC Jr, Charlton KH, Grod JP, et al. Subluxation: dogma or science? Chiropr Osteopat. 2005 Aug 10;13:17.
7. Homola S. Chiropractic: history and overview of theories and methods. Clin Orthop Relat Res 2006;444: 236–242.
8. Kelner M, Wellman B, Welsh S, Boon H. How far can complementary and alternative medicine go? The case of chiropractic and homeopathy. Soc Sci Med. 2006 Nov;63(10):2617–27. Epub 2006 Aug 22.
9. Tonelli MR. The limits of evidence-based medicine. Respir Care 2001;46(12):1435–1440 (discussion 1440–1441).
10. Khalsa PS, Eberhart A, Cotler A, Nahin R. The 2005 conference on the biology of manual therapies. J Manipulative Physiol Ther. 2006 Jun;29(5):341–6. Review.
11. Meeker WC, Haldeman S. Chiropractic: a profession at the crossroads of mainstream and alternative medicine. Ann Intern Med 2002;136(3):216–227.
12. DeVocht JW. History and overview of theories and methods of chiropractic: a counterpoint. Clin Orthop Relat Res 2006;444:243–249.
13. Nelson CF, Lawrence DJ, Triano JJ, et al. Chiropractic as spine care: a model for the profession. Chiropr Osteopat. 2005 Jul 6;13:9.
14. Druss BG, Rosenheck RA. Association between use of unconventional therapies and conventional medical services. JAMA 1999;282(7):651–656.
15. Shekelle PG, Adams AH, Chassin MR, Hurwitz EL, Brook RH. Spinal manipulation for low-back pain. Ann Intern Med. 1992 Oct 1;117(7):590–8. Review.
16. Mennell JM. The validation of the diagnosis "joint dysfunction" in the synovial joints of the cervical spine. J Manipulative Physiol Ther 1990;13(1):7–12.
17. Herzog W, Conway PJ, Kawchuk GN, Zhang Y, Hasler EM. Forces exerted during spinal manipulative therapy. Spine. 1993 Jul;18(9):1206–12.
18. Murphy D. 2000. In Dysfunction of the Cervical Spine, in Conservative Management of Cervical Spine Syndromes. Murphy D. Ed. McGraw Hill: New York.
19. Kulig K, Landel R, Powers CM. Assessment of lumbar spine kinematics using dynamic MRI: a proposed mechanism of sagittal plane motion induced by manual posterior-to-anterior mobilization. J Orthop Sports Phys Ther 2004;34(2):57–64.
20. Lee RY, McGregor AH, Bull AM, Wragg P. Dynamic response of the cervical spine to posteroanterior mobilisation. Clin Biomech (Bristol, Avon). 2005 Feb;20(2):228–31.
21. Ross JK, Bereznick DE, McGill SM. Determining cavitation location during lumbar and thoracic spinal manipulation: is spinal manipulation accurate and specific? Spine 2004;29(13):1452–1457.
22. Pickar JG. Neurophysiological effects of spinal manipulation. Spine J 2002;2(5):357–371.

23. Papageorgiou AC, Croft PR, Thomas E, et al. Influence of previous pain experience on the episode incidence of low back pain: results from the South Manchester Back Pain Study. Pain. 1996 Aug;66 (2–3):181–5.

24. Cramer GD, Fournier JT, Henderson CN, Wolcott CC. Degenerative changes following spinal fixation in a small animal model. J Manipulative Physiol Ther. 2004 Mar-Apr;27(3):141–54.

25. Wilder DG, Pope MH, Frymoyer JW. The biomechanics of lumbar disc herniation and the effect of overload and instability. J Spinal Disord 1988;1(1):16–32.

26. Wilder DG, Pope MH, Seroussi RE, Dimnet J, Krag MH. The balance point of the intervertebral motion segment: an experimental study. Bull Hosp Jt Dis Orthop Inst. 1989 Fall;49(2):155–69.

27. Cholewicki J, McGill SM. Lumbar posterior ligament involvement during extremely heavy lifts estimated from fluoroscopic measurements. J Biomech 1992;25(1):17–28.

28. Kang SW, Lee WN, Moon JH, Chun SI. Correlation of spinal mobility with the severity of chronic lower back pain. Yonsei Med J. 1995 Mar;36(1):37–44.

29. Dickey JP, Pierrynowski MR, Bednar DA, Yang SX. Relationship between pain and vertebral motion in chronic low-back pain subjects. Clin Biomech (Bristol, Avon). 2002 Jun;17(5):345–52.

30. Abbott JH, Fritz JM, McCane B, et al. Lumbar segmental mobility disorders: comparison of two methods of defining abnormal displacement kinematics in a cohort of patients with non-specific mechanical low back pain. BMC Musculoskelet Disord. 2006 May 19;7:45.

31. Seki K, Taniguchi Y, Narusawa M. Effects of joint immobilization on firing rate modulation of human motor units. J Physiol 2001;530(Pt 3):507–519.

32. Panjabi MM. The stabilizing system of the spine. Part I. Function, dysfunction, adaptation, and enhancement. J Spinal Disord 1992;5(4):383–389 (discussion 397).

33. Panjabi MM. The stabilizing system of the spine. Part II. Neutral zone and instability hypothesis. J Spinal Disord 1992;5(4):390–396 (discussion 397).

34. O'Sullivan P. Diagnosis and classification of chronic low back pain disorders: maladaptive movement and motor control impairments as underlying mechanism. Man Ther 2005;10(4):242–255.

35. Vicenzino B, Collins D, Benson H, Wright A. An investigation of the interrelationship between manipulative therapy-induced hypoalgesia and sympathoexcitation. J Manipulative Physiol Ther. 1998 Sep;21(7):448–53.

36. Melzack R, Wall PD. Pain mechanisms: a new theory. Science 1965;150(699):971–979.

37. Kristeva-Feige R, Rossi S, Pizzella V, et al. A neuromagnetic study of movement-related somatosensory gating in the human brain. Exp Brain Res. 1996;107(3):504–14.

38. Haas M, Groupp E, Kraemer DF. Dose–response for chiropractic care of chronic low back pain. Spine J 2004;4(5):574–583.

39. Winkelstein BA. Mechanisms of central sensitization, neuroimmunology & injury biomechanics in persistent pain: implications for musculoskeletal disorders. J Electromyogr Kinesiol 2004;14(1): 87–93.

40. Langevin HM, Sherman KJ. Pathophysiological model for chronic low back pain integrating connective tissue and nervous system mechanisms. Med Hypotheses 2007;68(1):74–80.

41. Giesecke T, Gracely RH, Clauw DJ, et al. [Central pain processing in chronic low back pain : Evidence for reduced pain inhibition.] Schmerz. 2006 Apr 4; [Epub ahead of print] German.

42. Giesecke T, Gracely RH, Grant MA, et al. Evidence of augmented central pain processing in idiopathic chronic low back pain. Arthritis Rheum. 2004 Feb;50(2):613–23.

43. Gracely RH, Geisser ME, Giesecke T, et al. Pain catastrophizing and neural responses to pain among persons with fibromyalgia. Brain. 2004 Apr;127(Pt 4):835–43. Epub 2004 Feb 11.

44. Maihofner C, Forster C, Birklein F, Neundorfer B, Handwerker HO. Brain processing during mechanical hyperalgesia in complex regional pain syndrome: a functional MRI study. Pain. 2005 Mar;114(1–2):93–103. Epub 2005 Jan 26.

45. Napadow V, Kettner N, Ryan A, et al. Somatosensory cortical plasticity in carpal tunnel syndrome–a cross-sectional fMRI evaluation. Neuroimage. 2006 Jun;31(2):520–30. Epub 2006 Feb 3.

46. Napadow V, Liu J, Li M, et al. Somatosensory cortical plasticity in carpal tunnel syndrome treated by acupuncture. Hum Brain Mapp. 2007 Mar;28(3):159–71.

47. Boal RW, Gillette RG. Central neuronal plasticity, low back pain and spinal manipulative therapy. J Manipulative Physiol Ther 2004;27(5):314–326.

48. Butefisch CM. Neurobiological bases of rehabilitation. Neurol Sci 2006;27(Suppl 1):S18–S23.

49. Le Bars D, Villanueva L, Bouhassira D, Willer JC. Diffuse noxious inhibitory controls (DNIC) in animals and in man. Patol Fiziol Eksp Ter. 1992 Jul-Aug;(4):55–65. Review.

50. Kemeny ME, Gruenewald TL. Psychoneuroimmunology update. Semin Gastrointest Dis 1999;10(1):20–29.

51. Pert CB, Dreher HE, Ruff MR. The psychosomatic network: foundations of mind-body medicine. Altern Ther Health Med 1998;4(4):30–41.

52. Hemingway H, Marmot M. Evidence based cardiology: psychosocial factors in the aetiology and prognosis of coronary heart disease. Systematic review of prospective cohort studies. BMJ 1999;318(7196):1460–1467.

53. McEwen BS. Stress, adaptation, and disease. Allostasis and allostatic load. Ann NY Acad Sci 1998;840:33–44.

54. Melzack R. 1999. Pain and stress. In Psychosocial Factors in Pain: Critical Perspectives. Gatchel R, Turk DC, Ed. New York: Guilford Press, pp 89–106.

55. Sapolsky RM, Romero LM, Munck AU. How do glucocorticoids influence stress responses? Integrating permissive, suppressive, stimulatory, and preparative actions. Endocr Rev 2000; 21(1): 55–89.

56. Hardy K, Pollard H. The organisation of the stress response, and its relevance to chiropractors: a commentary. Chiropr Osteopat 2006;14:25.

57. Budgell B, Hirano F. Innocuous mechanical stimulation of the neck and alterations in heart-rate variability in healthy young adults. Auton Neurosci 2001;91(1–2):96–99.

58. Budgell B, Polus B. The effects of thoracic manipulation on heart rate variability: a controlled crossover trial. J Manipulative Physiol Ther 2006;29(8):603–610.

59. Verhoef MJ, Page SA, Waddell SC. The Chiropractic Outcome Study: pain, functional ability and satisfaction with care. J Manipulative Physiol Ther 1997;20(4):235–240.

60. Haneline MT. Symptomatic outcomes and perceived satisfaction levels of chiropractic patients with a primary diagnosis involving acute neck pain. J Manipulative Physiol Ther 2006;29(4):288–296.

61. Gaumer G. Factors associated with patient satisfaction with chiropractic care: survey and review of the literature. J Manipulative Physiol Ther 2006;29(6):455–462.

62. Loney PL, Stratford PW. The prevalence of low back pain in adults: a methodological review of the literature. Phys Ther 1999;79(4):384–396.

63. Ernst E. Chiropractic spinal manipulation for neck pain: a systematic review. J Pain 2003;4(8): 417–421.

64. Ernst E. Chiropractic spinal manipulation for back pain. Br J Sports Med 2003;37(3):195–196 (discussion 196).

65. Ernst E. Manual therapies for pain control: chiropractic and massage. Clin J Pain 2004;20(1):8–12.

66. Ernst E, Canter PH. A systematic review of systematic reviews of spinal manipulation. J R Soc Med 2006;99(4):192–196.

67. Vernon HT, Humphreys BK, Hagino CA. A systematic review of conservative treatments for acute neck pain not due to whiplash. J Manipulative Physiol Ther 2005;28(6):443–448.

68. Bronfort G, Haas M, Evans RL, Bouter LM. Efficacy of spinal manipulation and mobilization for low back pain and neck pain: a systematic review and best evidence synthesis. Spine J. 2004 May-Jun;4(3):335–56. Review.

69. Bronfort G, Haas M, Moher D, et al. Review conclusions by Ernst and Canter regarding spinal manipulation refuted. Chiropr Osteopat. 2006 Aug 3;14:14.

70. Santilli V, Beghi E, Finucci S. Chiropractic manipulation in the treatment of acute back pain and sciatica with disc protrusion: a randomized double-blind clinical trial of active and simulated spinal manipulations. Spine J 2006;6(2):131–137.

71. Blaine E. Manipulative (chiropractic) dislocations of the atlas. JAMA 1925;85:1356–1359.

72. Hurwitz EL, Morgenstern H, Vassilaki M, Chiang LM. Frequency and clinical predictors of adverse reactions to chiropractic care in the UCLA neck pain study. Spine. 2005 Jul 1;30(13):1477–84.

73. Cagnie B, Vinck E, Beernaert A, Cambier D. How common are side effects of spinal manipulation and can these side effects be predicted? Man Ther. 2004 Aug;9(3):151–6.

74. Dvorak J, Orelli F. How dangerous is manipulation of the cervical spine? Man Med 1985;2:1–4.

75. Carey P. A report on the occurence of cerebral vascular accidents in chiropractic practice. J Can Chiropract Assoc 1993;37:104–106.

76. Klougart N, Leboeuf-Yde C, Rasmussen LR. Safety in chiropractic practice. Part I: The occurrence of cerebrovascular accidents after manipulation to the neck in Denmark from 1978–1988. J Manipulative Physiol Ther 1996;19(6):371–377.

77. Rosner AL. Chiropractic manipulation and stroke. Stroke 2001;32(9):2207–2208.

78. Haldeman S, Kohlbeck FJ, McGregor M. Stroke, cerebral artery dissection, and cervical spine manipulation therapy. J Neurol 2002;249(8):1098–1104.
79. Starfield B. Is US health really the best in the world? JAMA 2000;284(4):483–485.
80. Dabbs V, Lauretti WJ. A risk assessment of cervical manipulation vs. NSAIDs for the treatment of neck pain. J Manipulative Physiol Ther 1995;18(8):530–536.
81. Flynn T, Fritz J, Whitman J, et al. A clinical prediction rule for classifying patients with low back pain who demonstrate short-term improvement with spinal manipulation. Spine. 2002 Dec 15;27(24):2835–43.
82. Humphreys BK, Delahaye M, Peterson CK. An investigation into the validity of cervical spine motion palpation using subjects with congenital block vertebrae as a 'gold standard'. BMC Musculoskeletal Disord 2004;5:19.
83. Stochkendahl MJ, Christensen HW, Hartvigsen J, et al. Manual examination of the spine: a systematic critical literature review of reproducibility. J Manipulative Physiol Ther. 2006 Jul-Aug;29(6):475–85, 485.e1–10. Review.
84. Killinger LZ. Chiropractic and geriatrics: a review of the training, role, and scope of chiropractic in caring for aging patients. Clin Geriatr Med 2004;20(2):223–235.
85. Kaptchuk TJ, Miller FG. Viewpoint: what is the best and most ethical model for the relationship between mainstream and alternative medicine: opposition, integration, or pluralism? Acad Med 2005;80(3):286–290

17 Therapeutic Massage and Bodywork in Integrative Pain Management

Arthur Madore and Janet R. Kahn

CONTENTS

INTRODUCTION
A BRIEF HISTORY
AMERICANS' USE OF MASSAGE
WHAT IS THERAPEUTIC MASSAGE AND BODYWORK?
THE LITERATURE ON MASSAGE AND PAIN
CASE REPORTS
POTENTIAL MECHANISMS OF ACTION
ORGANIZATIONAL STRUCTURES OF INTEGRATION
ISSUES OF INTEGRATION

Summary

The role of massage in pain management undoubtedly predates recorded history. Today, while there is broad public acceptance and usage of therapeutic massage and a growing body of literature exploring its safety and efficacy, theory and research regarding possible mechanisms of action lag far behind.

This chapter explores the potential role of therapeutic massage and bodywork in contemporary integrative pain management. The range of methods that can collectively be called therapeutic massage and bodywork are described, the literature regarding their effect on pain is reviewed, and the little that is known about their mechanisms of action in relation to current theories of pain management is examined. Finally, case descriptions and suggestions about the beneficial use of therapeutic massage and bodywork in contemporary integrative pain management are offered.

Key Words: massage, bodywork, neuromuscular therapy, musculoskeletal pain, cancer pain

1. INTRODUCTION

The role of massage in pain management undoubtedly predates recorded history, as we can assume that early humans, like us, instinctively would rub a stubbed toe, a barked shin, or a tired muscle in order to ease the pain. Gate control theory of pain suggests that they were substituting one sensation for another—offering their neural pathways the sensation of touch, which travels to the brain at the rate of 35–75 miles per second and thus claims the brain's attention, leaving relatively powerless the sensations of pain, which travel at a mere 0.5–2 miles/second for dull pain or

From: *Contemporary Pain Medicine: Integrative Pain Medicine: The Science and Practice of Complementary and Alternative Medicine in Pain Management*
Edited by: J. F. Audette and A. Bailey © Humana Press, Totowa, NJ

5–35 miles/second for sharp or burning pain *(1,2)*. Of course, our ancestors did not think that way; they probably just noticed that it worked. In fact, things are not so different today in the field of therapeutic massage and bodywork. While there is broad public acceptance and usage of therapeutic massage, and a growing body of literature exploring its safety and efficacy, theory and research regarding possible mechanisms of action lag far behind.

This chapter will explore the potential role of therapeutic massage and bodywork in contemporary integrative pain management. We will describe the range of methods that can collectively be called therapeutic massage and bodywork, review the literature on their effect on pain, then examine the little that is known about their mechanisms of action in relation to current theories of pain management. Finally, we will offer case descriptions and suggestions about the beneficial use of therapeutic massage and bodywork in contemporary integrative pain management.

2. A BRIEF HISTORY

Given the tendency of humans to apply touch to injury, it is not surprising that some form of massage has been an integral part of every system of medicine humans have created in recorded history. The Asian roots reach back roughly 3,000 years to the origins of both Chinese and Ayurvedic medicine. Use of massage in many Asian countries has continued uninterrupted to the present time. The inclusion of therapeutic massage in Western medicine has been more erratic. Massage was a part of both Greek and Roman medical practices, with prescriptions for rubbing, friction, chest-clapping, and so forth found in the writings of Hippocrates, Galen, and Celsus *(3)*.

In the United States, interest in massage as an aspect of pain management heightened during World War I, when Americans became aware of the rehabilitation work available for soldiers (and civilians) among the allied nations. In 1918 the US Army created a Reconstruction Department that included physiotherapy and occupational therapy. Mary McMillan, a prominent figure in the development of physical therapy in England and founder of physical therapy in the United States, served as chief aide at Walter Reed Hospital and taught special courses in war-related reconstruction at Reed College Clinic during World War I. From 1921 to 1925 she was director of physiotherapy at Harvard Medical School, where she authored a textbook entitled *Massage and Therapeutic Exercise*. While massage continued as an important part of physical therapy treatment through World War II, its use declined throughout the late 1940s and 1950s in the face of increased availability of effective pharmaceuticals and technology in the fields of both physical therapy and nursing *(4)*.

In addition to these medical roots, contemporary US massage and bodywork is also influenced by the use of massage for athletes, from the original Olympians to the present time and by the exploration of touch in the human potential movement. In the 1960s and 1970s, this movement prompted investigation into the links between mental and bodily ease or distress, between human structure and consciousness *(5)*. This movement also brought increased attention to the role of the practitioner/client relationship in creating and maximizing therapeutic effects; an aspect of healing emphasized in integrative medicine that is still in need of systematic investigation *(6,7)*.

3. AMERICANS' USE OF MASSAGE

Massage is one of the most popular and fastest-growing forms of complementary and alternative medicine (CAM) in the United States. Between 1990 and 1997 the annual percentage of American adults using massage increased from 6.9% to 11.1% *(8)*. Eisenberg et al have estimated that 13.5 million Americans visited massage therapists in 1997, collectively making 114 million visits, which the American Massage Therapy Association has estimated cost between $4 and $6 billion. A 2003 survey sponsored by the American Hospital Association found that among the 1,007 hospitals responding, 82% of those offering CAM therapies included massage therapy among their healthcare offerings. This was the highest rate for any CAM therapy. Over 70% of those hospitals reported utilizing massage therapy for pain management and pain relief.

Treatment for pain appears to be the number one reason individuals go to massage therapists, according to a 1999 survey of licensed massage therapists in Washington and Connecticut. Cherkin et al. gathered systematic data on over 2,000 visits to these practitioners and found that 63% of the visits were for musculoskeletal concerns. One in five visits were made for back pain, 17% for neck pain, and 8% for shoulder pain *(9)*.

4. WHAT IS THERAPEUTIC MASSAGE AND BODYWORK?

In this chapter, we use the term *therapeutic massage and bodywork* to refer to a broad array of techniques, all of which involve purposeful manipulation of the soft-tissue and/or subtle energy (with or without active or passive movements and verbal cuing), done with the intention of alleviating pain and resolving structural imbalances or other abnormalities in the tissue or energy to restore health, well-being and ease. We have chosen to include forms of movement re-education such as Feldenkrais method and Alexander technique within this definition, although we recognize that this is a controversial issue. Many practitioners of these approaches quite reasonably do not want to come under massage licensure laws; and many regard themselves as educators rather than therapists. While respecting these views, we nonetheless include such forms of movement re-education in our definition because many massage therapists practice these techniques, considering education to be a key component of therapeutic massage treatment. Movement therapies can play a critical role in pain management, as we will illustrate later.

There is great variety in the forms of massage and bodywork currently employed. Some originated within Eastern understandings of anatomy and physiology that are relatively ecological or relational in view and focus on the healthy and balanced movement of energy (prana, chi, etc.) both within the patient and between the patient and his/her human and physical environments. Other forms are Western in origin and may be seen as more reductionist or scientific in their approach to assessment and exclusively focused on the material body. Even those therapists practicing within a Western framework, however, tend to hold a holistic view of the client and to see one's physical, spiritual, cognitive, and emotional aspects as essentially inseparable from one another. This has been beautifully stated by Deane Juhan, author of *Job's Body*, who said, "The skin is no more separated from the brain than the surface of a lake is separate from its depths...the two are different locations in a continuous medium... The brain is a single functional unit, from cortex to fingertips to toes. To touch the surface is to stir the depths." *(10)*

4.1. Frameworks To Consider

The field of therapeutic massage and bodywork is home to a plethora of techniques, many named for their founder and most of which are not absolutely new, but are combinations and re-combinations of the relatively limited number of ways in which one human can touch another with healing intent. These branding efforts can detract from our ability to see the forest in any meaningful way, and there is, to date, no definitive taxonomy of therapeutic massage and bodywork *(11)*.

In the absence of comprehensive taxonomy, we suggest three considerations when thinking about massage. First, the field can be viewed according to the physiological system or type of tissue most directly engaged. Andrade and Clifford have offered one such framework, clustering various massage techniques as superficial reflex techniques, superficial fluid techniques, neuromuscular techniques, connective tissue techniques, passive movement techniques, and percussive techniques *(12)*. The Massage Therapy Research Consortium has presented a somewhat different taxonomy that begins with a basic distinction between Western, Eastern, and hybrid forms *(13)*. They categorize the various Western methods as craniosacral, lymphatic, movement re-education, musculo-circulatory, myofascial, neuromuscular, and reflexive. The energetic forms familiar to most Americans appear either within the Eastern framework (e.g., Reiki) or within the hybrid designation (e.g., Therapeutic Touch, Healing Touch, Polarity, and Zero Balancing). Undoubtedly other schemas exist. One could, for instance, understand a variation of the above that locates all forms of movement re-education as neuromuscular approaches with a strong cognitive component. While other neuromuscular forms may use more touch and less talk, all forms in this category would share the goal of "re-programming" neuromuscular messaging.

A second approach to understanding massage is to focus on the intention of the therapist during treatment. The issue of therapist intent is just beginning to be explored in massage research. In fact, one sees studies in which an important aspect of the control or sham condition is asking the therapists to purposefully refrain from intending to heal the patient. In thinking about the application of intention to categorizations of massage or bodywork, we suggest that at all times the therapist is focused on one or more of the following:

- Promotion of relaxation or comfort,
- Promotion of structural or physiological change, or
- Encouragement of kinesthetic awareness, and/or somato-emotional awareness and repatterning.

Emphasizing the therapist's intention underscores the reality that the very same strokes or techniques may be used in efforts to produce these different results. Differences in those circumstances would include level of pressure, order of techniques, verbal cuing and, of course, therapist intention.

Finally, in the cases reported in this chapter you will find a framework of three types that relate to three stages of treatment. We classify those methods simply as gentle bodywork, structural bodywork, and movement education. These methods would typically be applied in that order. Within this framework, just as in selection of a conventional treatment, the first consideration is to utilize the least invasive and safest method likely to be effective.

Virtually all of contemporary massage shares an underlying view that the body tends toward self-healing and that a therapist's job is to initiate or support that tendency when the body seems to have forgotten or lost its way *(14)*. It should also be noted that specific strokes or techniques appear in a variety of massage forms. For instance, kneading actions are used in Swedish massage (which would be called musculo-vascular in our first framework), in a Chinese form called Tui'na, and as a component of myofascial work as well. Compression is a component of all but the non-touch or lightest touch forms. Compression takes on particular meanings and use in myofascial work, neuromuscular work (specifically in trigger point release), and musculo-vascular work.

4.2. Aspects of a Treatment

A therapeutic massage and bodywork treatment is more than simply the application of a particular manual technique, and some or all of the other components may be relevant to pain management. For example, the therapeutic relationship is built in part through the choice and sequencing of multiple techniques within one treatment. Most therapists in North America have received instruction in Swedish massage, and many use it as the bedrock upon which are built treatments utilizing additional forms. Therapists who specialize in neuromuscular or myofascial massage—forms that many refer to as "deep tissue"— nonetheless use Swedish massage to warm, soften, or otherwise prepare the tissue (and the person) before applying the deeper techniques. Utilizing gentle Swedish techniques to "open the conversation" allows the therapist more accurately to gauge the depth and timing of stronger strokes. The effect of therapeutic massage may also be a result of the verbal exchange between therapist and client, which may augment relaxation or serve as induction into a healing state. In addition, many therapists seek to extend the treatment through suggestion of self-care activities for the client. These might include specific stretches, exercises, breathing approaches, techniques to enhance somatic awareness and the like. In addition, environmental factors may, at the very least, enhance the relaxation effect. These include music, lighting, color schemes, aroma, temperature, and so on.

Finally, of course, the therapist's intention to heal, his or her manner, and the connection between therapist and client must also be viewed as aspects of treatment. For many therapists, and we suspect for many clients as well, the therapist's license to touch is viewed as a sacred trust. In this context, the relationship is at least as important as the physical aspect of the treatment. Tracy Walton has written of this quite eloquently.

> *By touching a body, we touch every event it has experienced. For a few brief moments we hold all of a client's stories in our hands. We witness someone's experience of their own flesh, through some of the most powerful means possible; the contact of our hands, the acceptance of the body without judgment, and the occasional listening ear. With these gestures, we reach across the isolation of the human experience and hold another person's legend. (15)*

5. THE LITERATURE ON MASSAGE AND PAIN

Research on therapeutic massage and bodywork is still rather limited. While a search of MEDLINE yields over 200 articles on massage published in the last three decades, with perhaps half of these being reports on clinical trials, many of the early studies and some current ones have serious limitations. In addition to small sample size, these include lack of randomization, adequate blinding, a meaningful comparison or control group, and/or clarity about the intervention (e.g., what kind and how much massage was used) *(16–19)*. In fact, many studies that purportedly examine effects of massage, in fact are looking at mixed interventions, of which massage is only one aspect. This makes it impossible to disentangle any specific massage effects. In addition, in some studies the intervention appears to have been delivered by someone who was not trained in massage, at least not to professional standards. In others, although the practitioners may have been seasoned professionals, the protocol appears to be substandard in terms of contemporary treatment patterns. That said, the good news is that some RCTs of sufficient power are now being conducted and, while the early literature looked at massage largely as a method of stress reduction, recent studies are also addressing the therapeutic effect of massage on musculoskeletal pain.

5.1. Musculoskeletal Pain

Cherkin et al.'s study of licensed CAM practitioners revealed that 20% of massage visits were made for back pain and 17% for neck pain *(20)*. Prior to 2000, there were no published RCTs evaluating the effectiveness of any types of massage for back pain. Since then, one medium-sized randomized clinical trial (78 massage subjects in a three-armed study) *(21)* and two small RCTs (12 and 25 massage subjects) *(22,23)* found therapeutic massage effective for subacute and chronic back pain, when assessed at the completion of the treatment intervention period. The larger of these trials, which compared massage with acupuncture and self-care educational material, also measured long-term outcomes and found that the benefits of 10 massage treatments were still evident 9–10 months after the completion of therapy *(23)*. Measures indicated that massage was more effective than acupuncture in reducing patients' assessments of the bothersomeness of symptoms ($p = 0.002$ at 52 weeks) and improving patient's Roland Disability Scores ($p = 0.01$ at 10 weeks and $p = 0.033$ at 52 weeks).

Regarding use of massage for treatment of neck pain, Haraldsson et al. conducted a systematic review of massage for mechanical neck pain that yielded 19 studies for consideration *(24)*. All studies were conducted prior to September 2004. They concluded that massage was safe for people with this condition, but that the data did not indicate that it was more effective than the treatments to which it was being compared, and there was a wide array of such comparative treatments across the included studies. Perhaps the strongest finding of this review, apart from the important issue of safety, is that the massage research literature does yet not lend itself well to such reviews. The authors note many shortcomings in the quality and rigor of the studies (e.g., small sample size) that might apply to early research in many areas. They also note an issue that is a special problem in massage research, *"Most studies lacked a definition, description, or rationale for massage, the massage technique or both. In some cases, it was questionable whether the massage in the study would be considered effective massage under any circumstance." (24)* They also noted that information on the credentials of those delivering the massage was frequently missing so there was no guarantee that "professional" massage had been tested in these studies.

One well-conducted study has been completed since publication of that review. This was a comparison of massage with a self-care book for the treatment of chronic neck pain *(25)*. In this RCT, 64 patients with neck pain of at least 3 months' duration were randomized to receive massage (up to 10 massages over 10 weeks) or a self-care book. Data were collected at 4, 10, and 26 weeks on outcomes that included dysfunction (Neck Disability Index—NDI), a 0–10 symptom bothersomeness scale, and medication usage. The investigator found that massage recipients were more likely than the self-education subjects to experience a clinically significant improvement on the NDI (48% vs. 18% of controls; RR = 2.7; 95% CI = 1.2–6.5) and on the bothersomeness scale (55% vs. 25% of controls; RR = 2.2; 95% CI = 1.1–4.5) at 10 weeks (end of treatment). At 26 weeks (16 weeks post end of treatment), the difference in symptom bothersomeness had evaporated, while the difference in function still favored massage, though it had been reduced (RR = 1.8; 95% CI = 1.1–3.3). Medication usage increased for the book group from 63% at baseline to 77% at 26 weeks, and decreased slightly for the massage group (56% at baseline, 53% at 10 and 26 weeks). While a single small study does not provide much data, this does suggest that massage is likely to provide some relief for those with chronic neck pain, and that further research is warranted.

Perlman et al. investigated the effects of 8 weeks of massage on pain and other symptoms associated with osteoarthritis (OA) of the knee. Adults (n = 68) with a diagnosis of OA of the knee and a pre-randomization score of 4 to 9 on the Western Ontario & McMaster Universities OA Index (WOMAC) and pain visual analog scale (0 = no pain, 10 = worst pain ever) were randomized to massage or usual care. A standard protocol of full-body Swedish massage was administered twice weekly in the first four weeks to build a loading dose, then once weekly for the next four weeks. The massage therapy group demonstrated significant improvements in the WOMAC Global Score (-21.15 ± 2.46 mm; p < .0001), Stiffness (-21.60 ± 26.99 mm; p < .0001), Physical Function domains (-20.50 ± 22.50 mm; p < .0001) and Pain (-17.62 ± 31.06 mm; p = 0.0023) at 8 weeks (end of treatment) as well as decreased pain (VAS) and time to walk 50 feet (p < 0.05). At 16 weeks (8 weeks post-treatment), improvements seen in the massage therapy group generally persisted (26).

Studies from Touch Research Institute (TRI) have shown decreased pain among subjects with various chronic pain conditions. Pediatric patients with juvenile rheumatoid arthritis massaged by their parents for 15 minutes/day for 30 days showed decreased cortisol levels, as well as decreased pain compared with subjects receiving relaxation therapy. Measurement of pain levels was based on reports from the patients, their parents, and the physicians (27). Researchers at TRI have also found reduced pain levels in subjects receiving massage for fibromyalgia (28,29).

Despite the paucity of high quality RCTs a number of systematic reviews have been attempted. Not surprisingly, authors of many of the reviews concluded that the available data constituted an inadequate basis for judgment (30–37). In fact, only two reviews found massage to be supported by the available data. Cherkin et al. conducted a review of the literature on three potential treatments for back pain—acupuncture, spinal manipulation, and massage (38). They examined the evidence of effectiveness, safety, and cost. The only RCTs on massage they found were the three we have mentioned above, and based on those data they concluding that, "Initial studies have found massage to be effective for persistent back pain …. Preliminary evidence suggests that massage, but not acupuncture or spinal manipulation, may reduce the costs of care after an initial course of therapy."

Two months after Cherkin's review, Van Tulder et al. published a review of CAM therapies for low back pain. While they noted that massage seemed to be more effective than sham treatments for persistent low back pain, they also noted that there was little data comparing massage to accepted conventional treatments (39). In general, then, the literature on massage as a treatment for musculoskeletal pain conditions is quite limited, with only back pain having received enough attention to warrant even tentative assessment. In the case of back pain the data are promising.

5.2. Cancer Pain

Apart from musculoskeletal conditions, perhaps the most frequent use of massage for pain control has been with cancer-related pain. One study by Weinrich and Weinrich, was a non-blinded, randomized trial, with two arms: massage and conversation control, that utilized a single outcome measure—a Visual Analogue Scale (VAS) of pain administered at baseline, post-treatment, 1 h post, and 2 h post *(40)*. The study population included 28 hospitalized cancer patients paired by medication prior to randomization. Treatment was a 10-minute Swedish back rub, administered by a nursing student. While the authors concluded that men had immediate short-term pain relief (p = 0.01) from massage, it should be noted that male subjects in the treatment group reported baseline pain levels twice that of the females. Thus pain intensity could easily be at least as relevant as gender in determining the effect of treatment.

Post-White and Kinney conducted a prospective two period crossover study with 230 (164 complete data) histologically documented adult cancer patients all of whom were receiving repeating cycles of the same chemotherapy. Subjects had all reported a score of at least three on a ten-point scale of pain, nausea, fatigue or anxiety. Randomization was to one of three arms – massage (MT), Healing Touch (HT), or presence. Pain-related outcomes included use of pain medication, self-reports of pain, and physiologic measures of relaxation (HR, BP, RR). Massage treatment consisted of a 45-minute full-body Swedish protocol; the HT was a 45-minute protocol of non-contact energetic healing; and the presence treatment consisted of 45 minutes of silence or conversation, depending upon the patient's choice. The study found that both MT and HT had significant short-term effects on pain (p = .001 for MT and .01 for HT) as well as on physiological outcomes and self-reports of relaxation measures (p = .01–.001). MT lowered subjects' use of NSAIDS over time. MT and HT both reduced total mood disturbance over the 4-week study period *(41)*. Perhaps the most important contribution of this study is the finding that there was no effect from presence alone when compared to the significant effects of both massage and healing touch in increasing relaxation and decreasing pain. It should be noted that the changes in pain were modest, only effecting scores of present pain.

An increasing number of hospitals are including massage as an aspect of their cancer care, prompting attention to both safety and efficacy. Perhaps most prominent among these hospitals is Memorial Sloan-Kettering Cancer Center (MSKCC) in New York, which has, for some years, also offered training in massage for cancer patients. By far the largest outcome study on massage for cancer patients was that done by Cassileth and Vickers, utilizing data on 1,290 patients treated at MSKCC Integrative Medicine Service over a 3-year period *(42)*. Pre- and post-massage data on symptom severity is routinely collected at MSKCC utilizing 0–10 scales gathering patients' reports of their pain, fatigue, stress/anxiety, nausea, depression, and "other" miscellaneous symptoms. For the 1,290 patients whose data were used in this analysis, symptom scores were reduced by approximately 50%, and it is reported that the benefits persisted with no return toward baseline scores for at least the 48 –hour follow-up period for which data are available. The authors note that the improvement was at least as marked for those patients with very high baseline pain scores. This finding echoes the earlier finding of Weinberg and Weinberg cited above.

Corbin conducted a recent review of the cancer and massage literature available through MEDLINE and CINAHL *(43)*. Regarding efficacy, he concluded that the data support the notion that massage is effective in reducing anxiety and stress among cancer patients. In terms of pain control the data were found to be promising but inconclusive. Regarding safety, Corbin concluded that massage can be considered a safe aspect of cancer care. Although there may be a slight increase in risk of adverse events among cancer patients over other populations, the general occurrence of those risks is quite slight.

5.3. Other Documented Effects of Massage

None of the studies cited thus far was designed to shed particular light on possible mechanisms of action through which therapeutic massage might mediate the experience of pain. This will be discussed later in this chapter. To cast the broadest possible net for that speculation, we should note the various physiological effects of massage that have been explored to date.

Changes have been recorded in subjects' neurochemistry as a result of massage. Uvnas has documented that the release of oxytocin can be prompted by "warm and rhythmic touch." *(44,45)* Her studies, carried out at the Karolinska Institute in Sweden, indicate that this neurohumeral response to touch is true for both men and women. Field's review of the massage literature, including many studies done at the Touch Research Institute that she founded at the University of Miami, indicates that massage reduces levels of cortisol, epinephrine, and norepinephrine *(46)*. However, Moyer's later meta-analysis of relevant data contradicted one aspect of Field's findings, indicating that cortisol levels were not significantly reduced *(47)*. Moyer did find evidence of significant reductions in heart rate and blood pressure, which had been reported by Meek and Fakouri, but not by Reed *(48–50)*.

The heart rate and blood pressure data are seen to indicate that massage promotes parasympathetic activity, which has long been claimed by massage therapists.

However, other areas of massage lore regarding long-held beliefs about the method of action and resultant therapeutic benefit have not been supported by recent studies. For example, a long-standing claim among massage therapists has been that massage "moves fluids" and that, among other effects, this increased circulation can prompt faster or more thorough elimination of metabolic waste from tissue, thereby reducing the degree of delayed onset muscle soreness (DOMS) in athletes. On the specific question of DOMS, Ernst found that there was not general support for this contention *(51)*. Regarding the more basic question of whether massage in fact moves fluids, two studies found that massage can prompt local increases in blood flow while two others found that it did not *(52–55)*.

Braverman and Schulman, in reviewing massage effects for rehabilitative contexts, cited evidence that massage can promote increased joint mobility, improved connective tissue pliability and mobility, and enhanced immune system function in addition to the reduction in stress hormones already cited *(56)*.

An often cited and sometimes disputed series of studies relate to the use of massage for pre-term infants. These studies, initiated by the Touch Research Institute, generally found that massage prompted increased weight gain in infants delivered prematurely, leading to earlier hospital release. Vickers et al, conducted two systematic reviews of these studies concluding each time that massage did improve daily weight gain by 5.1g (95% CI 3.5, 6.7g), and that gentle touch without movement (nonmassage) did not

(57,58). They also found that the massage intervention appeared to reduce length of stay by 4.5 days (95% CI 2.4, 6.5), although there were some methodological concerns regarding the blinding of this outcome. There was also limited evidence that massage interventions have a small positive effect on postnatal complications and weight at 4–6 months. However, again, there were serious concerns about the methodological quality of these studies.

Two studies have been conducted since the second Vickers review, both of which examine the role that vagal tone may play as a possible mechanism to explain the weight gain seen in premature infants. Both of these studies did, indeed, find increased vagal tone among the massaged infants but not among the control groups *(59,60)*. Diego et al, also found evidence of greater gastric motility *(59)*. Lee found greater awake state and motor activity among the massaged infants compared with the nonmassaged infants *(60)*. The intervention in these studies was a combination of simple Swedish massage strokes and passive limb movements. The total intervention time was 10–15 minutes, in some cases administered twice daily.

Massage has also been shown to improve sleep patterns in populations as disparate as cancer patients, young autistic children (ages 3–6), adults with low back pain, elderly residents known to have sleep disturbance, pregnant women, older men hospitalized in a critical care unit with a cardiovascular illness, and adolescents institutionalized for depression or adjustment disorder *(61–67)*. While some of these findings are based on simple self-reports, Chen utilized the Pittsburgh Sleep Quality Index (PSQI), Richards' study included use of polysomnagraphy and the Field study of institutionalized adolescents utilized time-lapse video and an actometer worn on the wrist that measures movement while asleep.

In summary, the early massage therapy literature is fraught with limitations that could lead to either type I or type II errors. They were typically small, underfunded, and underpowered studies that suffered from lack of rigorous controls including blinding and randomization. These problems could certainly lead to an overestimate of effects. At the same time, nontherapists often developed the protocols and graduate students or others who had been trained just for that study sometimes administered them. This lack of optimal treatment by qualified therapists could easily lead to an assumption that massage is ineffective in a situation in which proper treatment and dosage might yield another result. For that reason, we regard even the flawed studies as often offering promising suggestions for directions of future research. Among the more recent and more rigorous investigations there is suggestion that massage appears to be helpful in pain management in an array of circumstances that certainly warrant further investigation. However, serious investigations into possible mechanisms of action remain glaringly absent from the massage literature.

6. CASE REPORTS

The following case reports are drawn from the records of the first author. Therapy was based on the three phases of treatment system described earlier in this chapter (see Table 1). The first phase is termed *gentle bodywork*, which may include light pressure applications of Swedish massage, as well as modalities that include an energetic component such as Zero Balancing, Polarity, Therapeutic Touch, Craniosacral, Trager, Reiki, and Lomi Lomi. The mechanism of action is assumed to be indirect. The goal is to trigger natural homeostatic responses that in turn can positively affect the painful

Table 1
Three Phase Treatment System Recommended by First Author To Ensure a Sustained
Therapeutic Effect from Massage

Phases of treatment	Potential styles	Comments
Gentle bodywork	Light pressure applications of Swedish massage, Zero Balancing, Polarity, Therapeutic Touch, Craniosacral therapys, Trager, Reiki, and Lomi Lomi	The mechanism of action is assumed to be indirect. The goal is to trigger natural homeostatic responses that in turn can positively affect the painful condition; these types of massage are generally suitable for patients in significant pain as they are unlikely to aggravate the condition
Structural bodywork	Rolfing, Structural Integration, Neuromuscular therapy, Myofascial release, Hellerwork, and Tuina.	The goals of this phase include creating some direct change in the muscles, tendons, ligaments, and viscera that compose the soft tissue of the body; the pressure applied during this phase is usually greater than during the gentle bodywork phase, with a corresponding possibility for increased soreness and a short-term increase in pain
Movement therapy	Feldenkrais method, the Alexander technique, Hellerwork, and Trager Psychophysical Integration	A basic tenet of movement therapy is that no structural bodywork will be maintained if the person has a movement organization that causes a return of the pathological pattern of muscle strain; the best bodywork will be quickly undone by a person's habitual body usage

* For simplicity we have constracted one model of logical treatment sequencing. Experienced structural bodyworkers and movement therapists can adopt their skills to intervene at most levels of pain. The reality is that you do what works.

condition. These types of massage are generally suitable for patients in significant pain, as they are unlikely to aggravate the condition.

The baseline intention of the therapist using gentle touch is to induce in the patient a feeling of relaxation and safety. As the patient experiences the relaxation response, it is assumed that changes may be prompted that include reduction of cortisol and other stress hormones, increased production of serotonin, and activation of the parasympathetic nervous system. While no investigations have been done on biochemical responses to most of the modalities included in this category of gentle touch, they have been documented for Swedish massage in many of the studies from Touch Research Institute cited earlier as well as others (68). In addition to this basic intention, each of the above types of massage therapy has a specific approach to help facilitate the natural healing process. Although each of the specific techniques mentioned above during this gentle bodywork phase of treatment vary greatly, they share the view that the role of the therapist is to facilitate the patient's natural homeostatic healing mechanism. This gentle approach engages the patient's body in a way that reduces anxiety, depression, and the accompanying stress reactive hormones. These changes are particularly desirable in patients experiencing any type of chronic pain.

The second phase in this system is use of *structural bodywork*. As the term indicates, the goals of this phase include creating some direct change in the muscles, tendons, ligaments, and viscera that compose the soft tissue of the body. The pressure applied during this phase is usually greater than during the gentle bodywork phase, with a corresponding possibility for increased soreness and a short-term increase in pain. Many patients refer to this as "good pain," comparable to that produced by strenuous exercise. The first time a sedentary person jogs, there is a likelihood of short-term soreness that becomes non-existent after a few similar runs. While all practitioners can adjust their pressure and intention to accommodate the specific needs of the patient, structural work requires enough pressure to actively create physical change in tissues. An experienced massage therapist will use her skills to relax the patient and the tissue before using this more forceful approach. Structural bodywork might include Rolfing, structural integration, neuromuscular therapy, myofascial work, Hellerwork, and Tuina.

The author's (AM) primary modality for changing structure is neuromuscular therapy (NMT) as taught by Paul St. John. We mention the particular training because there are several schools of NMT that emphasize different facets of this modality. The developer of European NMT was Stanley Lief DO, DC. Raymond Nimmo, DC, developed the American version. Two massage therapists—Paul St. John and Judith Walker Delaney—adapted this work for the massage profession and have taught thousands of therapists over the past 20-plus years, making it one of the most commonly utilized massage modalities. The goal of this style of NMT is to balance the musculature to affect a relatively neutral posture. With a neutral or balanced skeleton, the muscles need far less tension to oppose gravity. Myofascial pain and trigger points are thus positively affected *(69,70)*. The pressure is strong and focused on changing the tonus of individual muscles that are pulling a person out of a relaxed, supported posture and into one of strain. The case discussed later will illustrate how it works.

The third phase in this approach is *movement therapy*. Some of the more popular forms of movement-based therapies are the Feldenkrais method, the Alexander technique, Hellerwork, and Trager Psychophysical Integration. A basic tenet of movement therapy is that no structural bodywork will be maintained if the person has a movement organization that causes a return of the pathological pattern of muscle strain. If you initiate bending forward to brush your teeth by arching your low back you will have more discomfort than achieving the same movement with a lengthened low back. The best bodywork will be quickly undone by a person's habitual body usage.

Perhaps the most familiar of these "bad" habits are those that so many of as use when at the computer. We typically have a forward head posture, a collapsed lower back, and raised shoulders that are disconnected from any support from our rib cage. Not only is the static position uncomfortable, but the computer user typically strains inappropriate muscles to type, answer the phone, and sit straight. The levator scapula muscle strains, as it not only holds the shoulder but then tries to help lift the hand on the keyboard. The lumbar muscles are either stretched taut in a slouch or strained as they try to hold the spine erect without any help from the larger muscles of the leg and pelvis. The case report that follows will illustrate how movement re-education can help such situations.

6.1. Case Report: CJ's Journey

While some cases of integrated care will involve both conventional and CAM treatments, our first example uses only CAM modalities. The patient CJ is a middle-aged office worker who presented with a high level of low back pain (9 on a 10 point scale). She injured herself when she fell off a ladder into some bushes. She had earlier injured her back when lifting a heavy object. She could not relax nor could she get any restful sleep. Her condition was making her anxious and somewhat fearful regarding her future.

CJ was referred by an internist to a craniosacral therapist, who was able to help her relax with this treatment approach. Craniosacral therapy is generally done with the patient passive in a supine position with very light touch. CJ reported that the resulting relaxation and ability to sleep, greatly improved her condition. Her pain level was cut in half by this gentle yet powerful treatment. It only took one session. There were no adverse effects.

Craniosacral therapy (CST), with its origins in osteopathic medicine (see Chapter 15), is one type of gentle bodywork approach. Craniosacral therapy is thought to influence autonomic tone because the origins of parasympathetic division of the autonomic nervous system are located in the craniosacral regions. CST, when practiced by massage therapists, is not always designed to treat specific medical conditions, but rather to improve the health and resilience of the human body. Just as full range breathing will affect the soft tissue directly attached to the ribs as well, so does a full range craniosacral rhythm affect the dura and other soft tissue, and ultimately perhaps the whole person. It can be a safe yet powerful approach for pain reduction.

After receiving CST, CJ went on to receive acupuncture and several sessions of chiropractic care. For her to drop her protective muscular splinting was an important first step in her rapid improvement. We believe that using high force techniques from whatever modality would have been counterproductive too early in her care. Not only would they risk increasing the pain, but they would likely not deliver all the benefits that come with the relaxation response and the engagement of intrinsic healing mechanisms. A goal of this three-phase approach is to avoid forcing tension out of a muscle, but rather to convince the CNS that it no longer needs to send the signal to contract it in the first place.

At this point CJ began to see the author (AM) to help deal with ongoing low back pain issues associated with activity. Palpation revealed hypertonic, tender, low back muscles and contracted anterior leg muscles, aggravating an abnormal pelvic position. This is a classic pattern seen frequently. To help understand the effect of muscle balance on the function of the pelvis, one can visualize the pelvis as a pulley, with the anterior muscles tilting it forward and the posterior muscles tilting it backward. In CJ's case, if the muscles on the front of the pelvis and spine had less tension there would be a more neutral pelvic tilt.

The treatment involved having CJ lie supine with a pillow under her knees. Using a variety of muscle-specific gliding massage strokes and myofascial release techniques, substantial pressure was applied to lengthen the muscles and fascia of the quadriceps, adductors, tensor fascia lata, and lower psoas. In NMT, the pressure is applied through the thumbs and forearm in contrast to the whole hand as done in a Swedish massage.

Such focused techniques can achieve a dramatic softening of the lumbar curve with consequent reduction in strain when the patient stands. After just a few minutes the lumbar spine dropped to a position about half its prior distance from the table. The patient reported less discomfort, and the low back muscles were soft to the touch even though no direct contact had been made with them. The hypertonic muscles that pulled them off the table were lengthened allowing the posterior tissues to rest comfortably. Another NMT technique is to use the leg as a lever to rotate the hip to a more posterior position in relation to the sacrum. A balanced pelvis both reduces the postural factor in muscle strain and disc compression, and reduces the creation and perpetuation of myofascial trigger points. According to NMT theory all structures that are supported by a balanced, stable pelvis will be less prone to develop muscular strain patterns. This treatment reduced one more contributing factor in CJ's saga of LBP. The excess lumbar curve was directly and quickly eliminated. The lumbar muscles were softer to the touch and her weight had moved to the middle of her feet without any conscious effort. She reported her pain level as a 1 of 10.

The second session with CJ was focused more on her sitting posture. Because CJ spent most of her day sitting, movement exercises were used to educate her in ways to use her pelvis other than those she has been using. The particular style of movement therapy used, Core Integration, originated with Josef Dellagrotte, PhD, a Feldenkrais trainer who simplified the Feldenkrais process along specific pathways of movement. The intention is the same: to have the patient learn modes of body organization that will produce pain free movement and posture.

In the case of CJ the emphasis was on improved use of her pelvis in relation to her low back when sitting. Moshe Feldenkrais used the term *acture* to describe the dynamic nature of sitting as well as standing positions *(71)*. The usual response to this lesson is that it works as long as the patient remembers to use it. The lesson can be recorded on videotape—so it can be reinforced on a daily basis. It may take several weeks of consistent practice for the patient to internalize this way of sitting. It does require a motivated person to dedicate a few minutes a day to retraining old habits. It is not a question of strength or flexibility but of the organization of the part into a fluid, integrated whole.

CJ's case illustrates how one patient used multiple modalities to achieve a dramatic improvement in low back pain in a relatively linear progression. CST and acupuncture were effective when the pain was at a severe level. Once it was down to a level 3, chiropractic and NMT were very effective in producing structural change. Feldenkrais-based Core Integration movement therapy then was successful in teaching CJ more comfortable and effective ways of doing the activities of her every day life without creating more pain. The whole process took only about a dozen treatments. There were no prescription medications or other conventional interventions used. By the end of the treatment the patient was excited about starting an exercise program along with a diet to lose weight.

6.2. Case History: The Firefighter

While CJ was treated in an integrated clinic and received only CAM treatments, massage can also be integrated with conventional pain management. SW was a 64-year-old disabled firefighter who presented with constant pain and burning in his neck and shoulder that referred to his arm, and was worsened by any activity which required movement of his hand. Even reading the paper would bother his neck. His diagnosis was cervical radiculopathy. His medical history included multiple cervical traumas dating back over 15 years. MRI showed multiple herniations with osteophyte formation impinging on exiting nerve roots but not on the spinal cord. His neurologist described his condition as chronic. By the time SW was referred to the author (AM), he had received multiple epidural injections at the C5–C6 level and trigger point injections to his shoulder muscles. The frequency of injections ranged from every 4 to 8 months. They were effective in relieving his symptoms, but he was limited in how much he used his neck and shoulders. He had also been taking 200 mg of Celebrex for about 5 years.

Although retired, SW was a very active man. He took pleasure in working around the yard. His radicular pain was aggravated if he mowed the lawn, painted, or raked leaves. He couldn't do anything that required lifting his hands over his head without a sharp pain. This pain would make him stop and could take several days to subside. His posture supported a forward head and a crimped thoracic outlet.

NMT techniques helped reduce the forward head and drop his shoulders allowing more room for the brachial nerves. This simply means that the myofascial tissue that was pulling his head forward was manually lengthened to help retract his head and reposition his thorax. It was also observed that each time he lifted or reached with his hand, he compressed his neck, which required movement reeducation to resolve. Over the course of about eight sessions, movement patterns that compressed his cervical spine were identified and replaced with neck lengthening movements. Once the pattern was identified, educational movements were taught and taped for home use.

By the end of his massage therapy treatment he was without pain and able to lift his arms comfortably over his head. He not only mowed his lawn but his neighbor's lawn as well. There was one instance of a return of symptoms following a motor vehicle accident 3 months after discharge. His recovery from this trauma took ten sessions of massage therapy with no need for any other intervention. The fact that SW was very compliant with his movement regimen was a key factor in this success story. One year post-discharge, SW reported that he had experienced no need for nerve blocks or trigger point injections and he had stopped Celebrex. He continued doing 15 minutes of movement exercises each day from those that had been taped for him during his treatment.

This approach has its limitations. If a person expects the therapist to fix him and assumes no responsibility for his condition, then he will not help himself. In screening a person for movement reeducation one must clarify that there is substantial motivation for self-care. To aid thinking about appropriate situations for referral to massage therapists, see Table 2 where we offer the suggestions regarding conditions for which we have found massage and bodywork to be effective.

7. POTENTIAL MECHANISMS OF ACTION

Perhaps the most neglected area in the generally under-researched field of therapeutic massage is the issue of how massage works when it does. As we consider the question of "mechanism of action," it is worth holding two thoughts in our minds. First, all massages are not the same and thus their effects may be prompted via different mechanisms. Second, a massage treatment is a complex mix of hands-on manipulation of tissue, verbal cuing for cognitive reframing, an interpersonal therapeutic relationship, and the full complement of nonspecific effects, including both patient and practitioner

Table 2
Conditions That Can Benefit from Therapeutic Massage Techniques and Other Therapeutic Modalities*

Condition	Alternative massage and therapeutic modalities	Goals
Acute low back pain	Craniosacral therapy (CST), Swedish massage, Reiki	Relaxation, generate endorphins, reduce cortisol, reduce excess anxiety
Chronic low back pain	Deep tissue massage, Rolfing, Movement therapy (Feldenkrais, Alexander), Neuromuscular therapy (NMT)	Release of muscles pulling pelvis out of neutral alignment, release trigger points, restore functional movement patterns
Occipital neuralgia & Cervicogenic headaches	CST, NMT, Swedish massage, Myofascial release (MFR)	Release of atlanto-occipital space, relax all cervical muscles, align head with spine, restore cervical biomechanics, release fascial pull of shoulders on occiput
Spinal stenosis	NMT, CST, Myofascial release, Rolfing	Release of muscle tension 360 degrees around affected spinal segment, teach non compressive movement patterns
Tension headaches	NMT, CST, Movement therapy, Swedish	Relieve muscular stress in the cervical and trapezius areas, release trigger points
Migraine headaches	CST, NMT, Alexander	Address cranial distortions and support system for the head and neck

Condition	Modalities	Goals/Description
Carpal tunnel syndrome	Deep tissue massage, NMT, MFR	Release brachial nerve entrapment along entire path from neck to hand; identify and correct overuse patterns
Fibromyalgia (mild)	Swedish massage, CST, Reiki, NMT	Balance asymmetries in posture such as a forward head posture, kyphosis, lordosis
Fibromyalgia (severe)	CST, Reiki, Movement therapy	Relaxations of CNS, identify and correct destructive movement patterns. These would include co-contractions, habitual holding, generalized tension
Post surgical pain,	MFR, Movement therapy, Deep tissue massage,	Release of scar tissue, restore comfortable movement, correct strain patterns
Sciatica	Deep tissue massage, NMT, MFR, Movement therapy	Decompress lumbar spine, release trigger points, restore normal gait and posture
Piriformis syndrome	Deep tissue massage, NMT, Rolfing, MFR, Movement therapy	Release piriformis and external rotators, correct postural and movement strain patterns
Osteoarthritis	All types of massage as tolerated	Release muscles that compress affected joints, teach gentler non-forceful methods of performing activities of daily living (ADLs)

*This table on massage therapy and pain conditions reflects the clinical experience of this author (AM) in an integrated pain management setting. It is not meant to be exhaustive or dogmatic. There are many gifted therapists with a wide array of modalities and techniques that can be very effective in the stated pain conditions. Use this table simply as an example of at least a few therapies that have proven effective in a limited number of cases. Future research will be needed to better refine the categories and the role of any given modality in any specific pain condition.

expectations and whatever enhanced or reduced therapeutic effect the patient may come to associate with massage per se and/or that particular treatment setting. Any number of these factors may be at play in the outcome of a given massage. Part of the power of massage may well be its ability to affect a number of these simultaneously, since as one researcher has said about low back pain, it has become "clear is that chronic LBP is a dynamic, fluctuating condition with multifactorial etiology and complex pathogenesis." *(72)* This could explain part of the power of massage as an isolated treatment, as well as its contribution to integrated pain management. That said, what are some of the explanatory variables regarding the effect of massage in relation to pain management?

In the cases described above, the therapist is designing the treatment with the assumption that at least one source of pain is specific identifiable postural distortions that can be located and corrected. Improved postural alignment allowing more efficient use of muscles is one explanation that massage therapists often offer to explain why massage is effective in relieving musculoskeletal pain. This explanatory model would be applicable to both the acute and long-term improvement seen with massage. The strength and duration of this avenue of effect is likely dependent upon the training and skill of the therapist and the follow-through of the patient to maintain these changes.

Some of the improved postural alignment is achieved through purposefully stretching the connective tissue in areas where a therapist believes it has become inappropriately constricted *(73)*. Connective tissue is notoriously pliable and can become "re-modeled" through via variations in mechanical stress including overuse, under use, or simply unusual use such as repetitive motions *(74)*. Connective tissue change can prompt alterations in the muscle(s) with which it is associated. For instance, shortening of muscle fibers due to immobilization has been shown to be preceded by shortening of the associated connective tissue which responds more quickly to the lack of movement *(75)*. Langevin (see Chapter 6) has hypothesized that " ... dynamic and potentially reversible plasticity of perimuscular connective tissue plays a key role in the pathophysiology of LBP as well as in the mechanism of therapies utilizing mechanical forces (e.g. massage, chiropractic manipulation, acupuncture) ...") *(76)*. We concur with this view.

Treatment design in our case reports also included movement re-education, with the underlying assumption being that "poor" or "incorrect" use of the body is at least partially responsible for maintaining the pain whether or not it was the source of it. Every day, therapists see clients who have, over time, developed surprisingly ineffi-cient and painful ways of moving – usually involving distortions that were employed originally to protect an injury that may have long since healed. In fact, avoidance of movement associated with pain-related fear has been suggested as a contributor to chronic pain *(77–79)*. Fear of pain has been associated with both decrease in and altered patterns of movement—changes that could easily be exacerbating the pain that is feared *(80)*. It is possible that movement re-education avoids the creation of chronic pain-inducing movement patterns especially when move re-education follows pain relieving soft tissue work.

It is generally assumed among massage therapists that relaxation itself eases pain. Or said another way, tension is a generally contracted state and this contraction is itself painful and can additionally lead to musculoskeletal injury and thus increased pain. From this view, inducing relaxation is a pain relief mechanism. Whether the pain reduction is a result of neurochemical shifts or release of muscular contraction or both is unknown. It is known that massage, or perhaps any form of soothing touch, can prompt decreases in production of stress hormones such as cortisol and epinephrine, as well as increases in the substances associated with well-being such as oxytocin and serotonin. It is possible that massage eases pain via shifts in neurochemistry, or by inducing overall muscular relaxation.

Given the power of therapeutic masage to induce relaxation, decrease cortisol levels and demonstrate other signs of stress reduction, it is possible that it at least modulates pain by preventing the kind of cumulative stress that underlies allostatic load (see Chapter 2). Allostatic load is defined as "a cumulative measure of the effects of multiple stressors and the process of responding to stressors on the soma." *(81,82)*. McEwan has hypothesized that "structural plasticity in response to repeated stress starts out as an adaptive and protective response, but ends up as damage if the imbalance in the regulation of the key mediators is not resolved. It is likely that morphological rearrangements in the hippocampus brought on by various types of allostatic load alter the manner in which the hippocampus participates in memory functions and it is conceivable that these may also have a role in chronic pain perception." *(83)* The notion that touching the skin can prompt changes in the brain is a central tenet of many massage therapists' worldview. As Deane Juhan has so eloquently stated, " *Skin and brain develop from exactly the same primitive cells ... The skin is the outer surface of the brain, or the brain is the deepest layer of the skin. The skin is no more separated from the brain than the surface of the lake is separate from its depths; to touch the surface is to stir the depths." (84)*.

It is also possible that the explanatory model with which we opened this chapter, the gate control theory of pain, is effective in short-term alleviation of pain. Given that this theory relies on one sort of sensation, e.g., tactile stimulation, to override another sensation, e.g., pain, one would not expect this to be a part of long-term pain reduction.

Finally, we suggest a mechanism of action less related to tissue manipulation. Kerr has suggested that what she calls touch healing therapies (TH) may be effective in chronic pain treatment through four features that jointly encourage neural plasticity, particularly the reformation of the somatosensory cortical map *(85)*. The four attributes could all be present in a series of massage treatments. They are light tactile stimulation, a behaviorally relevant and relaxed context, repeated sessions, and directed somatosensory attention. Many forms of massage work with a light touch. Craniosacral therapy, for instance, uses a nickel weight of pressure as the norm. Certainly the massage treatment room (omplete with table, dim lighting, warmth, music, etc.) is designed to induce relaxation and the expectation of healing. Typically a therapist will direct a client's attention—sometimes to the process of relaxation, sometimes just to become aware of where pain is centered.

Many instances of chronic pain are recognized as "centrally maintained" in that there is no obvious or no remaining damage to the tissue, thus no clear nociceptive generator to account for the pain sensation. Cortical dysregulation has been associated with centrally maintained pain *(86–88)*. Studies have indicated that remodeling is possible in the somatosensory maps of adults *(89,90)*. Body maps of chronic pain patients have shown enlargement in the areas related to the painful body regions, as well as increased fragmentation and neural activity *(91–93)*. Kerr et al. hypothesize that "TH modalities work to renormalize somatotopic maps via a therapeutic plasticity mechanism"*(85)*.

Clearly there is much opportunity for researchers interested in investigating possible mechanisms of action of therapeutic massage in relation to both chronic and acute pain.

8. ORGANIZATIONAL STRUCTURES OF INTEGRATION

We believe the literature supports the use of therapeutic massage as an important component of integrated pain management. It can be paired with physical, pharmaceutical and psychotherapeutic treatments. Such integration can happen either through referral among independent practitioners, or via integration in a clinical setting. There are three common arrangements through which massage therapists work as part of a hospital-based pain management program.

8.1. The Affiliated Practitioner

The affiliated practitioner is an independent practitioner delivering therapeutic massage to patients referred on an out patient basis by hospital physicians. The practitioner bills independently for the massage therapy services. The massage therapy office may be located either within the hospital, as in the case of the author's work (AM) at Caritas Carney Hospital in Boston, or outside.

8.2. MTs as Employees

An increasing number of hospitals have massage therapists on staff. Examples include Memorial Sloan Kettering mentioned earlier and St. Luke's Hospital in Cedar Rapids, Iowa, which employs 3 full time MTs, who divide their time between a women's wellness center, oncology, and the Ob-Gyn departments. When therapists are familiar with all services of the hospital, they can be helpful in guiding healthy patients who come for a relaxation massage to other important preventive services such as mammograms and skin screenings. The manager of St. Luke's Women's Health program reports that improved patient satisfaction and offsetting income from the outpatient program justifies the addition of MT to the Hospital budget.

8.3. The Contracted Service

Some hospitals contract with outside providers, sparing themselves the issues involved in credentialing massage therapists for work in the hospital. An example is Upper Chesapeake Health Services, which operates two hospitals in Maryland and employs a private company to provide MTs to both hospital staff and inpatients. The Maryland Hospital Massage, Inc. recruits, trains, and supervises massage therapists for work in hospital settings. There is a focus on safety and adaptation for the frail and elderly patient. Massage is part of the plan-of-care for all hip and knee replacement patients as well as for all new mothers. More recently it has been added to the plan of care for pain management. Patients fill out a pain assessment form daily. When the patient reports a 4 of 10 pain level (or higher) the supervising nurse can request a massage therapy treatment. In this way they can reduce the need for pain medication and improve patient satisfaction scores. They report a 49% reduction in self-reports of pain by 986 patients. The number of patient massages increased from 50 in 2002 to 1,922 in 2004 *(94)*.

9. ISSUES OF INTEGRATION

9.1. Safety

Therapeutic massage is an unusually safe treatment. In the context of over 114 million visits per year in the United States alone, very few adverse events have been noted. A 2003 review of the literature yielded 16 adverse events, the majority of which were the result of massage performed by non-professionals *(95)*. Ernst concluded that although massage therapy is not entirely risk free, serious adverse events are a true rarity. This conclusion is also supported by the number of liability claims against massage therapists. Studdert et al. studied claims from the insurance underwriter of the American Massage Therapy Association. The AMTA provides professional liability coverage for over 50, 000 members. From 1993 to 1996 claims against massage therapists were approximately fourteen times less than that of chiropractors per 1000 insured and the average claim was $6,384 for massage therapists compared with $57,120 for chiropractic *(96)*.

9.2. Contraindications

There are few absolute contraindications to massage therapy. Most conditions are easily accommodated by a combination of regional and pressure adaptations. A person with deep vein thrombosis of the leg, for instance, might still benefit from massage at upper body sites. Although it is wise to err on the side of caution, the fact that therapeutic massage has proven to be such a safe form of therapy indicates that massage therapists are making reasonable decisions regarding questionable sites and conditions to treat.

9.3. Licensing and Credentialing Standards

As of this writing, massage therapy is licensed (or otherwise regulated) in 37 states, the District of Columbia, and four Canadian provinces. Legislation is under consideration in 10 additional states. Typical licensure requirements include successful graduation from an accredited massage school with a minimal 500 hours of classroom instruction and passage of the National Certification Exam, or some other required exam. In 1993 the National Certification Board for Therapeutic Massage and Bodywork (NCBTMB) established a national exam for entry-level massage therapists. Included in licensure is acceptance of a professional code of ethics along with standards of practice. The NCBTMB also has a review process to revoke the license of a person found violating these standards. In 2001, the American Massage Therapy Association estimated that there were between 260,000 and 290,000 massage therapists and massage students in the U.S. That was almost about double the number estimated a mere five years earlier. More than 80,000 therapists have passed the national certification exam at some point, whether or not they have maintained their certification.

9.4. What To Look For in a Massage Therapist

Basic requirements for a massage therapist working in an integrated context should include graduation from an accredited school of massage therapy, licensure and passage of the national certification exam, liability and malpractice coverage, and active record of continuing education, membership in a professional association. Experience is important in working with difficult pain conditions. An employer might require a minimum of 3 years' clinical experience along with advanced postgraduate training. A bonus would be if the therapist teaches his/her modality. In the world of bodywork, it usually is true that instructors of manual skills have a working level of mastery of the techniques they teach.

9.5. Payment

Contemporary healthcare payment practices leave alternative therapies as largely fee for service, while medication, surgery, trigger point injections, and nerve blocks are covered services. The cost of healthcare leaves many patients deciding to pay out of pocket for uncovered costs only as a last resort. Sadly, this contributes to the creation of a class-based system of healthcare. While healthcare practitioners may seek to encourage their patients to pay for therapy that can relieve pain and improve their quality of life, the real issue is a healthcare policy issue. Clearly resources should be devoted to cost/benefit analyses of particular applications of therapeutic massage. The Cherkin study, for instance, comparing massage with acupuncture and self-help information as treatments for chronic low back pain found that subjects receiving massage tended to use other healthcare services less during the year post-treatment *(97)*.

A growing trend is for major health insurance companies to advertise that they cover alternative therapy. The reality is that they will create a network of alternative therapists who are credentialed and insured. The main requirement for acceptance into the network is that the alternative provider will offer a substantial discount of 20%–25%. The insurance company actually pays nothing. Although this may appear to be good for the consumer, participation in such networks is more appealing to newer practitioners who are more willing to discount their services in order to build a practice. The old adage "you get what you pay for" is probably operative in many cases.

9.6. Research and Education

The role that MT can play in acute and chronic pain is not yet well understood. As indicated earlier, research on massage for pain relief is relatively recent, and research into mechanisms of action is virtually nonexistent. Nonetheless, the data that do exist in this area are generally positive, and millions of Americans are employing massage for pain relief every day. Purposeful integration of massage with other pain treatments is a rarity, due in part to ignorance on both sides regarding the contributions to pain relief that can be made by the "other" therapy. This leaves the patient responsible for bushwhacking the path of integration, a sad commentary on healthcare education and delivery to date. Only the combination of education for integration and research on integrated delivery models can remedy this situation.

REFERENCES

1. Melzack R, Wall PD. Pain mechanisms: a new theory. Science 1965;150:971–19.
2. Dillard JN. 2002. The Chronic Pain Solution. New York: Bantam Books.
3. Tappan FM, Benjamin PJ. 1998. Tappan's Handbook of Healing Massage Techniques, Third Edition. Stamford, CT: Appleton and Lange.
4. Rubik B, Pavek R, Ward R, et al.1994. Manual Healing Methods. In Alternative Medicine: Expanding Medical Horizons. A Report to the National Institutes of Health on Alternative Medical Systems and Practices in the United States. NIH Pub No. 94–1066.
5. Johnson DH. 1995. Bone, Breath & Gesture: Practices of Embodiment. Berkeley, CA: North Atlantic Books.
6. Downing G. 1972. The Massage Book. New York: Random House.
7. Murphy M. 1992. The Future of the Body: Explorations into the Further Evolution of Human Nature. Los Angeles: Jeremy Tarcher.
8. Eisenberg DM, Davis RB, Ettner SL, et al. Trends in alternative medicine use in the United States, 1990–1997. Results of a follow-up national survey. JAMA 1998;280:1569–1575.
9. Cherkin D, et al. Characteristics of visits to licensed acupuncturists, chiropractors, massage therapists and naturopathic physicians. J Am Board Fam Pract 2002.

10. Juhan D. 1987. Job's Body: A Handbook for Bodywork. New York: Station Hill Press.
11. Sherman K, Dixon MW, Thompson D, et al. Development of a taxonomy to describe massage treatments for musculoskeletal pain. BMC Complement Alt Med 2006;6:24.
12. Andrade C, Clifford P. 2001. Outcome-Based Massage. Philadelphia, PA: Lippincott Williams & Wilkins.
13. Kahn J, Katomski J, Schmidt D. Taxonomy of therapeutic massage and bodywork. Massage Therapy Research Consortium Presentation at North American Research Conference on Complementary and Integrative Medicine, Edmonton, Alberta, May 2006.
14. Rubik B, Pavek R, Ward R, et al. Manual Healing Methods. In Alternative Medicine: Expanding Medical Horizons. A Report to the National Institutes of Health on Alternative Medical Systems and Practices in the United States. NIH Pub No. 94–066, December 1994, pp. 113–157.
15. Walton, T The Health History of a Human Being. Massage Ther J 1999;37:70–92
16. Field TM. Massage Therapy Effects. Am Psychol 1998;53:1270–281.
17. Crawley N. A critique of the methodology of research studies evaluating massage. Eur J Cancer Care 1997;6:23–31.
18. Ernst E. Massage Therapy for Low Back Pain: A Systematic Review. J Pain Symptom Manage 1999;17:65–69.
19. Ernst E, Fialka V. The clinical effectiveness of massage therapy—a critical review. Forsch Komplementarmed 1994;1:226–232.
20. Cherkin D, Deyo RA, Sherman KJ, et al, Characteristics of visits to licensed acupuncturists, chiropractors, massage therapists and naturopathic physicians. J Am Board Fam Pract 2002;15:463–472.
21. Cherkin DC, Eisenberg D, Sherman KJ, et al. Randomized trial comparing traditional Chinese medical acupuncture, therapeutic massage, and self-care education for chronic low back pain. Arch Intern Med 2001;161:1081–1088.
22. Hernandez-Reif M, Field T, Krasnegor J, et al. Lower back pain is reduced and range of motion increased after massage therapy. Int J Neurosci 2001;106:131–145.
23. Cherkin DC, Eisenberg D, Sherman KJ, et al. Randomized trial comparing traditional Chinese medical acupuncture, therapeutic massage, and self-care education for chronic low back pain. Arch Intern Med 2001;161:1081–1088.
24. Haraldsson BG, Gross AR, Myers CD, et al. Massage for mechanical neck disorders. Cochrane Database Systematic Reviews 2006, Issue 3. Art. No.:CD004871. DOI: 10.1002/14651858. CD004871, pub3.
25. Sherman KJ, Cherkin DC, Hawkes RJ, et al. Randomized trial of therapeutic massage versus self-care book for chronic neck pain. Presented at North American Research Conference on Complementary and Integrative Medicine, Edmonton, May 23—26, 2006.
26. Perlman A, Mojica E, Williams A-L, et al. Massage therapy for osteoarthritis of the knee: results of randomized controlled trial. Presentation at North American Research Conference on Complementary and Integrative Medicine, Edmonton, May 23–26, 2006
27. Field T, Hernandez-Reif M, Seligman S, et al. Juvenile rheumatoid arthritis: benefits from massage therapy. J Pediatr Psychol 1997;22:607–617.
28. Field T, Delage J, Hernandez-Reif M. Movement and massage therapy reduces fibromyalgia pain. J Bodywork Movement Ther 2003;7:49–52.
29. Field T, Diego M, Cullen C, et al. Fibromyalgia pain and substance P decrease and sleep improves after massage therapy. J Clin Rheumatol 2002;8:72–76.
30. Sellick SM, Zaza C. Critical review of 5 non-pharmacologic strategies for managing cancer pain. Cancer Prevent Control 1998;2:7–14.
31. Lafferty WE, Downey L, Mccarty RL, et al. Evaluating CAM treatment at the end of life: a review of clinical trials for massage and meditation. Complement Ther Med 2006;12:100–112.
32. Bisset L, Paungmali A, Vicenzino B, et al. A systematic review and meta-analysis of clinical trials on physical interventions for lateral epiconylalgia. Br J Sports Med 2005;39:411–422
33. Ernst E. Manual therapies for pain control: chiropractic and massage. Clin J Pain 2004;20:8–12.
34. Bondi DM. Physical treatments for headache: a structured review. Headache 2005;45:738–746.
35. Ernst E. Musculoskeletal conditions and complementary/alternative medicine. Best Pract Res Clin Rhematol 2004;8:539–556.
36. Wilson JJ, Best TM. Common overuse tendon problems: a review and recommendations for treatment. Am Fam Physician 2005;72: 811–818.
37. Fernandez-de-Las-Penas C, Alonso-Blanco C, Duadrado ML, et al. Are manual therapies effective in reducing pain from tension-type headache? a systematic review. Clin J Pain 2006;22:278–285.

38. Cherkin DC, Sherman KJ, Deyo RA, et al. A review of the evidence for the effectiveness, safety, and cost of acupuncture, massage therapy and spinal manipulation for back pain. Ann Intern Med 2003;138:898–906.

39. Van Tulder MW, Furlan AD, Gagnier JJ. Complementary and alternative therapies for low back pain. Best Pract Res Clin Rhematol 2005;19:639–654.

40. Weinrich SP, Weinrich MC. The effect of massage on pain in cancer patients. Appl Nurs 1990;3:140–145.

41. Post-White J, Kinney ME. The effects of therapeutic massage and healing touch on cancer patients. Presented at First Int'l Symposium on the Science of Touch, Montreal May 2002.

42. Cassileth BR, Vickers AJ. Massage therapy for symptom control: outcome study at a major cancer center. J Pain Symptom Manage 2004;28:244–249.

43. Corbin L. Safety and efficacy of massage therapy for patients with cancer. Cancer Cotnrol 2005;12:158–164.

44. Uvnas-Moberg K. 2003. The Oxytocin Factor: Tapping the Hormone of Calm, Love and Healing. Cambridge, MA: Da Capo Press.

45. Uvnas-Moberg K, Petersson M. Oxytocin, a mediator of anti-stress, well-being, social interaction, growth and healing. Z Psychosom Med Psychother 2005;51:57—80.

46. Field, F. Massage therapy effects. Am Psychol 1998a;53:1270–1281.

47. Moyer CA, Rounds J, Hannum JW. A meta-analysis of massage therapy research. Psychol Bull 2004;130:3–18.

48. Meek SS. Effects of slow stroke back massage on relaxation in hospice clients. Image J Nurs Sch 1993;25:17–21.

49. Fakouri C, Jones P. Relaxation Rx: slow stroke back rub. J Gerontol Nurs 1987;13:32–35.

50. Reed BV, Held JM. Effects of sequential connective tissue massage on autonomic nervous system of middle-aged and elderly adults. Phys Ther 1988;68:1231–1234.

51. Ernst E. Does post-exercise massage treatment reduce delayed onset muscle soreness? A systematic review. Br J Sports Med 1998;32:212–214.

52. Bell AJ. Massage and the physiotherapist. Physiotherapy 1964;50:406–408.

53. Hovind H, Nielsen SL. Effect of massage on blood flow in skeletal muscle. Scand J Rehabil Med 1974;6:74–77.

54. Shoemaker JK, Tiidus PM, Mader R. Failure of manual massage to alter limb blood flow: measures by Doppler ultrasound. Med Sci Sports Exerc 1997;29:610–614.

55. Tiidus PM. Shoemaker JK. Effleurage massage, muscle blood flow and long-term post-exercise strength recovery. Int J Sports Med 1995;16:478–483.

56. Braverman DL, Schulman RA. Massage techniques in rehabilitation and medicine. Phys Med Rehabil Clin N Am 1999;10:631–649.

57. Vickers A, Ohlsson A, Lacy JB, Horsley A. Massage for promoting growth and development of preterm and/or low birthweight infants. Cochrane Database Syst Rev 2000;(2):CD00390.

58. Vickers A, Ohlsson A, Lacy JB, Horsley A. Massage for promoting growth and development of preterm and/or low birthweight infants. Cochrane Database Syst Rev 2004;(2):CD000390.

59. Diego MA, Field T, Hernandez-Reif M. Vagal activity, gastric motility and weight gain in massaged preterm neonates. J Pediatr 2005;147:P50–P55.

60. Lee HK. The effect of infant massage on weight gain, physiological and behavioral responses in premature infants. Taehan Kanho Hakhoe Chi 2005;35:1451–1460.

61. Smith MC, Kemp J, Hemphill L, et al. Outcomes of massage therapy for cancer patients. J Nurs Scholarship 2002;34:257–262.

62. Escalona A, Field T, Singer-Strunck R, et al. Brief report: improvements in the behavior of children with autism following massage therapy. J Autism Dev Disord 2001;31:513–516.

63. Hernandez-Reif M, Field T, Krasnegor J, et al. Lower back pain is reduced and range of motion increased after massage therapy. Int J Neurosci 2001;106:131–145.

64. Chen ML, Lin LC, Wu SC, et al. The effectiveness of acupressure in improving the quality of sleep of institutionalized residents. Gerontol A Biol Sci Med Sci 1999;54:M389–M394.

65. Field T, Hernandez-Reif M, Hart S, et al. Pregnant women benfit from massage therapy. J Psychosom Obstet Gynaecol 1999;20:31–38.

66. Richards KC. Effects of a back massage and relaxation intervention on sleep in critically ill patients. Am J Crit Care 1998;7:288–299.

67. Field T, Morrow C, Valdeon C, et al. Massage reduces anxiety in child and adolescent psychiatric patients. J Am Acad Child Adolescent Psychiatry 1992;31:125–131.

68. Field T, Hernandez-Reif M. Cortisol decreases and serotonin and dopamine increase following massage therapy. Int J Neurosci 2005;115:1397–1413.
69. Travell J, Simons D. 1992. Myofascial Pain and Dysfunction: The Trigger Point Manual. Philadelphia, PA: Williams & Wilkins.
70. Kendall FP, McCreary EK. 1983. Muscle Testing and Function. Fourth edition. Philadelphia, PA: Williams & Wilkins.
71. Shafarman S. 1997. Awareness Heals: The Feldenkrais Method for Dynamic Health. New York, NY: Perseus Books.
72. Langevin H, unpublished manuscript and personal conversation. February 2006.
73. Barnes JK. 2004. Myofascial Release: The Missing Link in Traditional Treatment, in Complementary Therapies in Rehabilitation. Second Edition. Davis CM, Ed. New Jersey: SLACK Incorporated.
74. Cummings GS, Tillman LJ. 1992. Remodeling of dense connective tissue in normal adult tissues. In Dynamics of Human Biologic Tissues: Contemporary perspectives in rehabilitation. Currier DP, Nelson RM, Eds. Philadelphia, PA: F.A. Davis.
75. Williams PE, Goldspink G. Connective tissue changes in immobilised muscle. J Anat 1984;138: 343–350.
76. Langevin H, unpublished manuscript and personal conversation February 2006.
77. Hurwitz EL, Morgenstern H, Chiao C. Effects of recreational physical activity and back exercises on low back pain and psychological distress: findings from the UCLA Low Back Pain Study. Am J Public Health 2005 95:1817–1824.
78. Grotle M, Vollestad NK, Veierod MB, et al. Fear-avoidance beliefs and distress in relation to disability in acute and chronic low back pain. Pain 2004;112:343–352.
79. Swinkels-Meewisse IEJ, Roelofs J, Oostendorp RAB, et al. Acute low back pain: pain-related fear and pain catastrophizing influence physical performance and perceived disability. Pain 2006;120:36–43.
80. Moseley GL, Nicholas MK, Hodges PW. Does anticipation of back pain predispose to back trouble? Brain 2004;127:2339–2347.
81. Goldstein DS, McEwan B. Allostasis, homeostats and the nature of stress. Stress 2002;5:55–58.
82. Stewart JA. The detrimental effects of allostasis: allostatic load as a measure of cumulative stress. J Physiol Anthropol 2006;25:133–145.
83. McEwan B. 2001. Plasticity of the Hippocampus: Adaptation to Chronic Stress and Allostatic Load. In: Role of Neural Plasticity in Chemical Intolerance. Soyg BA, Bell IB, Eds. New York, NY: New York Academy of Sciences.
84. Juhan D. 1987. Job's Body: A Handbook for Bodywork. New York: Station Hill Press.
85. Kerr CE, Wasserman RH, Moore CI. Cortical Plasticity as a Therapeutic Mechanism for Touch Healing. Unpublished Manuscript.
86. Treede R, Kenshalo DR, Gracely RH, et al. The cortical representation of pain. Pain 1999;79:105–111.
87. Price D. Central neural mechanisms that interrelate sensory and affective dimensions of pain. Mol Intervent 2002;2:392–403.
88. Flor H. Cortical reorganization and chronic pain: implications for rehabilitation. J Rehabil Med 2003;41:66–72.
89. Pascual-Leone A, Torres F. Plasticity of the sensorimotor cortex representation of the reading finger in Braille readers. Brain 1993;116:39–52.
90. Wall J, Kass JH, Sur M, et al. Functional reorganization in somatosensory cortical areas 3b and 1 of adult monkeys after median nerve repair: possible relationships to sensory recovery in humans. J Neurosci 1986;6:218–233.
91. Flor H, Braun C, Elbert T et al. Extensive reorganization of primary somatosensory cortex in chronic back pain patients. Neurosci Lett 1997;224:5–8.
92. Flor H, Elbert T, Knecht S, et al. Phantom-limb pain as a perceptual correlate of cortical reorganization following arm amputation. Nature 1995;375:482–484.
93. Maihofner C, Handwerker HO, Neundorfer B, et al. Patterns of cortical reorganization in complex regional pain syndrome. Neurology 2003;61:1707–1715.
94. Creighton M. Massage benefits patients at Maryland hospital. Massage Magazine, January 2006.
95. Ernst E. The safety of massage therapy. Rhematol 2003;42:1101–1106.
96. Studdert DM, Eisenberg DM, Miller FH, et al. Medical malpractice implications of alternative medicine. JAMA 1998;280:1610–1615.
97. Cherkin DC, Eisenberg D, Sherman KJ, et al. Randomized trial comparing traditional Chinese medical acupuncture, therapeutic massage, and self-care education for chronic low back pain. Arch Intern Med 2001;161:1081–1088.

18 Acupuncture in Pain Management

David Wang and Joseph F. Audette

CONTENTS

Summary

Acupuncture is a system of treatment which involves the insertion of thin, solid needles into specific areas of the body known as acupuncture points, or acupoints, with the intention of positively affecting a patient's clinical condition or health status. In recent decades, the integration of the Western scientific model has provided novel means of furthering our understanding of acupuncture and its effects. Of all the complementary and alternative therapies, acupuncture is one of the best researched. Since the National Institute of Health Consensus Statement on Acupuncture, published in 1997, there has been a flood of high-quality randomized controlled clinical trials as well as a much broader investigation into the basic mechanisms of acupuncture. This chapter will define the various mechanisms by which acupuncture is believed to operate, both from traditional naturalistic and modern scientific contexts. A brief historical narrative will bridge the two approaches as they have flourished over different periods of time. An evidence-based review of the potential uses of acupuncture for various pain conditions will follow, along with discussions regarding acupuncture safety and its incorporation into a integrative pain management practice.

Key Words: acupuncture, pain, osteoarthritis, tendonitis, back pain traditional Chinese medicine

1. BACKGROUND

Acupuncture is a system of treatment which involves the insertion of thin, solid needles into specific areas of the body known as acupuncture points, or acupoints, with the intention of positively affecting a patient's clinical condition or health status. This

From: *Contemporary Pain Medicine: Integrative Pain Medicine: The Science and Practice of Complementary and Alternative Medicine in Pain Management*
Edited by: J. F. Audette and A. Bailey © Humana Press, Totowa, NJ

simple definition somewhat belies the intricately sophisticated and subtle nature of a therapeutic modality that has been developed over thousands of years. Acupuncture, in its original form, was based on observation and contemplation of the natural world and its forces; and how the interaction of these forces within the human being could manifest in wellness or illness. In recent decades, the integration of the Western scientific model has provided novel means of furthering our understanding of acupuncture and its effects, albeit from a distinctly different philosophical construct.

This chapter will define the various mechanisms by which acupuncture is believed to operate, both from traditional naturalistic and modern scientific contexts. A brief historical narrative will bridge the two approaches as they have flourished over different periods of time. An evidence-based review of the potential uses of acupuncture for various pain conditions will follow, along with discussions regarding acupuncture safety and its role in a integrative pain management practice.

2. CLASSICAL THEORY

In order to understand how acupuncture can be used for the management of pain, it helps to understand its theoretical underpinnings. Different from Western allopathic medicine, where the symptomatic presentation of pain is often treated via a medication or a procedure, traditional Chinese medicine (acupuncture and Chinese herbal formulas) treats the individual by focusing on the root cause of why the patient cannot heal. Traditional Chinese medicine (TCM) is tailored to the individual and not necessarily the disease, with the goal being to treat the root cause of the symptoms. The diagnostic methods used to find the cause of disease require a rudimentary understanding of the basis of TCM theory.

2.1. Yin-Yang: Eight Principal Patterns

Classic Chinese medical theory is rooted in the principle that the entire universe is in a dynamic state of balance between two opposing forces, known as yin and yang. Yin is characterized by such conditions as soft, dark, cold, lower, passive, nourishing, and still. Yang is the opposite of yin, and described as hard, bright, hot, upper, dominant, consuming, and active. As evident in the visual representation of yin and yang, which together are known as tai ji, (Grand Ultimate—see Figure 1), there is always a trace of yang within yin, and a trace of yin within yang. This allows for the dynamic transition from one state to another as yin and yang move and mix with one another. In traditional Chinese medicine, these two forces are subdivided into the eight principal patterns: yin and yang, interior and exterior, deficiency and excess, and cold and hot.

2.2. The Three Treasures: Qi, Jing, and Shen

Life itself is created through the interaction of yin and yang, which manifests as Qi (pronounced "chee"). Qi literally means steam (for example the steam coming from a rice pot) or breath, but is generally interpreted as vital energy and connects yin and yang together as the source of all movement. There are actually several different types of Qi with various functions within the body, including protection, nourishment, warmth, creation of blood, support of the organs, and condensation into jin (essence). Jin is subsequently converted into shen (spirit), and together these three vital substances of Qi, Jing, and Shen, known as the Three Treasures, are responsible for maintaining the health of body, mind, and emotions.

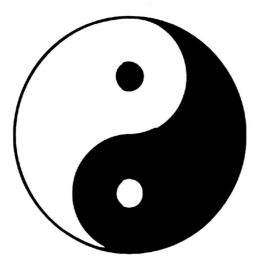

Fig. 1 The Grand Ultimate (太极拳) or yin and yang symbol.

2.3. The Five Phases

The Five Phases (or Elements) theory was integrated into Chinese medicine during the Song dynasty (960–1279 CE), and provides a way of adapting the principles of yin and yang to a more clinically relevant model. The Five Phases are metal, water, wood, fire, and earth; with each phase manifesting a yin and yang quality. The phases relate to one another through a productive or creative cycle and a destructive or controlling cycle (Figure 2). Each of the phases is associated with a set of characteristics, such as a unique color, season, direction, taste, odor, sound, and emotion. Within a clinical framework, each of the Five Phases relates to a paired yin/yang organ system: metal to lungs/large intestine, water to kidneys/bladder, wood to liver/gallbladder, fire to heart/small intestine, and earth to spleen/stomach. There is also a sixth yin/yang organ pair known as pericardium/triple warmer, which also corresponds to fire. Some of the functions of these organs are quite different from those defined in conventional anatomy and physiology, with the triple warmer embodying an organ function that is unique to Chinese medicine.

2.4. Meridians and Acupoints

Qi flows through the body constantly as it supports the functions necessary for life. This flow is concentrated along specific channels, called meridians, which course throughout the body. Classic Chinese medical theory has defined 14 main meridians: one for each of the six yin and six yang organs which run bilaterally along the extremities and trunk, and two extraordinary meridians which run along the midline of the body anteriorly (called the conception vessel) and posteriorly (called the governing vessel). There are numerous points located along these meridians which, when stimulated properly, are believed to have particularly significant effects on regulating the flow of Qi. The insertion and manipulation of needles into these points was developed over time as a method of Qi regulation, and thus the discipline of acupuncture was created. Classically, there are 361 points along the 14 main meridians (Figure 3). Modern nomenclature identifies the acupoints by number as they travel along the course of the meridian—Stomach 36 or Bladder 67, for example. In addition, a myriad

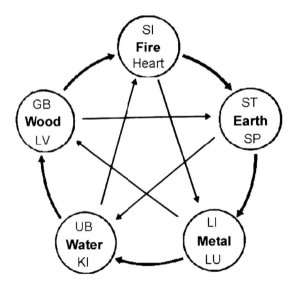

Fig. 2. Five Phases Creation and Control Cycle and its relationship to the relationships of the internal organs. The arrows on the circumference denote the creation cycle and the arrows within the circle indicate the control cycle (SI, Small Intestine; ST, Stomach, SP, Spleen/Pancrease; LI, Large Intestine; LU, Lung; UB, Urinary Bladder; KI, Kidney; GB, Gallbladder; LV, Liver).

of other meridians and points have been identified through the development of multiple styles of acupuncture, as described in a later section. When considering these additional points, the total number is in excess of 2000, although the average acupuncturist may be routinely familiar with only 150 acupoints (1). In traditional Chinese medicine teachings, proper needling technique involves manipulation of the needle (such as

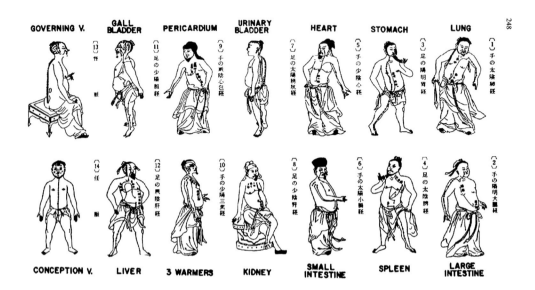

Fig. 3. Acupuncture meridians.

pecking, twirling, and flicking) after insertion until the patient feels a characteristic sensation of soreness, heaviness, and/or tingling—a phenomenon known as *de Qi*, which literally means *to acquire Qi*.

Modern applications of acupuncture include electroacupuncture (introducing small electrical currents at varying frequencies through inserted needles) and laser acupuncture (applying red or infrared monochromatic light in the 600–1000-nm-wavelength range to acupoints). Acupuncture is only one therapeutic modality employed in the practice of Chinese medicine. Other methods of point stimulation include moxibustion (burning small amounts of the herb *Artemisia vulgaris*) in order to induce a localized heating effect to a particular acupoint or body region, cupping (using special glass cups to apply a gentle vacuum), usually to the back, in order to draw out stagnant blood and Qi, and the prescription of herbal remedies.

The classic Chinese medical model synthesizes all of the above concepts to formulate a diagnosis based ultimately on the balance of yin and yang. For example, an individual may have a diagnosis of excess wind invading the lung, which describes a condition of wind coming from the exterior, as defined by the Eight Principal Patterns. In contrast, someone with a yin deficiency of the kidneys would demonstrate wind coming from the interior. Once these imbalances in Qi are identified, they can then be corrected by the appropriate application of acupuncture on specified points along the body's meridians to bring the yin-yang balance back into dynamic homeostasis. This lexicon is at once unfamiliar and complex, yet represents a well-defined and systematized philosophy that can guide clinicians practicing within this framework to provide a holistic treatment aimed at optimizing the health of the living being.

3. HISTORICAL BACKGROUND

The exact historical origins of acupuncture are unknown, and there continues to be debate regarding its inception and development *(2)*. However, many scholars believe that acupuncture was originally developed in China during the first few centuries BCE, with influences stemming from multiple sources *(1)*. What is commonly accepted as the earliest evidence of acupuncture practiced in an organized and codified manner is embodied in the *Huangdi Neijing*, or *Inner Classic of the Yellow Emperor* (often translated as the *Yellow Emperor's Classic of Internal Medicine*). This text has been dated to the Han dynasty, sometime between 200 and 100 BCE, depending on the historical reference *(3)*. The classic text has two parts; the Su Wen (Plain Questions) and the Ling Shu (Spiritual Pivot), each 81 chapters long. The *Neijing* contains discussions between the mythical yellow emperor and his chief physician Chi Po on a wide range of topics, including the theories of yin-yang and the five elements, diet, acupuncture, moxibustion, and blood letting. Several key texts were written over the next several hundred years which further refined the theory and practice of acupuncture within the context of Chinese medicine. These texts included the *Nanjing* (*Classic of Difficult Issues,* first or second century CE), *Zhen-jiu Da-cheng* (*Great Compendium of Acupuncture and Moxibustion*, 1601), and *Yizong jin jian* (*Golden Mirror of Medicine,* 1742), among many others.

The socioeconomic and political environment had a major impact on the status of acupuncture throughout its more recent history. Foreign trade between China and other

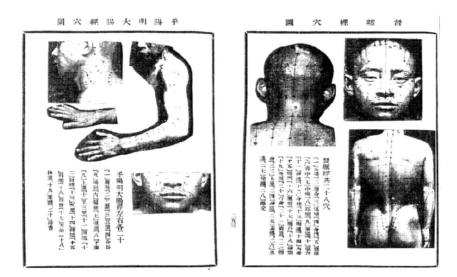

Fig. 4. Meridians precisely drawn on live human bodies for the first time by Cheng Dan'an in 1930 from *Chinese Acupuncture and Moxibustion Therapeutics.*

countries, including Japan, Korea, France, and Britain, opened avenues of communication that led to the gradual development of discrete systems of acupuncture within each country (see below). However, within China itself, the attitude toward acupuncture was becoming more disdainful. Because acupuncture was often practiced by the old and illiterate, it was seen as lower-class. Those who sought to modernize China regarded acupuncture as obsolete and superstitious *(4)*. Then in 1932, Cheng Dan'an, a Chinese physician educated in Western anatomy and physiology, published the *Zhongguo zhenjiu zhiliaoxue (Chinese Acupuncture and Moxibustion Therapeutics)*. Within this text he redefined acupuncture points and meridians to correlate more closely with peripheral nerve distributions (Figure 4), thereby returning credibility to a nearly lost art in the eyes of a rapidly modernizing country. During the 1960s and 1970s, acupuncture prospered as part of the Chinese Cultural Revolution *(4)*. In 1974, China invited President Nixon and the United States press core to witness and experience acupuncture therapy firsthand. This led to the first published American medical accounts on the use of acupuncture in pain management *(5,6)*.

4. ACUPUNCTURE STYLES

As a result of these cultural and historical influences, a multitude of different acupuncture styles have been developed. They are commonly differentiated by the country of origin, for example traditional Chinese medicine (TCM) versus Japanese versus French, and so on. There are also systems of acupuncture called microsystems, which are used to treat the entire body while only needling specific areas, such as the scalp, ear, or hand (Figure 5) *(1)*. These classic styles all have some differences in the specific locations of meridians and acupoints, as well as the rationale for their use. However, they all share the common principles of yin-yang balance and regulating Qi within a network of energetic meridians. In contrast, the modern development of Western acupuncture is based on a progressive scientific understanding of anatomy

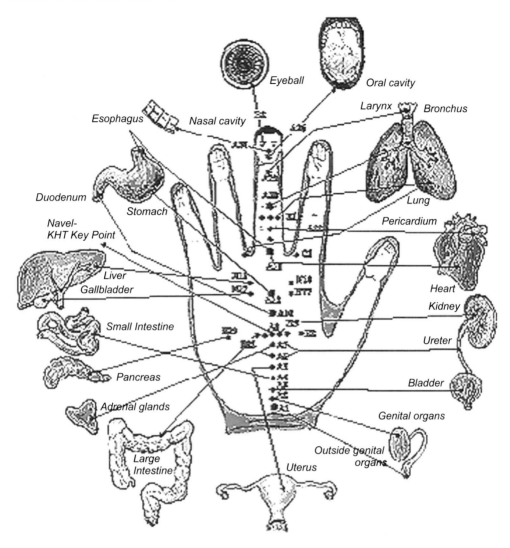

Fig. 5. Korean hand acupuncture montage illustrates the variety of clinical methods utilized both in the United States and around the world. This is a microsystem commonly used by Korean acupuncturist. Often these points would not be needled, but rather heated by burning a combustible herb, mugwort. This technique of heating points by burning mugwort is called moxibustion.

and physiology combined with a growing body of clinical research (see Table 1 for a summary of acupuncture styles).

5. MECHANISMS

Recent research on the basic physiologic mechanisms of acupuncture has generated several different theories to describe the nature of how acupuncture produces its observed clinical effects.

5.1. Neurochemical

Numerous studies have identified a host of different neurochemical mediators that are affected by acupuncture. Those which affect pain have received particular attention,

Table 1
Basic Characteristics of Several Major Styles of Acupuncture

Acupuncture style	*Basic characteristics*
Traditional Chinese Medicine (TCM)	Point selection often formulaic once diagnosis is made using a combination of history, pulse, and tongue diagnosis. Classically, aggressive needle twisting, thrusting and pulling methods are used to elicit the de Qi response. Electroacupuncture and herbal therapy are frequently used in conjunction with manual needling techniques.
Japanese	More meridian based with use of five-phase theory to guide point selection and palpatory methods to guide diagnosis. Strongly influenced by Chinese texts written in the Han dynasty (206 BC–220 AD). Moxabustion used frequently in addition to needles. Needle technique tends to be minimally invasive with more of a pecking style rather than needle twisting.
Korean	A combination of TCM and Japanese methods.
French	Energetic system with the body divided into different zones and point selection determined by the zone in which the pathology presents. Strongly influenced by the Vietnamese.
British	Five- phases theory as developed by Worsley common.
Ear (Auricular)	A microsystem where the whole body is represented in the ear. Distinct schools developed in France, Germany and China.
Scalp	Frequently used for neurological conditions with distinct schools that have developed in China and Japan.
Hand	A microsystem frequently used by Korean practitioners. Moxabustion rather than needle stimulation common.
Western	Often a combination of a number of styles with a strong foundation in TCM.

with early research focusing on the endogenous opioid system, and more recent discoveries elucidating the role of the cFos gene and its role in the maladaptive neuroplasticity seen in the central nervous system in chronic pain. Table 2 summarizes the effects of acupuncture on these various mechanisms.

5.1.1. Opioid Effects

Han has written an important review on the progression of our understanding about acupuncture's effects on the endogenous opioid peptide system *(7)*. Previous studies on the naloxone-reversibility of acupuncture analgesia had produced contradictory results regarding the influence of low versus high-frequency electroacupuncture (EA). Some studies suggested that only low frequency EA caused release of opioid neuropeptides

Table 2
Neurochemical Mechanisms Affected by Acupuncture

Mechanism affected	Functions	Location (of action)	Effect of acupuncture
Opioid B-Endorphin	Mixed m- and d-opioid-mediated analgesia	Periaqueductal gray, Arcuate nucleus of hypothalmus, nucleus accumbens, amygdala, nucleus caudatus	Increased release by low-frequency EA (2 Hz)*
Enkephalin	Mixed m- and d-opioid-mediated analgesia	Spinal cord	Increased release by low-frequency EA (2 Hz)*
Endomorphin	m-opioid-mediated analgesia		Increased release by low-frequency EA (2 Hz)*
Dynorphin	k-opioid-mediated analgesia	Spinal cord	Increased release by high-frequency EA* (100 Hz)
Neuronal nitric oxide synthase (nNOS)/ NADPH diaphorase (NADPHd)	Analgesia, sympathetically mediated cardiovascular effects (vasodilation) and somatosympathetic reflex activity	Gracile nucleus in dorsal medulla	Up-regulation by low-frequency EA*
GABA	May play role in attenuating Dopamine release	Cortico-striatal circuitry	Enhanced release with EA*
Epinephrine	Sympathomimetic	Paragiganto-cellularreticular nucleus	Variable effect
Cortisol		Variable effect	
Norepinephrine	Sympathomimetic, descending pain modulation in Dorsal Horn	Locus ceruleus, lateral tegmental area, (raphe magnus)	Decreased levels in brain, increased levels in spinal cord

(Continued)

Table 2
(Continued)

Mechanism affected	Functions	Location (of action)	Effect of acupuncture
Serotonin	Post-synaptic inhibition, modulates pain, mood, sleep, arousal, cognition	(Periaqueductal gray,) raphe magnus, medulla	Enhanced serotonin synthesis
Acetylcholine	May inhibit sensory response of thalamus	Caudate nucleus	Increased release
Dopamine	Involved in the reward response characteristic found in addiction	Nucleus accumbens	Abrogated by acupuncture
cFos gene	Activated after noxious peripheral stimulation and couples transient intracellular signals to long term changes in gene expression in the CNS	Second and third order neurons in CNS in pain pathway	Decreased expression

* Electroacupuncture

in the central nervous system, while Hokfelt hypothesized that this only occurred at high-frequency EA. Han et al. later discovered that both low- and high-frequency EA analgesia could be blocked by naloxone in a dose-dependent manner. Further confirmatory research demonstrated that 2 Hz EA increased met-enkephalin levels sevenfold but did not affect dynorphin. In contrast, 100 Hz EA produced a twofold increase in the release of dynorphin but not met-enkephalin. EA of 15 Hz produced a partial activation of both enkephalins and dynorphins. b-Endorphin and endomorphin have been shown to share similar release profiles as enkephalin to 2 Hz stimulation (Figure 6). This leaves dynorphin as the only opioid peptide responsive to high-frequency stimulation. From a clinical standpoint, the above studies have led to the common use of 3-second intervals of alternating 2- and 100-Hz EA, known as "dense and disperse mode" (DD mode), which has been shown to maximize the analgesic effect (7).

5.1.2. Neuronal Nitric Oxide Synthase (nNOS) and Nitric Oxide (NO)

Ma's review discusses the evidence that NO acts to attenuate the sympathetic nervous system (and possibly somatic and visceral pain) via the gracile nucleus and thalamus, and that this mechanism may be influenced by EA (8). NO is formed from arginine through a reaction catalyzed by nNOS. The gracile nucleus, located in the dorsal medulla, responds to excitatory somatosympathetic reflexes, some of which originate from somatosensory nociceptive afferents projecting from the hindlimb. This may explain in part why acupuncture at a distal point on an extremity can affect systemic functions. Chen and Ma (9) strengthened this notion by demonstrating that rat cardiac responses to EA at the Stomach (ST) 36 acupoint (located on the pretibial region of the lower extremity) can be affected by injection of lidocaine, L-arginine, and nNOS antisense oligos into the gracile nucleus. Another study has shown that in addition to

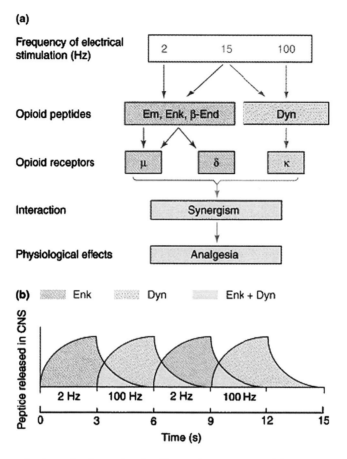

Fig. 6. Possible mechanisms for the analgesic effects of acupuncture. (a) Opioid peptides and opioid receptors involved in analgesia elicited by electroacupuncture of different frequencies. Opioids and receptors involved at 2 Hz and at 100 Hz. At 15 Hz, there is a partial involvement of components involved at both of the other two frequencies. Abbreviations: Dyn, dynorphin A; β-End, β-endorphin; Em, endomorphin; Enk, enkephalins. (b) Model for the synergistic analgesic effect produced by alternating low and high frequency stimulation (reproduced with permission from *(63)*).

ST36, low-frequency EA (3 Hz) at Bladder 64 and 65 on the hindlimb induces nNOS expression in the gracile nucleus. Ma further states that "the gracile nucleus–thalamic pathways are responsible for EA signal transduction, with NO playing an important role in the mediation of neuronal activities and therapeutics elicited by EA at ST36."

5.2. Neuromodulatory

The recent advent of increasingly sophisticated imaging techniques, particularly positron emission tomography (PET) and functional magnetic resonance imaging (fMRI), has provided a new and promising method of non-invasive analysis into the physiologic effects of acupuncture. Numerous studies have documented significant changes in brain activity after stimulation of various acupoints, which are often located on distal extremities. Lewith et al. published a systematic review in 2005, discussing the findings of 22 studies (4 PET and 18 fMRI) cited between 1997 and 2005 *(10)*.

5.2.1. Imaging in Non-Pain-Related Conditions

In one of the first functional imaging studies, Cho et al. discovered that stimulation of the vision-related acupoint Bladder 67 resulted in activation of the visual cortex in a pattern similar to that induced by shining a light into the eyes. These findings have been supported by the work of a number of other studies. Yoo et al. demonstrated that stimulation of Pericardium 6, a point commonly used in treating nausea, caused a consistent activation of specific areas in the left superior frontal gyrus, anterior cingulate gyrus, dorsomedial nucleus of the thalamus, and cerebellum, which did not occur with sham needling of a non-acupuncture point *(11)*. Yan et al. found that needling Large Intestine 4 and Liver 3 separately activated areas of the temporal lobe, cerebellum, middle temporal, and posterior cingulate gyrii, while simultaneously deactivating the middle and inferior frontal gyrii, anterior and posterior cingulate gyrii, inferior parietal lobule, and Broca's areas 8, 9, 17, 18, and 45 as compared to sham points *(12)*. All of these studies suggest that the verum points have a more specific effect on brain activity than sham points.

5.2.2. Imaging in Pain-Related Conditions

Lewith et al. subsequently reviewed several studies that elucidate the non-specific pain-related patterns of neural activation provoked by both real and sham acupuncture *(10)*. One particular experiment by Wu et al. *(13)* compared fMRI changes in brain activation of electroacupuncture, mock electroacupuncture, minimal acupuncture and sham electroacupuncture. Electroacupuncture caused a distinct activation pattern in the hypothalamus, primary somatosensory motor cortex and rostral anterior cingulate cortex. However, minimal electroacupuncture and sham electroacupuncture, and real electroacupuncture all induced non-specific activation of the superior temporal gyrus and medial occipital cortex. The effects of placebo and expectation were examined by Wager et al., who found that anticipation of pain resulted in increased activity within the thalamus, insula and anterior cingulate cortex, whereas the expectation of pain relief from placebo caused decreased activity in these same regions *(14)*. These studies indicate that there is considerable overlap between the regions of the brain that are affected by placebo, expectation and true acupuncture (see Chapter 4). Pariente et al. has found that verum acupuncture also stimulates the *ipsilateral* insula in patients with pain secondary to osteoarthritis. This finding is contrary to our conventional understanding of neuroanatomy in which the spinothalamic tract, which transmits pain and temperature sensation and presumably the sensations related to acupuncture stimulation, crosses over to the *contralateral* side, usually at the spinal level superior to the level of stimulation *(10)*. There are a number of possible explanations for this finding; the brain can become sensitized and activate in response to sensory input in a more diffuse way in chronic pain states (see Chapter 4), but the ipsilateral activation pattern could also suggest a yet undefined neural pathway which may be uniquely activated by acupuncture stimulation.

Lewith et al. conclude their review by suggesting that there may be noteworthy differences in the specificity of the neural response of acupuncture points used for painful versus non-painful indications. Studies that involved the needling of *non-pain*-related acupoints, such as Pericardium 6 used for nausea, have shown more consistent and specific locations of brain activation than pain studies. In contrast, both real and sham acupoint stimulation *in studies of pain* have resulted in a more non-specific pattern of brain activation. This lack of specificity may explain the non-specific clinical effects of sham acupuncture, as described in several studies which are reviewed in the following section.

5.3. Acupuncture and the Fascia

The connective tissue or fascia envelops and invests the entire body, with multiple interconnecting planes running throughout the muscles, tendons, ligaments, and viscera. The neurovascular supply to the various organs and muscles also lie within the fascia. Myofascial pain syndrome (MPS) is thought to be a complex dysfunction of the central nervous system and the muscle and fascia characterized by four clinical features: *(1)* a tight band of muscle which is palpable on examination, *(2)* localized point tenderness within this tight band (the myofascial trigger point (MTrP)), *(3)* a specific pattern of referred pain reproduced with pressure on the trigger point, and *(4)* a local twitch response (LTR) within the muscle with snapping palpation of the trigger point *(15)*. Conventional treatment of MPS involves hyperstimulation analgesia of MTrP regions by various methods, including dry needling, intense cooling or heating, or chemical stimulation to the skin. As such, pain relief through hyperstimulation can be explained by the gate control theory of pain *(16)*; however, recent advances in understanding the underlying biochemical milieu in the fascia surrounding the muscle suggest alternative mechanisms (see Chapter 5).

With regard to acupuncture correlations, Dr. Sun Si Miao of the Tang Dynasty (618–907 CE) developed the principle of *ah shi points*, which are local sites of soreness or pressure representing active acupoints *(16)*. The Japanese and German traditions have also noted these nodularities within the fascia and have called them *kori* and *myogeloses* respectively. These areas of hyperirritability can be needled regardless of whether they are on a defined meridian or not, and may represent focal areas within the fascia that have become sensitized in a way that is similar to the process of peripheral and central sensitization that has been suggested by Shah et al. *(17)* to cause the development of an active MTrP (see Chapter 5). Palpation of these areas will often reveal not only mechanical hyperalgesia (enhanced sensitivity to deep pressure) but even signs of allodynia (enhanced sensitivity to light touch). Such points are called *active points* to distinguish them from acupuncture points that may be less effective in a particular individual. In 1977, Melzack *(18)* reported a 77% correspondence between locations of acupoints and MTrPs. More recently, Kao and colleagues *(19)* demonstrated by needle electromyography of normal human volunteers that there were significantly more endplate noise (EPN) loci at the Stomach 36 acupoint region than at nearby non-acupoint control regions. Furthermore, the needle always elicited an unpleasant sensation when nearing an EPN locus, which was rarely the case when no EPN was recorded, whether from an acupoint or non-acupoint region. This study provides additional evidence supporting the similarity between acupoints and MTrPs.

The theory that *active points* have become sensitized may explain why even minimal needle stimulation methods, such as is found in some of the Japanese styles of acupuncture or in research protocols (where the sham treatment involves minimal acupuncture stimulation), can still have profound effects on the CNS because of signal amplification (see Chapters 2 and 5). The pattern of acupoint activation may in part be a result of neurogenic inflammation in response to either organ or musculoskeletal pathology. Grigg et al has shown lowering of activation thresholds for muscle nociceptors adjacent to the joint in an animal model of knee arthritis *(20)*. There is similar evidence that peripheral sensitization of cutaneous nociceptors occurs in the

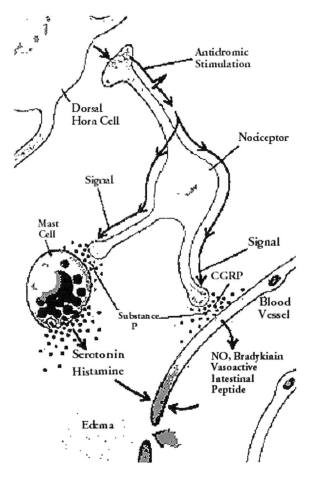

Fig. 7. Diagram illustrates the neurosecretory actions of peripheral nociceptors and the role the release of substance P plays in causing mast cell degranulation and peripheral sensitization.

L1–L2 dermatome of the pelvis in response an experimental model of uterine inflammation *(21)*. Both of these phenomenon can be explained by the concept of dorsal horn reflexes (see Chapter 2). The initiating event is that with either joint or organ pathology an afferent, nociceptive barrage enters the dorsal horn alerting the organism of injury or disease. This information will typically synapse at wide dynamic range (WDR) neurons in the dorsal horn that receive convergent input from multiple sources including viscera, muscle, skin and joint. This WDR neuron responds by not only transmiting that information cephalad along the spinal thalamic tract, but also by causing a retrograde depolarization back out the primary afferent that then leads to peripheral neuropeptide release and a phenomenon called neurogenic inflammation. This is called a dorsal horn reflex. The peripheral release of these neuropeptides (substance P (SP) and calcitonin gene-related peptide (CGRP)), then leads to a cascade of events including degranulation of mast cells and the release of histamine, vasodilation and swelling, the release of bradykinin from endothelium, and so on eventually leading to a sensitized peripheral nociceptor (Figure 7). This response of the nervous system to pathology provides us with an explanatory model of acupoint activation within the fascia in response to disease or injury and can help us understand the physical findings of an *active point* (i.e., erythema, trophedema, hyperalgesia, and allodynia).

A complementary theory explaining the physiologic effect of acupuncture needle manipulation via connective tissue stimulation has been proposed by Langevin *(22)*. She has found that needle twirling in both an animal model and in humans caused winding of the connective tissue around the needle that increased its pull-out force. This allows for greater tensile forces to be generated at the acupoints through needle manipulation. This manipulation results in mechano-transduction through the connective tissue and fascia which ultimately stimulates a cellular response, potentially at sites distant to the acupoint (see Chapter 6).

6. METHODOLOGY IN ACUPUNCTURE RESEARCH

Although acupuncture has been used to treat disorders of every system in the human body, modern scientific research was virtually nonexistent before the 1970s *(23)*. Since that time, hundreds of studies have been performed on a myriad of conditions. Unfortunately, the majority of these studies suffer from numerous methodological flaws, including insufficient numbers of subjects, poor or nonexistent blinding of patients, inappropriate or no control groups, inappropriate outcome measures, and multiple sources of bias. Several systematic reviews of this early literature have generally drawn tepid conclusions due to these methodological flaws. In recent years, however, several high quality randomized controlled trials (RCT's) have been published which have paid much greater attention to these methodological issues.

6.1. Evaluating Methodological Quality

The latest systematic reviews have examined the influence of study design on clinical outcomes. White et al. *(24)* provided an in-depth discussion of the various pitfalls in conducting such reviews, and identified at least 26 different quantitative scales for rating methodological quality. The most commonly used is the five-point Jadad scale (Table 3), which was designed specifically to assess the scientific "quality, defined as the likelihood of the trial design to generate unbiased results and approach the therapeutic truth." However, despite its relative ease of use, inter-rater reliability of this scale has been shown to be poor. There are a number of modified

Table 3
The Jadad Scale

Methodologic question	Points*
1. Was the study described as randomized?	1
2. Was the randomization scheme described and appropriate?	1
3. Was the study described as double blind?	1
4. Was the method of double blinding appropriate?	1
5. Was there a description of dropouts and withdrawals?	1

* Scoring for Jadad scale: 5 possible points; 0–2 = low quality; 3–5 = high quality.

versions of the Jadad scale which attempt to address the issue of practitioner blinding, as discussed in the following section.

6.2. Blinding and Sham Control

As with any complex physical intervention, acupuncture trials are inherently very difficult to blind effectively. Clinician blinding is virtually impossible, since experienced acupuncturists cannot be ignorant of whether they are performing real or sham acupuncture, just as surgeons cannot be blinded to whether they are performing real surgery or not. As for subject blinding, there is no consensus regarding the best type of sham or placebo control. Various procedures have been employed, each with specific advantages and disadvantages (Table 4). As discussed in the neuromodulatory section above, both real and sham acupuncture have been associated with positive outcomes, both apparently greater than placebo alone. The recent design of a placebo acupuncture needle, which only touches the skin superficially, but mimics the appearance of an actively inserted needle has allowed for even greater control of the placebo effect *(24–27)*. One design by Streitberger utilizes a needle that has a blunt-tip whose shaft telescopes into the handle upon application without penetrating the skin. The Park

Table 4
Acupuncture Controls used in Various Studies *(62)*

Control	Definition	Comments
No additional treatment	No therapeutic intervention	Controls for regression to the mean
Active control	Active standard of treatment, such as physical therapy, massage, ultrasound, or medication	Allows direct comparison between acupuncture and an accepted standard or alternative intervention
Sham acupuncture	Needling to the same depth with the same stimulation technique as real acupuncture but at non-acupoints or points felt to be non-influential for the condition treated	Controls for specificity of needle location (real vs. non-acupoint); often mistakenly used as a placebo equivalent, as non-specific needling has been shown to have physiologic effects
Minimal acupuncture	Similar to Sham acupuncture but with more superficial needling	Mimics real acupuncture, but may still have a physiologic effect similar to sham
Placebo acupuncture	Special blunt-tipped needle whose shaft telescopes into handle upon application without penetrating the skin, applied to real acupoints	Mimics insertion of a real needle, but even blunt stimulation of the cutaneous afferents over an acupoint may not be inert
Sham laser acupuncture	A laser acupuncture device is used on real acupoints, but not turned on	Used as placebo because it is considered inert
Sham TENS	Attaching surface electrodes and equipment without application of current	Used as placebo because it is completely inert, but may not preserve blinding of study participants

needle is similar to the Steitberger needle, in that the design utilizes a blunt needle that is free to telescope into the handle rather than penetrate the skin, but it has the addition of an adhesive tube that sticks to the skin of the subject (see Figure 8) *(24)*. Other strategies used to minimize the influence of bias among study participants include recruiting acupuncture-naïve subjects, blindfolding subjects during treatments, and assessing the effectiveness of blinding via participant questionnaire.

6.3. Acupuncture Point Selection

It is inherently difficult to standardize acupuncture treatment protocols for any particular condition. Inclusion and exclusion criteria for clinical study cohorts are based on Western diagnoses of pathology and comorbidity. Evidence-based methodology emphasizes a reductionist approach, with point standardization designed to minimize inter-subject variability. However, because the classical principles of acupuncture treatment are based largely on constitutional factors that may be unique to an individual; patients with identical Western diagnoses may have different constitutional patterns, and therefore require different treatment points. This principle-versus-protocol dilemma presents a fundamental challenge in interpreting clinical outcomes. More recent studies have adopted a semi-standardized treatment approach, combining the use of certain common acupoints with a number of additional points based on individual need. Although this strategy attempts to combine the best of both rationales, its actual impact on outcome has yet to be determined.

6.4. Acupuncture Dosing

Another fundamental hurdle in acupuncture research is the lack of consensus on appropriate acupuncture dosing. There are currently insufficient data to draw strong conclusions regarding number of needles, duration, frequency, or total number of treatments required for therapeutic effect. Many experienced acupuncturists recommend 20–30-minute treatment sessions, with frequency generally varying between 1 and 3 treatments per week depending on the condition, with a few studies recommending 6–10 treatments using 6–11 needles each time as a minimum for a positive outcome *(24)*. Unfortunately, acupuncture dosing used in clinical studies is incredibly variable, using anywhere between 2 and over 20 needles per session, with treatment duration ranging

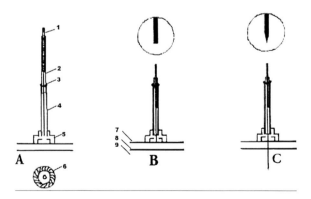

Fig. 8. The Park placebo needle (**A**) has a blunt needle that is free to telescope into the handle (**B**), which does not penetrate the skin. The verum needle (**C**) looks exactly like the placebo needle except it holds a sharpened needle that penetrates the skin as would a normal acupuncture needle.

from 4 to 30 minutes, frequency ranging from three times per week to bi-weekly, and total treatments ranging from a single session to a series of over 40 sessions.

7. CLINICAL EVIDENCE

In 1997, the National Institutes of Health convened a 12–member panel to review the current scientific literature and expert opinion of 25 authorities in the field *(28)*. They formulated a consensus statement regarding the potential indications for acupuncture and stated that there was sufficient evidence for efficacy in postoperative and chemotherapy nausea and vomiting and in postoperative dental pain. Furthermore, they concluded that acupuncture may be useful in addiction, stroke rehabilitation, headache, menstrual cramps, tennis elbow, fibromyalgia, myofascial pain, osteoarthritis, low back pain, carpal tunnel syndrome, and asthma. This consensus statement seemed to motivate the scientific medical community to focus its efforts in acupuncture research, leading to a great increase in the recent number of studies and systematic reviews. The following review of the scientific literature will focus on the most recent evidence from well-controlled trials, and discuss the findings of systematic reviews which have critically evaluated the older studies.

7.1. Fibromyalgia

Despite numerous publications since the late 1970s, there has been only one systematic review by Berman et al. *(29)* that examined acupuncture alone in the treatment of fibromyalgia. They identified seven studies for review out of 67 articles, with only one RCT by Deluze and colleagues *(30)* being deemed of high methodologic quality. Their trial compared 36 patients receiving real electroacupuncture vs. 34 patients receiving sham acupuncture involving superficial needling at non-acupoints. Fifteen patients (21%) dropped out during the 3-week treatment course. Eight outcome measures were evaluated, including pain threshold, number of analgesic tablets used, regional pain score, pain recorded on visual analogue scale, sleep quality, morning stiffness, and patient's and evaluating physician's appreciation. The electroacupuncture group had significant improvement over baseline in seven of the eight measures, and significant improvement in five measures compared to the sham group. Deluze et al. concluded that electroacupuncture is effective in relieving symptoms of fibromyalgia. However, the effectiveness of patient blinding was not assessed, which has been a major criticism of the study. The reviewers decided to use the Deluze trial as the basis for recommendations on efficacy, and use the other studies to generate hypotheses rather than conclusive statements. They concluded that the limited evidence suggests that real acupuncture is more effective than sham acupuncture for improving symptoms of patients with fibromyalgia. However, this conclusion is based only on a single high-quality study, and that more high-quality RCTs were needed.

There have been two recent high-quality, randomized, single-blind studies published in 2005 whose results were somewhat less promising. Assefi et al. *(31)* randomized 96 patients to receive either directed acupuncture (n = 25), or one of three sham controls: *(1)* simulated acupuncture at the same fibromyalgia acupoints using a toothpick to mimic needle insertion without puncturing the skin (n = 23), *(2)* acupuncture on different acupoints for an unrelated condition (n = 24), or *(3)* sham needling on non-acupoints (n = 24). Every intervention arm received two 30-minute treatment sessions per week for 12 weeks. Blinding was assessed to be effective across all groups at week 12. The primary outcome was subjective pain, and secondary outcomes included fatigue, sleep quality, overall well-being, physical and mental functioning, and total number of pain medications used during the treatment period. All groups improved; however, there were no statistically significant differences between the directed acupuncture results and pooled results of the three control groups for any of the outcome measures. Assefi and colleagues concluded that directed acupuncture for fibromyalgia was no better than sham acupuncture at relieving pain. However, they did concede that sham needling may induce the same physiologic changes as real acupuncture, and that a usual-care control group could have more clearly defined the nonspecific response.

Similar results were achieved in a study by Harris and colleagues (32), which examined 114 fibromyalgia patients each receiving one of four interventions: either real or sham acupuncture both with and without manual stimulation. The subjects received one 20-minute intervention a week for 3 weeks followed by two per week for 3 weeks, then three per week for 3 weeks for a total of 18 treatments, with a 2-week wash-out period in-between each 3-week session. After accounting for a 33% patient dropout rate, no statistically significant differences in pain were found among any of the four intervention groups, nor were there any clinically significant changes in the secondary outcome measures of fatigue and function. However, when data for the groups were combined, a statistically significant improvement in pain was noted while subjects were receiving three treatments per week as compared to one treatment per week, suggesting a frequency-dependent response. Given that it is unlikely that 3 weeks of acupuncture would have enough cumulative benefit for a patient with a chronic disease like fibromyalgia, the study design does not test the question of whether a more sustained trial of acupuncture unbroken by the wash out periods would have had a more significant effect on the outcomes measured.

7.2. Myofascial Pain Syndrome (MPS)

There are far fewer well-controlled studies on acupuncture in the treatment of MTrPs and MPS. One RCT by Irnich et al. (33) involved a crossover design comparing three treatment arms for chronic neck pain: (1) non-local acupuncture, (2) dry needling of local MTrPs, and (3) sham laser acupuncture. Thirty-six subjects were divided equally into six groups, and every group received all three interventions in different orders with a one-week washout period between each crossover. The non-local acupuncture group received an average of 7.1 needles to individualized distant points according to the TCM theory. The dry needling group had an average of 7.4 needles inserted into cervical MTrPs, with at least one LTR elicited per muscle. The sham laser group had an inactivated laser applied for two minutes to each acupoint (average of 6.8 points), with the identical point selection process as the acupuncture group. Each patient had a single 30-minute session, with three outcome measures assessed immediately before and after treatment. Motion-related pain on 100 mm visual analogue scale (VAS) decreased by 11.2 mm with acupuncture compared to sham laser (p = 0.00006), while dry needling resulted in a 1.0 mm decrease compared to sham laser (p = 0.7). Cervical ROM in the acupuncture group improved by 3.6° over sham laser (p = 0.016) and the dry needling group improved by 1.7° over sham laser (p = 0.032). Patient rating of general complaints on an 11-point scale improved 1.5 points between acupuncture and dry needling (p = 0.008) and 1.7 points between acupuncture and sham (p = 0.0001). The study conclusion was that a single session of acupuncture is superior to both dry needling and sham laser in immediate improvement of motion-related cervical pain and ROM, while dry needling is not immediately effective for motion-related pain.

In contrast, a RCT of 35 consecutive outpatients (25 women, 10 men; age range: 65–81 years) with non-radiating low back pain for at least six months and normal neurological examination, were randomized to one of three groups over 12 weeks *(34)*. Each group received two treatments with an interval between (9 patients dropped out during the course of the study). The standard acupuncture group (n = 9) received treatment at traditional acupuncture points for low back pain, while the other acupuncture groups received superficial dry needling (n = 9) or deep dry needling (n = 9) treatments on trigger points. Outcome measures were VAS pain intensity and Roland Morris Questionnaire. Although the study was not sufficiently powered to detect between group differences, there was a significant within group change in pain intensity between the treatment in the group that received deep needling to trigger points (p < 0.01), that was not found in the standard acupuncture group or the group that received superficial needling to trigger points.

Ceccheerelli's group has studied the difference between superficial (SDN) and deep dry needling (DDN) of MTrP in low back pain (LBP) abnd shoulder pain, both showing significantly greater benefit from DDN. In the LBP trial, 42 patients with lumbar myofascial pain were randomized to receive 8 sessions of either SDN, where the needle was introduced in the skin at a depth of 2 mm, or to DDN, where the needle was placed deeply into muscular tissue using a trigger point method of needling. Outcome measures included the McGill Pain Questionnaire before and after treatment and at the 3-month follow-up examination. Although at the end of the treatment there was no evidence of significant statistical differences between the two different groups, pain reduction was greater in the group treated with DDN. This benefit was more sustained in the DDN group, and a statistical difference did develop between the two groups at the 3-month follow-up *(35)*. A similar result was found in a RCT of 44 subject with myofascial shoulder pain *(36)*. A statistically significant difference rose between the two needling techniques at the end of the treatment and at the follow up after one and three months. DDN was shown to be better at all times and this underlines the importance of the muscular afferent drive in acupunctural stimulation in the control of pain.

7.3. Rheumatoid Arthritis (RA)

In 2005, Casimiro et al. *(37)* performed a follow-up to their comprehensive review from 2001. This updated search identified five new articles in addition to the original eight; however, none met the inclusion criteria. Thus, the two RCTs by Man and Baragar *(38)* and David et al. *(39)* from the original 2001 review stood as the only studies that met inclusion criteria on acupuncture and RA. In the Man trial, 20 subjects that had RA present for at least 5 years with bilateral knee pain were randomized into an electroacupuncture group, which received a single 15-minute treatment to one knee using three needles, and a control group, which had electroacupuncture to one knee on three non-acupoints. The study was of a parallel design, so in both groups the other knee was injected with 50 mg of hydrocortisone. The electroacupuncture group reported a significant reduction in subjective pain over the control group both at 24 hours and four months post-treatment, as measured by a 0–4 pain reduction scale.

In the randomized, crossover study by David and colleagues, subjects were placed in either an acupuncture group (n = 29) or a placebo group (n = 27). The acupuncture group had five weekly treatments where a single needle was inserted into each foot at the Liver 3 point for only four minutes. The two needles were each manipulated for five seconds after they had been left in for two minutes. The placebo group had the needle guide tubes placed on the skin over the Liv 3 points for four minutes without actual needle insertion. After the first 5-week treatment phase, a six-week washout period took place before the cross-over for the second 5-week phase. Outcome measures included erythrocyte sedimentation rate (ESR), C-reactive protein level (CRP), number of swollen joints, number of tender joints, pain score on the visual analogue scale (VAS P), global assessment score on the visual analogue scale (VAS G), score on the general health questionnaire (GHQ), score on the modified disease activity scale (DAS) and analgesic medication intake. These measures were assessed before and after each of the two 5-week treatment phases, then at six weeks post treatment. The investigators found no statistically significant differences between groups for any of the outcome measures at any time point.

Casimiro et al.'s review concluded that electroacupuncture may be beneficial to reduce symptomatic knee pain in patients with RA, and that needle acupuncture has no effect on the numerous outcome measures as assessed in David et al.'s study mentioned above. The two included studies were later criticized for their inappropriate treatment algorithms, specifically, "well qualified acupuncture practitioners would never use such a simple protocol as that used by David et al (1999) to treat pain in RA. Both studies that met the inclusion criteria for this review used an approach to acupuncture which would be unacceptable to appropriately qualified acupuncture practitioners."

7.4. Headache

In 2005, Melchart and coworkers updated their 2001 review of acupuncture in the treatment of headache *(40)*. Twenty-six out of the 102 trials identified were reviewed, including 16 for migraine, six for tension-type headache, and four for various types of headache. A combined total of 1151 patients were studied, with a median of 37 per trial (range 10–150). The median treatment dose was eight treatment sessions (range 6–12) over eight weeks (range 6–26), with a median follow-up time of 26 weeks (range 3–104). The median Jadad score was 1.5 (range 1–5), with seventeen of the 26 studies being placebo-controlled. Of those studies with sham control groups involving patients with migraine, five demonstrated statistically significant improvement favoring acupuncture, three showed trends favoring acupuncture over sham, and two showed no differences. Hesse and colleagues found acupuncture and metoprolol to be equally effective in treating migraine. Three sham-controlled studies examined tension-type headaches, with one only reporting significantly improved headache indices compared to sham *(41)*. The two trials that found no significant differences between verum acupuncture and sham had small sample sizes *(10,30)*. As for acupuncture vs. massage, the review authors' reanalysis of Wylie et al.'s study suggested that massage and relaxation had a greater effect on patients with tension-type headache, while acupuncture had a greater effect on migraine patients. The review authors concluded that the evidence does support the value of acupuncture for the treatment of idiopathic headaches, although trials were generally small and many had methodologic flaws. Two rigorous trials examining tension-type headache and migraine compared to placebo have been published since this 2005 review.

7.4.1. TENSION-TYPE HEADACHE

Melchart et al. *(42)* randomized 270 patients with tension-type headache for at least 12 months into three groups via previously defined acupuncture randomized trial (ART) protocols *(43)*. The true acupuncture group (n = 132) received a maximum of 25 needles—a set of three standardized bilateral acupoints plus additional acupoints selected individually—with achievement of de Qi. The minimal acupuncture group (n = 63) had at least 10 needles inserted superficially into predefined distant non-acupoints bilaterally without eliciting de Qi. The waiting list group (n = 75) received no treatment for 12 weeks, followed by the true acupuncture protocol. All true and minimal acupuncture treatments involved twelve 30–minute sessions over eight weeks. The primary outcome of number of days with headache between baseline and weeks 9–12 decreased by 7.2 ± 6.5 in the acupuncture group, compared to 6.6 ± 6.0 in the minimal acupuncture group ($p = 0.58$) and 1.5 ± 3.7 in the waiting list group ($p < 0.001$). Likewise, with all secondary outcomes, including pain diary records and questionnaires on pain, disability and depression, the true acupuncture group had statistically significant improvement over the waiting list control, but differences between true and minimal acupuncture groups were not significant. Regarding assessment of blinding, subjects in the true acupuncture group successfully guessed their allocation at 24 weeks slightly more often than those in the minimal acupuncture group, but the difference was not statistically significant ($p = 0.08$). The authors concluded that patients with tension-type headache had benefits from acupuncture that were comparable to other accepted headache treatments, but minimal acupuncture had a similar effect.

7.4.2. MIGRAINE HEADACHE

A methodologically similar ART study by Linde et al. *(42)* recruited 302 patients diagnosed with migraine with or without aura; 145 were assigned to the true acupuncture group, 81 to sham acupuncture, and 76 to waiting list. Again, the true acupuncture group had twelve 30-minute sessions over 8 weeks of semi-standardized acupoint treatment with de Qi, while the minimal acupuncture group had superficial needling without de Qi to predefined distant non-acupoints. The number of days with headache between baseline and weeks 9–12 decreased by 2.2 ± 2.7 in both the true and sham acupuncture groups ($p = 0.96$) and by 0.8 ± 2.2 in the waiting list group (difference vs. acupuncture, $p < 0.001$). Secondary outcomes with similar pain diaries and questionnaires also showed that true acupuncture resulted in statistically significant improvements over waiting list, but not over sham acupuncture. Blinding was deemed less effective in this ART trial, as a significantly greater number of subjects in the true acupuncture cohort correctly guessed their group allocation as compared to those in the sham acupuncture group. These authors concluded that acupuncture reduced migraine headache attacks compared with no treatment, but similar effects were observed with sham acupuncture, and may be due to nonspecific physiological and/or placebo effects. It is important to note that in both of these German ART trials, physician acupuncturists were performing the interventions, many of whom had only completed a 140-hour basic course in acupuncture.

7.5. Neck Pain

White and Ernst *(44)* published a comprehensive systematic review that included 14 RCT's of needle acupuncture, electroacupuncture, or laser acupuncture in the treatment of neck pain. Three studies comparing acupuncture to physiotherapy found acupuncture to be either equal or superior. Of the three trials that tested laser acupuncture, the verum laser was found to be superior to sham laser in two studies but no different in the third study. Yet four out of five trials that compared needle with a sham acupuncture control did not find any significant differences in efficacy. As such, the authors suggested that precisely administered acupuncture is no more effective than the generalized physiological response resulting from random needling. However, it is important to note that three of the four negative studies provided only three or fewer treatment sessions. In comparison, all three trials that averaged 12 or more treatments yielded positive outcomes. Overall, of the 15 studies, seven were in favor of acupuncture and eight were equivocal as compared to controls. Eight higher quality studies, scoring at least three points on the modified Jadad scale, showed three in favor and five equivocal. The authors admitted that the results of the negative studies may not have been conclusive because they all showed positive trends with small sample sizes.

A recent large-scale RCT performed by White et al. *(45)* assigned 135 patients with chronic mechanical neck pain to receive either verum needle acupuncture (n = 70) or mock TENS as a control (n = 65). All acupuncture treatments were performed by a single acupuncturist with 7 years of experience in western acupuncture, who needled an average of six acupoints per side, including at least one distal point, until de Qi was achieved. Patients who received mock TENS had electrodes attached to the skin over the same acupoints, however, the connecting cables were decommissioned and unable to transmit any electrical current from the stimulator. Treatment sessions lasted 20 minutes and were given twice a week for four weeks. At one week post-treatment, both groups had statistically significant decreases in pain scores from baseline, as recorded for seven consecutive days using the 100-mm VAS. In comparing between groups, the acupuncture group improved 6.3 mm more than the placebo group on the 100-mm VAS, which was statistically significant ($p < 0.01$), but not clinically significant. There were no statistically significant between-group differences for any of the secondary outcomes, which included the Neck Disability Index and SF-36 Physical and Mental Component Summary scores. Blinding was deemed successful as assessed by the Borkovec and Nau credibility scale.

In another large-scale German trial of neck pain, 14,161 patients with chronic neck pain (duration >6 months) were randomly allocated to either an acupuncture group or a control group receiving no acupuncture *(46)*. Patients in the acupuncture group received up to 15 acupuncture sessions over 3 months. Patients who did not consent to randomization received acupuncture treatment immediately. All subjects were allowed to receive usual medical care in addition to study treatment. Outcomes were assessed with the Neck pain and Disability (NPAD scale at treatment cessation and after three months *(47)*. Of 14,161 patients (mean age 50.9 ± 13.1 years, 68% female) 1,880 were randomized to acupuncture and 1886 to control, and 10,395 included into the non-randomized acupuncture group. At 3 months, neck pain and disability improved by 16.2 (SE: 0.4) to 38.3 (SE: 0.4) and by 3.9 (SE: 0.4) to 50.5 (SE: 0.4), difference 12.3 ($p < 0.001$) in the acupuncture and control group, respectively. These effects were maintained at 6-month follow up. Although this trial shows that treatment with acupuncture when added to routine care in patients with chronic neck pain can have a sustained and significant effect on neck pain over usual care, it is not possible to know, given the study design, whether this benefit was due to nonspecific effects of acupuncture.

7.6. Low back pain

Manheimer and colleagues *(48)* recently performed an exhaustive meta-analysis evaluating the effect of needle acupuncture in the treatment of low back pain with regard to pain, functional status, overall improvement, return to full work, and analgesic consumption. The primary outcome was quantitative synthesis of the short-term effectiveness of acupuncture on pain. The quality of every study examined was rated using both the modified Jadad scale as well as a 10-point system employed by the Cochrane Back Review Group. Thirty-three studies were included in this review, with 22 RCTs (all testing Chinese acupuncture for chronic low back pain) incorporated in the meta-analysis. With regard to the short-term effectiveness in chronic low back pain, the pooled data showed that acupuncture is statistically significantly more effective than sham acupuncture, sham TENS, and no-additional-treatment controls. In specifically comparing acupuncture to sham acupuncture, the reviewers calculated an overall effect size of 0.58, which corresponded with a clinically important improvement of 14.5 mm on the VAS. However, acupuncture was not found to be more effective than other active treatments (medication, true TENS and massage) and was actually statistically significantly less effective than spinal manipulation on the basis of two studies, both by Giles and Muller. In terms of long-term pain relief, acupuncture was found to be significantly better than no-additional-treatment and sham TENS. Among the secondary outcome measures, acupuncture was significantly more effective than the no-additional-treatment control for short-term functional improvement (overall effect size 0.62). In addition, acupuncture was significantly more effective than the sham and no-additional-treatment controls for short- and long-term overall improvement. The reviewers cited two studies that assessed return to work and three that assessed analgesic use, but stated that no definitive conclusions could be drawn. Manheimer et al. remarked that the results of this meta-analysis were different from those of a previous Cochrane Review by van Tulder and colleagues', which did not conclude that acupuncture was effective for LBP. Their reasoning was that five high-quality RCTs had been published since the Cochrane Review in 1999, with four of them in favor of acupuncture. Furthermore, Manheimer et al.'s review included 33 RCTs, which is more than twice as many as any of the previous reviews on back pain, and specifically compared acupuncture to numerous controls and active treatments, allowing for more specific and stronger conclusions to be drawn.

7.7. Shoulder Pain/Impingement Syndrome

Green and colleagues *(49)* performed a comprehensive database search through December 2003 for randomized and quasi-randomized acupuncture trials in adults with shoulder pain lasting longer than 3 weeks which was not due to rheumatoid arthritis, polymyalgia rheumatica, cervically referred pain, or fracture. Nine studies were discussed—sample sizes were generally small, with a median of 44 subjects (range of 18–150). The outcomes assessor was blinded in seven of the nine trials, but the subjects were blinded in only two. Interventions were poorly described in all studies and a wide range of placebo controls were used. Acupuncture was of benefit over placebo in improving the Constant Murley Score (a measure of shoulder function) in one study. However, by 4-month follow-up, the difference between the acupuncture and placebo groups, while still statistically significant, was no longer considered clinically significant. Acupuncture in combination with exercise was more effective than exercise alone in one small trial. One of the larger trials found nerve blocks to be more effective than acupuncture on a range of outcome measures, but no follow-up data were reported. The authors of the review concluded that because there were only a few trials testing a variety of interventions in various populations against differing controls, it was difficult to interpret the evidence regarding the value of acupuncture for shoulder disorders.

However, a recent high-quality RCT by Guerra de Hoyos et al. *(50)* provides strong evidence for the effectiveness of acupuncture. They randomly assigned 130 acupuncture-naïve subjects with shoulder soft tissue lesions (rotator cuff tendonitis, capsulitis, bicipital tendonitis, or bursitis) equally between active electroacupuncture treatment and placebo acupuncture control groups. The treatment cohort had needles inserted into four points (two on the affected shoulder and two on the opposite leg) with elicitation of de Qi. Electrical current was then applied at a frequency of 5–10 Hz with a strong enough intensity to induce light muscle twitching. The placebo acupuncture cohort had Park placebo needles placed on the same four acupoints, which were connected to an electroacupuncture device that did not deliver any current. Both groups had 15-minute interventions every week for seven weeks, performed by two licensed acupuncturists both with more than four years of experience. At 7-week, 3-month, and 6-month follow-up, the acupuncture group showed statistically significant improvements over placebo in the primary outcome measure of pain intensity on 0–10 VAS (difference of 1.5–2.0, $p < 0.0005$), as well as nearly all secondary outcome measures ($p < 0.0005$), including pain intensity (Lattinen index), range of motion (goniometer), functional ability (SPADI), quality of life (COOP-WONCA charts), and diclofenac consumption. This well-designed study indicates that acupuncture can be safe and effective in the treatment of soft tissue shoulder pain.

7.8. Lateral Epicondyle Pain

A 2004 systematic review by Trinh et al. *(51)* concluded via a best-evidence synthesis approach that "there is strong evidence suggesting that acupuncture is effective in the short-term relief of lateral epicondyle pain." They identified 6 out of 53 studies which were all randomized or quasi-randomized, involved needle acupuncture as the primary intervention, and evaluated patients with any pain originating from the common extensor tendon at the lateral epicondyle. The studies were performed between 1990 and 2002 with sample populations ranging from 17 to 82. The quality of each paper was evaluated, also using the Jadad scale, and all six were rated as high-quality, with the Fink et al. 2002 study scoring a perfect 5 out of 5 *(52)*. All six studies demonstrated statistically significant pain relief of the acupuncture groups over baseline levels. Five studies indicated statistically significant improvement compared to control groups, with four of the five using sham acupuncture controls. Limitations cited among the studies included inconsistent definitions of lateral epicondyle pain, differences in outcome measures with respect to the definition and duration of pain relief, variations in the style and dosing of acupuncture treatment protocols, and appropriate selection of sham acupuncture type for control.

7.9. Knee Osteoarthritis (OA)

A comprehensive systematic literature review was performed by Ezzo et al. in 2001 *(53)*. They reported on seven randomized or quasi-randomized studies involving actual needle insertion into acupuncture points on patients with knee OA exclusively. The seven articles were published between 1981 and 1999 and had study sizes between 14 and 103 subjects. Four of the seven trials were of low methodologic quality per evaluation using a modified Jadad scale, but there was no association between the quality of the trial and its subsequent results. The studies were also evaluated for adequacy of treatment dose; five of the studies were determined to have adequately treated the subjects with four yielding positive results for improving pain. The studies were categorized into short-term (<1 month after treatment completion), intermediate-term (1–3 months after treatment completion), and long-term follow-up (>3 months after treatment completion). With regard to short-term follow-up, two low-quality studies compared acupuncture against wait-list or treatment-as-usual controls, and provided limited evidence that acupuncture was more effective for improving both pain and function in patients with OA of the knee. Two out of three high-quality studies using sham acupuncture as a control indicated that there is strong evidence in favor of true over sham acupuncture for the treatment of OA pain, but inconclusive evidence for improvement of function. Two studies evaluated acupuncture as compared to physical therapy and rendered inconclusive evidence for improvement of pain or function. Four trials had intermediate-term follow-up; one demonstrated maintenance of benefit from acupuncture at 3 months, two indicated benefit attenuation at 1 month, and one showed no benefit for acupuncture at any time point. None of the studies had strictly controlled long-term follow-up.

There have been two subsequent large RCTs assessing the benefit of acupuncture in knee OA. In 2004, Berman and Lao reported the results of an NIH sponsored trial where 570 subjects with chronic knee OA (mean age 65.5) were randomized to either Chinese acupuncture, sham acupuncture, or a patient education control group *(54)*. Each acupuncture group received 23 treatment sessions over 26 weeks while the control group received six 2-hour education sessions over 12 weeks. Primary Outcomes included the Western Ontario and McMasters Universities Osteoarthritis Index (WOMAC) pain and function scores. By 8 weeks there was a significant improvement in the function score in the verum acupuncture group (p = 0.01) that continued through 26 weeks (p = 0.009), with a 40% improvement from baseline. The pain score did not show separation from sham until 14 weeks (p = 0.02) and then continued to be significant through 26 weeks (p = 0.003), with a 40% improvement from baseline. There was a 25% dropout in both verum and sham groups, and a 50% dropout in the education group. The study utilized a novel sham intervention; the needles were touched on the actual points in the leg after which they were taped flat to the skin and then a mock electroacupuncture stimulator was hooked up to the needles. A curtain was used to prevent the patients from seeing their knees, however visible needles were placed subcutaneously off meridian in the abdomen to strengthen the patient belief that they were getting verum acupuncture.

In 2005, Witt et al. published another German trial that randomized chronic knee OA patients into true acupuncture (N = 150), minimal acupuncture (n = 76), or waiting list control (n = 74) groups *(55)*. The patients in the true acupuncture group had an average of 17 local and distant acupoints (along with occasional trigger points) needled and manipulated to achieve de Qi. Patients who received minimal acupuncture had an average of 12 needles inserted superficially into distant non-acupuncture points without manipulation or de Qi. Both the true and minimal acupuncture groups had twelve 30-minute treatment sessions over 8 weeks, while the waiting list group had

Table 5
Summary of Clinical Efficacy for Acupuncture Treatment of Painful Conditions

Condition	*Overall efficacy*	*Comments*
Fibromyalgia	True acupuncture appears to be no more effective than sham acupuncture as tested against various sham controls	Sham acupuncture may not have been an inert placebo; recent high-quality studies did not have no-treatment control comparisons
Myofascial pain	Non-local may provide greater initial improvement in pain and ROM compared to local DDN for neck pain. DDN however is superior to SDN for LBP and Shoulder pain at long term follow-up.	Only a few low-powered studies have been published; more information needed about technique of needling
Rheumatoid arthritis	Electroacupuncture may reduce knee pain in RA; a brief single-needle technique of acupuncture has no significant effect on numerous clinical and laboratory measures	Based on 2 studies identified from a systematic review, both of which were criticized for unacceptably brief treatment periods
Headache (tension-type and migraine)	True acupuncture is more effective than no treatment, but not more effective than sham acupuncture	Sham acupuncture used in these high-quality studies may not have been an inert placebo
Neck pain	Studies suggest that true acupuncture is more effective than both sham acupuncture and no treatment, but data are inconclusive	Effectiveness seems dose-dependent—studies with a greater total number of treatments yielded more positive results
Chronic low back pain	*Short-term*: Acupuncture is significantly more effective than sham acupuncture, sham TENS, and no-additional-treatment controls. *Long-term*: Acupuncture is significantly more effective than sham TENS and no-additional-treatment controls.	Based on comprehensive meta-analysis of 33 studies, including 22 RCT's
Shoulder pain	Electroacupuncture is more effective than placebo needle for improving pain, ROM, and function	Based on a single high-quality RCT; previous studies were of lower quality and less conclusive
Lateral epicondylitis	Effective in the short-term relief of lateral epicondyle pain	Based on a systematic review of 6 high-quality RCT's
Knee osteoarthritis	True acupuncture is more effective than both sham acupuncture and no treatment for short-term pain relief	Based on several studies of varying quality; few data on long-term outcomes

an 8-week period of no treatment, followed by a course of true acupuncture. Patient assessment of treatment credibility after three sessions and at the end of the study indicated proper subject blinding. The primary outcome measure was the WOMAC index. The mean baseline-adjusted WOMAC index at the end of eight weeks of treatment was 26.9 in the true acupuncture group compared with 35.8 in the minimal acupuncture group ($p = 0.0002$) and 49.6 in the waiting list group ($p < 0.0001$). However, the differences were no longer significant at 26 or 52 weeks post-treatment ($p = 0.063$ and 0.080, respectively). The true acupuncture group also had statistically significant improvements compared to the two other groups at eight weeks for nearly all secondary outcome measures, including all WOMAC subscales (pain, stiffness, and physical function), the Pain Disability Index, SF-36, and SES questionnaire on emotional aspects of pain. The authors concluded that acupuncture had statistically and clinically significant short-term effects when compared to minimal or no acupuncture treatment controls in patients with osteoarthritis of the knee.

7.10. Summary

In summary, a number of clinical trials covering a broad range of pain conditions have been published (see Table 5). Trials that study a more homogenous population of patients such as knee OA, soft tissue shoulder pain, and lateral epicondylitis tend to favor verum acupuncture over sham treatment. Trials that study more heterogenous conditions that are often associated with significant co-morbid psychiatric issues such as tension type headaches (TTH), fibromyalgia, and low back pain (LBP) tend show equal benefit from verum and sham acupuncture. For example, in studies of OA of the knee, there are accepted, objective criteria to establish the diagnosis, which is not the case in conditions like fibromyalgia or non-specific LBP, which depends much more on a subjective complaint of pain.

8. SAFETY

Like many systems of complementary and alternative medicine, acupuncture has long been touted as safe. However, only in the last several years have large-scale prospective studies actually been performed in order to characterize the types and rates of incidence of adverse events associated with acupuncture. Table 6 summarizes the incidence rates of adverse events related to acupuncture treatment as reported in various prospective safety studies. These reports indicate that most of the adverse events observed are quite rare, occurring in only a fraction of a percent of treatment encounters. Only two prospective studies *(56,57)* were able to quantify any serious, potentially life-threatening adverse events, which included pneumothorax, asthma exacerbation with angina and hypertension, and acute hypertensive crisis. These serious events only occurred in 0.001 to 0.002% of treatment encounters—representing a very low risk of occurrence. For several of the above listed adverse events there is a wide range of incidence rates. Multiple factors may contribute to this range, including methodological differences in defining, identifying and reporting data, the probability of some amount of underreporting *(58)*, large differences in sample size, and difficulty in establishing explicit cause-and-effect relationships between acupuncture and occurrence of the adverse events *(59)*.

Furthermore, the above studies have not been able to characterize how these incidence rates are affected by the different needling techniques among various styles of acupuncture. For example, Japanese acupuncture employs a relatively superficial

Table 6
Summary of Adverse Events as Reported in Prospective Acupuncture Safety Trials *(58)*

Adverse event	% incidence (least to most frequent)
Constitutional	
Fatigue/exhaustion/lethargy	0.0031^2, 0.012^3, 0.027^1, 2.3^7, 3.3^{10}
Nausea	0.0063^2, 0.01^8, 0.015^3, 0.2^{11}, 0.25^7
Vomiting	0.0029^3, 0.0031^2
Worsening of symptoms	0.12^1, 0.96^2, 1.8^7, 2.8^3
Local pain, bleeding, Or bruising	
Pain upon needling	0.2^6, 0.9^{11}, 1.10^2, 1.23^3, 3.28^1, 4.2^7, 13^{10}
Prolonged pain at needle site	0.0087^3, 0.0094^2, 2.3^{10}
Ecchymosis/Hematoma	0.03^8, 0.33^7, 1.6^4, 1.71^3, 2.2^{11}, 3.19^1, 7.6^{10}
Bleeding	0.4^3, 1.38^1, 2.9^{11}, 3.10^2, 38^{10}
Dermatologic	
Local skin irritation	0.18^1
Burn	0.0029^3, 0.0031^2, 0.01^8
Psychiatric/emotional	
Disorientation	0.0031^2
Exacerbation of depression	0.0010^1
Anxiety and panic/anger	0.0031^2, 0.012^3
Neurologic	
Headache	0.0029^3, 0.0031^2, 0.039^1
Drowsiness	0.0029^3, 0.0063^2
Seizure	0.0031^2
Cardiovascular	
Feeling faint/dizziness	0.0029^3, 7^4, 0.25^7, 0.02^8, 0.02^9, 1^{11}
Fainting/vasovagal reaction	0.0010^1, 0.012^3, 0.019^2, 0.14^{11}, 0.19^5, 0.3^4
Orthostatic problems	0.46^1
Acute hypertensive crisis	0.0010^1
Respiratory	
Pneumothorax	0.0014^4, 0.0020^1
Asthma exacerbation/angina	0.0010^1
Allergic/immunologic	
Needle allergy	0.0063^2
Iatrogenic/technical	
Forgotten needles	0.0058^3, 0.016^2, 0.04^8, 0.25^1
Needle fracture	0.0014^4

1. Melchart; 2. White; 3. MacPherson; 4. Umlauf; 5. Chen; 6. Melchart; 7. Melchart; 8. Yamashita; 9. Yong; 10. Yamashita; 11. Ernst.

depth of needling whereas Chinese acupuncture tends to involve deeper needle insertion and manual stimulation of the needles after insertion. As such, the risk of direct trauma and systemic reactions may be lower in Japanese as compared to Chinese style acupuncture *(58)*. Other factors to consider are the thickness of the needle—where larger-gauge needles may cause more local pain on insertion and thinner needles may be more likely to break, and needle quality—where less solid construction or the use of less malleable metals may result in more breakable needles.

8.1. Case Reports

Prior to these recent prospective studies, case reports were a primary method of citing adverse events related to acupuncture. Lao and colleagues *(60)* published perhaps the most comprehensive systematic review of all case reports of adverse events resulting from acupuncture. They identified 202 cases described in 98 reports that were published in English between 1965 and 1999. This amounted to less than six cases per year among 22 countries over the course of 35 years. A recent MEDLINE search of adverse events or complications related to acupuncture yielded additional case reports since Lao's study as outlined in Table 7.

8.2. Contraindications, Precautions, and Interactions

In general, safety measures for acupuncture are the same as those for any needle procedure such as injection or venipuncture. Some acupuncturists also advocate for certain treatment-specific contraindications, particularly regarding acupuncture during pregnancy. However, there do not appear to be any detailed scientific data regarding these particular contraindications. Table 8 summarizes the generally accepted standards for safety in acupuncture practice as discussed by Sierpina *(23)* and Rampes and James *(61)*.

In summary, acupuncture is a very safe therapeutic intervention in which the risk of significant adverse events is quite small compared to many conventional therapeutic interventions. The more common types of adverse events, such as pain, bleeding, and hematoma formation, are akin to those seen in any therapeutic needle intervention.

Yet despite the low risk of complications related to acupuncture, the clinician must always be vigilant regarding the signs and symptoms of a possible negative outcome from acupuncture, and continue to integrate his or her knowledge of anatomy and potential contraindications into regular practice.

9. MODELS OF INTEGRATION IN CLINICAL CARE

There are a number of ways acupuncture can be successfully integrated into a pain practice. If a physician in the practice has an interest in this treatment modality, then they would need to seek further training. The standard in the United States for basic training in acupuncture that would allow the physician to practice acupuncture in most states and/or be credentialed at most hospitals is 300 continuing medical education (CME) hours (physicians are encouraged to check with their local state medical board to determine the local requirements). There are a number of clinical training programs in acupuncture for physicians that provide this basic training, including the Harvard CME Course *Structural Acupuncture for Physicians* and the UCLA CME Course *Medical Acupuncture*, both of which have long-distance learning systems. Physicians within a pain practice that want to start providing this service would have better success if they

Table 7

Case Reports of Adverse Events Related to Acupuncture: Prior to 1999 (*60*) and from 1999 to 2005

Complication reported: Prior to 1999	Cases	Complication reported: 1999–2005	Cases
Infections[1]	118	**Infections**	16
Hepatitis	94	Mycobacterium chelonae infection	2
Auricular infections	9	Mycobacteriosis	1
Staphylococcal septicemia	3	Prosthetic valve endocarditis	1
Endocarditis	3	Infected left atrial myxoma	1
Pseudoaneurysm	1	Infectious aneurysm formation	1
HIV infection	1	Multiloculated pleural empyema	1
Bacterial meningitis and epidural hematoma	1	Pyoderma gangrenosum	1
Chronic osteomyelitis	1	Intraabdominal abscess	1
Spinal infection	1	Retroperitoneal abscess	1
Cervical spinal epidural abscess	1	Subcutaneous staph abscess	1
Posterior tuberculous spondylitis	1	Soft tissue abscess & osteomyelitis	1
Peritemporomandibular abcsess	1	Inflammatory granuloma	1
Glenohumeral pyarthrosis	1	Infected compartment syndrome	1
		Necrotising fasciitis	1
		Lumbar facet septic arthritis	1
Internal organ or tissue injury[2]	60	**Internal organ or tissue injury**	21
Pneumothorax[3]	26	Pneumothorax	8
Spinal cord injury[4]	13	Cardiac tamponade	3
Cardiac tamponade	5	Aortic pseudoaneurysm	1
Lipoatrophy	2	Popliteal artery pseudoaneurysm	1
Retroperitoneal hematoma	1	Rectus sheath hematoma	1
Needles in soft tissue	1	Acute intracranial hemorrhage	1
Needle imbedded in chest wall	1	Needle migration to medulla	1

Needle in bladder	1
Renal lithiasis	1
Foreign needle stone in ureter	1
Foreign body in kidney	1
Foreign body in ureter	1
Lesion of the medulla oblongata	1
Median nerve injury	1
Drop foot	1
Factitial panniculitis	1
Multiple lymphocytoma cutis	1
Argyria (blue macules)	1
Other COMPLICATIONS	**11**
Acute asthmatic attack	2
3rd degree burns from moxibustion	2
Eschar and scarring (from hot needles)	1
Bleeding	1
Compartment syndrome of lower leg	1
False aneurysm of the popliteal artery	1
Deep vein thrombophlebitis of leg	1

Peroneal nerve palsy	1
L5 radiculopathy by broken needle	1
Acute pancreatitis	1
Other COMPLICATIONS	**9**
Galactorrhea	2
Convulsive syncope	2
Triggering of ICD shocks	1
Facial erysipelas	1
Localized argyria (blue macules)	1
Auricular cartilage calcification	1
Bilateral hand edema	1

(Continued)

Table 7
(Continued)

Complication reported: Prior to 1999	Cases	Complication reported: 1999–2005	Cases
Posttraumatic sympathetic dystrophy	1		
Tingling in right arm and bilateral hands	1		
Minor adverse effectS	13	Total	46
Contact dermatitis[5]	7		
Electromagnetic interference with pacemaker	1		
Hypotension	1		
Recurrent fainting, vomiting, and sweating	1		
Fainting with seated treatment	1		
Cutaneous herpes	1		
Petechiae	1		
Total	202		

[1] Of note, only eight of the 118 cases of infection were reported after 1988, with no cases of hepatitis or auricular infection. This is presumably due to the widespread institution of sterile disposable needles and clean needle technique from 1989 onward. [2] For the non-pneumothorax incidents of organ and tissue injury, the time of symptom onset ranged from immediately after needle insertion to 30 years post-treatment. Interestingly, the majority of the spinal cord injuries and some of the "other" cases involved a particular Japanese style of acupuncture called Okibari, in which multiple needles are permanently embedded in the subcutaneous paraspinal tissue. These time-lapsed cases indicate that possible needle migration into critical organ systems is a potentially worrisome cause of severe adverse events. [3] Twenty-four of the 26 pneumothorax episodes reported outcomes, with 23 recoveries and one death (the patient had a history of severe emphysema). [4] Upon examination, needles were found in the cervical region in nine patients, in the lumbar region in two patients, and in two patients no needles found. [5] Six of these cases involved positive metal allergies to nickel sulfate, chromium, zinc sulfate, or potassium dichromate which are all used in the various types of acupuncture needles.

Table 8
Summary of Acupuncture Contraindications, Precautions, and Interactions

Contraindications

Absolute return
- Allergy to metal used in needles (metal varies with the type of needle, but include nickel sulfate, chromium, zinc sulfate, and potassium dichromate)
- Severe fear of needles
- Septic patients
- Delusions/hallucinations/paranoia
- Local infections (cellulitis)
- Loss of skin integrity (burns, ulcers)
- Severe bleeding disorders/hemophilia
- Electroacupuncture over heart, brain or implanted electrical device (pacemaker or pump)

Relative

- Anticoagulation and minor bleeding disorders (with deep needling)
- Prosthetic or damaged heart valves (risk of endocarditis with infection)
- Pregnancy (can stimulate uterine contractility)
- During menses (acupuncture may be ineffective)
- Overt fontanelles in an infant

Precautions

- Anticoagulation (with superficial needling)
- Treatment in the seated position (due to possible vasovagal reactions)
- Immunosuppressed patients (use careful aseptic technique)
- DRIVING immediately after receiving treatment (due to possible drowsiness)

Interactions

- The effectiveness of acupuncture may be reduced if initiated while a patient is taking corticosteroids, benzodiazepines, or narcotics (presumably due to medication effects on neuropeptides that are influenced by acupuncture)

initially carved out 4 hours per week of clinical time devoted to acupuncture (this time block could grow as the practice increases in volume). A minimum of two rooms are needed to remain efficient with patient flow, with three rooms being better to allow scheduling of a patient every 20 to 30 minutes. Typically a patient treatment will last from 30 to 45 minutes. Acupuncture is, for the most part, a non-covered service by most third-party payers. The typical charge can vary depending on the overhead of the practice from $75 to $125 per session. Physicians that incorporate this modality into their practice should contact their malpractice insurance provider to determine if a change in coverage is needed (see Chapter 1).

Alternatively, a pain practice could hire a non-physician acupuncturist to provide this service. Generally, payment would be on a fee-for-service basis. Typically, the acupuncturist would not be salaried, but would either be charged rent for the use of the rooms, or have a pre-arranged percentage (15–30%) of the total fee to cover overhead. If space is an issue, the acupuncturist could work during off-hours, for example, in the evening or on weekends. Another approach would be to develop a referral relationship with an off-site acupuncturist; however, for this to be effective, there should be regular communication with the acupuncturist to coordinate patient care. Non-physician acupuncturists should meet the following basic standards to ensure the highest quality of care:

- Successful completion of examinations the National Certification Committee for Acupuncture and Oriental Medicine (NCCAOM) written and oral examination (completion to be verified by the NCCAOM examination board), the Clean Needle Technique course, and state oral and/or practical examination if required by relevant local medical board rules and practices.
- Valid, active state acupuncture license
- Evidence of at least 3 consecutive years of clinical experience since licensure (with an average of at least 500 patient visits per year).
- Three letters of recommendation from peer practitioners.
- Three letters of recommendation from physicians with whom the clinician has co-managed patients.

10. RESOURCES

10.1. American Academy of Medical Acupuncture (AAMA)

This is the United States training organization for medical acupuncture—a system of primarily western acupuncture that is taught only to physicians. There are five training programs in the United States, which aim to integrate the conventional biomedical model into the practice of acupuncture. Most of the programs have a heavy focus on the treatment of pain conditions. The Academy's website is www.medicalacupuncture.org.

10.2. National Certification Commission of Acupuncture and Oriental Medicine (NCCAOM)

This is the primary non-physician acupuncture organization of the United States. They oversee the traditional acupuncture training programs, which consist of 3–4-year accredited schools that vary widely in the scope of their instruction, with many including coursework in herbs, bodywork, tai-chi, meditation, and Eastern philosophy. The website is www.nccaom.com.

11. CONCLUSIONS

In summary, the past several years have shown an increase in the quality of trials examining the clinical efficacy of various CAM modalities for pain conditions. There is still need to raise the quality of the studies from a scientific and methodological point of view in many areas of CAM research by randomization, appropriate sample size, blinding, and developing more sophisticated sham procedures. However, much work still has to be done to find ways to preserve the clinical authenticity of CAM treatment methods when brought into the light of a research protocol. Recent attempts have been made to find a method of maintaining the standardization and reproducibility of a research protocols while allowing the kind of flexible treatment that would normally be applied in a clinical setting. Other questions that should be answered with future studies include understanding how treatment length influences outcome, if maintenance treatments are needed for chronic conditions, and cost and risk comparisons with standard pharmacological treatment. Providing this kind of detail will assist both with reproducibility as well as help us gain a better understanding about whether certain treatment paradigms are superior to others for specific clinical conditions. Finally, physicians who have an interest in pursuing CAM research should educate themselves both about the methodological issues inherent with the particular area of interest as well as about ways to maintain the authenticity of the CAM treatment protocols so that the literature is not populated with more poorly designed studies.

With the emerging interest in integrative medicine, there is a growing interest in collaboration and a greater number of physicians are interested in obtaining training in CAM modalities to help bridge this gap between CAM and conventional clinicians. For example, the American Academy of Medical Acupuncturists (AAMA) has been formed to help as both an educational and research forum for physician acupuncturist and the American Holistic Medical Association provides educational exposure to a broader range of Integrative and CAM modalities. The future of medicine will likely be Integrative and the more health care providers can educate themselves about this area of medicine, the better they will be able to provide the highest quality of care to their patients.

REFERENCES

1. Kaptchuk TJ. Acupuncture: theory, efficacy, and practice. *Ann Intern Med.* Mar 5 2002;136(5): 374–383.
2. Ramey DW. Inaccurate acupuncture history. *Rheumatology (Oxford).* Dec 2004;43(12):1593; author reply 1593–1594.
3. White A, Ernst E. A brief history of acupuncture. *Rheumatology (Oxford).* May 2004;43(5):662–663.
4. Andrews BJ. History of Pain: Acupuncture and the Reinvention of Chinese Medicine. *APS Bulletin.* May/June 1999;9(3).
5. Bonica JJ. Anesthesiology in the People's Republic of China. *Anesthesiology.* Feb 1974;40(2): 175–186.
6. Bonica JJ. Therapeutic acupuncture in the People's Republic of China implications for American medicine. *Jama.* Jun 17 1974;228(12):1544–1551.
7. Han JS. Acupuncture and endorphins. *Neurosci Lett.* May 6 2004;361(1–3):258–261.
8. Ma SX. Neurobiology of Acupuncture: Toward CAM. *Evid Based Complement Alternat Med.* Jun 1 2004;1(1):41–47.
9. Chen S, Ma SX. Nitric oxide in the gracile nucleus mediates depressor response to acupuncture (ST36). *J Neurophysiol.* Aug 2003;90(2):780–785.
10. Lewith GT, White PJ, Pariente J. Investigating acupuncture using brain imaging techniques: The current state of play. *Evidence-Based Complementary and Alternative Medicine.* 2005;2(3):315–319.
11. Yoo SS, Teh EK, Blinder RA, Jolesz FA. Modulation of cerebellar activities by acupuncture stimulation: evidence from fMRI study. *Neuroimage.* Jun 2004;22(2):932–940.
12. Yan B, Li K, Xu JY, et al. Acupoint-specific fMRI patterns in human brain. *Neuroscience Letters.* Aug 2005;383(3):236–240.
13. Wu MT, Hsieh JC, Xiong J, et al. Central nervous pathway for acupuncture stimulation: localization of processing with functional MR imaging of the brain–preliminary experience. *Radiology.* Jul 1999;212(1):133–141.
14. Wager TD, Dagfinn MB, Casey KL. Placebo effects in laser-evoked pain potentials. *Brain Behavior and Immunity.* May 2006;20(3):219–230.
15. Audette JF, Wang F, Smith H. Bilateral activation of motor unit potentials with unilateral needle stimulation of active myofascial trigger points. *American Journal of Physical Medicine & Rehabilitation.* May 2004;83(5):368–374.
16. Audette JF, Blinder RA. Acupuncture in the management of myofascial pain and headache. *Curr Pain Headache Rep.* Oct 2003;7(5):395–401.
17. Shah JP, Phillips TM, Danoff JV, Gerber LH. An in-vivo microanalytical technique for measuring the local biochemical milieu of human skeletal muscle. *J Appl Physiol* Nov 2005;99(5):1977–1984.
18. Melzack R, Stillwell DM, Fox EJ. Trigger points and acupuncture points for pain: correlations and implications. *Pain.* Feb 1977;3(1):3–23.
19. Kao MJ, Hsieh YL, Kuo FJ, Hong CZ. Electrophysiological assessment of acupuncture points. *Am J Phys Med Rehabil.* May 2006;85(5):443–448.

20. Grigg P, Schaible HG, Schmidt RF. Mechanical Sensitivity of Group-Iii and Group-Iv Afferents from Posterior Articular Nerve in Normal and Inflamed Cat Knee. *Journal of Neurophysiology.* Apr 1986;55(4):635–643.

21. Wesselmann U, Lai J. Mechanisms of referred visceral pain: uterine inflammation in the adult virgin rat results in neurogenic plasma extravasation in the skin. *Pain.* Dec 1997;73(3):309–317.

22. Langevin HM, Churchill DL, Wu J, et al. Evidence of connective tissue involvement in acupuncture. *Faseb J.* Jun 2002;16(8):872–874.

23. Sierpina VS, Frenkel MA. Acupuncture: a clinical review. *South Med J.* Mar 2005;98(3):330–337.

24. Park J, White A, Stevinson C, Ernst E, James M. Validating a new non-penetrating sham acupuncture device: two randomized controlled trials. *Acupunct Med.* Dec 2002;20(4):168–174.

25. Kleinhenz J, Streitberger K, Windeler J, Gussbacher A, Mavridis G, Martin E. Randomised clinical trial comparing the effects of acupuncture and a newly designed placebo needle in rotator cuff tendinitis. *Pain.* Nov 1999;83(2):235–241.

26. Streitberger K, Friedrich-Rust M, Bardenheuer H, et al. Effect of acupuncture compared with placebo-acupuncture at P6 as additional antiemetic prophylaxis in high-dose chemotherapy and autologous peripheral blood stem cell transplantation: a randomized controlled single-blind trial. *Clin Cancer Res.* Jul 2003;9(7):2538–2544.

27. Streitberger K, Kleinhenz J. Introducing a placebo needle into acupuncture research. *Lancet.* Aug 1 1998;352(9125):364–365.

28. Acupuncture. *NIH Consens Statement.* Nov 3–5 1997;15(5):1–34.

29. Berman BM, Ezzo J, Hadhazy V, Swyers JP. Is acupuncture effective in the treatment of fibromyalgia? *J Fam Pract.* Mar 1999;48(3):213–218.

30. Deluze C, Bosia L, Zirbs A, Chantraine A, Vischer TL. Electroacupuncture in fibromyalgia: results of a controlled trial. *Bmj.* Nov 21 1992;305(6864):1249–1252.

31. Assefi NP, Sherman KJ, Jacobsen C, Goldberg J, Smith WR, Buchwald D. A randomized clinical trial of acupuncture compared with sham acupuncture in fibromyalgia. *Ann Intern Med.* Jul 5 2005;143(1):10–19.

32. Harris RE, Tian X, Williams DA, et al. Treatment of fibromyalgia with formula acupuncture: investigation of needle placement, needle stimulation, and treatment frequency. *J Altern Complement Med.* Aug 2005;11(4):663–671.

33. Irnich D, Behrens N, Gleditsch JM, et al. Immediate effects of dry needling and acupuncture at distant points in chronic neck pain: results of a randomized, double-blind, sham-controlled crossover trial. *Pain.* Sep 2002;99(1–2):83–89.

34. Itoh K, Katsumi Y, Kitakoji H. Trigger point acupuncture treatment of chronic low back pain in elderly patients–a blinded RCT. *Acupunct Med.* Dec 2004;22(4):170–177.

35. Ceccherelli F, Rigoni MT, Gagliardi G, Ruzzante L. Comparison of superficial and deep acupuncture in the treatment of lumbar myofascial pain: a double-blind randomized controlled study. *Clin J Pain.* May-Jun 2002;18(3):149–153.

36. Ceccheerelli F, Bordin M, Gagliardi G, Caravello M. Comparison between superficial and deep acupuncture in the treatment of the shoulder's myofascial pain: a randomized and controlled study. *Acupunct Electrother Res.* 2001;26(4):229–238.

37. Casimiro L, Barnsley L, Brosseau L, et al. Acupuncture and electroacupuncture for the treatment of rheumatoid arthritis. *Cochrane Database Syst Rev.* 2005;(4):CD003788.

38. Man SC, Baragar FD. Preliminary clinical study of acupuncture in rheumatoid arthritis. *J Rheumatol.* Mar 1974;1(1):126–129.

39. David J, Townsend S, Sathanathan R, Kriss S, Dore CJ. The effect of acupuncture on patients with rheumatoid arthritis: a randomized, placebo-controlled cross-over study. *Rheumatology (Oxford).* Sep 1999;38(9):864–869.

40. Linde K, Jonas WB, Melchart D, Willich S. The methodological quality of randomized controlled trials of homeopathy, herbal medicines and acupuncture. *Int J Epidemiol.* Jun 2001;30(3):526–531.

41. Hesse J, Mogelvang B, Simonsen H. Acupuncture versus metoprolol in migraine prophylaxis: a randomized trial of trigger point inactivation. *J Intern Med.* May 1994;235(5):451–456.

42. Melchart D, Streng A, Hoppe A, et al. The acupuncture randomised trial (ART) for tension-type headache–details of the treatment. *Acupunct Med.* Dec 2005;23(4):157–165.

43. Melchart D, Linde K, Streng A, et al. Acupuncture Randomized Trials (ART) in patients with migraine or tension-type headache–design and protocols. *Forsch Komplementarmed Klass Naturheilkd.* Aug 2003;10(4):179–184.

44. White AR, Ernst E. A systematic review of randomized controlled trials of acupuncture for neck pain. *Rheumatology (Oxford)*. Feb 1999;38(2):143–147.
45. White P, Lewith G, Prescott P, Conway J. Acupuncture versus placebo for the treatment of chronic mechanical neck pain: a randomized, controlled trial. *Ann Intern Med*. Dec 21 2004;141(12): 911–919.
46. Witt CM, Jena S, Brinkhaus B, Liecker B, Wegscheider K, Willich SN. Acupuncture for patients with chronic neck pain. *Pain*. Nov 2006;125(1–2):98–106.
47. Goolkasian P, Wheeler AH, Gretz SS. The Neck Pain and Disability Scale: Test-retest reliability and construct validity. *Clinical Journal of Pain*. Jul-Aug 2002;18(4):245–250.
48. Manheimer E, White A, Berman B, Forys K, Ernst E. Meta-analysis: acupuncture for low back pain. *Ann Intern Med*. Apr 19 2005;142(8):651–663.
49. Green S, Buchbinder R, Hetrick S. Acupuncture for shoulder pain. *Cochrane Database Syst Rev*. Apr 18 2005;2:CD005319.
50. Guerra de Hoyos JA, Andres Martin Mdel C, Bassas y Baena de Leon E, et al. Randomised trial of long term effect of acupuncture for shoulder pain. *Pain*. Dec 2004;112(3):289–298.
51. Trinh KV, Phillips SD, Ho E, Damsma K. Acupuncture for the alleviation of lateral epicondyle pain: a systematic review. *Rheumatology (Oxford)*. Sep 2004;43(9):1085–1090.
52. Fink M, Wolkenstein E, Karst M, Gehrke A. Acupuncture in chronic epicondylitis: a randomized controlled trial. *Rheumatology*. Feb 2002;41(2):205–209.
53. Ezzo J, Hadhazy V, Birch S, et al. Acupuncture for osteoarthritis of the knee: a systematic review. *Arthritis Rheum*. Apr 2001;44(4):819–825.
54. Berman BM, Lao LX, Langenberg P, Lee WL, Gilpin AMK, Hochberg MC. Effectiveness of acupuncture as adjunctive therapy in osteoarthritis of the knee - A randomized, controlled trial. *Annals of Internal Medicine*. Dec 2004;141(12):901–910.
55. Witt C, Brinkhaus B, Jena S, et al. Acupuncture in patients with osteoarthritis of the knee: a randomised trial. *Lancet*. Jul 2005;366(9480):136–143.
56. Melchart D, Weidenhammer W, Streng A, et al. Prospective investigation of adverse effects of acupuncture in 97 733 patients. *Archives of Internal Medicine*. Jan 2004;164(1):104–105.
57. Umlauf R. Completion of Research into the Feasibility and Implementation of Acupuncture for Trauma Care and Medical First-Aid. *American Journal of Acupuncture*. 1991;19(2):192–192.
58. Ernst E, White AR. Prospective studies of the safety of acupuncture: a systematic review. *Am J Med*. Apr 15 2001;110(6):481–485.
59. Birch S, Jamison RN. Controlled trial of Japanese acupuncture for chronic myofascial neck pain: assessment of specific and nonspecific effects of treatment. *Clin J Pain*. Sep 1998;14(3):248–255.
60. Lao LX, Hamilton GR, Fu JP, Berman BM. Is acupuncture safe? A systematic review of case reports. *Alternative Therapies in Health and Medicine*. Jan-Feb 2003;9(1):72–83.
61. Rampes H, James R. Complications of acupuncture. *Acup Med*. May 1995;13(1):26–33.
62. Lee TL. Acupuncture and chronic pain management. *Ann Acad Med Singapore*. Jan 2000;29(1): 17–21.
63. Han JS. Acupuncture: neuropeptide release produced by electrical stimulation of different frequencies *Trends Neurosci*. January 2003;26(1):17–22.

19 Nutrition and Supplements for Pain Management

Maria Sulindro-Ma, Charise L. Ivy, and Amber C. Isenhart

CONTENTS

Summary

This chapter discusses dietary guidelines and nutritional supplements that have been proven to be beneficial in the treatment of pain. First, a strong foundational diet is presented, including anti-inflammatory ingredients. Next, several key supplements that are helpful for pain conditions are discussed. The chapter is completed with a discussion of some of the most common chronic pain conditions, with specific dietary guidelines and nutritional supplement selections for each condition.

Key Words: pain, nutrition, diet, supplements, vitamins, inflammation, osteoarthritis (OA), rheumatoid arthritis (RA), premenstrual syndrome (PMS), osteoporosis, pelvic inflammatory disease (PID), migraine, fibromyalgia, chronic fatigue syndrome (CFS)

1. INTRODUCTION

Complementary and Alternative Medicine (CAM) covers a wide range of treatment options including diet and nutrition *(1)*. Many individuals living with chronic pain seek CAM treatments in addition to or instead of allopathic medicine. The healthcare costs associated with unsuccessfully treated pain total $61.2 billion per year *(2)*. The foundation of good nutrition along with exercise and stress reduction can greatly contribute to improving a chronic pain sufferer's quality of life *(3)*. This chapter will focus on nutrition as a treatment modality, and will look at how the foods we eat play a powerful role in pain management.

The cellular membrane theory teaches us that the absorption of necessary molecules into a cell and its mitochondria depends on the bioavailability of nutrients from food

From: *Contemporary Pain Medicine: Integrative Pain Medicine: The Science and Practice of Complementary and Alternative Medicine in Pain Management*
Edited by: J. F. Audette and A. Bailey © Humana Press, Totowa, NJ

and supplements in the diet. Each cell, tissue, organ, and system of our bodies depends on the nutritional signals we send. Although it has been practically ignored by allopathic medicine for many decades, nutrition is truly the foundation of medicine and healing. Without a proper foundation, any structure will be weak and ultimately ineffective. Food *is* medicine!

Pain is the common denominator in many of the most common disabling conditions such as cancer, cardiovascular disease, osteoporosis, osteoarthritis, rheumatoid arthritis, diabetic neuropathy, fibromyalgia, premenstrual syndrome, and pelvic inflammatory disease. But even when the pain described by different people arises from the same underlying condition, or the same body region, nutritional management needs to be personalized to the individual.

No two patients are the same in the field of nutritional medicine. Each individual's body is different in its chemistry and nutritional needs. Each is therefore unique in its sensitivities and susceptibilities to various deficiencies and clinical conditions, and each individual requires different nutrients to maintain proper balance.

Before prescribing dietary changes or supplements, it is especially important to consider objective laboratory findings that may indicate a nutritional deficiency or give other helpful information. The philosophy of care is then fairly simple. If a nutritional deficiency is found, replenish it. If a toxin is found, remove it. The ultimate goal is to provide positive balance and health.

Nutritional medicine for pain also requires an understanding of the pathogenesis of the disease process. The practitioner can then prescribe ingredients with specific roles in mitigating the disease process, such as reduction of inflammation, or with specific effects on other factors contributing to pain, such as stress and insomnia. The combined treatment of the primary cause and the secondary contributing factors helps the patient to be more comfortable and to have patience to observe the benefit of nutritional treatment which is usually slower than pharmacological pain control.

The goal of this chapter is to present guidelines for foods and supplements that can help in managing pain. First, the basics of a strong foundational diet, including anti-inflammatory ingredients, will be presented. Then, several key supplements that have been shown to be helpful for pain conditions will be covered. The chapter concludes with a discussion of some of the most common chronic pain conditions, with specific dietary guidelines and supplement selections for each condition.

2. DIETARY GUIDELINES FOR MANAGING PAIN

Scientific evidence shows that certain foods are as effective at treating or managing disease as medications. More specifically, eating a balanced diet of whole foods such as fresh fruits and vegetables, whole grains, and lean meats, while eliminating processed sugars, manufactured foods, and unhealthy fats, helps reduce pain and inflammation. In addition, omega-3 fatty acids, B vitamins, and antioxidants have been recognized as having properties that assist in the reduction of pain and inflammation. The anti-inflammatory and pain-reducing properties of vitamin D are also being studied.

Inflammation and pain are closely related physiologic mechanisms. Typically inflammation, a marker for fighting disease, results in pain. While medications provide relief, foods can provide additional relief without side effects. Providing the body with disease-fighting ammunition in a healthy diet is a great foundation.

To begin, it is important to consume a diet high in green leafy vegetables and brightly colored fruits and vegetables. Fruits and vegetables are high in antioxidants and contain anti-inflammatory phytochemicals. Antioxidants are compounds that protect cells against the effects of damaging free radicals and other reactive oxygen species. An overload of reactive oxygen species leads to oxidative stress and subsequent cellular damage. Oxidative stress has been linked to cancer, aging, atherosclerosis, inflammation, and neurodegenerative diseases such as Parkinson's disease and Alzheimer's dementia *(4)*.

Flavonoids are antioxidant plant compounds that lessen inflammation and strengthen the connective tissue in joints. Broccoli, blueberries, grapefruit, onions, apples, oranges, soybeans, chocolate, pomegranates, limes, lemons, tomatoes, carrots, red wine, and tea are high in flavonoids. Quercetin is an antioxidant flavonoid that is found in apples, red onions, grapes, and green tea. Quercetin has also been studied for its ability to decrease inflammation *(5)*.

Vitamins C and E, selenium, and carotenoids are antioxidants that have the capability to decrease inflammation. Food sources high in vitamin C include cabbage, red potatoes, strawberries, tangerines, red bell peppers, oranges, and kiwis. The antioxidant properties of vitamin E are thought to protect joint cells from free radical damage. According to research, low levels of vitamin E have been found in the joint fluid of rheumatoid arthritis patients. Great food sources of vitamin E include almonds, peanut butter, avocados, olive oil, peanuts, and sunflower seeds *(6)*.

Brightly colored fruits and vegetables are not alone in their pain and inflammation-fighting properties. Foods from each category (carbohydrates, protein, and fat) also provide unique anti-inflammatory and pain reduction properties.

The human body requires carbohydrates for energy. Some of the best sources of carbohydrates are whole grains such as slow-cooked oatmeal, 100% whole-wheat bread, and brown rice. Whole grains contain the outer bran and inner germ layers of the grain, which provide fiber and also energy-rich starch. The body breaks down whole grains more slowly than it does refined carbohydrates such as white flour and sugar. The slow digestion of these high-fiber foods maintains more stable glucose and, therefore, insulin levels in the bloodstream. Better control of blood glucose and insulin can help prevent the development of type-2 diabetes and the potential chronic pain that can accompany diabetes-related conditions. Refined sugars, found in candy and sweets, white rice, white bread, and white pasta should be eliminated, as these carbohydrates may increase the susceptibility to pain and inflammation.

Protein choices can also affect inflammation and pain in the body. Protein is needed to build healthy body tissues. Good protein choices include lean poultry, seafood, nuts, legumes, and seeds. Certain fish have the added benefit of being rich in omega-3 fatty acids as well as being high in protein. A wealth of research suggests that consuming certain types of fish that contain omega-3 fatty acids may help to reduce pain and inflammation. Omega-3 fatty acids are discussed in more detail later in this chapter. In addition, derivatives of soybeans such as tofu, as well as the soybeans themselves, have anti-inflammatory properties due to the antioxidants isoflavones. Nuts, seeds, and legumes are excellent sources of protein and are also good sources of omega-3 fatty acids.

Some protein foods have fewer anti-inflammatory properties due to their high concentration of arachidonic acid, an omega-6 fatty acid. Even though arachidonic acid is essential for proper body functioning, too high an intake has been shown to trigger inflammatory responses. Arachidonic acid can be found in protein foods such as red meats and eggs.

Fats are an integral part of our diets and provide an alternative way to manage pain and inflammation. Fats are either saturated, polyunsaturated or monounsaturated. The healthier fats are monounsaturated, followed by polyunsaturated fats. Saturated fats are labeled as "bad fats" due to their inflammatory properties and potential damage to the cardiovascular system. Monounsaturated fats are "good fats" because they have been shown to improve lipid profiles by increasing the good cholesterol (HDL) and decreasing the bad cholesterol (LDL) in our blood.

Classes of fats called essential fatty acids, omega-3 (alpha-linolenic) and omega-6 (linoleic), are especially important in the role of preventing inflammation and pain. The omega-3 fatty acids are made up of eicosapentaenoic acid (EPA) and docosahexaenoic acid (DHA). Omega-6 fatty acids are well known for their ability to increase hormone-like substances that are capable of suppressing inflammation. One preliminary study showed that the administration of gamma-linolenic acid (an omega-6 fatty acid derivative) to patients with chronic joint inflammation reduced pain symptoms (7).

Omega-3 and omega-6 fatty acids are referred to as essential fatty acids because they cannot be synthesized in the human body and are only obtainable from the foods we eat. Although omega-6 fatty acids have some anti-inflammatory properties on their own as mentioned above, a diet too high in omega-6 fatty acids produces inflammatory metabolites, such as arachidonic acid, that reduce the production of omega-3 fatty acids. The *ratio* of omega-3 to omega-6 fatty acids in the body is more important in the anti-inflammatory process. In general, a higher intake of omega-3 fatty acids is the key for reduction of inflammation, but most people consume very few omega-3 fatty acids, and too many omega-6 fatty acids. In the United States, the average dietary intake of omega-3 fatty acids is approximately 1.6 g per day with comsumption of omega-6 fatty acids being roughly 10–20 times this amount.

The ratio of omega-6 to omega-3 fatty acids in the US diet has increased due to the introduction of processed foods, hydrogenated vegetable oils, and food preservation. In order to reduce the amount of saturated fats in our diet and increase the shelf life of foods, food manufacturers created more stable polyunsaturated fats in the form of hydrogenated oils. This alteration of oil, however, created trans fats. The United States Food and Drug Administration (FDA) and other regulatory entities now state that trans fats are more damaging to the cardiovascular system and produce more inflammatory agents than saturated fats.

To increase the intake of omega-3 fatty acids, the American Heart Association recommends consuming fish at least two times per week for healthy adults with no history of heart disease. In particular, fatty fish such as anchovies, bluefish, carp, catfish, halibut, herring, lake trout, mackerel, pompano, salmon, striped sea bass, tuna (albacore), and whitefish are recommended due to their higher levels of omega-3 fatty acids. The FDA states that intake of up to 3 g per day of omega-3 fatty acids from fish is "Generally Regarded As Safe" (labeled GRAS)(8). Omega-3 content varies from fish to fish ranging from 0.6 g for trout to 2.2 g for mackeral. Omega-3 fatty acids can also be found in flax seeds and walnuts. In addition, olive oil, grapeseed oil, primrose oil, borage oil, and walnut oil contain high amounts of omega-3 fatty acids and have the same anti-inflammatory properties.

Recent research indicates that adequate vitamin D intake is important in reducing chronic pain as well, and reversely that inadequate vitamin D may actually contribute to chronic pain *(9,10)*. Vitamin D is also vital for calcium absorption in bones and to improve muscle strength.

In one study performed at the University of Minnesota, 93% of subjects with non-specific musculoskeletal pain were found to be deficient in serum levels of vitamin D. The authors recommended regular screening of individuals with persistent musculoskeletal pain for vitamin D deficiency. In a second study that included children, as well as adults, the researchers found 100% of African-American, East African, Hispanic, and Native American subjects were vitamin D deficient based on serum levels of 25-hydroxyvitamin D measured by radioimmunoassay. In addition, study subjects under age 30 were vitamin D deficient. Of these, 55 percent were severely deficient, and five patients were completely vitamin D deficient. According to the authors, this study supports additional routine testing for deficiencies of vitamin D in patients with persistent, nonspecific musculoskeletal pain.

Vitamin D is found in foods such as fortified milk and in slight amounts in cheese. Other food sources include egg yolk, cod liver oil, oysters, canned salmon and tuna, fortified soy beverages, and fortified cereals. Additionally, UV rays from sunlight trigger the synthesis of vitamin D in the skin.

The B vitamins, thiamin (B1), pyridoxine (B6), and cyanocobalamin (B12), have shown some clinical effectiveness in managing pain particularly of neuropathic origin. The conditions researched include lumbago, sciatica, trigeminal neuralgia, facial paralysis and optic neuritis *(11–13)*. B vitamins are found in whole grains, beans, dried peas, lean meats, legumes, green leafy vegetables and eggs.

See Table 1 for concrete recommendations for patients wishing to adopt a more anti-inflammatory and pain reducing diet.

Table 1
Patient Recommendations for an Anti-Inflammatory Diet

Breakfast	Oatmeal or other whole grain minimally processed cereal served with fresh berries, ground flaxseed and a cup of soy milk
Lunch	Fiber-rich salad loaded with colorful vegetables and topped with grilled salmon
Dinner	Whole grain pasta with pesto or rice dish with soy nuts and grilled tofu or chicken
Snacks	Focus on fresh fruits, vegetables, nuts, and seeds instead of cookies, chips, and candy
Miscellaneous	• Fish should be consumed more frequently than saturated fat-rich red meat • Avoid deep-fried foods high in trans fats; instead bake or sauté your meals with olive oil • Choose green, orange, red, and yellow vegetables everyday for your side dishes • Fruits and vegetables known as "nightshade" (tomatoes, potatoes, egg plant, peppers, and tobacco) have higher sugar contents and promote water retention; these can be decreased or eliminated in people wanting to take extra measures to decrease inflammation • Drink plenty of water and herbal and green teas; avoid sodas and other sweetened drinks • Maintain a healthy weight

3. NUTRITIONAL SUPPLEMENTS IN THE MANAGEMENT OF PAIN

On a physiological level, nutritional supplements can decrease pain through a variety of mechanisms. They can reduce inflammation and muscle fatigue from overexertion, help support joint function, maintain joint range of motion, protect bone, and stimulate the formation of cartilage *(14,15)*. The following is an alphabetical list of key nutritional supplements with analgesic and anti-inflammatory properties.

3.1. Bromelaine

Bromelaine, also called Bromelin, is a proteolytic enzyme sulphydryl from the pineapple family Ananas Comosus (Bromelainceae). The pure form of bromelaine, from the stem of the plant, has a high pH of 9.5–10.0, which results in an average pH of 5.0–8.0 when activated. Bromelaine from the fruit of the plant has an acidic pH of 4.0–5.0 *(16)*.

This enzyme assists in the digestion of protein. It also stimulates the production of prostaglandins, reduces inflammation, and decreases blood platelet aggregation.

Because it relaxes skeletal muscle, it can be used to avoid muscle strain and prevent injury, such as in preparation for athletic competition *(17)*. Due to the high pH, it also can prevent gastric ulcer exacerbation and enhance wound healing. For many people it helps relieve sinus problems, likely due to its anti-inflammatory effect.

Because of these anti-inflammatory properties, bromelaine has important roles in pain management *(18)*:

- Activates proteolytic activity at the site of inflammation
- Reduces kininogen, activates plasmin and reduces kinin
- Inhibits pro-infammatory prostaglandins and induces accumulation of the anti-inflammatory prostaglandin E1, which then inhibits the release of polymorphonuclear (PMN) leukocytes and lysosomal enzymes
- Induces fibrinolysis
- Inhibits the mobilization of arachidonic acid, decreasing joint inflammation and atherogenesis factors

Dose: 1,800–2,500 mg orally per day, or 500–1,500 mg in three divided doses between meals.

Clinical applications:

1. Athletic injury; muscle strain
2. Premenstrual syndrome; dysmenorrhea *(19)*
3. Angina
4. Arthritis
5. Pancreatic insufficiency
6. Cellulitis
7. Sinusitis
8. General edema
9. Thrombophlebitis *(20)*

Toxicity: No negative side effects have been reported. Long-term use is well tolerated. In people sensitive to pineapple, bromelaine may cause a temporary allergic reaction, including rash, urticaria, nausea, and diarrhea. There are no reported cases of anaphylaxis.

3.2. Cartilage Factors

Many European studies have supported the use of hydrolyzed collagen peptides to support joints and protect cartilage *(21)*. One of the observed mechanisms of these peptides is the stimulation of the collagen matrix restructuring process *(22)*. They also maintain healthy enzyme function and aid in nutrient and energy consumption. Bovine cartilage specifically contains enzymes for proteolysis that may build and maintain cartilage in joints.

Dose: Load 5–10 g orally per day for 6 months.

Clinical applications:

1. Decreases joint inflammation
2. Promotes build-up of cartilage
3. Strengthens collagen
4. Supports chondrocytes in cartilage

Toxicity: No negative side effects have been reported.

3.3. Cayenne Pepper (Capsicum frutescens)

Other common names for cayenne pepper are capsaicin, chili pepper, American pepper and red pepper. This fruit, which is technically a berry, is native to tropical America, but it is now located throughout the world. It is particularly used in the foods of Southeast Asia, Italy, and Mexico.

Cayenne pepper decreases pain by depleting the neurotransmitter substance P, the chemical mediator of pain, from the periphery of the body. Substance P activates inflammatory mediators such as those that occur in joint tissue in patients with osteoarthritis and rheumatoid arthritis. Cayenne pepper also contains vitamins A and C and volatile oils *(23)*.

When taken internally, cayenne pepper can reduce cholesterol and triglycerides and decrease platelet aggregation, thus reducing the likelihood of developing arthrosclerosis *(24)*.

Dose:

- 0.025% or 0.075% capsaicin cream or ointment; apply topically three to four times per day to the painful area.
- As a food spice, cayenne pepper can be used as tolerated.

Clinical Applications:

1. Asthma
2. Fever
3. Sore throat
4. Digestive disturbance *(25)*
5. Cancer *(26)*
6. Diabetic neuropathy *(27,28)*
7. Cluster headache
8. Rheumatoid arthritis
9. Other arthritis
10. Psoriasis *(29)*
11. Post-herpetic neuralgia *(30,31)*

12. Trigeminal neuralgia *(32)*
13. Post-surgical mastectomy pain
14. Mouth sores and pain from chemotherapy or radiation

Toxicity: No negative side effects have been reported. Cayenne pepper has been used liberally in cuisine without complications. It has a grade of GRAS (Generally Recognized as Safe) in the United States. When applied topically or taken internally, it may produce a temporary burning sensation, which can feel severe, but there is increased tolerance with increased use. Contrary to popular belief, it does not cause gastric ulcer, and can even have a positive effect as a digestant and carminative *(25)*.

3.4. Chondroitin Sulfate

Bovine chondroitin sulfate is an ingredient that is responsible for building and supporting cartilage. Chondroitin is also commonly formulated as chondroitin hydrochloride *(33)*.

Dose: 500–1,000 mg orally per day in two to three divided doses. Use in combination with glucosamine.

Clinical applications:

- Osteoarthritis *(34)*
- Anti-inflammatory

Toxicity: No negative side effects have been reported.

3.5. CMO (Cetyl-myristoleate)

This is an ester of the fatty acid myristoleic acid *(35,36)*. There is some support for the use of this ingredient for joint and collagen health *(37)*. It maintains a healthy immune response at the cellular level and promotes joint lubrication. It also acts as an immune system modulator, mediating the histamine and leukotriene response *(38)*.

Dose: 1,000–1,500 mg orally per day in two divided doses.

Clinical Applications:

1. Osteoarthritis *(39,40)*
2. Rheumatoid arthritis *(41,42)*
3. Fibromyalgia
4. Temperomandibular joint dysfunction

Toxicity: No negative side effects have been reported.

3.6. Cucurmin

Cucurmin is the yellow pigment of the *Cucurma longa* or Turmeric plant, which is both a spice and a medicinal plant. Cucurmin contains diferuloyl methane, which has anti-inflammatory and antioxidant effects. It inhibits the formation of leukotrienes and other inflammatory mediators. It has the ability to stimulate the formation of adrenal corticosteroids, potentiating the action of cortisol and also preventing the breakdown of cortisol *(43)*.

Cucurmin is reported to be as effective as cortisone, or the potent anti-inflammatory drug phenylbutazone, in models of acute inflammation, with no major side effects.

A dosage of 1,200 mg per day of cucurmin has been shown to have comparable anti-inflammatory efficacy to 300 mg per day of phenylbutazone *(44)*. In people with rheumatoid arthritis, there was reduction of joint swelling, decrease in the duration of morning stiffness, and improvement in walking time with use of cucurmin *(45)*.

Turmeric is a fabulous spice for a wide variety of foods. One can also receive the benefits of cucurmin by taking it as a supplement.

Dose: 1,500–2,000 mg orally per day in three divided doses, for anti-inflammatory effect. (This is equivalent to 8,000–60,000 mg per day of turmeric.) The absorption of cucurmin is improved if taken with bromelaine 20 minutes before a meal or on an empty stomach. Fish oil, lecithin, or essential fatty acids may also help to increase absorption.

Clinical Applications:

1. Rheumatoid arthritis (especially in an acute exacerbation)
2. Osteoarthritis
3. Joint inflammation
4. Pelvic inflammatory disease
5. Temperomandibular joint disorder
6. Cancer pain
7. Postoperative inflammation

Toxicity: No negative side effects have been reported. No toxicity has been observed in animals fed with high doses of cucurmin up to 3 g per kg body weight.

3.7. Devil's Claw

Harpagophytum procumbent is a plant indigenous to South Africa. It is known as devil's claw due to its claw-like extensions. Other common names are grapple plant and wood spider. Its health benefit is connected to the tuberous root extension. Devil's claw maintains healthy interleukin and leukocyte activity. It relieves pain and inflammation. Clinical studies have supported its properties in the promotion of musculoskeletal flexibility and function *(46,47)*. Studies in Europe have found that it increases flexibility of the neck, back and shoulders, and promotes better hip and knee function *(48)*. Devil's claw can also be used as a diuretic.

Dose: 500–1500 mg orally per day in two divided doses with meals.

Clinical Applications:

1. Osteoarthritis
2. Rheumatoid arthritis
3. Allergies
4. Liver detoxification
5. Gall bladder and kidney disorders
6. Lumbago
7. Gout
8. Menopausal symptoms

Toxicity: Devil's claw enhances gastric juice production and is therefore contraindicated with stomach and intestinal ulcers. It should not be used in pregnancy.

3.8. Ginger (**Zingiber officinalis**)

Ginger is native to Asia, but it is also available in other tropical areas such as India, Jamaica, Nigeria, and Haiti. The root of the plant is used for culinary and medicinal purposes. It has been used in China to treat numerous conditions since the fourth century BC.

Ginger has many pharmacological properties. It has an analgesic effect by inhibiting the release of substance P (similar to the action of capsaicin in red pepper) *(49,50)*. It inhibits the synthesis of prostaglandins, thromboxane and leukotriene, and inhibits platelet aggregation. It has an antioxidant effect. It helps to lower cholesterol. It can calm diarrhea, improve cardiac muscle function, and raise metabolic rate. It has some natural antibiotic activities. It can also be used to decrease the risk of gastric ulcers in those who are sensitive to indomethicin, aspirin, or other common ulcerogenic medications *(51,52)*.

Dose: For acute inflammation, 5–10 g per day orally of a powdered form, in two to three divided doses. (One gram of powder is equivalent to 10 g of fresh ginger root or maintenance or chronic use, 500–1,000 mg per day orally in three divided doses for ginger extract (20% gingerol and shogaol)).

Clinical Applications:

1. Inflammatory conditions such as rheumatoid arthritis
2. Migraine headaches
3. Osteoarthritis
4. Muscular discomfort
5. Nausea and vomiting
6. Motion sickness

Toxicity: No negative side effects have been reported. Some people experience gastrointestinal discomfort with high doses of 6 g per day or more.

3.9. Glucosamine

The failure of our body to manufacture enough glucosamine to maintain joint cartilage has been suggested as a major contributing factor to osteoarthritis *(53–55)*. Supplementation of glucosamine is currently being used all over the world in the treatment of arthritic conditions. It has the ability to block enzymes that degrade cartilage *(56)*.

For many years glucosamine has been the most widely sold over the counter supplement due to its endorsement by many physicians as an alternative for joint pain. *(57)*. Commercially it is sold as glucosamine sulfate, and this form has been extensively studied for clinical efficacy. Glucosamine is often combined with chondroitin to build up proteoglycan and connective tissue in the joint cartilage *(58–60)*.

There is no food source of glucosamine. The supplement is usually derived from chitin, a substance in the shells of shrimp, lobster, or crabs.

Dose: 1,000–2,500 mg orally per day in two divided doses.

Cinical Applications:

1. Osteoarthritis
2. Use as alternative to non-steroidal anti-inflammatory medications.

Toxicity: No negative side effects have been reported. It is well tolerated by most people. Some light gastrointestinal problems can occur in highly sensitive individuals. If this occurs, glucosamine should be taken with meals. There are recent case reports of a possible increase in total cholesterol.

3.10. Hyaluronic Acid

This denatured low molecular weight type 2 collagen supports joints by promoting cartilage and synovial fluid synthesis, enhancing the integrity and motility of joints. Hyaluronic acid also supports the elasticity and firmness of skin. It attracts water, promoting hydration and moisture retention within the dermal matrix. This function leads to its use in skin therapeutic care to diminish fine lines and wrinkles.

Hyaluronic acid is available in an oral powdered form, and an injectable form for intraarticular use *(61,62)*.

Dose: 100–200 mg orally per day in one to two divided doses. For intraarticular use the dose varies depending on the manufacturer.

- Intra-articular—dose varies depending on the manufacturer.

Clinical Applications:

1. Knee osteoarthritis (intraarticular form) *(63–66)*
2. Fibromyalgia
3. Gout
4. Temperomandibular joint dysfunction
5. Lumbago

Toxicity: No significant toxicity. There is a very high L-50 (lethal dose) level. Doses higher than 300–400 mg per day can cause a detoxification crisis syndrome from rapid detoxification. Excess medication is completely removed by the liver and kidneys.

3.11. MSM (Methylsulfonylmethane)

Methylsulfonylmethane is a well-known nutrient for the support of cartilage and connective tissue strength, and is used to decrease joint pain. The sulfur helps to enhance the structure and integrity of proteoglycans *(67)*.

MSM is the major metabolite of DMSO (dimethylsulfoxide), a sulfur-based compound known to help maintain connective tissue and support the collagen and keratin in skin, nails and hair. It is essential to methionine, cysteine, and protein metabolism. It also supports the immune and respiratory systems *(68)*.

Dose: 1,000–3,000 mg per day orally in two to three divided doses. Start with a low dose and increase as tolerated to avoid rapid detoxification.

Clinical Applications:

1. Osteoarthritis *(69)*
2. Rheumatoid arthritis *(70)*
3. Premenstrual syndrome *(71)*
4. Fibromyalgia
5. Gout
6. Allergies
7. Gastrointestinal disturbances / disorders
8. Gastroesophageal reflux disease

9. Migraine headaches
10. Muscle aches and pains

Toxicity: May cause insomnia with long-term use. If taken in very large doses, may cause a detoxification crisis that is reversible *(72)*.

3.12. Omega-3 Fatty Acids (Fish Oil)

It is well known and accepted that consumption of fish oil is beneficial to general health. In terms of pain management, studies have reported that omega-3 fatty acids can ameliorate the signs and symptoms of psoriasis *(73)* and rheumatoid arthritis due their efficacy in reconditioning cellular membranes and their antiinflammatory effects.

The omega-3 fatty acids are eicosapentaenoic acid (EPA) and docosahexaenoic acid (DHA). They are also called polyunsaturated fatty acids and are found in shellfish, sea mammals, phytoplankton, and fish, specifically herring, cod liver, salmon, mackerel and sardines. Commercial fish contain less DHA and EPA than wild fish.

Dietary omega-3 fatty acids are also found in foods such as tofu, canola oil, black currant oil, flaxseed oil, nuts, and soybeans. However, these sources can contain more omega-6 fatty acids than omega-3, which can neutralize many of the therapeutic benefits. (See above section Dietary Guidelines for Managing Pain.)

Dose:

- 5,000–15,000 mg orally per day of EPA and DHA for at least three months per year for reconditioning of the cell membranes
- 1,000–3,000 mg orally per day for maintenance.

Clinical Applications:

1. Reconditioning of cellular membranes to improve absorption of nutrients
2. Cardiovascular disease *(74)*
3. Angina pectoris (reduces frequency of attacks) *(75–77)*
4. Migraine headache (changes prostaglandin synthesis; reduces platelet serotonin release; reduces cerebral vasospasm)
5. Hyperlipidemia *(78)*
6. Hypertension
7. Rheumatoid arthritis (decreases morning stiffness and joint tenderness)

Toxicity:

- 1.8 g of EPA daily is safe for long-term use.
- Omega-3 fatty acids are commonly formulated with vitamins A and D, both of which can cause vitamin toxicity if taken in high doses. Omega-3 alone is safer and more beneficial.
- Some studies indicate an effect in prolongation of bleeding time due to inhibition of platelet aggregation and a decrease of thromboxane A2 production. Caution should be taken when a person is also taking aspirin or warfarin.

4. NUTRITION AND SUPPLEMENTS FOR SPECIFIC PAIN-RELATED CONDITIONS

4.1. Osteoarthritis

Osteoarthritis is a universal condition of "wear and tear" degeneration of intra-articular cartilage, and is commonly viewed as a marker of aging. More than 75%

of Americans over the age of 50 are reported to have osteoarthritis, also known as degenerative joint disease (DJD).

Interestingly, this condition has been documented in prehistoric animals including reptiles and birds. However it is not found in bats or sloths, animals that spend a significant amount of time hanging upside down, suggesting that gravity and steady mechanical force upon joint tissue may be the primary contributing factors. However it is difficult to blame gravity alone because osteoarthritis also affects some non-weight-bearing joints, such as the patellofemoral joint.

The disease process may be triggered by intraarticular chondrocyte proliferation causing proteoglycan degradation and the presence of increased protease and collagenases in the joint. The end result is deterioration of the intraarticular cartilage and increased friction between bones.

Osteoarthritis is a primary cause of disability. Signs and symptoms usually appear after the age of 60, but can appear as early as the thrid decade of life. There is an increased incidence in women and people with diabetes. The knees, hips, and spine are the most commonly involved areas, but it also frequently affects joints in the hands. Treatment is primarily aimed at mitigating the symptoms.

Characteristic symptoms:

1. Joint pain and stiffness, especially in the morning
2. Joint swelling
3. Joint deformity
4. Restriction in range of motion
5. Crepitus (crackling noises with movement of the joint)

Possible causes:

1. Wear and tear on the joint over time
2. Poor diet
3. Lifestyle
4. Excess weight
5. Bacterial, viral, or fungal infection
6. Joint trauma

Dietary guidelines:

1. Optimize complex carbohydrate and fiber intake; limit simple carbohydrates
2. Eliminate fruits and vegetables known as nightshade (tomatoes, potatoes, egg plant, peppers, and tobacco) that cause fluid retention and can increase inflammation
3. Eating all berries is encouraged to open cell membranes for better absorption of nutrients and supplements
4. Reduce excess weight

Nutritional supplements:

1. Glucosamine sulfate 1,000 mg orally twice per day or 500 mg orally four times per day *(79–82)*
2. Chondroitin HCl 250–500 mg orally twice per day
3. Bromelaine 250–500 mg orally twice per day
4. Other: Look for hormone imbalance, particularly estradiol and thyroid hormones. Balance vitamins, enzymes, and antioxidants (vitamins A, C, E, and selenium) *(83)*
5. S-adenosyl methionine (SAM) *(84,85)*

6. Vitamin B5 (pantothenic acid) to reduce joint inflammation 500 mg orally per day *(86–88)*

Note: Most glusosamine sulfate and chrondroitin HCl are bound with other supplements as co-factors (e.g., niacin amide, superoxide dismutase, zinc, magnesium, and boron) *(84,89)*.

4.2. Rheumatoid Arthritis

Rheumatoid arthritis (RA) is an autoimmune disorder in which the immune system improperly identifies the synovial membrane of joints as foreign and attacks it, causing excessive inflammation in joints. With time, bone can be destroyed, cartilage damaged, and soft tissues destroyed. RA can be very painful and disabling. It is usually diagnosed early in life, before the age of 40. It affects predominantly females, with a 3:1 ratio of females to males *(90,91)*.

Characteristic symptoms and signs:

1. Inflamed, stiff, painful joints (can affect any synovial joint)
2. Joint deformity
3. Muscle atrophy and weakness
4. Physical or emotional stress, fatigue, low-grade fever, and generalized weakness
5. Anemia
6. Lymphadenopathy
7. Irritable bowel syndrome
8. Erosion of cartilage on x-ray
9. Rheumatoid factor antibody in blood
10. Antinuclear antibody is found in 20–60% of cases
11. Ferritin, C-reactive protein, and sedimentation rate might also be elevated

Possible causes:

1. Genetic factors are strong; 70% have the HLA-DRW4 antigen
2. Poor diet *(92)*
3. Bacterial infection
4. Microorganisms such as amoeba
5. Mycoplasma, Epstein Barr virus, and rubella are hypothesized causes

Dietary guidelines: *(93–96)*

1. Eliminate fruits and vegetables known as nightshade (tomatoes, potatoes, egg plant, peppers, and tobacco) that cause fluid retention and can increase inflammation
2. Increase other fruits (especially berries) and vegetables
3. Avoid wheat, corn, milk or dairy products, and beef

Nutritional supplements:

1. Omega-3 fatty acids (EPA and DHA) 1,000 mg orally per day for maintenance, with reconditioning protocol of 5,000 mg orally per day three months of the year (to recondition cell membranes)
2. Antioxidants (vitamins A, C, E, and selenium) *(97)*
3. Pantothenic acid 100 mg orally twice per day
4. Niacin amide 2000 mg orally twice per day
5. Curcumin (turmeric) 600 mg orally twice per day

6. Bromelaine 250–500 mg orally twice per day *(98,99)*
7. Ginger extract 100 mg orally three to four times per day
8. Dihydroepiandosterone (DHEA) (a precursor hormone) 50–200 mg orally per day

4.3. Premenstrual Syndrome

Premenstrual syndrome (PMS) is estimated to affect 40% of menstruating women, among whom 10% suffer severe uterine pain and cramping. It is believed that PMS is due to a decreased production of progesterone from the corpus luteum in the luteal phase of the menstrual cycle, three weeks after the previous menstruation. The decreased progesterone causes hormone imbalance and subsequent cramping of the uterus. Some also speculate that PMS is connected to low thyroid function.

For PMS it is valuable to test hormone levels (estradiol, estriol, progesterone, testosterone, DHEA, and cortisol) in serum. A thyroid function panel in serum and a magnesium level in packed red blood cells should also be tested. *(100)* Magnesium plays a very important role in hormone balance for women. It can also be helpful to test for heavy metal toxicity.

There are four types of PMS patients: *(101)*

1. Type A is linked to anxiety. Symptoms include anxiety, irritability, and emotional imbalance. There is a decrease in adrenal androgen or progesterone secretion.
2. Type C is linked to carbohydrate and sweet cravings. This is often due to low magnesium and prostaglandin levels.
3. Type D is linked to depression. These women are commonly found to have low estrogen. It is also related to stress. There is an increase in adrenal androgen or progesterone secretion (opposite from type A).
4. Type H is linked to hyperhidration. These women experience weight gain of more than 3 lbs, bloating of the abdomen, and breast tenderness and congestion. In severe cases, they have edema and swelling of the face, hands, or ankles. The fluid retention is due to excess aldosterone. This type is also linked to magnesium deficiency and estrogen excess.

Characteristic symptoms:

1. Uterine cramps
2. Breast pain
3. Irritability
4. Depression
5. Headache
6. Altered libido

Dietary guidelines:

1. Avoid milk and dairy products
2. Decrease meat and increase vegetables (ratio of 1:3)
3. Reduce or avoid saturated fat and sugar
4. Increase soy-based foods
5. Avoid foods treated with hormones, herbicides, or pesticides (look for organic foods)
6. Eliminate caffeine completely
7. Minimize salt

Nutritional supplements:

1. High-potency mutivitamins and amino acids are helpful for most women to balance nutrients *(102,103)*
2. Probiotic acidophilus 20–30 billion units orally per day
3. Magnesium (organic forms bound with maleate, citrate, or aspartate are better absorbed and have less of a laxative effect than the non-organic forms.) Start with 200 mg orally three times per day and increase or decrease as tolerated. Avoid watery stools.
4. An oral detoxification agent such as the B vitamins and malic acid
5. Bioidentical natural progesterone soy or yam based cream 100–200 mg topically once per day has no observed side effects or toxicity. It is recommended to monitor progesterone levels for follow up during the luteal phase of the menstrual cycle *(104,105)*.
6. Thyroid glandular extract 50–100 mg orally per day can be used for a subclinical hypothyroid patient with normal or borderline TSH, T4 or T3 levels.
7. Calmplex homeopathic treatment, St. John's Wort, or 5-hydroxytryptophan (5-HTP), a direct precursor to serotonin, can be helpful for stress management and anxiety *(106)*.
8. Vitamin B6 (pyridoxine) intramuscular injection is an option when PMS symptoms are severe, especially when accompanied by depression. Oral Vitamin B6 can also be used at a dose of 50–100 mg per day in divided doses *(107)*.
9. An additional 100 mg orally per day of calcium and manganese will help those who experience severe cramping.
10. Zinc picolinate 50 mg orally per day to suppress excessive prolactin secretion.
11. Chromium polynicotinate 400–800 mg orally per day in divided doses helps decrease carbohydrate and sweet cravings by regulating sugar metabolism.
12. Other well-known herbal medicines for PMS include dong quai (*Angelica sinensis*), licorice root (*Glycyrrhiza glabra*), black cohosh (*Cimifuga racemosa*) and chaste berry (*Vitex agnus castus*) *(108)*.

4.4. Osteoporosis

Osteoporosis has become the most common orthopedic diagnosis in the United States. It most often affects postmenopausal women. Bone loss decreases by about 2% every year after the age of 40. Many factors contribute to bone loss, but the most prominent factor is hormone imbalance. Osteoporosis commonly affects the spine and hips, and hip fracture is the eventual cause of death in 20% of cases.

Eating soy-based foods can help to decrease the destruction of bone caused by hormone imbalance. Soy foods, such as soybeans, miso, tempeh, and tofu, contain isoflavonoids like genestin and diadzein that enhance the effects of calcitonin on calcium metabolism to prevent bone destruction *(109)*.

In addition to hormone imbalance, postmenopausal women also frequently have an elevated homocysteine level. Homocysteine interferes with collagen cross-linking, leading to a defect in bone matrix formation, and subsequent osteoporosis. Directing treatment at this mechanism is one way to treat osteoporosis nutritionally. Folic acid, vitamin B6, and vitamin B12 are the best weapons against an elevated homocysteine level.

With osteoporosis, prevention is much more effective than treatment. Choosing a healthy diet and avoiding food and drinks that reduce bone formation (see Dietary Guidelines below) is important in the prevention of osteoporosis. Weightbearing and resistance exercise is the best preventive and therapeutic exercise program. It is crucial to avoid smoking.

In the formation of collagen strands, and the building of the bone matrix, calcium and other mineral factors are carried to their receptor sites by magnesium. Silicon prepares the receptor sites to accept the minerals. Strontium then acts like a glue to add minerals into the bone matrix. All these minerals (calcium, magnesium, silicon, and strontium) are therefore crucial to the maintenance of a strong bone matrix.

Characteristic symptoms and signs:

1. Low back pain is often the first symptom
2. Pain can be in any bone or joint
3. Fracture
4. X-rays show demineralization of the bone, and also show fractures if present
5. Dexa scan bone density test confirms a diagnosis of osteoporosis

Dietary guidelines: *(110)*

1. Avoid high-protein diets that encourage calcium loss from the bones
2. Maximize intake of green leafy vegetables
3. Avoid refined sugar
4. Minimize salt intake
5. Avoid drinks with low calcium and high phosphorous content such as coffee, caffeinated teas, alcohol, and all sodas *(111)*
6. Avoid very acidic foods and drinks

Nutritional supplements:

1. A 1:2:1 ratio of 300 mg calcium to 600 mg magnesium to 300 mg strontium is very important. Increase the dose as tolerated, maintaining this ratio *(112,113)*.
2. Vitamin D 400–700 IU orally per day *(114)*.
3. Vitamin B6 (50–100 mg daily), folic acid (800 µg–5 mg daily), and vitamin B12 (1–3 mg daily) to encourage methionine to form cysteine rather than homocysteine *(115)*.
4. Phytoestrogen (ipriflavone) 200 mg orally three times per day *(116)*.
5. In severe cases (very low bone density, severe pain, or limited function) start a bisphosphanate. This helps to reduce symptoms in the first year while the supplements begin to work *(117)*.
6. An intramuscular injection of a combination of 100 mg vitamin B6, 1,000 µg vitamin B12, and 2,000 mg magnesium sulfate can be initiated two times per week for about 20 weeks while the patient is starting to take the supplements.

4.5. Pelvic Inflammatory Disease

Many women suffer from pelvic inflammatory disease (PID) with infertility, ectopic pregnancy, chronic abdominal pain, and pain during sexual intercourse.

The etiology of PID is still unknown. Infection with *Neisseria gonorrhoeae* has been thought to be the cause. Other organisms speculated include *Chlamydia trachomatis*, *Mycoplasma pneumoniae*, *Escherichia coli*, *Haemophilus influenzae*, anaerobic organisms, and *Streptococcus* species *(118)*.

Fifteen percent of women with PID fail antimicrobial therapy *(119–122)*. Nutritional supplements that inhibit anaerobic bacteria can be helpful. All foods and supplements with strong anti-inflammatory properties are useful. The fat-soluble vitamin ascorbyl palmitate is a good anti-inflammatory vitamin. Beta-carotene is also a good supplement option. Beta-carotene is naturally found in high levels in the ovaries, but it decreases in PID, likely from the presence of anaerobic bacteria.

Maintaining the body at a basic pH of 7.4–7.8 discourages the growth of many microorganisms causing PID, including *Mycoplasma* and *Candida*. Yam-based or soy-based transdermal bioidentical natural progesterone can also be used to inhibit bacterial growth, but a blood level should be monitored to prevent uterine hyperplasia.

Characteristic symptoms and signs:

1. Pain during sexual intercourse
2. White vaginal discharge
3. Elevated body temperature
4. Cramping lower abdominal pain with tenderness to palpation
5. Elevated white blood cell count

Diagnostic tests: *(123)*

1. Serum or urine beta-HCG to detect pregnancy
2. Abdominal ultrasound may be needed to detect ectopic pregnancy
3. Urinalysis can differentiate PID from a urinary tract infection

Dietary guidelines:

1. Avoid foods treated with hormones, herbicides, or pesticides (look for organic foods)
2. Maximize intake of green leafy vegetables (aim for a 3:1 ratio of vegetables to meat)
3. Avoid citrus
4. Avoid coffee and caffeinated tea

Nutritional supplements:

1. Beta carotene 100,000 IU orally per day for 3 months
2. Vitamin E 400 IU orally per day for 3 months
3. Ascorbyl palmitate (C-palmitate) 500–1,000 mg orally per day
4. Soluble chlorophyll 40–50 mg orally per day in three to four divided doses
5. Bromelaine 1,500–2,000 mg orally per day in three to four divided doses
6. MSM 100 mg orally per day in the morning
7. pH balancing formula (any strong mixture of greens) orally per day

Lifestyle adjustments and therapies:

1. Do not use an internal uterine device (IUD), to decrease bacterial colonization
2. Avoid douching due to vaginal flora imbalance
3. Condoms are the preferred sexual barrier
4. Avoid intercourse during menses to avoid spreading the infection through broken mucous membranes *(122)*
5. Avoid tobacco
6. Sitz baths of a hot temperature (100 °F) for 3 minutes, followed by a cold temperature (60°F) for 30 seconds, one to two times per day
7. Suprapubic diathermy or heat therapy *(124)*

4.6. Migraine Headaches

Migraine headaches affect 10–20 % of the population. Women are affected three times as often as men. Characteristic migraine headaches are often described as paroxysmal and recurrent pounding unilateral head pain increased by stimuli such as light, sound, or smells. Many patients report prodromal symptoms such as blurry vision, anxiety, or fatigue prior to the headache.

Treatment of migraine headaches focuses on finding and eliminating the underlying causes, including food and environmental triggers. Common causes are food allergies, stress, medications and drugs, heavy metal toxicity, toxicity in the gastrointestinal tract, insomnia, mineral imbalances, hormone imbalances and poor nutrition. Consider testing for food allergies with a delayed reaction allergy test, an assay used to test for an allergic reaction of greater than six months, rather than acute symptoms.

Dietary guidelines:

1. Eliminate food allergens. Foods that are commonly found to induce migraines are cow's milk, wheat, chocolate, carrots, melons, strawberries, bananas, potatoes, yeast, sugar cane, corn, pork, peanuts, coffee, walnuts, and eggs.
2. Eliminate sodas, chocolate, alcohol (especially red wine), caffeine, cheese, citrus fruits, shellfish, and chemical nitrates (MSG, nitroglycerine).
3. High intake of vegetables
4. Low intake of animal fats that activate an amine reaction in the vascular system and induce platelet aggregation
5. Consume fish oil, fish, garlic, and onions.

Nutritional supplements:

1. 5-HTP in high doses of up to 400–600 mg per day
2. Omega-3 fatty acids (EPA and DHA) 5,000 mg orally per day for three months per year, then maintenance of 3,000 mg orally per day for the rest of the year, until a significant reduction in headaches is noticed
3. Magnesium (organic forms bound with maleate, citrate, or aspartate are better absorbed and have less of a laxative effect than the non-organic forms.) Start with 200 mg orally three times per day and increase or decrease as tolerated. Avoid watery stools. *(125)*
4. Vitamin B1 (100 mg orally per day), vitamin B6 (25–50 mg orally per day) and vitamin B12 (2–3 mg orally per day) to improve the absorption of magnesium
5. Intravenous or intramuscular injection of magnesium can be used for an acute migraine headache *(126,127)*
6. Intravenous gluthatione can be helpful for people with food allergies and sensitivities, due to its detoxifying effect
7. Oral chelation agents, mineral or chemical detoxifiers, such as EDTA (ethylenediaminetetraacetic acid) 1,200–1,800 mg, DMSA (dimercaptosuccinic acid) 100–300 mg, DMPS (dimercapto-propane sulfonate) 100–300 mg, or activated zeolite 30–60 g can be used, if necessary, based on blood toxicity studies
8. Enzyme therapy (non animal-based) can be helpful for people with a toxic colon and constipation
9. Ginger 500–1,000 mg orally per day decreases pain by decreasing inflammation
10. Some people benefit from a chemical therapeutic combination of propanolol (50–100 mg per day), aspirin 600–1,500 mg per day in several divided doses), clonidine (0.2–0.6 mg per day), egonovine maleate (0.6–2 mg per day), and / or calcium channel blockers (80–60 mg per day).

Lifestyle adjustments and therapies:

1. Reduction of muscle spasm and tension in the upper back and neck muscles through isometric exercises 15–20 minutes two to three times per day
2. Cervical manipulation can be helpful to reduce intradiscal pressure
3. Evaluation for temporomandibular joint (TMJ) dysfunction, and correction of the problem

4. TENS therapy below the precipitation threshold is a good option for home care
5. Acupuncture is helpful for many people
6. Hydrocolonic therapy can correct bowel patterns and relieve toxic colon syndrome
7. Biofeedback treatment, training in relaxation therapy, and home meditation for stress reduction *(128)*
8. Evaluation and adjustment of prescription medications such as blood pressure medications and pain medications
9. Review of over-the-counter medications which can cause sensitivity: aspirin, codeine, ergotamine, acetaminophen, propoxyphene, nasal decongestants, and antihistamines

4.7. Chronic Fatigue Syndrome and Fibromyalgia

Chronic fatigue syndrome and fibromyalgia are fairly newly named, and sometimes controversial, syndromes. They are not specific disease entities, but rather combinations of symptoms that may be caused by underlying diseases. In clinical practice, the two syndromes are often referred to together, because of significant symptom overlap *(129–132)*. Fibromyalgia is diagnosed when the patient's predominating complaint is musculoskeletal pain. If fatigue is predominant, the diagnosis of chronic fatigue syndrome (CFS) is given. However, many patients experience both pain and fatigue.

The estimated prevalence of these syndromes in the United States is 12,000–12 million, and 75% of those affected are female. There are no accepted diagnostic laboratory tests or specific treatments. Patients often look to CAM practitioners, supplements, and modalities for treatment. It is interesting to note that similar diagnostic and therapeutic controversies also initially occurred with lupus, rheumatoid arthritis, polio, multiple sclerosis, Lyme disease, and many other disorders.

Patients with fibromyalgia and chronic fatigue syndrome are often very complicated and their treatment needs to be personalized. A detailed medical history and review of all body systems is necessary to identify the many symptoms and contributing factors. Both the mind and the body need to be addressed, and a strong, trusting relationship between the patient and the treating clinician is critical. Due to the wide range of possible causes, a full laboratory workup can be expensive. It is acceptable to start a therapeutic trial before investigating all possible causes.

Many other names have been used to describe these syndromes, including chronic fatigue and immune dysfunction syndrome, post-viral fatigue syndrome, yuppie flu, chronic mononucleosis-like syndrome, chronic Epstein-Barr syndrome, and neurasthenia.

The American College of Rheumatology has made diagnostic criteria for Fibromyalgia (see below) *(133)*. In 1988, the United States Center for Disease Control (CDC) also formalized chronic fatigue syndrome with diagnostic criteria (see below) *(134)*.

CDC diagnostic criteria for chronic fatigue syndrome:

Major criteria

1. New onset fatigue, causing a 50% reduction in activity for at least 6 months
2. Exclusion of other illnesses than can cause fatigue

Minor criteria: The presence of 8 of the 11 symptoms listed below, or 6 of the 11 symptoms and 2 of the 3 signs listed below.

Symptoms:

1. Mild fever
2. Recurrent sore throat
3. Painful lymph nodes
4. Muscle weakness
5. Muscle pain
6. Prolonged fatigue after exercise
7. Recurrent headache
8. Migratory joint pain
9. Neurological or psychological complaints:

   - Sensitivity to bright light
   - Forgetfulness
   - Confusion
   - Inability to concentrate
   - Excessive irritability
   - Depression

10. Sleep disturbance (hypersomnia or insomnia)
11. Sudden onset of symptoms

Signs:

1. Low-grade fever
2. Non-exudative pharyngitis
3. Palpable or tender lymph nodes

American College of Rheumatology Fibromyalgia Criteria: A person can be classified as having fibromyalgia if he or she has

(i) a history of widespread pain, steady or intermittent, for at least 3 months,
(ii) the pain must have been present—

   - on both the right and left sides of the body
   - both above and below the waist
   - mid-body (For example, in the head, neck, middle chest, or middle back)

(iii) pain with pressure over at least 11 of 18 recognized tender points

   Possible causes:

1. Hypothalamic dysfunction altering sleep, hormones, autonomic nervous system, and temperature. Hypothalamic dysfunction is multifactorial, but is often associated with depression or stress.
2. Impaired liver function from a variety of causes such as poor diet, obesity, diabetes, gallstones, alcohol, bacterial toxins in the gastrointestinal tract, medications, viral insult, and environmental toxins *(131)*.
3. Chronic candida infection
4. Food allergies
5. Hypothyroidism *(135)*
6. Hypoglycemia
7. Hypoadrenalism *(136)*
8. Systemic viral infection (i.e., Epstein–Barr virus) *(137–139)*

9. Other proposed organisms: human herpes virus-6, cytomegalovirus, enterovirus, retrovirus, brucella, giardia
10. Deficient immune system (i.e., decreased natural killer cells) *(140)*

Dietary guidelines:

1. Avoid caffeine *(141)*
2. Minimize sugar
3. Maximize fruits and vegetables
4. Maximize water
5. Small, frequent, low-calorie meals and snacks throughout the day (as opposed to three large meals)
6. Refer to guidelines for an anti-inflammatory diet at the beginning of this chapter

Nutritional supplements:

1. Vitamin C 3,000 mg orally per day in divided doses to boost immune and adrenal function
2. Bioflavonoids 500 mg orally per day for blood vessel integrity
3. Magnesium aspartate or citrate 600–1,500 mg orally per day in divided doses. Gradually increasing the dose will improve compliance. Magnesium can cause loose stools due to difficulties with absorption, so some patients may benefit from intramuscular injections of magnesium sulfate 1,000 mg/ml, 2 ml (2,000 mg) two times per week for 20 weeks *(142–144)*.
4. Malic acid 900–2,000 mg orally per day to increase energy
5. NAC (N-acetyl-cysteine) 650 mg orally per day for three months to facilitate glutathione
6. Glutamine 1,000–4,000 mg orally per day in divided doses to facilitate glutathione
7. Glycine 500–1,000 mg orally per day to facilitate glutathione
8. Lysine 500 mg orally per day to facilitate carnitine and suppress arginine
9. Arginine can be supplemented to increase growth hormone, but it must be given and monitored carefully, because it can stimulate herpes
10. Taurine 500 mg orally per day for energy
11. Tyrosine 500 mg orally per day to increase dopamine and norepinephrine
12. Calcium 500 mg orally per day with 400 IU of vitamin D, especially if the patient has altered thyroid function
13. Pantothenic acid 50 mg orally per day to support adrenal function
14. Vitamin E 100 IU orally per day as an antioxidant and to thin the blood
15. Vitamin A 35,000 IU orally per day for mucosal immunity and to facilitate the use of zinc
16. Vitamin D at least 400 IU orally per day for cognition, bone strength, vision, and immune function
17. Iodine 150 μg orally per day for thyroid support and temperature control
18. Thymus extract
19. Adrenal blend
20. Glutathione (see glycine, cysteine, and glutamine above)
21. Zinc 15 mg orally per day for immune function and wound healing
22. Selenium 200 μg orally per day as an antioxidant and to boost immune function
23. Chromium polynicotinate 400–800 mg orally per day for sugar regulation and to reduce sugar cravings
24. Molybdenum 250 mg orally per day for allergies and chemical sensitivities (e.g., sulfites)
25. Inositol 750 mg orally per day to decrease anxiety and support nerve function

26. Vitamin B12: If laboratory value is less than 500, give intramuscular injections (3000 mg of hydroxycobalamine) 3–7 times per week for 30 doses, then as needed every month
27. Vitamin B1 (thiamine) 75 mg orally per day for cognition and muscle and heart function
28. Vitamin B2 (riboflavin) 75 mg orally per day
29. Niacin 50 mg orally per day for energy
30. Vitamin B6 (pyridoxine) 85 mg orally per day for energy and nerve function
31. Folic acid 800 mcg orally per day to boost immune function
32. Plant-based enzymes 3–8 tablets orally per day
33. Omega-3 essential fatty acids (EPA and DHA) 5,000–10,000 mg orally per day for 3 months to recondition cellular membranes and allow for better nutritional absorption, then 3,000 mg orally per day for maintenance. EPA and DHA are helpful to reduce inflammation and support all cellular functions.
34. Lipoic acid 600–2,000 mg orally per day to protect the liver and prevent neuropathy
35. L–Lysine 1,000–3,000 mg orally per day to reduce or suppress cold sores or genital herpes
36. Coenzyme Q-10 200 mg orally per day to reduce LDL and total cholesterol, and to boost cellular mitochondrial function
37. Iron *only* if Fe saturation and ferritin laboratory values are low
38. Potassium chloride if laboratory value is low
39. Options for sleep (take orally at night):
    Valerian root 200 mg (note this can energize some people)
    Passion flower 90 mg
    L-theanine 50 mg (green tea)
    Hops 30 mg
    Piscidia 12 mg
    Wild lettuce 28 mg
    5-HTP 100–400 mg (or less than 200 mg if taken with an antidepressant)
    Melatonin 0.5–1 mg (time release)
    Magnesium and calcium taken at bedtime have a relaxant effect
    Kava-kava 30% extract 250 mg capsule, 1–3 capsules
    Note: a prescription medication is sometimes needed for sleep

Lifestyle adjustments and therapies:

1. Exercise: Exercise can improve mood and decrease stress, and has specifically been shown to have a positive effect in chronic fatigue syndrome *(145)*. Exercise should be started with caution however, because it can make pain symptoms worse in some patients *(146)*. Start with routine daily stretching and range of motion, or light to moderate exercise for 15–20 minutes per day for the first 8–10 weeks, until you can see the benefit of this recommendation for your particular patient.
2. Stress management: It is helpful to discuss and encourage a patient's personal method of stress relief. Ideas include exercise, yoga, use of a hot bath or jacuzzi, social events, prayer meetings and spiritual support, breathing and posture exercises, laughter, or drinking hot teas such as chamomile or valerian root.
3. Detoxification: Detoxification has taken a very important role in the treatment of CFS and fibromyalgia. Hepatic detoxification, gastrointestinal detoxification (hydro-colonic treatments), and systemic detoxification have been found to be beneficial *(147,148)*.
4. Sleep hygiene:
    Avoid caffeine and other stimulants in the afternoon and evening
    Enjoy a small meal for dinner

Eat foods with low glycemic indexes
Avoid television in the evening
Avoid drinking fluids after 6:00 P.M. for bladder control
Follow a relaxing nightly pre-sleep routine
Establish good mattress and pillow support for the spine
Sleep alone if partner is disruptive
Sleep in total darkness

5. Hormonal support and balance:

Thyroid hormone
Estradiol / Estriol
Progesterone
Testosterone
DHEA
Cortisol
Melatonin

5. CONCLUSIONS

There are currently many supplements and nutritional options available for patients with painful disorders. Depending on the condition and the individual patient, nutritional treatments may be used in isolation or to complement other therapies. Despite the disorder and other individual factors, the basics of a nutritious diet as described in the first section of this book may help decrease pain symptoms and improve function and quality of life.

When prescribing complementary and alternative treatments to your patients, including nutritional supplements, it is imperative to be candid that you are practicing alternative medicine. It is also important to explain and offer any traditional treatments available (the current standard of care), making sure your patient has the ability to choose their own course of treatment. You should explain any risks associated with alternative nutritional supplements, as well as with traditional pharmaceuticals. Your conversation with the patient should be well documented.

For further training in complementary, alternative, and integrative medicine, there are a variety of educational and certification programs available to physicians and other healthcare practitioners. Further information on programs, as well as other resources, can be found on the American College for Advancement in Medicine website, www.acam.org.

REFERENCES

1. Nahleh Z, Tabbara IA. Complementary and alternative medicine in breast cancer patients. Palliat Support Care 2003;1(3):267–273.
2. DeAngelis CD. Pain Management JAMA 2003;290(18):2480–2481.
3. Dillard JN, Knapp S. Complementary and alternative pain therapy in the emergency department. Emerg Med Clin North Am 2005;23(2):529–549.
4. http://lpi.oregonstate.edu/f-w00/flavonoid.html.
5. https://www.amsa.org/healingthehealer/antiinflam.cfm.
6. https://www.wholehealthmd.com.
7. Iiev E, Tsankov N, Broshtilova V. Omega-3 omega-6 fatty acids in the improvement of psoriatic symptoms. Semin Integrative Med 2003;1(4):211–214.

8. Capodice JL, Bemis DL, Buttyan R, Kaplan SA, Katz AE. Complementary and alternative medicine for chronic prostatitis/chronic pelvic pain syndrome. Evid Based Complement Alternat Med 2005;2(4):495–501.

9. Plotnikoff GA, Quigley JM. Prevalence of severe hypovitaminosis D in patients with persistent, nonspecific musculoskeletal pain. Mayo Clin Proc 2003;78:1463–1470.

10. People with undetermined muscle/bone pain tend to be severely vitamin D deficient. Public release: 9 Dec 2003. Minneapolis, St. Paul. Contact: ashleyb@umn.edu, University of Minnesota.

11. http://www.intelihealth.com B-vitamins prove effective in relieving chronic pain. April 10, 2003.

12. Zhang J, Song X, LaMotte R. Enhanced excitability of sensory neurons in rats with cutaneous hyperalgesia produced by chronic compression of the dorsal root ganglion. J Neurophysiol 1999;82:3359–3370

13. Medina-Santillan R, Reyes-Garcia G, Rocha-Gonzalez HI, Granados-Soto V. B vitamins increase the analgesic effect of ketorolac in the formalin test in the rat. Proc West Pharmacol Soc 2004;47:95–99.

14. Balch PA, Balch JF. 2000. Prescription For Nutritional Healing. Third edition. New York: Penguin Putnam, Inc.

15. Compston J. Bone densitometry in clinical practice. BMJ 1995;310:1570.

16. Tussig SJ, Batkin S. Bromelaine, the enzyme complex of pineapple and its clinical application. An update. J Ethonopharm 1988;22:191–203.

17. Masson M. Bromelaine in the treatment of blunt injuries to the musculoskeletal system. A case observation by an orthopedic surgeon in private practice. Fortschr Med 1995;133:330–336.

18. Seligman B. Bromelaine. An anti–inflammatory agent. Angiology 1962;13:508–510.

19. Hunter RG, Hebry GW, Henicke RM. The action of papain and bromelin on the uterus. Am J Obgyn 1957;73:887–880.

20. Seligman B. Oral bromelaines as adjuncts in treatment of acute thrombophlebitis. Angilogy 1969;20:22–26.

21. Moskowitz RW. Role of collagen hydrolyzed in bone and joint disease. Semin Arthritis Rehum 2000;30(2):87–99.

22. Snowden JM. The stabilization of in vivo assembled collagen fibrils by proteoglycans/glycosaminoglycans. Biochem Biophysics Acta 1982;703(1):21–25.

23. McCarthy GM, McCarty DJ. Effect of topical capsaicin in the therapy of painful osteoarthritis of the hands. J Rheumatol 1992;19:604–607.

24. Visudhiphan S, Poolsuppasit S, Piboonnukarintr. The relationship between high fibrinolytic activity and daily capsicum ingestion in Thais. Am J Clin Nutr 1982;35:1452–1458.

25. Horowitz M, Wishart J, Maddox A. The effect of chili on gastrointestinal transit. J Gasterol Hepatol 1992;7:52–56.

26. Nelson C. Heal the burn. Pepper and lasers in cancer pain therapy. J Nat Canc Inst 1994;86:1381.

27. Pfeiffer MA, Ross DR, Scharge JP. A highly successful and novel model for treatment of chronic painful diabetic peripheral neuropathy. Diabetes Car 1993;16:1003–1115.

28. The Capsaicin Study Group. Effect of treatment with capsaicin on daily activities of patients with painful diabetic neuropathy. Diabetic Care 1992;15:159–165.

29. Ellis CN, Berberian B, Sulica VI. A double blind evaluation of topical capsaicin in puritic psoriasis. J Am Acad Dermatol 1993;29:438–442.

30. Bjerring P, Arendt-Nielsen L, Soderberg U. Argon laser induced cutaneous sensory and pain thresholds in post herpetic neuralgia. Quantitative modulation by topical capsaicin. Acta Derm Venereol 1990;70:121–125.

31. Piekert A, Hentrich M, Ochs G. Topical 0.025% capsaicin in chronic post herpetic neuralgia. Efficacy, predictors of response and long term course. J Neurol 1991;238:452–256.

32. Fusco BM, Alessandri M. Analgesic effect of capsaicin in idiopathic trigeminal neuralgia. Aneth Analg 1992;51:365–379.

33. Garg AK, Berg RA, Silver FH, Garg HG. Effect of proteolysis on type 1 collagen fiber formation. Bio Mater 1989;10(6):413–419.

34. Mazieres B, Combre B, Phan Van A, Tondut J, Grynfelt M. Chondroitin sulfate in osteoarthritis of the knee: a prospective, double blind, placebo controlled multi-center clinical study. J Rheumatol 2001;28(1):173–181.

35. Diehl HW, Fletcher HG. A simplified preparation of 2–deoxy-D-ribose based on treatment of a D-glucose monohydrate with solid calcium hydroxide. Archiv Biochem Biophys 1958;78(2).

36. Diehl HW. Cetyl myristoleate. U.S. Patent #4,049,824.

37. Murray MT. 1996. Encyclopedia of Nutritional Supplements. Rocklin, CA: Prima Publishing, 237.

38. Siemandi H. The effect of *cis*-9-cetyl myristoleate (CMO) and adjunctive therapy on arthritis and auto-immune disease: a randomized trial. Townsend Lett Doctors Patients 1997;(Aug/Sept):58–63.
39. Diehl HW, May EL. Cetyl myristoleate isolated from Swiss albino mice: an apparent protective agent against adjuvant arthritis in rats. J Pharm Sci 1994;83(3):296–299.
40. Diehl HW. Method for the treatment of osteoarthritis. U.S. Patent #5,569,676.
41. Sobel D, Klein AC. Arthritis: What Works. New York: St. Martins Press, pp 221–225.
42. Diehl HW. Method of treating rheumatoid arthritis. U.S. Patent #4,113,881.
43. Srimal R, Dhawan B. Pharmacology of diferuloyl methane (cucurmin), as non steroidal anti-inflammatory agent. J Pharm Pharmac 1973;25:447–452.
44. Satoskar RR, Shah SJ, Shenoy SG. Evaluation of anti-inflammatory property of cucurmin (diferuloyl methane) in patients with post-operative inflammation. Int J Clin Pharmacol Ther Toxicol 1986;24:651–654.
45. Deodhar SD, Sethi R, Srimal RC. Preliminary studies on anti-rheumatic activity of cucurmin diferuloyl methane. Int J Med Res 1980;71:632–634.
46. Davidson, P. 1985. Are You Sure It's Arthritis? New York: Macmillan Publishing Co.
47. Walker, L. 1998. Nature's Pharmacy. Paramus, NJ: Reward Books.
48. Wegener T, Lupke NP. Treatment of patients with arthrosis of hip or knee with aqueous extract of Devil's Claw. Phytother Res 2003;17(10):1165–1172.
49. Altman RD, Marcussen KC. Effects of a ginger extract on knee pain in patients with osteoarthritis. Arthritis Rheum 2001;44(11):2531.
50. Onogi T, Minami M, Kurhaishi Y, Staoh M. Capsaicin-like effect of 6-shagoal on substance P containing primary afferents of rats. A possible mechanism of its analgesic action. Neuropharmacology 1992;31:1165–1169.
51. Al Yahya MA, Rafatullah S, Moss JS. Gastro protective activity of ginger, zingiber officinale rosc., in albino rats. Am J Chin Med 1989;17:51–56.
52. Yamaha J, Mochizuki M, Rong HQ. The anti-ulcer effect in rats of ginger constituents. J Ethnopharmacol 1988;23:299–304.
53. Braham R, Dawson B, Goodman C. The effect of glucosamine supplementation on people experiencing regular knee pain. Br J Sports Med 2003;37(1):45–49.
54. Bruyere O, Palvelka K, Rovati LC, Deroisy R, Olejarova M, Gatterova J, Glacovelli G, Reginster JY. Glucosamine sulfate reduces osteoarthritis progression in postmenopausal women with knee osteoarthritis: Evidence from two 3-year studies. Menopause 2004;11(2):138–143.
55. Drovanti A, Bignamini AA. Rovati Al. Therapeutic activity of oral glucosamine sulfate in osteoarthritis. A placebo controlled double blind investigation. Clin Ther 1980;3:260–272.
56. Lippiello L. Glucosamine and chondroitin sulfate: biological response modifiers of chondrocytes under simulated conditions of joint stress. Osteoarthritis Cartilage 2003;11(5):335–342.
57. Muller-Fass Bender H, Bach GL, Haase W. Glucosamine sulfate compared to ibuprofen in osteoartritis of the knee. Osteoartritis Cartilage 1994;2:61–69.
58. Noack W, Fischers M, Foster KK. Glucosamine sulfate in osteoarthritis of the knee. Osteoarthritis Cartilage 1994;2:51–59.
59. Philippi AF, Leffler SG, Mosure JC, Kim PD. Glucosamine, chondroitin and manganese ascorbate for degenerative joint disease of the knee or low back: a randomized, double blind, placebo controlled pilot study. Mil Med 1999;164(2):85–91.
60. Zupanets JA, Benzdetto NV, Dedukh NV, OStrishko JA. Experimental study of the effect of glucosamine hydrochloride on metabolic and repair processes in connective tissue structures. Eksp Klin Farmakol 2002;65(6):67–69.
61. Peyron JG. Intraarticular hyaluronan injections in the treatment of osteoarthritis: state-of-the-art review. J Rheumatol Suppl 1993;39:10–15.
62. Rosner IA, Boja BA, Malemud CJ, Moskowitz RW, Goldberg VM. Intraarticular hyaluronic acid injection and synovial prostaglandins in experimental immune synovitis. J Rheumatol 1983;10(1): 71–78.
63. Bunyaratavej N, Chan KM, Subramanian N. Treatment of painful osteoarthritis of the knee with hyaluronic acid. Results of a multicenter Asian study. J Med Assoc Thai 2001;84(Suppl 2): S576—S581.
64. Jubb RW, Piva S, Beinat L, Dacre J, Gishen P. A one-year, randomized, placebo (saline) controlled clinical trial of 500–730 kDa sodium hyaluronate (Hyalgan) on the radiological change in osteoarthritis of the knee.Int J Clin Pract 2003;57(6):467–74.

65. McHughes M, Lipman AG. Managing osteoarthritis pain when your patient fails simple analgesics and NSAIDs and is not a candidate for surgery. Curr Rheumatol Rep 2006;8(1):22–29.
66. Novaes AC, Schaiquevich P, Nasswetter G; The Latin American Group of Quality of Life in Rheumatology. Multicenter study of hyaluronic acid obtained by biotechnology to evaluate clinical efficacy and safety in knee osteoarthritis. Int J Clin Pharmacol Res 2005;25(1):1–7.
67. Herschler RJ. Methysulfonylmethane in dietary products. United States Patent No: 4,616,039; October 7, 1986.
68. Barrager E, Veltman JR, Schauss AG, Schiller RN. A multicentered open label trial on the safety and efficacy of methylsulfonylmethane in the treatment of seasonal allergic rhinitis. J Altern Complement Med 2002;8:167–174.
69. Lawrence RM. MSM (Methysulfonylmethane): A double blind study of its use in degenerative arthritis. Int J Anti Aging Med 1998;1(1):50.
70. Emery P, Bradley H, Gough A. Increased prevalence of poor sulphoxidation in patients with rheumatoid arthritis: effect of changes in acute phase response and second line drug treatment. Ann Rheum Dis 1992;51:318–320.
71. Herschler RJ. Use of methysulfonylmethane to relieve pain and nocturnal cramps and to reduce stress induced deaths in animals. United States patent No 4,973,605; November 27, 1990.
72. Hovarth K, Noker PE, Somfai-Relle S. Toxicity of methysulfonylmethane in rats. Food Chem Toxicol 2002;40:1459–1462.
73. Kragballe K, Fogh K. A low fat diet supplemented with dietary fish oil (max EPA) results in improvement of psoriasis and in formation of leukotriene B5. Acta Derm Venereol 1989;69:23–28.
74. Lorenz R, Spengler U, Fisher S. Platelet function, thromboxane formation and blood pressure control during supplementation of the Western diet with cod liver oil. Circulation 1983;67:504–511.
75. Myerburg RJ. Epidemiology of ventricular tachycardia / ventricular fibrillation and sudden cardiac death. Pacing Clin Electrophysiol 1986;9:1334–1338.
76. Neutse JM, Starling MB. Fish oil and coronary heart disease. NZ Med J 1986;99:583–585.
77. Solomon SA. A placebo-controlled, double blind study of eicosapentaenoic acid-rich fish oil in patients with stable angina pectoris. Curr Med Res Opinion 1990;12:1–10.
78. Sperling RI. Dietary omega-3 fatty acids. Effect of lipid mediator on inflammation and rheumatoid arthritis. Rheum Dis Clin North Am 1991;17:373–389.
79. Crolle G, D'Este E. Glocosamine sulfate and management of arthrosis; A controlled clinical investigation. Curr Med Res Opin 1980;7:104–109.
80. Drovanti A, Bignamini AA, Rovati AL. Therapeutic activity or oral glucosamine in outpatients with arthrosis. Clin Ther 1981;3:260–272.
81. Noak W. Glucosamine sulfate in osteoarthritis of the knee. Osteoarthritis Cartilage 1994;2:51–59.
82. Setnikar I, Palimbo R, Canali S. Pharmacokinetics of glucosamine in man. Arzneim Forsch 1993;453:1109–1113.
83. Schwartz ER. The modulation of osteoartritic development by vitamin C and E. Int J Vit Nutr Res Suppl 1984;26:141–146.
84. Konig B. A long term (two year) clinical trial with S-adenosylmethyonine for treatment of osteoarthritis. Am J Med 1987;83:89–94.
85. Muller-Fasbender H. Double blind clinical trial of S-adenosylmethyonine versus ibuprofen in treatment of osteoarthritis. Am J Med 1987;83:81–83.
86. A report from the General Practitioner Research Group. Calcium pantothenate in arthritis conditions. Pract 1980;224:208–211.
87. Anand JC. Osteoartritis and pantothenic acid. J Coll Gen Pract 1963;5:136–137.
88. Anand JC. Osteoartritis and pantothenic acid. Lancet 1963;ii:1168.
89. Kulkani RR, Patki PS, Jog VP. Treatment of osteoarthritis with a herbomineral formulation. A double blind, placebo controlled, cross over study. J Enthopaharmacol 1991;33:92–95.
90. Benner JC, Plum F, Eds. 1996. Cecil Textbook of Medicine. Philadelphia: WB Saunders, pp 1459–1466.
91. General Practitioner Research Group. Practitioner 1980;224:208–211.
92. McCrae F, Veerapen K, Dieppe P. Diet and arthritis. Practitioner 1986;230:359–361.
93. Buchanan HM, Preston SJ, Brooks PM. Is diet important in rheumatoid arthritis? Br J Rheumatol 1991;30:125–134.
94. Darlington LG, Ramsey NW, Mansfield JR. Placebo-controlled, blind study of dietary manipulation therapy in rheumatoid arthritis. Lancet 1986;i:236–238.

95. Hicklin JA, McEwen LM, Morgan JE. The effect of diet in rheumatoid arthritis. Clin Allergy 1980;10:463–467.

96. Kejdsen-Kragh J. Controlled trial of fasting and one year vegetarian diet in rheumatoid arthritis. Lancet 1991;338:899–902.

97. Tarp U, Overvad K, Thorling EB. Selenium treatment in rheumatoid arthritis. Scand J Rheumatol 1984;53:103.

98. Herger I. Enzyme therapy in multiple rheumatoid diseases. Therapieoche 1983;33:3948–3957.

99. Taussig S, Batkin S. Bromelaine: the enzyme complex of pineapple (Ananas comosus) and its clinical application. An update. J Ethonopharmacol 1988;22:191–203.

100. Abraham G. Nutritional factors in the etiology of the premenstrual tension syndromes. J Reprod Med 1983;28:446–464.

101. Banhart KT, Freeman EW, Sondheimer SJ. A clinician's guide to the premenstrual syndrome. Med Clin North Am 1995;79:1457–1472.

102. Collins A, Landgren BM. Essential fatty acids in treatment of premenstural syndrome. Acta Obstet Gynecol 1993;81:93–98.

103. (a) Piesse JW. Nutritional factors in the premenstrual syndrome. Int Clin Nutr Rev 1984; 4:54–81.
(b) Piesse JW. Nutritional factors in the premenstrual syndrome. Int Clin Nutr Rev 1984;4:54–81.

104. Dinnerstein L. Progesterone treatment of premenstrual syndrome. A double blind cross over trial. Br Med J 1985;290:1617–1621.

105. Facchinetti F, Nppi G, Petralgia F. Oestradiol/progesterone imbalance and the premenstrual syndrome. Lancet 1983;2:1302.

106. Harada M, Suzuki M, Ozzaki Y. Effect of Japanese Anglica root and peony root on uterine contraction in the rabbit in situ. J Pharm Dyn 1984;7:304–311.

107. Klienjnen J, Ter Riet G, Knipschild P. Vitamine B6 in the treatment of premenstrual syndrome – a review. Br J Obstet Gynacol 1990;97:847–852.

108. Yoshiro K. The physiology actions of tang kuei and cenidium. Bull Oriental Healing Arts Inst USA 1985;10:269–278.

109. Brandi ML. New treatment strategies. Irpiflavone, strontium, vitamin D metabolites and analogs. Am J Med 1993;95(suppl 5A):69S–74S.

110. Block G. Dietary guidelines and results of food consumption surveys. Am J Clin Nutr 1991;53:356S–357S.

111. Mazzatiegos-Ramos E, Guerrero-Romero F, Rodriguez-Moran M. Consumption of soft drinks with phosphoric acid as risk factor for the development of hypocalcaemia in children: a case control study. J Pediatric 1995;126:940–942.

112. Carr CJ, Shangraw RF. Nutritional and pharmaceutical aspects of calcium supplementation. Am Pharm 1987;27:49–57.

113. Saltman PD, Strausse LG. The role of trace minerals in osteoporosis. J Am Coll Nutr 1993;4:384–389.

114. Rude RK, Adams JS, Ryzen E. Low serum concentration of 1,25–dihydroxyvitamin D in human magnesium deficiency. J Clin Endo Metabol 1985;61:933–940.

115. Brattstorm LE, Hultberg BL, Hardebo JE. Folic acid responsive postmenopausal homocysteinemia. Metabolism 1985;34:1073–1077.

116. Agnisdei D, Crepaldi G, Isaia G. A double blind, placebo controlled trial of ipriflavone for prevention of post menopausal spinal bone loss. Calcif Tissue Int 1997;61:142–147.

117. Fessenden RJ, Fessenden JS. The biological properties of silicon compounds. Adv Drug Res 1987;4:95.

118. Holmes K, Eschenbach D, Knapp J. Salpingitis: overview of etiology and epidemiology. Am J Ob Gyn 1980;138:893–900.

119. Hemsell D, Heard M, Nobles B. Single agent therapy for women with acute polymicrobial pelvic infections. Am J Obstet Gyn 1987;157:488–490.

120. Mattingly R. Office management of acute pelvic and urinary tract infections. Clin Obstet Gyn 1962;5:275–285.

121. Trehearne JD, Ripa KT, Mardh PA. Antibodies to Chlamydia trachomatis in acute salpingitis. Br J Vener Dis 1979;55:26–29.

122. Eschenbach D, Buchanan T, Pollock H. Polymicrobial etiology of acute pelvic inflammatory disease. Am J Obstet Gyn 1975;122:166–177.

123. Burnham RC. Therapy for acute pelvic inflammatory disease. A critique of recent treatment trials. Am J Obstet Gyn 1984;148:235–240.

124. Gelhorm G. Diathermy in gynecology. JAMA 1982;Mar:1005–1008.
125. Ramadan NM, Halvorson H, Vande-Linde A. Low brain magnesium in migraine. Headache 1989;29:590–593.
126. Mauskop A, Altura BT, Cracco RQ. Intravenous magnesium sulfate rapidly alleviates headaches of various types. Headache 1996;36:154–160.
127. Pfaffenrath V, Wessely P, Meyer C. Magnesium in the prophylaxis of migraine; A double blind placebo controlled study. Cephalgia 1996;16:436–440.
128. Benson H. 1975. The Relaxation Response. William Morrow.
129. Komaroff AL, Goldenberg D. The chronic fatigue syndrome: definition, current studies and lessons for fibromyalgia research. J Rheumatol 1989;16:23–27.
130. Buchwald D, Garrity DL. Comparison of patients with chronic fatigue syndrome, fibromyalgia and multiple chemical sensitivities. Arch Int Med 1994;154:2049–2053.
131. Shafran SD. The chronic fatigue syndrome. Am J Med 1991;90:731–739.
132. Kyle DV, Deshazo RD. Chronic fatigue syndrome. A conundrum. Am J Med Sci 1992;303:28–34.
133. Wolfe F. ACR 1990 criteria for FMS. Arthritis Rheum 1990;33:160–172.
134. Holmes GP, Kaplan J, Gantz N. Chronic fatigue syndrome: a working case definition. Ann Intern Med 1988;108:387–389.
135. Gold M, Pottash A, Extein I. Hypothyroidism and depression, evidence from complete thyroid function evaluation. JAMA 1981;245:1919–1922.
136. Demitrack MA. Evidence for impaired activation of hypothalamic-pituitary-adrenal axis in patients with chronic fatigue syndrome. J Clin Endocrinol Metab 1991;73:1224–1234.
137. Komaroff AL. Chronic Fatigue Syndrome: relationship to chronic viral infections. J Virol Meth 1988;21:3–10.
138. Starus SE, Tosato G, Amstrong G. Persisting illness and fatigue in adults with evidence of Epstein–Barr virus infection. Ann Intern Med 1985;102:7–16.
139. Holmes GP, Kaplan J, Stewart J. A cluster of patients with a chronic mononucleosis-like syndrome. Is Epstein–Barr virus the cause? JAMA 1987;257:2297–2302.
140. Caligiuri M, Murray C, Buchwald D. Phenotypic and fictional deficiency of natural killer cells in patients with chronic fatigue syndrome. J Immunol 1987;139:3306–3313.
141. Greden JF, Fontaine P, Lubetsky M. Anxiety and depression associated with caffeine among psychiatric inpatients. Is J Psychiatry 1978;135:963–966.
142. Cox IM, Campbell MJ, Dowson D. Red blood cell magnesium and chronic fatigue syndrome. Lancet 1991;337;757–760.
143. Gullestad L, Oustein, Dolve L, Birkeland K. Oral versus intravenous magnesium supplementation in patients with magnesium deficiency. Magnes Trace Elem 1991;10:11–16.
144. Linberg JS, Zobitz MM, Poindexter JR. Magnesium bioavailability from magnesium citrate and magnesium oxide. J Am Coll Nutr 1990;9:48–55.
145. Flatiron MA, Morley JE, Bloom ET. The effect of exercise on natural killer cells activity in young and old subjects. J Gerontol 1989;44:37–45.
146. Fitzgerald L. Exercise and the immune system. Immunol Today 1988;9:337–339.
147. Bland JS, Barrager E, Reedy RG, Bland K. A medical food supplemented detoxification program in the management of chronic health problems. Altern Ther 1995;1:62–71.
148. Rigden S. Entero-hepatic resuscitation program for CFIDS. CFIDS Chron 1995;Spring:46–49.

20   Botanicals in the Management of Pain

Tieraona Low Dog

CONTENTS

Summary

Interest in botanical medicine is steadily growing in the United States. When compared to all other complementary and alternative medicine (CAM) practices, the greatest relative increase in the United States between 1997 and 2002 was for botanical medicine. Many of the top-selling herbs in the Uniteds States have been subjected to clinical trials in Europe and are recognized for numerous health conditions by authoritative groups such as the World Health Organization, The European Scientific Cooperative on Phytomedicine and the German Commission E. Their growing popularity has spurred research inquiries into their potential benefits, as well as concerns over product quality, long-term safety, herb-drug interactions, and use in specific populations (e.g., pediatrics, pregnancy). The National Center for Complementary and Alternative Medicine and the Office of Dietary Supplements are focusing considerable time and money on botanical research. Surveys indicate that CAM use is high in patients with chronic pain conditions, and back pain, in particular, is the single most common condition for which Americans use CAM. There is a great deal of historical evidence that reveals the extensive use of botanicals for the relief of pain. Plants with analgesic, anti-inflammatory and/or anti-spasmodic activities were widely employed and continue to be used. This chapter reviews the current data on botanical medicines that may be useful in the management of various painful conditions.

Key Words: botanical medicine, herbal medicine, pain, alternative medicine, arthritis, rheumatology

1. INTRODUCTION TO BOTANICAL MEDICINE

The history of botanical medicine is universal, as plants have been used to heal the sick since antiquity. Fossil records date the human use of medicinal plants to at least the Middle Paleolithic age some 60,000 years ago. Although botanical medicine is

From: *Contemporary Pain Medicine: Integrative Pain Medicine: The Science and Practice of Complementary and Alternative Medicine in Pain Management*
Edited by: J. F. Audette and A. Bailey © Humana Press, Totowa, NJ

considered part of "complementary and alternative medicine" in the West, it remains a primary source of medicine in many parts of the world including present day China, India and many countries in South America and Africa.

Interest in botanical medicine is steadily growing in the United States. Between 1990 and 1997, the use of these remedies increased by 380% *(1)*. In fact, when looking across all CAM practices, the greatest relative increase in the Unites States between 1997 and 2002 was for botanical medicine (12.1% vs.18.6%, respectively; representing 38 million adults) *(2)*. Many of the top-selling herbs in the United States (e.g., garlic, saw palmetto, echinacea, ginkgo, black cohosh, St. John's wort) are those that have been subjected to clinical trials in Europe and are recognized for numerous health conditions by authoritative groups such as the World Health Organization, The European Scientific Cooperative on Phytomedicine, and the German Commission E. Their growing popularity has spurred research inquiries into their potential benefits, as well as concerns over product quality, long-term safety, herb–drug interactions, and use in specific populations (e.g., pediatrics, pregnancy). The National Center for Complementary and Alternative Medicine ($122 million budget for fiscal year 2005) and the Office of Dietary Supplements, both under the umbrella of the National Institutes of Health, are focusing considerable time and money on botanical research. This includes improving standards for identification and characterization of raw material, developing innovative technologies for determining bioactivity, conducting basic science and funding phase I, II and III clinical trials.

2. THE USE OF BOTANICALS IN PAIN MANAGEMENT

Surveys indicate that CAM use is high in patients, both pediatric and adult, with chronic pain conditions *(3–6)*. Back pain is the single most common condition for which Americans use CAM. There is a great deal of historical evidence that reveals the extensive use of botanicals for the relief of pain. Plants with analgesic, anti-inflammatory and/or anti-spasmodic activities were widely employed.

2.1. Botanical History of Opiates in Pain Management

Most healthcare professionals are well aware of the powerful role that opiates play in the management of pain. Historical documents reveal that opium was well-known by the early physicians in Egypt, Rome and Greece. In 1680, the English physician Thomas Sydenham wrote, "Among the remedies which it has pleased Almighty God to give man to relieve his sufferings, none is so universal and efficacious as opium." Morphine was isolated in 1802 by Frederick Serturner, so named after Morpheus, the Greek god of sleep. With the creation of the hypodermic needle in 1853, the use of morphine and heroin for the relief of pain was taken to a new level, as was the growing problem of addiction and abuse. The proper use of opiates in the management of pain remains the subject of debate today amongst both healthcare providers and regulatory bodies.

2.2. Anti-Inflammatory Agents in History

The history of willow (*Salix* spp) and other salicin-rich plants is another example of the powerful role botanicals have played in the management of pain. The analgesic and antipyretic properties of willow were noted by ancient Egyptian, Greek, Indian, and Roman civilizations. *Salix* species contain several prodrugs of salicylate, principally salicin, which was isolated in 1828 by the French chemist Henri Leroux but its use as an analgesic was limited by severe gastric irritation. Various chemists continued to work on developing a product that was gentler on the stomach and in 1899 Bayer went to market with acetylsalicylic acid under the trade name of aspirin, one of the most successful drugs in history.

There are numerous botanical medicines that continue to be utilized for the management of pain both in the United States and abroad. Pain conditions commonly treated with botanical remedies include arthritis, back pain, headache, and irritable bowel syndrome. Botanicals contain a vast array of compounds that have wide-ranging physiological effects, including anti-spasmodic, analgesic and ant-inflammatory activity, however, unlike their pharmaceutical counterparts, plants generally work through a number of pathways and mechanistic explanations for their observed effects are still being developed. For instance, ginger inhibits cyclooxygenase (COX) 1 and 2 and 5-lipoxygenase (5-LOX) but also inhibits inducible genes that encode for inflammatory cytokines and chemokines. This broad range of activity may, in part, explain the milder therapeutic activity seen with ginger but also its lower risk of serious adverse effects. Since there are many herbs that could be included in chapter on pain, in order to make things more manageable, this chapter will primarily focus on botanicals studied for the relief of back pain and arthritis, with a brief review of the most popular botanicals used for sleep and depression, given how commonly these problems occur in patients with chronic pain.

3. SELECTED BOTANICALS

3.1. Boswellia (Boswellia serrata Roxb. ex Colebr.)

The resinous gum obtained from the *Boswellia serrata* tree, commonly known as Indian frankincense, has been used as fragrant incense and medicinal agent since ancient times and the extracts remain popular in India for the treatment of numerous inflammatory disorders. Boswellia resin is composed of fatty acids, volatile oils and four pentacylic triterpenes, collectively referred to as boswellic acid that are thought to account for much of the extracts activity *(7)*. Boswellic acid is an inhibitor of 5-lipoxygenase *(8)* but does not appear to have any significant activity on cyclooxygenase. There is preliminary evidence that boswellia extract may be beneficial in inflammatory bowel disease *(9)* and asthma *(10)*.

Clinical trial data are limited for boswellia in the management of pain disorders. A randomized, double blind, placebo-controlled crossover study assessed the efficacy, safety and tolerability of 1000 mg/d *Boswellia serrata* extract (Cap WokVel, containing 333 mg boswellia extract per capsule with minimum 40% total boswellic acids, Pharmanza, Gujrat, India) in 30 patients of osteoarthritis of knee for 8 weeks, followed by a washout and then the groups were crossed over to receive the opposite intervention for eight weeks *(11)*. After the first intervention, the decrease in pain intensity and swelling and the improvements in knee function were clinically and statistically significant ($p < 0.001$) in the active group. After the crossover, the group who had received boswellia extract during the first 8 weeks showed a worsening of symptoms while taking the placebo. No radiological differences between the BSE and placebo interventions were observed, though this would be unlikely after only 8 weeks of any intervention. Adverse events were minor and included diarrhea, epigastric pain and nausea in two patients in the active arm.

A review by Etzel *(12)* reported positive findings from several small studies for a particular boswellia extract (H-15: chloroform/methanol extract) in patients with rheumatoid arthritis. However, a more recent double-blind, placebo-controlled study of 78 patients with active RA failed to show any significant benefit for 3,600 mg/d boswellia extract (nine tablets/d each containing 400 mg chloroform/methanol extract) over placebo daily when given in addition to their current medical therapy *(13)*. Efficacy parameters included Ritchies Index for swelling and pain, erythrocyte sedimentation rate (ESR), C-reactive protein (CRP), pain on VAS and NSAID dose, which were documented at baseline and 6 and 12 weeks after initiation. There was no subjective, clinical or laboratory parameter showing a significant or clinically relevant change from baseline or difference between both groups at any time point of observation. Only 37 patients were included in the final analysis, significantly limiting any firm conclusions that can be drawn from the study.

In many traditional medical systems, combination herbal formulae are more the rule than the exception. Many herbal practitioners individualize formulations and hold that combinations of plants may work together in a synergistic fashion, though this area has not been the subject of much scientific research. An Ayurvedic herbal mixture of *Withania somnifera*, *Boswelia serrata*, *Z. officinale*, and *Curcuma longa* was tested in a double-blind RCT with 182 patients suffering from chronic RA *(14)*. Patients were given either the herbal mixture or placebo for 16 weeks. Out of multiple end-points, only joint swelling showed a significant inter-group difference in therapeutic response. The total daily dose was purported to be 444 mg of herbal mixture, but the source and quality of the extract was not given.

Boswellia extracts are typically standardized to 37.5–65% boswellic acids with a daily dose of 900–3,600 mg of extract. Boswellia has been well tolerated in most studies, though some may experience nausea, heartburn, epigastric pain or diarrhea. The safety of boswellia in pregnancy and lactation is not known.

While there is impressive historical, in vitro, and animal data attesting to the anti-inflammatory activity of B. serrata, there are limited clinical data to support its use in patients with rheumatic complaints.

*3.2. Capsicum (*Capsicum frutescens L.*)*

The resinous compound capsaicin is extracted from the fruit of chili peppers (*C. frutescens* and others). Capsaicin binds to the vanilloid receptor subtype 1 (VR1) that is expressed in primary sensory neurons and vagal nerves, where it stimulates the release of substance P, a chemical involved in the transmission of pain, from nerve terminals. Eventually, the nerve terminals become depleted of substance P, leading to the loss of pain sensation and the desensitization of sensory neurons after prolonged administration *(15)*.

A meta-analysis of capsaicin for the treatment of pain by Mason et al. *(16)* reported that topical capsaicin is better than placebo for the treatment of chronic pain from neuropathic and musculoskeletal disorders. Six double-blind placebo controlled trials (656 patients) for neuropathic pain and three trials (368 patients) for musculoskeletal pain were included and were considered of moderate to high quality. For neuropathic conditions, the mean treatment response rate at eight weeks for capsaicin 0.075% was 60% (range 20–75%) and 42% for placebo (range 10–65%), while for musculoskeletal conditions, the mean treatment response rate at four weeks for capsaicin 0.025% cream or plaster was 38% (range 34–42%) versus 25% for placebo (range 17–37%).

The FDA and Health Canada approve capsaicin as an over-the-counter drug. Various commercial creams are available, generally in 0.025% and 0.075% strengths, which are applied 3–4 times per day. A single-application, very-high-dose capsaicin patch is currently undergoing phase II clinical trials for neuropathic pain (NeurogesX NGX-4010).

Adverse events are fairly common with topical capsaicin. Overall in clinical trials, 54% of patients using capsaicin experienced at least one local adverse event, compared to 15% using placebo, and adverse-event-related withdrawals occurred in 13% patients using capsaicin compared to 3% using placebo *(16)*. Patients should be instructed to wash their hands thoroughly with soap and water after applying capsaicin to avoid accidentally coming into contact with sensitive mucous membranes.

The FDA approves capsaicin topical cream as an over-the-counter medicine. Evidence supports its use for relief of neuropathic and musculoskeletal pain.

3.3. Cat's Claw (**Uncaria tomentosa** *(Willd.) DC*, U. guianensis *(Aubl.) Gmel.*)

Cat's claw, known as *una de gato* in Spanish, is a large woody vine that is a member of the Uncaria genus. The botanical name, *Uncaria*, is from the Latin *uncus*, for "hook," while its common name is derived from the curved thorns that grow along the vine, which resemble the claws of a cat. There are numerous species used around the globe as medicinal agents. The most heavily researched is *Uncaria tomentosa*, which is found only in the tropical areas of Central and South America, followed by *U. guianensis*, which grows both in the Amazon and in the areas of Bangladesh and Burma, and *U. rhynchophylla*, which is found in China and Japan *(17)*. Indigenous peoples have long used the root and bark for the treatment of arthritis, fever, asthma, ulcers and cancer. The botanical is promoted in the United States primarily as an agent to support the immune system.

An extract *U. tomentosa* was studied in 40 patients with active RA taking sulfasalazine or hydroxychloroquine for 52 weeks *(18)*. Patients were randomized to receive either 60 mg/d extract (20 mg root extract per capsule standardized to 1.3% pentacyclic oxindole alkaloids and free of tetracyclic oxindole alkaloids; IMMODAL Pharmaka GmbH, Austria) or placebo for 24 weeks, followed by an additional 28 weeks in which all participants took the extract. During the first 24-week double-blind period of the trial, 53% of patients receiving the extract and 24% on placebo experienced a reduction in the number of tender joints and severity of pain (p = 0.044) but there was no significant effect on laboratory indicators of inflammation. Those who received *Uncaria* only during the second phase of the trial had a reduction in the number of painful (p = 0.003) and swollen joints (P = 0.007) and the Ritchie Index (p = 0.004) when compared with values after 24 weeks of placebo. This extract was unique in that it did not contain any tetracyclic oxindole alkaloids, which are thought to interfere with immunomodulating activity of the pentacyclic oxindole alkaloids.

An extract of *U. guianensis* was studied in 45 patients with osteoarthritis of the knee *(19)*. Thirty patients were administered 100 mg freeze-dried *U. guainensis* (no further description of extract was provided) and 15 received placebo capsules. Subjects were assessed at baseline for pain at rest, at night, and during exercise using a 4-point scale. Liver function tests, hematocrit and hemoglobin were assessed at baseline and the conclusion of the study. The extract significantly improved pain with exercise, as compared to placebo (p< 0.001) but had no effect on pain at rest or at night. There was no change noted in any laboratory parameters. The lack of extract specifications limits the conclusions from the study.

The oxindole alkaloids present in the root bark of cat's claw are thought to account for much its anti-inflammatory activity, though other constituents likely play a role *(17)*. While *U. tomentosa* is higher in total oxindole and pentacyclic alkaloid content, one study found it to have considerably less anti-inflammatory activity than *U. guainensis (20)*. Solvents used in the extraction process may also affect the therapeutic activity of cat's claw. Ethanolic extracts of *U. tomentosa* were superior to aqueous extracts in anti-inflammatory activity *(21)*. There is a tremendous need for basic science research to determine which species, solvent and dose would be most effective for specific rheumatic disorders. A review of the safety data found a low potential for acute and subacute oral toxicity *(22)*. Safety in pregnancy is not known.

There is evidence from a single study that a unique extract prepared from *U. tomentosa* is of benefit for patients with rheumatoid arthritis.

3.4. Devil's Claw (**Harpagophytum procumbens** *(Burch.) DC ex. Meisn.*)

Devil's claw is a perennial plant belonging to the family Pedaliaceae that grows in the southern and eastern parts of Africa. Most of the world's supply comes from Namibia, with lesser amounts from Botswana and South Africa. The dried, secondary tubers have been used in the traditional medical systems of southern Africa as a digestive stimulant, anti-pyretic and analgesic. Devil's claw has been available for more than 50 years in Europe and is approved by the German Commission E (health authority) as a "supportive therapy for degenerative disorders of the locomotor system" *(23)*. Harpagoside, an iridoid glycoside, is a key player in the plant's pharmacologic activity, though other constituents may be important for the plant's medicinal effects as suggested by one animal study that found the aqueous extract more active than isolated, pure harpagoside *(24)*. Harpagoside remains an important marker compound and the European Pharmacopoeia requires a minimum content of 1.2% (2004). *Harpagophytum* extracts inhibit both the cyclooxygnase (COX) and 5-lipoxygenase (LOX) mediated pathways of the arachidonic acid cascade *(25)*.

Devil's claw is one of the better-studied botanicals for the treatment of pain conditions. A review by Gagnier, et al *(26)* included 12 trials in its analysis; six osteoarthritis, four low back pain, and three for mixed pain conditions. Methodological quality was assessed using guidelines developed by Van Tulder *(27)* for the Cochrane Collaboration Back Review Group for Spinal Disorders. Of the 12 controlled trials reviewed, eight were rated as high quality. The reviewers concluded that the evidence is consistent for a benefit from aqueous extracts of devil's claw delivering a daily dose of 50 mg or more of harpagoside per day, particularly for acute episodes of nonspecific low back pain. There was limited evidence for the efficacy of ethanolic extracts in the treatment of osteoarthritis.

The research suggests that Devil's claw extracts are well tolerated. Devil's claw contains bitter compounds purportedly stimulate gastric acid production. Both the German Commission E and European Scientific Cooperative on Phytotherapy (ESCOP) list gastric and duodenal ulcers as contraindications for use *(23,28)*. Devil's claw may potentiate the activity of warfarin *(29)*. Safety in pregnancy and lactation is not known.

There is strong and consistent evidence for a benefit from aqueous extracts of devil's claw delivering a daily dose of 50 mg or more of harpagoside per day, particularly for acute episodes of nonspecific low back pain.

3.5. Feverfew (Tanacetum parthenium (L.) Schultz-Bip.)

Feverfew has a long history of use for fever, headache and rheumatic complaints and is very popular as a preventive therapy for migraine headaches in the United States, Europe and Australia. A systematic review of five clinical trials (343 patients total) concluded that there is insufficient evidence to suggest an effect of feverfew over and above placebo for preventing migraine (30). The review, however, is limited as the trials evaluated diverse products (dried leaf, ethanolic extract, supercritical CO2 extracts) and different doses (18.75–250 mg/d). There is evidence to suggest that dried feverfew leaf is more effective than placebo for prevention of classic migraine and that the supercritical CO2 extracts are superior to placebo for reducing migraine frequency.

Optimal doses for prevention of migraine have not been established and there are no German Commission E, ESCOP or WHO monographs for review, Doses vary from 50 to 250 mg/d dried leaf (common dose is 125 mg/d standardized to 0.2% parthenolide, (though it remains uncertain if this an "active" or simply a marker compound) to two fresh leaves/day (approximately 60 mg/d) taken with food. If the CO_2 extracts become available in the United States, the dose of 6.25 mg TID was found to be most effective in randomized studies (31,32). Feverfew tincture is recommended by many herbalists in the United States and the UK, often in combination with other herbs. The one study conducted with an ethanol extract failed to find any benefit and no trials using combinations have been investigated at this time.

Though there is historical use of feverfew for arthritic conditions, there has been very little clinical research in this area. A double-blind, placebo-controlled study of dried feverfew leaf (70–86 mg/d) in 41 women with active rheumatoid arthritis found no difference between the active and placebo groups in stiffness, pain, grip strength, erythrocyte sedimentation rate (ESR), C-reactive protein (CRP), or functional capacity at the end of the 6-week study (33).

Withdrawal syndrome can occur after abrupt discontinuation of feverfew by long-term users; symptoms include headache, abdominal pain, diarrhea, fatigue, and joint pain (34). Mouth ulceration and gastric disturbance can occur in a small percentage of patients (35). Allergic reactions are theoretically possible in those sensitive to members of the Asteraceae family (ragweed, marigolds, daisies, etc). There is a potential inter-action with warfarin and other anticoagulant therapies (29). Feverfew is contraindicated during pregnancy due to possible uterine-stimulating activity (36).

A single trial does not the support the use of dried feverfew leaf in rheumatoid arthritis. There is mixed evidence in the literature to support the use of feverfew in migraine, with some evidence to support that CO2 extracts are superior to placebo and that dried feverfew leaf may be more effective for classical migraine than common migraine.

3.6. Ginger (Zingiber officinale Roscoe)

Ginger is a popular spice and the world production is estimated at 100,000 tons annually, of which 80% is grown in China. Ginger is a member of the Zingiberaceae family, which consists of 49 genera and 1300 species. In addition to its long history of use as a spice, references to ginger as a medicinal agent can be found in ancient Chinese, Indian, Arabic and Greco-Roman texts. Ginger has been used to treat a variety of conditions, but it is chiefly known as an anti-emetic, anti-inflammatory, digestive aid and diaphoretic. In the year 2000, ginger sales ranked 17th among all herbal supplements sold in U.S. mainstream retail stores. Research demonstrates that some compounds in ginger inhibit 5-LOX, while others are potent inhibitors of COX-2 *(37)*.

Three clinical trials evaluating the use of ginger in arthritis have been published. Ginger extract (170 mg 3 times/d EV.EXT 33; standardized ethanol extract of dry *Z. officinale* rhizomes, Eurovita A/S, Denmark) was compared to placebo and ibuprofen (400 mg 3 times/d) in 67 patients (56 completed) with osteoarthritis of the hip or knee in a controlled, double-blind, crossover study with a wash-out period of 1 week followed by 3 treatment periods in a randomized sequence, each of 3 weeks duration *(38)*. Acetaminophen was used as rescue medication throughout the study. The ranking of efficacy was ibuprofen > ginger extract > placebo for visual analog scores (VAS) on pain and the Lequesne index, but no significant difference was seen when comparing ginger extract and placebo directly.

A 6-week double-blind, placebo-controlled study randomized 261patients with OA of the knee to receive 255 mg BID "ginger" extract (EV.EXT 77, extracted from 2500– 4000 mg of dried ginger rhizomes and 500–1500 mg of dried galanga rhizomes; Eurovita A/S, Denmark) or matching placebo *(39)*. The primary efficacy variable was the proportion of responders experiencing a reduction in "knee pain on standing". A responder was defined by a reduction of 15 mm on VAS. Of the 247 patients who finished the study, the percentage of responders experiencing a reduction in knee pain on standing was superior in the ginger extract group compared with the control group (63% vs. 50%; p = 0.048). Reduction in the WOMAC composite index was not statistically significant (12.9 mm vs. 9.0 mm; *p*=0.087). Gastrointestinal adverse events were more common in the ginger group [116 events in 59 patients (45%)] compared with the placebo group [28 events in 21 patients (16%)], though none were considered serious by the investigators. It should be noted that this ginger extract is actually a combination of ginger and greater galangal (*Alpinia galanga* L.). Though greater galangal is a member of the Zingiberaceae family, this product is very different than the one used in the Bliddal, et al study *(38)* making any direct comparison of outcomes impossible.

A 6-month double blind, placebo-controlled crossover study randomized 29 patients with symptomatic gonarthritis (knee arthritis) to 250 mg ginger extract four times daily (Zintona® EC, Dalidar Pharma Ltd, Israel) or placebo for three months and then patients were crossed-over to the other treatment arm for an additional 3 months *(40)*. There was no statistically significant difference between groups at the crossover. The study suffered from small sample size and significant attrition, as eight dropped out due to inefficacy and 2 dropped out due to heartburn while on the ginger extract.

Heartburn is a bothersome adverse effect in a number of patients taking higher doses of ginger, as was seen in the trial by Altman et al *(39)*. Due to its cholagogue effect (stimulates bile secretion), those with active gallstone disease should avoid ginger supplements. The USP-DI suggests that patients with an increased risk of hemorrhage or those taking anti-coagulants should use ginger with caution *(41)*. The German Commission E contraindicates the use of ginger during pregnancy *(23)*. Two controlled experimental rat studies evaluated the effect of ginger on fetal development and found no evidence of maternal or developmental toxicity at daily doses up to 1000 mg/kg of body weight *(42,43)*. A prospective observational study of 187 pregnant women who used some form of ginger in the first trimester reported that the risk of these mothers having a baby with a congenital malformation was no higher than the control group *(44)*. Follow-up of 4 randomized controlled trials consistently showed that there were no significant side effects or adverse effects on pregnancy outcomes *(45)*. The currently recommended anti-emetic dose for nausea and vomiting of pregnancy (1,000 mg of dried ginger powder per day) is likely safe.

Overall, the evidence for ginger extracts for arthritis is inconclusive. The three trials used different types of extracts with varying doses, making any definitive statement about the efficacy of "ginger" for arthritis impossible.

3.7. Phytodolor ®

The majority of research is conducted on single botanical products; however, a combination formulation has been the subject of numerous controlled studies for the treatment of musculoskeletal pain. Phytodolor® is a standardized ethanolic herbal extract of common ash bark (*Fraxinus excelsior* L.), aspen bark (*Populus tremula* L.), and goldenrod aerial parts (*Solidago virgaurea* L.) in a 1:3:1 ratio. This German formula (Steigerwald Arzneimittel GmbH) is standardized to contain salicin (0.75 mg/ml), salicylic alcohol (0.042 mg/ml), isofraxidin (0.015 mg/ml) and rutin (0.06 mg/ml). A systematic review by Ernst *(46)* included 10 randomized controlled trials conducted from 1988 through 1992 with a total sample size of 1035 patients. Six were placebo-controlled trials and seven were conducted against other active medications (three of these studies also had a placebo control group). The reviewer concluded that Phytodolor® is more effective than placebo for the symptomatic treatment of musculoskeletal pain and equally as effective as the medications diclofenac 3 × 25 mg/day and indomethacin 2 × 50 mg/day. Most trials examined standard doses (30–40 drops (1.5–2 ml) three times/day) for 2–4 weeks. Limitations of the studies include the heterogenous nature of patient groups and the low dose of comparative medications. Clinical trials found the extract relatively devoid of adverse effects.

Evidence from a systematic review suggests that the combination herbal formulation Phytodolor® is superior to placebo and equally as effective as 75 mg/d diclofenac and 100 mg/d indomethacin for the symptomatic relief of musculoskeletal pain.

3.8. St. John's Wort (Hypericum perforatum L.)

St. John's Wort is the most heavily studied of the botanical remedies for depression and is widely used and recognized by health authorities in Europe as a treatment for anxiety, nervous unrest, and mild-to-moderate depression in both adult and pediatric populations. It is one of the top=selling botanical remedies in the United States, but practitioners of natural medicine and scientific researchers are divided regarding its effectiveness. The recent meta-analysis by Linde et al. *(47)* reflects this uncertainty with the following conclusion reached after reviewing 37 clinical trials: "Current evidence regarding hypericum extracts is inconsistent and confusing. In patients who meet criteria for major depression, several recent placebo-controlled trials suggest that the tested hypericum extracts have minimal beneficial effects while other trials suggest that hypericum and standard antidepressants have similar beneficial effects." Unfortunately, this type of conclusion does little to help the practitioner counseling her patient regarding the use of St. John's wort.

When looking at the risk/benefit of a particular therapy, safety and tolerability must also be heavily weighted. Systematic reviews have verified that St. John's wort has fewer adverse reactions when compared to prescription antidepressants; 26.3% for St. John's wort vs. 44.7% for standard antidepressants *(48)* Side effects are generally mild and include headache, gastrointestinal upset, dizziness, insomnia, and palpitations.

Pruritis and exanthema occurred in 17 of 3,250 patients (0.52%) taking 900 mg/d St. John's wort extract *(49)*. Phototoxicity is extremely rare but can occur in light-skinned individuals who are prone to sunburns *(50)*.

The main concern with St. John's wort is not its side effect profile but the fact that it can interact with numerous prescription medications. Numerous drug interactions have been reported in the literature. There is sufficient evidence from interaction studies and case reports to demonstrate that St. John's wort induces the cytochrome P450 (CYP) 3A4 enzyme system and the P-glycoprotein drug transporter in a clinically relevant manner, reducing the efficacy of co-medications *(51)*. Medications that are metabolized via both CYP3A4 and P-glycoprotein pathways are most likely to produce an herb–drug interaction. These include certain HIV protease inhibitors, HIV non-nucleoside reverse transcriptase inhibitors (only CYP3A4), the immunosuppressants cyclosporine and tacrolimus, and the antineoplastic agents irinotecan and imatinib mesylate.

Extracts of St. John's wort are generally standardized to 0.3% hypericin, 2–5% hyperforin, or both. There is no current scientific consensus on which constituent(s) to standardize and to what level. The dose used in the clinical trials is 600–1,800 mg/d. Two studies in pediatrics have shown good tolerability with 900 mg/d *(52)* and up to 1800 mg/d *(53)*.

While the studies are not entirely consistent, the weight of the evidence suggests that St. John's wort extract is beneficial for mild forms of depressive mood.

3.9. Thunder God Vine (Tripterygium wilfordii Hook)

Thunder god vine, or *lei gong teng*, is a perennial vine that grows in China and Myanmar (formerly Burma). It has been used in traditional Chinese medicine for more than 2000 years to treat a variety of ailments ranging from fever to leprosy. More recently, it has been used to treat a number of inflammatory conditions, including lupus and RA. *T. wilfordii* extract has been shown to inhibit the production of cytokines and block the up-regulation of a number of pro-inflammatory genes, including TNFα, COX2, interferon-γ, IL-2, prostaglandin, and iNOS. This fascinating botanical is currently the subject of NIH sponsored research.

An open-label, dose-escalation phase I NIH study of 13 patients with RA found that doses of up to 570 mg/d of an ethyl alcohol/ethyl acetate extract of *T. wilfordii* were well tolerated. The greatest improvement in both clinical response and laboratory findings was seen in the group receiving 360 mg/d extract (8 of 9 patients), one patient met the American College of Rheumatology criteria for remission *(54)*.

A double-blind placebo controlled study randomized 35 patients with long-standing RA to receive low dose (180 mg/d) or high dose (360 mg/d) ethanol/ethyl acetate extract of *T. wilfordii* or placebo for 20 weeks, followed by an open-label period *(55)*. Clinical response was defined as at least a 20% improvement in disease activity according to the American College of Rheumatology criteria. Of the 21 patients who completed the study, a therapeutic benefit was noted in the high dose group when compared with placebo (p = 0.0001). Less effectiveness was seen in the low-dose group but it was still superior to placebo (p = 0.0287). The most common adverse effect was diarrhea. Another RCT reported that thundergod vine increases the efficacy of methotrexate and reduces adverse effects *(56)*.

A 24-week phase II multi-center trial sponsored by the National Institute of Arthritis and Musculoskeletal and Skin Diseases (NIAMS) is currently underway (clinical-trials.gov). Approximately 157 patients with RA will be assigned to one of two drug-treatment groups, *T. wilfordii* extract or sulfasalazine. During the clinic visits, investigators will obtain multiple blood samples; give physical exams; assess swollen, tender, and painful joints; and administer x-rays. Patients will be allowed to continue stable doses of NSAID therapy and/or low dose corticosteroids but will discontinue any Disease-Modifying Anti-Rheumatic Drugs (DMARDs).

The extract used in the studies by Tao et al. was well tolerated at doses of 360 mg/d for up to 20 weeks; however, side effects reported for *T. wilfordii* include diarrhea, nausea, vomiting, hair loss, dry mouth, headaches, leukopenia, thrombocytopenia, rash, skin pigmentation, angular stomatitis, oral ulcers, gastritis, abdominal pain, weight loss, diastolic hypertension, and vaginal spotting *(57)*. Classical Chinese texts carefully describe the preparation of the medicine. The root is peeled and the bark discarded, only the root pulp is used. Infertility was an unexpected side effect noted in men using *T. wilfordii*. Low doses of the extracts have been shown to reduce sperm density and motility in both animals and humans *(58)*. Researchers are currently investigating the possibility of developing a male contraceptive agent from isolated compounds in the root. Amenorrhea is a reversible side effect in women younger than 40 years of age and if present for less than 2 years. Follicle-stimulating hormone (FSH) and luteinzing hormone (LH) levels being to rise within 2–3 months of use and reach menopausal levels within 5 months, while estradiol levels fall to very low levels *(59)*. Long-term administration of *T. wilfordii* has been shown to decrease bone mineral density (BMD) in women with systemic lupus erythematosus who were treated with the extract for > 5 year,, though the loss of BMD was less severe than that induced by prednisone *(60)*.

Despite its long history of use in traditional Chinese medicine and impressive preliminary research, given the potentially significant adverse effects and lack of well characterized extracts in the marketplace—it is premature for practitioners to recommend the use of *T. wilfordii*.

*3.10. Valerian (***Valeriana officinalis** *L.)*

People suffering with acute and/or chronic pain often have difficulty sleeping and many turn to over-the-counter remedies. Valerian is the most prominent herbal remedy for insomnia, alone or in combination with other sedative herbs. The genus name, *Valeriana*, comes from the latin *valere*, meaning a "state of being well or happy." There are numerous species of valerian; the one most commonly researched and utilized in the herb industry is *Valeriana officinalis*. Valerian is recognized by the German Commission E, the European Scientific Cooperative on Phytotherapy (ESCOP) and the World Health Organization as a sleep-promoting agent and mild sedative. A systematic review of nine randomized, placebo-controlled, double-blind clinical trials of valerian for sleep disorders found that the evidence for valerian in the treatment of insomnia is inconclusive, though, the three highest-rated studies (5 out of 5 for quality) were all positive *(61)*.

There are also positive studies for the combination of valerian/lemon balm and valerian/hops/lemon balm *(62)*.

Valerian is generally quite safe when taken appropriately. The crude herb is generally taken in doses of 2–3 grams approximately 1 hour before bedtime. Extracts are often standardized to contain 0.3–0.8% valerenic acid and the dose varies according to manufacturer specifications. Individuals may need to take valerian for several weeks to achieve maximum effect. The German Commission E lists no contraindications. ESCOP contraindicates the use of valerian in children under 3. The World Health Organization contraindicates the use of valerian during pregnancy and lactation due to lack of studies. A small number of individuals experience stimulation and restlessness even at normal doses—valerian should be discontinued in these patients. A study in human volunteers found that neither single nor repeated evening administrations of 600 mg of valerian root extract have a relevant negative impact on reaction time, alertness and concentration the morning after intake *(63)*.

There is moderate evidence to suggest that valerian is effective as a mild, non-habit-forming sleep-promoting agent.

3.11. Willow (Salix spp)

The analgesic and antipyretic properties of willow were well known by ancient Egyptian, Greek, Indian, and Roman civilizations. *Salix* species contain salicin, a prodrug of salicylate. Though aspirin is easily accessible and relatively inexpensive, there has been a resurgence of interest in willow bark for the treatment of chronic pain conditions. White willow (*Salix alba* Kern.) is the species most commonly used for medicinal purposes, though crack willow (*Salix fragilis* L.), purple willow (*Salix purpurea* L.), and violet willow (*Salix daphnoides* Vill.) all contain salicin and are sold under the name "willow bark." While salicin is thought to be the primary analgesic in willow bark, other components such as tannins, flavonoids, and salicin esters likely contribute to its overall effect *(64)*. Willow bark is recognized by the German Commission E for the treatment of "diseases accompanied by fever, rheumatic ailments and headaches" (Blumenthal 1998) in a daily dose equivalent to 60-120 mg salicin. The ESCOP monograph recommends an equivalent of up to 240 mg/d salicin *(65)*.

There are five published controlled trials for willow bark extract (WBE). Two trials evaluated the extract in patients with acute exacerbation of low back pain, one placebo controlled and the other a comparative study with rofecoxib. Two trials evaluated the extract in patients with osteoarthritis, both had a placebo arm but one also had a comparative arm with diclofenac. One placebo-controlled study was conducted in patients with active RA (see Table 1).

Two studies of WBE in patients with low back pain were positive, both conducted by the same lead researcher. One study by Chrubasik et al. (compared two different strengths of WBE in 210 patients with exacerbation of chronic lower back pain, reporting at least 5 of 10 on the visual analog scale *(66)*. Patients received either 120 mg/d or 240 mg/d of salicin per day or placebo as twice a day dosing (product contained 0.153 mg of salicin per mg of extract; Plantina GmbH Munich, Germany). The principal outcome measure was the number of patients who responded to treatment by being pain-free without tramadol (a synthetic opioid) for at least 5 days during the last week of the study. Thirty-nine percent of those in the high-dose group, 21% in the low-dose group, and 6% of those receiving placebo achieved this endpoint (p < 0.001). The second study was a 4-week randomized, controlled, open trial of 228 patients comparing 12.5 mg/day of rofecoxib with 240 mg/day of salicin (Assalix®, dry extract from willow bark with 15% salicin; Bionorica AG, Neumarkt, Germany) in patients

Table 1
Controlled Clinical Trials of Willow Bark Extract

Author (year)	Design	Control	Treatment	Outcome measures	Results
Chrubasik (2000)	RDBCT (n = 210) acute exacerbation NSLBP 4 weeks	Placebo	WBE; providing 120 mg/d or 240 mg/d salicin	Number pain-free, without tramalol 5 days of 7.	39% high-dose group, 21% low-dose group, 6% placebo (p < 0.001)
Chrubasik (2001)	RCT, open. (n = 228) acute exacerbation NSLBP 4 weeks	Rofecoxib 12.5 mg/d	WBE; providing 240 mg/d salicin	Improvement ≥30% of the Total Pain Index from baseline.	No difference between groups
Schmid (2001)	RDBCT (n=78) OA hip or knee2 weeks	Placebo	WBE; providing 240 mg/d salicin	Primary outcome: pain dimension of WOMAC OA Index	Significant reduction in pain dimension (d = 6.5 mm, 0.2–12.7 mm; p = 0.047)
Biegert (2004)	RDBCTOA hip or knee (N=127) 6 weeks	Placebo or diclofenac 100 mg/d	WBE; providing 240 mg/d salicin	Pain subscore of WOMAC OA Index	Pain scores decreased: 23 mm (47%) diclofenac, 8 mm (17%) willow 5 mm (10%) placebo. No statistical difference between willow and placebo (p = 0.55)
Biegert (2004)	RDBCT Active RA (n=26) 6 weeks	Placebo	WBE; providing 240 mg/d salicin	VAS	Pain reduction: –8 mm (15%) willow –2 mm (5%) placebo (p = 0.93)

RDBCT: randomized, double blind, controlled trial. RCT: randomized, controlled trial.
WBE: willow bark extract. VAS: visual analog scale. WOMAC: Western Ontario and McMaster University Osteoarthritis Index.

with acute exacerbations of low back pain *(67)*. After 4 weeks, 60% of patients in both groups experienced a positive response to treatment, as determined by an improvement of ≥30% of the Total Pain Index from baseline, suggesting that this willow bark extract at a dose of 240 mg per day of salicin was as effective as the COX-2 inhibitor.

Trials of WBE in patients with osteoarthritis were contradictory. The study by Schmid et al. *(64)* randomized 78 patients with osteoarthritis of the hip or knee to receive WBE corresponding to 240 mg salicin/day (340 mg extract per tablet of *Salix purpurea* and *S. daphnoides* corresponding to 60 mg salicin; Salus Haus GmbH, Germany) or placebo for 2 weeks after a washout period of 4 to 6 days with placebo. Additional NSAIDs, corticosteroids, and analgesics were not allowed at any point of the study. A moderate analgesic effect was found: the Western Ontario and McMasters University Osteoarthritis Index (WOMAC) pain score was reduced by 14% after 2 weeks of active treatment, compared with an increase of 2% in the placebo group. The patient diary visual analog scale also demonstrated efficacy for willow bark extract (investigator's assessment, p = 0.0073; patients' assessment, p = 0.0002). However, a randomized, double blind, 3-arm study by Biegert et al. *(68)* failed to note any significant effect for willow bark extract providing 240 mg/d salicin (ethanol 70% v/v, drug-extract ratio: 8-14:1, Finzelberg, Andernach, Germany) in 127 patients with osteoarthritis of the hip or knee over placebo. Over the 6 week study, WOMAC pain scores decreased by 8 mm (17%) in the willow bark group, by 5 mm (10%) in the placebo group, and by 23 mm (47%) in the diclofenac group, showing clear superiority for diclofenac over placebo (p = 0.0002). The difference between willow bark extract and placebo did not reach statistical significance (p = 0.55).

This study also failed to note any benefit in 26 patients with active rheumatoid arthritis when compared to placebo. The mean reduction of pain on the VAS was −8 mm (15%) in the willow bark group compared with −2 mm (4%) in the placebo group. The difference was not statistically significant (p = 0.93).

Roughly 3% of participants suffered allergic skin reactions in clinical trials, which disappeared soon after stopping treatment. The incidence of other adverse events was 11%, less than, or similar to, placebo *(67)*. Unlike aspirin, willow bark does not seem to be associated with gastrointestinal irritation. Theoretically, the risks of willow bark may be similar to aspirin, thus many authorities contraindicate the its use in febrile children to avoid the risk of Reye's syndrome, those with aspirin allergies, or those taking anticoagulant medications. While there is some impact on platelets, oral consumption of 240 mg/d of willow bark extract was found have a lesser effect on platelet aggregation than 100 mg/d aspirin (*p* = 0.001) *(69)*.

There is strong historical evidence for willow bark and the endorsement of its use for rheumatic complaints by both the German Commission E and ESCOP; however, the clinical trial data are contradictory regarding its benefit in LBP, OA and RA.

4. CONSIDERATIONS WHEN EVALUATING BOTANICAL RESEARCH

Due to the complex nature of botanicals, variation in constituents between species, plant part and preparation - it is essential that authors of research articles clearly provide an adequate description of the product used in their clinical trial. Descriptions

Table 2
Summary of Botanical Substances, Indications, Dose Ranges, and Safety Issues

Botanical substance	Therapeutic indications	Common dose ranges	Safety issues of concern
Boswellia (*Boswellia serrata* Roxb. ex Colebr.)	Osteoarthritis,* rheumatoid arthritis*	900–3600 mg/d of extract (standardized to 37.5–65% boswellic acids)	Boswellia well-tolerated in most studies. Some may experience nausea, heartburn, epigastric pain or diarrhea; safety in pregnancy and lactation is not known
Capsicum (*Capsicum frutescens* L.)	Relief of neuropathic and musculoskeletal pain***	Capsaicin creams: 0.025% and 0.075% strengths, applied 3–4 times per day.	Burning and worsening of pain common initially when applying topical cream; patients should be instructed to wash their hands thoroughly with soap and water after applying to avoid contact with sensitive mucous membranes.
Cat's claw (*Uncaria tomentosa* (Willd.) DC, *U. guianensis* (Aubl.) Gmel.)	Osteoarthritis,* rheumatoid arthritis *	Extract *U. tomentosa*—60 mg/d extract (20 mg root extract per capsule standardized to 1.3% pentacyclic oxindole alkaloids and free of tetracyclic oxindole alkaloids	Low potential for toxicity (Valerio 2005); safety in pregnancy and lactation is not known
Devil's claw (*Harpagophytum procumbens* (Burch.) DC ex. Meisn.)	Acute back pain,*** osteoarthritis,** mixed pain conditions*	Aqueous extracts of devil's claw providing 50 mg or more harpagoside per day	Contraindicated in gastric and duodenal ulcers. May potentiate activity of warfarin; safety in pregnancy and lactation is not known
Feverfew (*Tanacetum parthenium* (L.) Schultz-Bip.)	Migraine,** osteoarthritis*	125–250 mg per day of dried feverfew leaf, sometimes standardized to 0.2% parthenolide; clinically tested CO_2 extract is not currently available in United States	Withdrawal syndrome can occur after abrupt discontinuation by long-term users; mouth ulceration and gastric disturbance can occur in a small percentage of patients; allergic reactions theoretically possible in those sensitive to members of the Asteraceae family (ragweed, marigolds, daisies, etc); there is a potential interaction with warfarin and other anticoagulant therapies; feverfew is contraindicated during pregnancy

Table 2
(Continued)

Botanical substance	Therapeutic indications	Common dose ranges	Safety/issues of concern
Ginger (*Zingiber officinale* Roscoe)	Osteoarthritis**	Varied dosage and preparations used in clinical trials	Heartburn with higher doses not uncommon; contraindicated in those with active gallstone disease; possibly an increased risk of hemorrhage in those using > 4 g/d dried ginger and taking anticoagulants
St. John's wort (*Hypericum perforatum* L.)	Mild-to-moderate depression **	900–1800 mg per day extract generally standardized to 0.3% hypericin, 2–5% hyperforin or both.	Generally well-tolerated in clinical trials; rare cases of phototoxicity. Herb-drug interactions due to induction of CYP3A4 and P-glycoprotein drug transporter
Thunder god vine (*Tripterygium wilfordii* Hook)	Rheumatoid arthritis**	Not recommended at this time, as standardized product is not readily available in United States	Diarrhea, nausea, vomiting, hair loss, dry mouth, headaches, leukopenia, thrombocytopenia, rash, skin pigmentation, angular stomatitis, oral ulcers, gastritis, abdominal pain, weight loss, diastolic hypertension, vaginal spotting and amenorrhea have all been reported; loss of bone mineral density with long-term use
Valerian (*Valeriana officinalis* L.)	Insomnia**	2–3 g of crude root or equivalent as an extract; sometimes standardized to 0.3–0.8% valerenic acid as a marker compound	Generally well-tolerated; contraindicated by some authorities for children under 3 years and pregnancy; some patients experience stimulation at normal doses—valerian should be discontinued in these cases
Willow (*Salix* spp)	Acute back pain,** osteoarthritis,** rheumatoid arthritis*	Willow bark extract providing 120–240 mg/d salicin	Theoretically, the risks are similar to aspirin, though this is not well-supported by adverse event reporting or clinical trial data

*Strong support in the literature for use of botanical in this condition.
**Moderate or mixed support in the literature for use of the botanical in this condition.
***Commonly used for this condition, but little evidence in the literature at this time.

should include identification (Latin binomial and authority), plant part (root, leaf, seed, etc.) and type of preparation (tea, tincture, extract, oil, etc.). Tincture and extract description should include the identity of the solvent, and the ratio of solvent to plant material. If the preparation is standardized to a chemical constituent, then that information should also be included. Precise and clear dose and dosage form should be provided *(70)*. A number of trials reviewed for this chapter did not provide any information for the botanical product beyond the Latin binomial and dose, making it difficult to draw any firm conclusions about the outcomes.

A growing number of meta-analyses and systematic reviews on botanical remedies are being published in the medical literature; however, it is important to point out one potentially serious problem with this approach in the field of botanical medicine—the "pooling" of different products to reach a conclusion about one particular herb. When comparing products that differ in extraction technique, plant part, delivery system and dose—it makes the question of equivalency a very valid one. For example, it is difficult to make any definitive conclusion about the efficacy of "cat's claw" in rheumatologic disorders when different species were studied using different extraction techniques at different doses? Pharmacologic and biological equivalency between products cannot simply be presumed.

5. QUALITY OF BOTANICAL PRODUCTS

Given the dramatic increase in the use of botanical remedies and the sheer number of products, it is understandable that consumers and healthcare professionals alike have difficulty navigating the supplement marketplace. Questions such as which botanical product should I take? at what dose? will it interact with my medications? is it safe? and will it work,? plague everyone who has ever looked down a supplement aisle. In addition to questions of efficacy and safety concerns inherent to the plant, there has also been growing concern about the quality of dietary supplements in general, and botanical remedies in particular. There have been numerous reports in the popular media and professional literature regarding adulteration and contamination of products, as well as variation between what is printed on the label and what is actually present in the bottle. While many manufacturers produce quality botanical products, the unscrupulous and/or incompetent have, unfortunately, tarnished the industry and it relatively difficult for consumers to recognize the good companies from the bad.

The implementation of new good manufacturing practice (GMP) guidelines proposed by the FDA that specifically addresses the unique challenge of using botanical ingredients will be a significant step forward in assuring the public of higher quality dietary supplements. In the meantime, groups such as the United States Pharmacopoeia (USP) and NSF International have launched dietary supplement quality verification programs to help ensure the public that the brand they are purchasing has been made to high and rigorous standards. These are voluntary programs that require manufacturers who use the quality seal on their label to undergo a rigorous auditing of manufacturing sites for good manufacturing practice (GMP) compliance, laboratory testing of product samples, label review and periodic off-the-shelf testing of products. Other independent testing groups, such as Consumer Labs, have begun to randomly test dietary supplements for quality and release their findings to the public. See the resource section at the end of the chapter for more information.

6. TALKING WITH PATIENTS

The concomitant use of botanical remedies with prescription or over-the-counter medications may lead to adverse interactions, especially in the elderly who are more likely be experiencing rheumatic complaints and also be using multiple drugs. A national survey noted that 16% of prescription drug users also reported use of one or more herbals/supplements within the prior week *(71)*. Thus, it is important that we dialogue with our patients about their use of botanical medicines and other dietary supplements. There is such a wide variety of herbal practices and products available in the United States that generalizations are difficult; however, by asking a few open-ended questions, you should be able to assess your patient's beliefs, cultural practices, and use of botanical remedies.

- When you were growing up did you, or your family, ever use any medicinal plants or herbal remedies to improve your health or treat an illness?
- If you and I were to walk around your house and look for containers of herbs or vitamins, what would we find?
- Are you taking any herbs or herbal medicines now? If so, what are you trying to treat and do you think the herbs are working?

Document all patient responses in the medical chart and be alert for potential adverse effects and herb-drug interactions. If you suspect a possible adverse effect, report it to FDA Medwatch (see FDA website in Resource section at end of this chapter) or your local Poison Control Center.

7. RESOURCES

7.1. Information on Testing Dietary Supplements and Botanical Products

United States Pharmacopeia (USP) Website: www.uspverified.org

The USP established a rigorous third-party testing program to verify the quality of dietary supplements. Manufacturers who meet USP quality specifications (including on-site good manufacturing practices (GMP) inspections, product testing and ongoing monitoring) can put the USP quality seal on their label. The website provides a list of companies that have passed quality testing.

NSF International Website: www.nsfconsumer.org/food/dietary_supplements.asp

NSF International is a nonprofit public health organization that provides a certification service for dietary supplement manufacturers that can meet their quality specifications (including on-site good manufacturing practices (GMP) inspections, product testing and ongoing monitoring). The website also provides some very useful consumer handouts.

Consumer Labs Website: www.consumerlabs.com

Consumer Labs evaluates commercially available dietary supplement products for composition, potency, purity, bioavailability, and consistency of products. They also have a certification program that allows manufacturers to have their products voluntarily tested. Approved products can bear the CL seal. An annual individual subscription of $27 allows complete access to test results for hundreds of dietary supplements.

7.2. Government Websites

The National Center for Complementary and Alternative Medicine (NCCAM) Website: www.nccam.nih.gov

NCCAM provides information on complementary and alternative medicine for consumers, healthcare providers and researchers. Services include fact sheets, on-line newsletter, clinical trial information, and health information available in both English and Spanish.

CAM on PubMed Website: www.nlm.nih.gov/nccam/camonpubmed.html.

CAM on PubMed, a database on the Web developed jointly by NCCAM and the National Library of Medicine, offers citations to (and in most cases, abstracts of) articles in scientifically based, peer- reviewed journals on complementary and alternative medicine. Most citations include abstracts, and some link to the full text of articles.

Food and Drug Administration (FDA) Dietary Supplements Page Website: vm.cfsan.fda.gov/~dms/supplmnt.html.

This website provides an overview of dietary supplement regulations, warnings and safety information, information on adverse event reporting and current topics and policies in the field.

Office of Dietary Supplements (ODS) Website: ods.od.nih.gov/index.aspx.

Under Quick Links you can access dietary supplement fact sheets and the link to the International Bibliographic Information on Dietary Supplements (IBIDS). This database is coordinated by the Office of Dietary Supplements, National Institutes of Health, Food and Nutrition Information Center, National Agricultural Library, and the United States Department of Agriculture and contains bibliographic records on dietary supplements.

Health Canada Website: www.hc-sc.gc.ca.

The Canadian government regulates natural health products in Canada by licensing products with evidence of safety and efficacy. This website lists products licensed in Canada, as well as providing a limited number of monographs.

7.3. Other Useful Websites

American Botanical Council Website: http://www.herbalgram.org/.

Established in 1988, the American Botanical Council is a nonprofit, international member-based organization providing education using science-based and traditional information on herbal medicine. The website offers an excellent on-line bookstore featuring premiere botanical texts, an Herb Clip service summarizing current research articles in the field and an educational resource section offering continuing education credits for healthcare professionals.

AltMedDex® Website: http://www.micromedex.com/products/altmeddex.

Contains several hundred evidence-based monographs and patient handouts on dietary supplements and medical conditions, updated semiannually. This is a component of the larger Micromedex product, published by Thomson. A hand-held version is also available. (Subscription required).

Cochrane Collaboration Complementary Medicine Field Website: www.compmed. umm.edu/cochrane/index.html.

The Cochrane Collaboration Complementary Medicine Field is an international group that provides systematic reviews of randomized clinical trials in topic areas such as acupuncture, massage, chiropractic, herbal medicine, homeopathy and mind-body therapy. Abstracts are free; there is a $235.00 annual subscription fee for full access to the research.

Natural Medicines Comprehensive Database Website: http://www.naturaldatabase.com/.

Created by the publishers of the Pharmacist's Letter, this fee-based database includes evidence based dietary supplement monographs with safety and efficacy information, as well as potential herb-drug interactions and recommended dose ranges. You can also search by medical condition or commercial dietary supplement product name. Continuing education credits are available. The annual cost for an individual subscriber is $92.

Natural Standard Website: www.naturalstandard.com.

This fee-based database created by an international research collaboration to evaluate and summarize scientific data on complementary and alternative therapies. The monographs use a grading scale for the evidence and each is highly referenced. The database can be searched by medical condition or therapy/product. Continuing education credits available. A hand-held version will be available soon. Annual individual subscription is $99.

Longwood Herbal Task Force Website: www.longwoodherbal.org.

This is free website that provides a limited number of well-done peer-reviewed herb and dietary supplement monographs, clinician summaries, and patient information sheets. The website also contains links to reputable websites providing information about vitamins, minerals, supplement-drug interactions, etc.

HerbMed Website: www.herbmed.org

HerbMed is a free herbal database that provides hyperlinked access to scientific data on 45 herbs. HerbMedPro is an enhanced version of the site with information on 128 herbs with continuous updates available with a subscription.

8. CONCLUSION

When reviewing the historical data and contemporary research, it is clear that plants have played a role in easing the suffering of humankind and assisted researchers in their understanding of the transmission of pain. Given the vast number of botanicals that have yet to be explored for their medicinal effects, it is likely that plants will continue to contribute to our understanding and management of pain. However, there is much work to be done from "bench to bedside" to determine which are the most efficacious and how they are best used in clinical practice. Although there are many botanical remedies that are purported to be efficacious for specific pain conditions, the research literature reflects only a small percentage of these plant products and there is definitely a need for more rigorous and creative research in this area. Of those botanicals that have been the subject of controlled clinical trials, there is evidence that devil's claw extract, the combination product Phytodolor®, and topical capsaicin preparations are effective for certain pain conditions. There is limited evidence of benefit for a unique cat's claw extract (*U.tomentosa*) in rheumatoid arthritis. While the preliminary research for *T. wilfordii* extract in RA is impressive, it is currently premature to recommend its use given the potentially significant adverse effects and lack of well-characterized extracts in the marketplace. The clinical trial data are contradictory for willow bark extract in the treatment of OA and RA and for boswellia extract in RA. A single trial does not the support the use of dried feverfew leaf in rheumatoid arthritis.

In spite of the lack of rigorous research for many botanicals, it is highly likely that many patients will continue to seek out these therapies as a means of self-treatment and a way to maintain additional life control *(72)*. Healthcare providers must be able to dialogue with patients about a wide variety of treatment options, including those that fall outside what was learned during their formal training. Clinicians who face the challenge of working with people living with chronic pain are keenly aware that treatments must often be tailored to individual patients and that there is often not a simple answer.

REFERENCES

1. Eisenberg DM, Davis RB, Ettner SL, et al. Trends in alternative medicine use in the United States, 1990–1997: results of a follow-up national survey. JAMA 1998;280:1569–1575.
2. Tindle HA, Davis RB, Phillips RS, Eisenberg DM. Trends in use of complementary and alternative medicine by US adults: 1997–2002. Altern Ther Health Med 2005;11(1):42–49.
3. Quandt SA, Chen H, Grzywacz JG, Bell RA, Lang W, Arcury TA. Use of complementary and alternative medicine by persons with arthritis: results of the National Health Interview Survey. Arthritis Rheum 2005;53(5):748–755.
4. Tsao JC, Zeltzer LK. Complementary and alternative medicine approaches for pediatric pain: a review of the state-of-the-science. Evid Based Complement Alternat Med 2005;2(2):149–159.
5. Foltz V, St Pierre Y, Rozenberg S, et al. Use of complementary and alternative therapies by patients with self-reported chronic back pain: a nationwide survey in Canada. Joint Bone Spine 2005;72(6):571–577.
6. Ernst E. Musculoskeletal conditions and complementary/alternative medicine. Best Pract Res Clin Rheumatol. 2004;18(4):539–556.
7. Schauss AG, Milholland RBR, Munson SE. Indian frankincense (Boswellia serrata) gum resin extract: a review of therapeutic applicatiosn and toxicology. Nat Med J 1999:February:16–20.
8. Schweizer S, von Brocke AF, Boden SE, Bayer E, Ammon HP, Safayhi H. Workup-dependent formation of 5-lipoxygenase inhibitory boswellic acid analogues. J Nat Prod 2000;63(8):1058–1061.
9. Gerhardt H, Seifert F, Buvari P, Vogelsang H, Repges R. Therapy of active Crohn disease with *Boswellia serrata* extract H 15. Z Gastroenterol. 2001;39(1):11–17.
10. Gupta I, Gupta V, Parihar A, et al. Effects of Boswellia serrata gum resin in patients with bronchial asthma: results of a double-blind, placebo-controlled, 6-week clinical study. Eur J Med Res 1998;3(11):511–514.
11. Kimmatkar N, Thawani V, Hingorani L, Khiyani R. Efficacy and tolerability of *Boswellia serrata* extract in treatment of osteoarthritis of knee—a randomized double blind placebo controlled trial. Phytomedicine 2003;10(1):3–7.
12. Etzel R. Special extract of *Boswellia serrata* (H 15) in the treatment of rheumatoid arthritis. Phytomedicine 1996;3:91–94.
13. Sander O, Herborn G, Rau R. Is H15 (resin extract of *Boswellia serrata*, "incense") a useful supplement to established drug therapy of chronic polyarthritis? Results of a double-blind pilot study. Z Rheumatol 1998;57(1):11–16.
14. Chopra A, Lavin P, Patwardhan B, Chitre D. Randomized double blind trial of an ayurvedic plant derived formulation for treatment of rheumatoid arthritis. J Rheumatol 2000; 27:1365–1372.
15. Sasamura T, Kuraishi Y. Peripheral and central actions of capsaicin and VR1 receptor. Jpn J Pharmacol 1999;80(4):275–280.
16. Mason L, Moore RA, Derry S, Edwards JE, McQuay HJ. Systematic review of topical capsaicin for the treatment of chronic pain. BMJ 2004;328(7446):991.
17. Heitzman ME, Neto CC, Winiarz E, Vaisberg AJ, Hammond GB. Ethnobotany, phytochemistry and pharmacology of Uncaria (Rubiaceae). Phytochemistry 2005;66(1):5–29.
18. Mur E, Hartig F, Eibl G, Schirmer M. Randomized double blind trial of an extract from the pentacyclic alkaloid-chemotype of *Uncaria tomentosa* for the treatment of rheumatoid arthritis. J Rheumatol 2002;29:678–681.
19. Piscoya J, Rodriguez Z, Bustamante SA, Okuhama NN, Miller MJ, Sandoval M. Efficacy and safety of freeze-dried cat's claw in osteoarthritis of the knee: mechanisms of action of the species *Uncaria guianensis*. Inflamm Res 2001;50(9):442–448.

20. Sandoval M, Okuhama NN, Zhang XJ, et al. Anti-inflammatory and antioxidant activities of cat's claw (*Uncaria tomentosa* and *Uncaria guianensis*) are independent of their alkaloid content. Phytomedicine 2002;9:325–337.

21. Aguilar P, Rojas A, Marcelo A, et al. Anti-inflammatory activity of two different extracts of *Uncaria tomentosa* (Rubiaceae). J Ethnopharmacol 2002;81:271–276.

22. Valerio LG, Jr., Gonzales GF. Toxicological aspects of the South American herbs cat's claw (*Uncaria tomentosa*) and Maca (*Lepidium meyenii*) : a critical synopsis. Toxicol Rev 2005;24(1):11–35.

23. Blumenthal M, Busse WR, Goldberg A, et al., Eds. 1998. The Complete German Commission E Monographs: Therapeutic Guide to Herbal Medicines. Austin: American Botanical Council and Boston: Integrative Medicine Communications.

24. Lanhers MC, Fleurentin J, Mortier F, Vinche A, Younos C. Antiinflammatory and analgesic effects of an aqueous extract of *Harpagophytum procumbens*. Plant Med 1992;58:117–123.

25. Loew D, Möllerfeld J, Schrödter A, Puttkammer S, Kaszin M. Investigations on the pharmacokinetic properties of *Harpagophytum* extracts and their effects on eicosanoid biosynthesis in vitro and ex vivo. Clin Pharmacol Ther 2001;69:356–364.

26. Gagnier JJ, Chrubasik S, Manheimer E. *Harpgophytum procumbens* for osteoarthritis and low back pain: a systematic review. BMC Complement Altern Med 2004;4:13.

27. VanTulder MW, Assendelft WJ, Koes BW, Bouter LM. Method guidelines for systematic reviews in the Cochrane Collaboration Back Review Group for Spinal Disorders. Spine 1997;22: 2323–2330.

28. European Scientific Cooperative on Phytotherapy (ESCOP). 1996. Harpagophyti radix: Devil's claw. Monographs on the Medicinal Uses of Plant Drugs. Fascile 2. Exeter, UK: European Scientific Cooperative on Phytotherapy.

29. Heck AM, DeWitt BA, Lukes AL. Potential interactions between alternative therapies and warfarin. Am J Health Syst Pharm 2000;57(13):1221–1227.

30. Pittler MH, Ernst E. Feverfew for preventing migraine. Cochrane Database Syst Rev 2004;(1):CD002286.

31. Diener HC, Pfaffenrath V, Schnitker J, Friede M, Henneicke-von Zepelin HH. Efficacy and safety of 6.25 mg t.i.d. feverfew CO2-extract (MIG-99) in migraine prevention—a randomized, double-blind, multicentre, placebo-controlled study. Cephalalgia 2005;25(11):1031–1041.

32. Pfaffenrath V, Diener H, Fischer M, et al. The efficacy and safety of *Tanacetum parthenium* (feverfew) in migraine prophylaxis—a double-blind, multicentre, randomized, placebo-controlled dose–response study. Cephalalgia 2002;22:523–532.

33. Pattrick M, Heptinstall S, Doherty M. Feverfew in rheumatoid arthritis: a double-blind; placebo controlled study. Ann Rheum Dis 1989;48:547–549.

34. Johnson ES, Kadam NP, Hylands DM, Hylands PJ. Efficacy of feverfew as a prophylactic treatment of migraine. BMJ 1985;291(6495):569–573.

35. Bradley PR. 1992. British Herbal Compendium Vol. 1. Dorset: British Herbal Medicine Association.

36. Newall CA, Anderson LA, Phillipson JD. 1996. Herbal Medicines: A Guide for Health-Care Professionals. London: The Pharmaceutical Press.

37. Chrubasik S, Pittler MH, Roufogalis BD. *Zingiberis rhizoma*: a comprehensive review on the ginger effect and efficacy profiles. Phytomedicine 2005;12(9):684–701.

38. Bliddal H, Rosetzsky A, Schlichting P, et al. A randomized, placebo-controlled, cross-over study of ginger extracts and ibuprofen in osteoarthritis. Osteoarthritis Cartilage 2000;8:9–12.

39. Altman RD, Marcussen KC. Effects of a ginger extract on knee pain in patients with osteoarthritis. Arthritis Rheum 2001;44:2531–2538.

40. Wigler I, Grotto I, Caspi D, Yaron M. The effects of Zintona EC (a ginger extract) on symptomatic gonarthritis. Osteoarthritis Cartilage 2003; 11:783–789.

41. United States Pharmacopoeia/Drug Information. 1998. Botanical monograph series: Ginger. Rockville, MD: The United States Pharmacopoeial Convention, Inc.

42. Wilkinson JM. Effect of ginger tea on the fetal development of Sprague-Dawley rats. Reprod Toxicol 2000;14:507–512.

43. Weidner MS, Sigwart K. Investigation of the teratogenic potential of a *Zingiber officinale* extract in the rat. Reprod Toxicol 2001;15:75–80.

44. Portnoi G, Chng LA, Karimi-Tabesh L, Koren G, Tan MP, Einarson A. Prospective comparative study of the safety and effectiveness of ginger for the treatment of nausea and vomiting in pregnancy. Am J Obstet Gynecol 2003;189:1374–1377.

45. Borrelli F, Capasso R, Aviello G, Pittler M, Izzo AA. Effectiveness and safety of ginger in the treatment of pregnancy-induced nausea and vomiting. Obstet Gynecol 2005;105(4):849–856

46. Ernst E. The efficacy of Phytodolor® for the treatment of musculoskeletal pain—a systematic review of randomized clinical trials. Nat Med J 1999;2:14–17.

47. Linde K, Berner M, Egger M, et al. St John's wort for depression—meta-analysis of randomised controlled trials. Br J Psychiatry 2005;186:99–107.

48. Linde K, Mulrow CD. 2001. St. John's Wort for depression (Cochrane Review). In The Cochrane Library, Issue 1. Oxford: Update Software. This update was made on July, 9, 1998.

49. Woelk H, Burkard G, Gruenwald J. 1994. Benefits and risks of the *Hypericum* extract LI 160: drug monitoring with 3250 patients. J Geriatr Psychiatry Neurol 1994;7(suppl 1):534–538.

50. Brockmoller J, et al. Hypericin and pseudohypericin: pharmacokinetics and effects of photosensitivity in humans. Pharmacopsychiatry 1997;30(Suppl 2):94–101.

51. Mannel M. Drug interactions with St John's wort : mechanisms and clinical implications. Drug Saf 2004;27(11):773–797.

52. Findling RL, McNamara NK, O'Riordan MA, et al. An open-label pilot study of St. John's wort in juvenile depression. J Am Acad Child Adolesc Psychiatry 2003;42(8):908–914.

53. Hubner WD, Kirste T. Experience with St John's Wort (*Hypericum perforatum*) in children under 12 years with symptoms of depression and psychovegetative disturbances. Phytother Res 2001;15(4):367–370.

54. Tao X, Cush JJ, Garret M, Lipsky, PE. A phase I study of ethyl acetate extract of the chinese antirheumatic herb *Tripterygium wilfordii* Hook F in rheumatoid arthritis. J Rheumatol 2001;28:2160–2167.

55. Tao X, Younger J, Fan FZ, Wang B, Lipsky PE. Benefit of an extract of Tripterygium wilfordii Hook F in patients with rheumatoid arthritis a double-blind, placebo-controlled study, Arthritis Rheum 2002;46:1735–1743.

56. Wu YJ, Lao ZY, Zhang ZL. Clinical observation on small doses *Tripterygium wilfordii* polyglycoside combined with methotrexate in treating rheumatoid arthritis (In Chinese). Zhongguo Zhing Xi Yi Jie He Za Zhi 2001;21:895–889.

57. Setty AR, Sigal LH. Herbal medications commonly used in the practice of rheumatology: mechanisms of action, efficacy, and side effects. Semin Arthritis Rheum 2005;34(6):773–784.

58. Lopez LM, Grimes DA, Schulz KF. Nonhormonal drugs for contraception in men: a systematic review. Obstet Gynecol Surv 2005;60(11):746–745.

59. Gu CX. Cause of amenorrhea after treatment with *Tripterygium wilfordii*. Zhongguo Yi Xue Ke Xue Yuan Xue Bao. 1989;11(2):151–153 (Article in Chinese).

60. Huang L, Feng S, Wang H. Decreased bone mineral density in patients with systemic lupus erythematosus after long-term administration of *Tripterygium wilfordii* Hook, F. Chin Med J 2000;113:159–161.

61. Stevinson C, Ernst E. Valerian for insomnia: a systematic review of randomized clinical trials. Sleep Med 2000;1:91–99.

62. Blumenthal M. The ABC clinical guide to herbs. Am Bot Council Austin, TX 2003;351–64.

63. Kuhlmann J, Berger W, Podzuweit H, et al. The influence of valerian treatment on "reaction time, alertness and concentration" in volunteers. Pharmacopsychiatry (Germany), 1999;32(6): 235–241.

64. Schmid B, Ludtke R, Selbmann HK, et al., Efficacy and tolerability of a standardized willow bark extract in patients with osteoarthritis randomized placebo-controlled, double blind clinical trial. Phytother Res 2001;15:344–335.

65. European Scientific Cooperative on Phytotherapy. Salicis cortex. Exeter, UK: ESCOP; 1996–1997:2. Monographs on the Medicinal Uses of Plant Drugs, Fascicule 4. European Pharmacopoeia. 2004. Devil's Claw Root Chapter 4.3;2997.

66. Chrubasik S, Eisenberg E, Balan E ,et al. Treatment of low back pain exacerbations with willow bark extract a randomized double-blind study. Am J Med 2000;109:9–14.

67. Chrubasik S, Kunzel O, Model A, et al., Treatment of low back pain with a herbal or synthetic anti-rheumatic a randomized controlled study. Willow bark extract for low back pain. Rheumatology 2001;40:1388–1393.

68. Biegert C, Wagner I, Ludkte R, et al. Efficacy and safety of willow bark extract in the treatment of osteoarthritis and rheumatoid arthritis: results of 2 randomized double-blind controlled trials. J Rheumatol 2004;31(11):2121–2130.

69. Krivoy N, Pavlotzky E, Chrubasik S, Eisenberg E, Brook G. Effect of salicis cortex extract on human platelet aggregation. Planta Med 2001; 67:209–212.

70. Low Dog T. 2004. Clinical Trial Reviewer's Guidance and Checklist. In The Handbook of Clinically Tested Herbal Remedies. Volume 1. Barrett M, Ed. New York: The Haworth Herbal Press.

71. Kaufman DW, Kelly JP, Rosenberg L, et al. Recent patterns of medication use in the ambulatory adult population of the United States: the Slone survey. JAMA 2002;287(3):337–344.

72. Dillard JN, Knapp S. Complementary and alternative pain therapy in the emergency department. Emerg Med Clin North Am 2005;23(2):529–549.

21 Chinese Herbal Medicine for Pain

David Euler

CONTENTS

Summary

The rising cost of treating chronic pain is a significant public health problem, and given the aging of our population, one that will continue to grow. Unfortunately, many of the conventional medical interventions that we have to treat pain are better designed to deal with acute pain conditions. As a result, there is an expanding interest by patients in the use of complementary and alternative medicine (CAM) treatments for pain. Recent national surveys indicate that more and more patients are paying out of pocket for CAM treatments and the most common reason for seeking these treatments is persistent pain. Unfortunately, little is known about the appropriate care for patients with chronic pain using any type of treatment, whether with CAM or conventional options. As a result, patients are frequently treated symptomatically with medications that can be addictive in nature and procedures that often are not proven to be effective, all of which can cause a barrage of unwanted side effects. It is in this pain management setting that the growing research that is developing in Chinese herbal treatments among other CAM therapies can provide a perfect counterbalance to conventional approaches to help reintroduce a model of care that is more process oriented and helps move the patient from passive therapies to a more active role in their self-care.

Key Words: traditional chinese medicine, herbal medicine, alternative medicine, botanicals, Ayurvedic medicine

1. INTRODUCTION

Herbal medicine is the use of various parts of plants for medicinal purposes. Since the beginning of history all indigenous cultures in the world have used natural substances (especially plants and animal parts) to promote healing and alleviate pain. In the modern Western clinic, the most common approaches in herbal medicine include Western

From: *Contemporary Pain Medicine: Integrative Pain Medicine: The Science and Practice
of Complementary and Alternative Medicine in Pain Management*
Edited by: J. F. Audette and A. Bailey © Humana Press, Totowa, NJ

herbal approaches, traditional Chinese herbal formulas and Ayurvedic medicine (traditional medicine from India). This article will emphasize the Western and Chinese approaches.

The main difference in the various approaches to herbal medicine, besides the terminology used, lies in the differential diagnosis and the clinical strategies for prescribing specific herbs. While in the Western approach the strategy for prescribing herbs is more symptom-oriented and leans toward single herbs for specific alignments, the Ayurvedic and traditional Chinese approaches rely on prescribing herbal combinations (formulas) for syndromes that are individualized for the different types of patients. An herbal pain treatment for a "hot patient" that presents with a red face, feeling warm, and elevated blood pressure would be quite different than that used for a "cold patient," who might present with a pale face and body, feeling cold, and the tendency for low blood pressure. This unique difference between approaches can be bridged in clinical practice by using the best of both worlds. For example, if a patient complains of coughing and wheezing with copious thick yellow sputum, and labored breathing, and is found to have a greasy yellow tongue coat, slippery rapid pulse, with fever and chills, one can recommend a Western herbal combination such as inhalations of the essential oils from eucalyptus (bronchodilator) and pine (expectorant) together with a traditional Chinese herbal formula Ding-Chuan-Tang *(1)*, which acts according to Chinese theory to expand Lung & push down rebellious Lung Qi, arrest wheezing, clear Heat, and transform Phlegm. In this example the Chinese formula addresses not only the symptomatic presentation, but also the constitution of the patient.

In this chapter, we will outline the basic theory of Chinese medicine to help motivate a better understanding of the formulation of a differential diagnoses and prescription for pain in Chinese herbal medicine. We will then give case examples for particular pain conditions and end by discussing safety issues and methods of integrating Chinese herbal medicine into a pain clinic.

2. HISTORY

The written history of Chinese materia medica dates back from the Eastern Han dynasty of China (AD 25–220), with the *Shen Nong Ben Cao Jing* (*Divine Husbandman's Classic of the Materia Medica*). This book is also known as *The Canon of Materia Medica,* or *Shen-nong's Herbal Classics*. The book contains 365 entries, one for each day of the year. The entries include botanical (252 entries), zoological (67 entries), and mineral (45 entries) substances. The herbal literature developed by continuous addition of new drugs, together with a re-evaluation and addition of new uses for existing drugs in subsequent dynasties. The Xin Xiu Ben Cao (*Newly Revised Materia Medica,* AD 659) was the first official book compiled and issued by the government, and much later the classic *Ben Cao Gang Mu* (*Compendium of Materia Medica,* 1596) was written by Li Shi Zhen. This tradition has continued up to the present day, with the publication in 1977 of Zhong Yao Da Ci Dian (*Encyclopedia of Traditional Chinese Medicinal Substances*). It contains 5,767 entries, with 4,773 substances from plants, 740 from animals, 82 from minerals, and 172 products made from these sources *(2)*.

3. TRADITIONAL CHINESE MEDICINE THEORY

As one can see from the example mentioned in the introduction, the differential diagnosis needed to prescribe a traditional Chinese herbal formula is complex and requires further exploration of whether certain conditions exist in the patient that go beyond the symptoms of cough and wheezing (e.g., greasy yellow tongue coat, slippery rapid pulse), in order for the practitioner to make the decision to use this specific formula.

It is often the case that there will be a multitude of traditional Chinese herbal formulas for one specific Western medical condition. The choice of which formula to use depends on a variety of factors that are often discounted in Western medicine, such as the constitution of the patient and other subtle symptomatic presentations and complaints that help to contribute to the differential diagnosis. When reading the indications for Chinese herbal formulas, it quickly becomes apparent that the language used for the differential diagnosis differs from that used in modern Western, allopathic medicine: for example, whether a patient is hot or cold, damp or dry, or whether the symptoms reside mainly in the upper body or lower body, can all matter with this herbal approach.

In traditional Chinese medicine (TCM), the patient is evaluated through a set of questions to help develop an individualized diagnosis:

1. Did the condition originate primarily from the inside or outside of the body?
2. Where is the major symptomatic presentation (upper or lower body)?
3. What is the patient's individual response to the pathogenic factor (i.e., do they have fever, chills, cold, dampness, etc.)?
4. What is the nature of the syndrome (wind, heat, cold, damp, dryness, fire, etc.)?

The different words used to describe the collection of symptoms that make up a syndrome are heavily borrowed from the natural world, such as would be used to describe the weather. Such Chinese medical descriptions include concepts of wind, dampness, dryness, heat, and cold. The parallel use of words to describe human health and external natural phenomenon such as the weather speaks to a core philosophical premise of TCM, namely, that there is an inter-relatedness of human health and disease with the world around us. Although sometimes intuitive, correct application of these descriptions can get quite complex when several conditions or a more complicated and/or multi-system problem appears in one patient.

To better understand how Chinese herbs are used for the management of pain, one has to learn some of the basic theories of TCM. In contrast to Western allopathic medicine, where the symptomatic presentation of pain is often treated via a medication or a procedure, TCM (acupuncture and Chinese herbal formulas) treats the individual by focusing on the root cause of why the patient cannot heal. TCM is tailored to the individual and not necessarily the disease.

3.1. Qi

One of the most important concepts in TCM is the concept of Qi (Chee). Qi has been loosely translated into English as vital energy; however, this does not really do justice to the term, given that Qi can imbue both animate and inanimate objects. It is a force that allows for movement, growth, warmth, and development in the body and the universe. In good health, Qi flows freely through the meridian system. An obstruction in the flow of Qi can lead to the manifestation of disease and pain. According to traditional Chinese medicine, acupuncture points are used to bring the body back into a state of equilibrium by balancing the flow of Qi in the meridian system and through the organs. There are 14 major meridians in the body; these meridians can be understood as virtual lines along the body's surface on which acupuncture points are found.

3.2. Yin and Yang

The concept of Yin and Yang is a unique binary understanding of opposites that is used for differential diagnosis and treatment strategy planning. All existing phenomena can be described, explained and further divided into the Yin–Yang concept. The basic properties of heat, brightness, activity, moving outward, moving upward, and hyper-function belong to the concept of Yang. The basic properties of coldness, darkness, stillness, moving inward, moving downward, and hypo-function belong to the concept of Yin. Yin and Yang oppose each other and at the same time have an interdependent relationship. Physically, the upper parts of the body, the exterior and dorsal aspects of the body are all considered as Yang. The lower parts of the body, the interior and ventral aspects of the body are all Yin. Physiologically, Yin can be viewed as cholinergic, parasympathetic, as well as the solid aspect of the body, while Yang can be viewed as adrenergic, sympathetic, as well as the functional aspect of the organism.

3.3. Blood

Oriental medicine views Blood as a fluid manifestation of Qi. The Spleen and Stomach are considered the primary sources of Qi and Blood, as they are the starting point of the transformation process that turns food and water intake into Blood. After the stomach receives the food, the Spleen extracts the Qi from the food and sends it upward to the Lung where it mixes with the Qi from the air and is then sent to the Kidney to be mixed with the Jing (Jing is a term used in traditional Chinese medicine to describe the genetic potential of an individual) and the body's primary Qi to produce the end result: Blood. Blood circulates throughout the body from the five Zang and six Fu organ system in the interior to the skin, muscle, tendons, and bone at the exterior level. It is Blood that nourishes and moistens those organs and tissues. Blood is also viewed as the material foundation of mental activity.

3.4. The Organ System

In traditional Chinese medicine, the organ system is organized somewhat differently than in Western bio-medical systems. Each organ is considered a concept or a system that is in charge of specific physiological functions and corresponds to a variety of aspects of the body. The Zang organs are "solid" and are Yin in nature, the Fu organs are hollow and considered Yang in nature. Organ concepts according to traditional Chinese medicine are written with a capital letter (such as Spleen, Triple Warmer, Heart, etc.); organs and functions according to Western understanding and terminology are written in lowercase. Tables 1 and 2 provide an overview of the correlations between the Zang-Fu organs, their main functions, area of control, and diagnostic meaning. The extraordinary organs do not actually fall under the Zang-Fu organ system and have functions outside the scope of this monograph. They are Brain, Marrow, Bones, Blood Vessels, and Uterus.

Table 1
The Five Zang Organs

Zang (yin) organ	Related Fu (yang) organ	Main function	Opens into—	Manifests on—	Related function
Liver	Gallbladder	Maintaining potency and free flow of Qi	Eyes	Nails	Controls tendons, stores the blood
Heart	Small Intestine	Dominates the vessels	Tongue	Face	Houses the Mind, controls blood vessels
Spleen	Stomach	Governs digestion and assimilation	Mouth	Lips	Muscles of the four limbs and the muscles
Lungs	Large Intestine	Circulates Qi and controls respiration	Nose	Body hair and skin	Dominates water dispersing, descending, water passages, hair, skin, and pores
Kidney	Urinary Bladder	Stores essence, regulates development and reproduction	Ear	Head hair	Dominates water metabolism, bone, teeth and the anterior and posterior orifices; manufactures marrow

3.5. Pathogenic Causes of Disease

The main categories for the differential diagnosis of a clinical presentation are called *pathogenic factors*. These borrow their metaphors from nature and describe the manner in which a disease invades the body as well as the way it manifests in the individual patient. The actual symptomatic presentation of a disease is the interaction between

Table 2
The Six Fu Organs

Fu (Yang) organ	Related Zang organ	Main function
Gallbladder	Liver	Storing bile
Small intestine	Heart	Separates the pure from the turbid
Stomach	Spleen	Receives and decomposes food
Large Intestine	Lung	Receives waste material sent down from the small intestine, absorb its fluid content, and form the remainder into feces for excretion
Urinary bladder	Kidney	Temporary storage of urine
San-Jiao*	Pericardium	Governs various forms of Qi and assists in the passage of Yuan Qi and body fluid

*This organ system (also called "Triple Warmer") comprises functions without any form. The Triple Warmer also refers to the division of the body into three sections: upper section (chest), middle section (epigastric region to umbilicus), and lower section (pelvic organs).

Table 3
Summary of Potential Pathological Factors

Six external factors	The seven emotions	Miscellaneous Factors
Wind	Joy	Improper diet
Cold	Anger	Over strain
Summer-heat	Worry	Stress
Dampness	Pensiveness	Lack of exercise
Dryness	Sadness	Excessive sexual activity
Fire	Fear	Phlegm retention
	Shock	Blood stasis

the individual's constitution and the pathogenic factor (see Table 3). Understanding these categories helps devise an herbal and/or acupuncture treatment.

3.5.1. WIND

Wind is a primary pathogenic factor as well as a carrier of other pathogens into the body as it invades. Because of its Yang nature, it tends to attack the posterior aspect and outer surfaces of the body first. However, it may quickly penetrate more deeply and progress into serious diseases if it is not expelled when it first attacks. Diseases caused by Wind are usually associated with external conditions, i.e., colds and flu, intermittent symptoms, and migrating symptoms, such as rheumatic arthritis, or abdominal pain that moves from one location to another. Wind diseases are usually rapid in onset; however, Wind can linger in the body for long periods of time and progress if it was undiagnosed or treated improperly. Wind can carry Heat, Cold, and Dampness. Wind-Heat is a syndrome associated with an external pathogen. This is another way of saying the patient has a virus, like the common cold, or most commonly a bacterial infection. Wind-Cold is also an external pathogen, but in modern Western terms is more likely to be a viral attack. Generally speaking, it is not common for bacterial infections from an external influence to cause diseases of a cold nature. The patient with Wind-Cold will have predominant chills, a milder fever than seen with Wind-Heat that is associated with a strong headache and body aches. Wind-Cold is differentiated from Wind-Heat by the patient's longing for hot drinks and warm covers. Wind-Damp is usually represented by arthritic disorders because the Wind combines with Dampness and it settles in the joints. Arthritis disorders are then further differentiated between Wind-Damp, Wind-Damp-Cold, and Wind-Damp-Heat. Wind can be external as well as internal in origin. Internal Wind may be internally generated from a deficiency of Yin and/or Blood, or excessive Fire in the body. A few examples of internally generated Wind are epilepsy, convulsions, abnormal eye movements such as nystagmus, hypertension, tremor, or fitful movements.

3.5.2. COLD

Cold is a Yin pathogenic factor. If overly predominant, coldness can injure Yang, as Yang is hot and moving in nature; therefore, too much coldness can slow down the body's metabolic rate, create stagnation and pain as well as fatigue and an actual feeling of coldness. Coldness can be generated from an external influence, such as exposure to excessively cold conditions, or from an internal influence, such as eating or drinking too many cold (and raw) substances. Conversely, an excessive amount of Cold can accumulate from a deficient amount of Qi and Yang in the body.

3.5.3. HEAT

Heat is a Yang pathogenic factor. If overly predominant, Heat can injure Yin and cause dryness, inflammation, and pain. As Yin is lubricating and cooling in nature, deficiency of Yin ("Empty Heat") can stem from chronic disease, medications (and/or radiation), improper nutrition, too much processed sugar, and lack of hydration.

3.5.4. DAMPNESS

Dampness is heavy and turbid in nature. It therefore creates a blockage of energy wherever it settles in the body. This kind of blockage creates a heavy sensation. It may be a sensation of denseness, dullness, aching, or even numbness. Dampness may also create the turbid fluids in, or discharged from, the body; for example, excessive phlegm, discharge from the eyes, edema, mucous in the stools, or oozing infections. These discharges will often have a heavy, foul odor. The patient with this pathogen will feel sluggish, and if the digestion is affected, abdominal distention and bloating will occur.

3.5.5. DRYNESS

Dryness consumes body fluids. This condition may be contracted by external forces (if accompanied by Wind) but is more commonly seen as a result of a deficiency of fluids in the body due to chronic diseases, inflammation and dehydration. Conditions that may be associated with excess Dryness include vascular disease, burning pain, wounds, and sores. Heat may come from dryness and include chapped lips, dry skin, dry hair, excessive thirst, dry eyes, and dry cough.

3.5.6. FIRE

Fire is a Yang pathogenic factor often contracted in summer or as a result of being exposed to heat and dryness. Fire may also be generated from a longer-term pathological condition known as Yin deficiency if left untreated. In the latter case, it may affect the blood and create serious illness. Fire tends to flare up and cause symptoms that tend to appear in the upper portion of the body, usually with complaints of high fever, mouth ulceration or swellings, and in severe cases even, coma. If it is left untreated long enough, the condition tends to effect the blood and may cause bleeding anywhere in the body, including the lower parts of the body.

3.5.7. EMOTIONS

Emotions may have an effect on the corresponding organs, or, conversely, may be an expression of the disease in an organ system. The concept of emotional factors causing illness is common to both Western and Eastern traditions, but in Chinese medicine, emotionally based diseases are not considered less real when compared to the organ-based pathology that we tend to focus on in the West. Clinically it is interesting to see that most patients' dominant emotion corresponds to the organ that is unbalanced (see Table 4). Generally speaking, the more severe the organ pathology or imbalance, the more expressive or strong the correspondent emotion may be.

4. CHINESE HERBAL FORMULAS

The unique approach and genius of TCM herbal formulas is that the formulation combines a number of herbs that work synergistically with one another, in an attempt to both address all the various symptoms and signs that present within the constitutional complex of the patient and protect the patient from possible side effects. This is a complicated mission that requires a very thorough differential diagnosis. Thankfully, there are a few "shortcuts" made possible through herbal companies that work with the clinician to achieve this goal (a list of reputable herbal companies with their contact numbers is provided at the end of this article), as well as computer programs that help the clinician to find the exact herbal formula for the individual patient. Ready manufactured formulas (patent formulas) in the form of pills, powders and tinctures that are organized according to the main complaint (low back pain, for example) as well as the accompanying syndrome (heat and dampness with a rapid pulse and scanty urination) are also designed to help the clinician find the correct formula. These finished products also make it possible for the patient to take the herbs without the need to cook and prepare them, a process that might take an hour or more.

Usually Chinese herbal formulas should be taken for 4–12 weeks (depending on the complexity of the syndrome) before the patient is reevaluated. The goal is to improve or modify the constitutional nature of the patient with the herbal formula and thus the attempt is to heal from the inside out. Often the patient will feel symptomatic relief in a shorter time.

4.1. Herbal Treatment of Low Back Pain

The following is an example that might shed some light on the differential diagnosis and the different prescriptions given to patients that present complaining of the same medical problem (lower back pain) but who have in essence very different constitutions that require substantially different herbal formulas.

Three patients come to the clinic complaining of chronic lower back pain (LBP) associated with mild degenerative disc disorder and tight paravertebral muscles but no damage to the facet joints, disk protrusion, or stenosis. All three patients have tried non-steroidal anti-inflammatory drugs without significant relief.

The first patient was given an herbal formula Qiang Huo Sheng Shi Tang (Notopterygium & Tuhuo combination) to expel pathogenic wind and dampness in the upper body. In this case the complaint of LBP was associated with symptoms of a heavy and painful feeling in the head, difficulties rotating or bending the trunk, and a mild fever with a floating pulse and a white coating on the tongue.

The second patient was given Du Huo Ji Shen Tang (meridian circulation pills) to tonify the Liver, Qi and Blood as well as expel Wind and Dampness from the lower body. This patient complained of heavy and painful sensations at fixed locations in the lower back and lower extremities with weakness and stiffness, aversion to cold, palpitations, shortness of breath, and presented with a pale tongue with a white coating, and a thin, weak and slow pulse.

The third patient was given Jia Wei Er Miao San (Augmented Two Marvel Powder) to clear Damp-Heat. This patient also complained that rainy or hot weather and warm compresses made the pain worse and that he was thirsty all the time. He presented with heat at the painful area, a yellow coating on the tongue, rapid pulse, and a red face.

4.2. Herbal Hierarchy

Chinese herbal formulas are often composed of several herbs that work with each other to strengthen the effect on the main pathology, treat related secondary aspects of the illness, as well as limit each other's action to prevent side effects. For example, if an herbal remedy is supposed to warm the body and promote circulation, it will also contain some cooling and moistening herbs to prevent the formula from becoming too hot and dry, which could create a set of side effects arising from internal heat and dryness (such as bitter taste in the mouth and stomach pain, rapid pulse, and nervousness).

One commonly used template for designing traditional Chinese herbal formulas is based on the monarchical form of government. At the top is the king or emperor. Next are the ministers or deputies. Last are the assistants or adjutants with usually one guide or messenger herb. Any herb can fill any of these roles depending on the desired effect of the entire formula.

The King or Emperor herb is directed toward and has the strongest effect on the most important imbalance or pathology. For example, in the formula Qiang Huo Sheng Shi Tang (Notopterygium & Tuhuo combination) that was given to the first patient with LBP, the herb Qiang Huo (Notopterygium) is the Emperor and its main action is to release or open the exterior and disperse cold (for chills, low-grade fever, headache, and the heavy sensation in the body). This herb also alleviates or disperses difficult, chronic pain conditions that are felt to arise from cold (wind) and dampness, such as chronic shoulder tendinosis. Here the rational was that the patient was not healing due to the existence of cold trapped in the body.

The Minister herb is directed to both the main and secondary imbalance and pathology. In our example this would be Du Huo (Radix angelicae pubescentis), which is warming, dispels wind, resolves dampness and relieves pain.

There are three kinds of assistant herbs:

1. Helpful assistants that strengthens the effect of the King.
2. Corrective assistants that reduces or eliminates the harsh or toxic effects of the King and/or Minister herbs to prevent side effects.
3. Opposing assistants that decrease the effects of the King. This role is mostly used in complex combinations as well as to prevent side effects.

The Guide, Envoy, or Messenger herb focuses the actions of all other herbs on a particular organ, channel, or region of the body, usually where the pathology or imbalance occurs.

4.3. Herbal Strategies for Stagnation

According to traditional Chinese medicine, the factor that is most likely to cause a pain syndrome is stagnation. Several forms of stagnation exist, such as stagnation of Qi, blood, or dampness and phlegm. The differential diagnosis is based on the nature and quality of the pain *(3)*. Qi stagnation is the mildest form of pain and blood stagnation the most severe. Acupuncture and Chinese herbal medicine are geared toward alleviating the stagnation and reducing the pain.

4.3.1. QI STAGNATION

Qi stagnation is often caused by emotional stress, anger, frustration, sloth, or lack of movement. The pain that results from such stagnation can be alleviated, at least briefly, with heat, movement, or rubbing the affected area. Although this type of pain is often chronic, it can be treated with relative ease because the stagnation is still on an energetic level. When emotions are blocked or not correctly channeled, like any form of energy, they will stagnate and cause pathology. When Qi is stagnant in a particular organ (see Table 4) the resulting emotion correlates with the nature and location of the painful condition. For example, Liver Qi stagnation may result in or be caused by excessive anger, and the blocked energy tends to collect and then periodically escape and rise up, resulting in headache. In contrast, the energies that are associated with the emotions of sadness, fear, or excessive worry tend to sink and cause lower back pain (in addition to the symptoms associated to the specific organ where the stagnation has occurred). The herbal formula prescribed should cause movement and warming of Qi as well as address the organ involved.

Another cause of Qi stagnation is the invasion of Cold or Dampness into the acupuncture channels (meridian system), causing a slower flow of Qi and pain. This can happen after an exposure to external cold and dampness or due to excessive consumption of cold foods or foods that are considered to cause dampness in TCM (such as ice cream and other dairy products). This kind of painful condition will also be exacerbated by cold or damp weather; for example, this pattern is typically found in osteoarthritis. A very effective herbal formula for this is called Du Huo Ji Sheng Tang. Also called Meridian Circulation Pills, this formula is used to strengthen or tonify Liver, Kidney, Qi and Blood, and expel Wind and Dampness, especially from the lower limbs. However, this formula is only appropriate if the problem is aggravated by cold or damp weather.

Mechanical injuries (blunt trauma or surgery) can produce Qi stagnation and pain; and if it is not treated immediately, Blood stagnation will occur, causing a more fixed, stabbing pain that is difficult to treat. Prescribing the patient herbal formulas that move Qi after an accident or surgery can prevent Blood stagnation and chronic pain. Beneficial patent herbal formulas (these are ready-made Chinese formulas in the form of pills) for this case are Recovery pills by ITM, Qiang Jin 1 (LI485) by Sun Ten, Tieh Ta Formula (Die Da Wan) by Golden Flower (Seven Forests/ITM , Sun Ten, and Golden Flower, are some of the recommended herbal companies listed at the end of this chapter), and a traditional Chinese formula Da Huo Dan (traditional Chinese herbal formulas are prepared as decoctions, tea, and powder by traditional Chinese herbalists).

Spinal misalignment may cause Qi stagnation. Early massage and hot compresses may be applicable and might help some patients. In other, more severe and chronic

Table 4
Organ-Related Emotions

Emotion	Affected Zang organ	Related Fu organ
Anger	Liver	Gallbladder
Joy (anxiety)	Heart	Small Intestine
Worry & pensiveness (obsessive thinking)	Spleen	Stomach
Sadness (grief & melancholy)	Lungs	Large intestine
Fear, fright & shock	Kidney	Urinary bladder

cases, the person may need to see a good manual physical therapist, chiropractor, or a doctor of Osteopathy. Sometimes Cold that has invaded the meridian system can cause the paraspinal muscles to contract and pull the spine out of alignment. If this condition is prolonged, stagnation of Qi may turn to stagnation of Blood as well as heat and cause severe chronic back pain. Hence the herbal strategy to prevent stagnation of Blood and fixed stabbing pain should be in the form of combinations that move Qi, warm the channels, and expel Cold. Such patented formulas include AC Q Tabs™ and Head Q™ (Feverfew with Chinese aromatics) by Health Concerns, AR125 (Juan Bi 1), PA623 (Shu Jin 2), and MU543 (Jie Jing) by Sun Ten, Tian MA Formula (Zhui feng tou gu wan) by Golden Flower, and Meridian Circulation by Jade pharmacy. Two traditional Chinese formulas can also be considered: The first is Shang Shi Bao Zhen Gao, which eliminates Wind Dampness, warms the meridians, removes stagnation in the muscles (Wind Cold, Dampness) to treat aching muscles, shoulder pain, back pain, traumatic injuries to muscles and/or tendons, neuralgia, rheumatism (acute or chronic), osteoarthritis or rheumatoid arthritis. The other is Da Huo Luo Dan, which promotes smooth circulation of Blood and Qi to relax muscles and tendons, expels Wind and Cold, stops spasm, and relieves pain.

Patients that suffer from Qi deficiency (these patients are pale, tired, often short of breath, and feel cold) frequently also suffer from Qi stagnation. There is not enough Qi to convert food and promote good circulation; this leads to stagnation and chronic pain. This type of patient needs to receive herbal formulas that tonify Qi as well as relieve pain due to Qi stagnation. For example, these patients may suffer from arthritis in the joints, chronic lower back pain, cold back and knees, sciatica, pain in the legs and knees, stiff joints, and difficulty walking. This is also often seen as a sequelae of poliomyelitis, with atrophy in the lower limbs and fatigue (these

Table 5
Differential Diagnosis of Pain

Type of pain	Etiology	Differential diagnosis
Dull, achy, fixed	Stagnation of Qi	Alleviated by warmth and/or movement
Sharp, fixed	Stagnation of Blood & Heat	Worsens with heat and pressure, alleviated with cold, swelling
Sharp, fixed	Stagnation of Blood & Cold	Worsens with cold and pressure, alleviated with heat, swelling
Migrating	Wind	Moves from one area of the body to another
Either sharp or achy, usually fixed, can be migrating	Cold	Worsens with cold application, alleviated with heat
Either sharp or achy can be fixed or migrating	Heat	Worsens with heat application, alleviated with cold
Either sharp or achy, usually fixed, can be migrating	Damp	Swelling, sensation of fullness

patients may also complain of shortness of breath and palpitations). Formulas suited to treat this condition include the patented formulas Tonify Qi and Ease the Muscles, Radio-Support (postradiation pain) by The Three Treasures, and the traditional Chinese formula Du Huo and Loranthus formula (Du Huo Ji Sheng Tang) by Golden Flower.

Wind is usually the primary environmental energy to invade the body, while the other environmental energies (Cold, Heat, and Dampness) are typically carried by this Wind. Wind refers to any unseen pathogenic factor invading the body from outside. However, it also describes the pattern of the complaint it creates. Pain due to Wind comes and goes, it moves around the body just as Wind moves about the earth, affecting one joint and then another. Wind blocks the free flow of Qi, so the pain is achy. When Wind blocks the channels, swelling of the joints may occur as seen in rheumatic diseases. The swelling and redness are also called Dampness and Heat (carried by Wind). The patented formulas used for these conditions include Tian Ma Wan (Gastrodia Teapills) and Guan Jie Yan Wan (Joint Inflammation Teapills) both by Plum Flower Brand. Tian Ma Wan can also be very effective for Bell's palsy. If the arthritic pain becomes more severe in cold weather the main objective is to dispel wind and Cold with patented formulas such as Mobility 3™ by Health Concerns.

4.3.2. BLOOD STAGNATION

If the condition called stagnation of Qi is not treated or is not treated correctly, it may lead to a more serious condition called "stagnation of Blood" (Blood stasis). What was a dull ache that radiates outward from the central location can become a very sharp, more disabling, fixed pain.

The most common cause of Blood stagnation is as a result of local trauma that can occur with surgery, lifting too much weight, or a sport's injury. Any specific trauma such as a "sprain and strain" or "pulled muscle" will give rise to Blood stagnation. The treatment principle is the same as Qi stagnation; once the Blood and Qi move, the pain will stop.

In more severe or chronic cases, where the pain syndrome was not addressed correctly, it is necessary to use formulas that dispel the Blood stasis. Blood stasis is more palpable and visible than is Qi stagnation and in Western terms it is manifest by the local inflammation, bruising, and purple, thick blood that can be found at the site of the trauma. The usual formula used for back pain due to a pulled muscle, for example, is called Huo Luo Xiao Ling Dan (Fantastically Effective Pill to Invigorate the Collaterals) modified slightly for back pain.

When lower pack pain is due to chronic Blood stagnation the herbal formula should strengthen or tonify the Kidneys as well as move Blood. Such a remedy is "Kidney Mansion" (Shen Fu Zhu Yu Tang by Blue Poppy Enterprises; see Resources at end of chapter). This formula is for the treatment of chronic low back pain due to a combination of the following:

1. Kidney deficiency: The signs and symptoms associated with Kidney deficiency include low back pain (soreness and weakness), knee pain, advanced age, frequent urination dizziness, hearing problems, as well as tinnitus. Not all of the signs and symptoms must exist in order to diagnose this condition.
2. Blood stagnation: The signs and symptoms associated with Blood stagnation include a fixed and localized pain, enduring pain, pain that is worse at night, pain that is worse

with pressure, varicose veins, dark facial complexion, purple lips, and nails. Not all of the signs and symptoms must exist in order to diagnose this condition
3. Lingering Wind Dampness factors
4. It may also be used to treat postmenopausal osteoporosis.

4.4. Herbal Strategies for Cold and Dampness

When cold settles into the channels, the pain tends to be in a fixed location and is sharp and severe. Cold congeals the flow of blood, thus resulting in blood stasis. Pain due to cold gets worse with cold and feels better with warmth.

Pain due to dampness is usually fixed, sharp, and associated with swelling. Damp Heat is a syndrome associated with more inflammation in the joints as well as Heat signs in the clinical presentation. Damp Cold is associated with swelling and or edema with less inflammation but more signs of Cold in the clinical presentation. In both cases, the herbal formula should remove the dampness and the accompanying factor (Cold, Heat, Wind, etc.).

For example, if a patient presents with fixed pain in the lower back and lower extremities associated with weakness and stiffness as well as an aversion to cold, shortness of breath, palpitations, the herbal formula best suited would be Du Huo Ji Sheng Tang (Tuhuo and Loranthus combination). If used as a patented formula in the form of pills, one may find this formula under the names: "Solitary Hermit Teapills" or "Meridian circulation". This formula tonifies the Liver and Kidney as well as the general state of Qi and Blood but also expels dampness. This formula is designed to concentrate on symptoms at the lower limbs. The Secara Company enhances this formula's effectiveness as a pain reliever and anti-inflammatory by adding Boswellia standardized extract. Clinical trials have demonstrated this phyto-medicine effective in reducing pain and inflammation due to arthritis (see Chapter 20).

If one needs to expel Wind and Dampness from the upper body or upper limbs, the formula Qiang Huo Sheng Shi Tang is recommended (Notopterygium and Tuhuo combination). The herbal company Health Concerns has a modified version of this formula by the name of Head Q™. This variation of the formula is suited to treat and prevent Wind and Damp headaches as well as treat TMJ, neck, shoulder, and upper back pain.

Qiang Sheng Huo Xue Plus by Secara Company is a variation suited to treat repetitive strain disorders and tendonitis as well as trauma to the upper limbs. To enhance this traditional pain relief formula, white willow bark extract has been added, which contains a natural form of salicylic acid, and has been demonstrated effective in human clinical trials at reducing pain and inflammation, without causing digestive distress. Patient symptoms to support use of this formula include heavy and painful head, generalized feeling of heaviness, upper and middle back pain, especially when associated with difficulty rotating the trunk.

A very effective formula for the treatment of Damp Heat is Dang Gui Nian Tong Tang (Dang Gui and Anemarrhea Blue Poppy Enterprises) for joint or muscle pain accompanied by redness, swelling and heat, which is aggravated by warmth and decreased by cold. This formula is for the treatment of Wind-Damp-Heat associated with joint pain and Spleen Qi deficiency. This is a commonly encountered pattern in rheumatoid arthritis, systemic lupus erythamotosus, and dermatomyositis/ polymyositis. It is also a common pattern in fibromyalgia and chronic fatigue immune deficiency syndrome.

Another option for certain presentations of osteoarthritis and rheumatoid arthritis is Bi Tong Ling Tang (Impediment Magic, Blue Poppy Enterprises). This formula is designed for the treatment of chronic, enduring pain due to a combination of Wind-Cold-Damp invasion and Blood stagnation.

The following is a summary of effective traditional Chinese herbal formulas for the treatment of low back pain. This example can serve as a reference as well as a guide for differential diagnosis of any pain syndrome.

Acute Low Back Pain
Cold-Damp—Gan Jiang Ling Zhu Tang + Du Huo Ji Sheng Tang
Damp-Heat—Jia Wei Er Miao San
Wind-Damp—Qiang Huo Sheng Shi Tang
Wind-Cold—Jing Fang Bai Du San
Wind-Heat—Xiao Chai Hu Tang
Blood stagnation—Huo Luo xiao Ling Dan

Chronic Low Back Pain
Liver Qi Stagnation—Tian Tai Wu Yao San
Spleen deficiency—Bu Zhong Yi Qi Tang
Spleen deficiency with Dampness—Ping Wei San
Spleen deficiency with knee pain and sweating—Fang Ji Huang Qi Tang
Spleen Yang deficiency with cold symptoms and edema—Shi Pi Yin
Kidney Yang deficiency—You Gui Wan
Kidney Yin deficiency—Zuo Gui Wan

5. CLINICAL LITERATURE

The scientific literature has a paucity of articles on using Chinese herbal preparations for pain conditions. In one review, a single constituent of many herbal preparations, *Tripterygium wilfordii* (also known as Thunder God Vine), which is believed to have an immunosuppressive effect, was evaluated as a treatment of rheumatoid arthritis (RA). The study authors included only randomized and controlled studies and of the 16 studies found, only two RCTs met the inclusion criteria. Both found that *T. wilfordii* TwHF has beneficial effects on the symptoms of RA. In both of these studies, no toxic or adverse effects other than diarrhea were observed in patients receiving the highest dose. In other studies, the most common side effects of TwHF were vomiting, hair loss, diarrhea, headaches, dryness, abdominal pain, and vaginal spotting. (TwHF) usage can also lead to the development of amenorrhea, which is reversible if present for <2 years in patients <40 years of age but irreversible in perimenopausal women patients *(4)*. However, the association of *T. wilfordii* with adverse events in other studies led the authors of the review to state that the risk–benefit analysis for this herb is unfavorable. Unfortunately, no information is available to better understand whether these adverse side effects could be ameliorated if the herb was used as part of a multi-herb formulation, as would typically be the case in TCM *(5)*. Both treatment groups showed a significant decrease in the number of tender and swollen joints and improvement in the physician's global assessment.

The blood-nourishing and hard-softening (BNHS) capsule is a traditional Chinese patent formula used in the symptomatic treatment of inflammation and pain that contains an extract from Bai Shao (radix paeoniae alba), Qin Jiao (radix gentianae macrophyllae), and Gan Cao (radix glycyrrhizae). A randomized controlled trial of 120 patients compared the efficacy of BNHS with a commonly prescribed Western herbal preparation used in Europe. The intervention was carried out over a period of 4 weeks (6). Primary outcome measures included self-reported pain level, and changes in stiffness and functional ability as measured by the Western Ontario McMaster Universities Osteoarthritis (WOMAC) index. Substantial improvements in disease-specific symptoms were observed, after 4 weeks of treatment, in patients taking BNHS capsules. As assessed by the WOMAC index, the pain level of the BNHS group decreased by 57% (95% confidence interval (CI) = 50, 63), stiffness by 63% (95% CI = 55, 71), and functional ability increased by 56% (95% CI = 50, 63). No significant differences were found in any of the outcome measures between the BNHS group and either of the comparison groups, although the BNHS was substantially cheaper. No severe adverse effects were reported.

Duhuo Jisheng Wan (DJW) means pill of pubescent angelica root and Mulberry mistletoe combination, and it was mentioned in the book *Bei Ji Qian Jing Yao Fang* compiled by *Sun Simiao* in the *Tang* Dynasty (652 AD). It is a widely used Chinese herbal recipe for arthralgia. A study of this combination was performed: a randomized, double-blind, double-dummy, controlled trial of 200 patients suffering from OA of the knee, comparing DJW and diclofenac 25mg 3 times a day (7). The patients were evaluated after a run-in period of one week (week 0) and then weekly during 4 weeks of treatment. The clinical assessments included visual analog scale (VAS) score that assessed pain and stiffness, Lequesne's functional index, time for climbing up 10 steps, as well as physician's and patients' overall opinions on improvement. Ninety-four patients in each group completed the study. In the first few weeks of treatment, the mean changes in some variables (VAS, which assessed walking pain, standing pain and stiffness, as well as Lequesne's functional index) of the DJW group were significantly lower than those of the diclofenac group. Afterward, these mean changes became no different throughout the study. Most of the physicians' and patients' overall opinions on improvement at each time point did not significantly differ between the two groups. Approximately 30% of patients in both groups experienced mild adverse events.

Finally, a study was performed in Japan using the herbal medicines Shakuyaku-kanzo-to (SK) and Toki-shakuyaku-san (TS) for dymenorrhia. SK is a commonly used Japanese herbal combination and is a Kampo formula made up of a blend of two crude drugs: Shakuyaku (peony root) and Kanzo (glycyrrhiza root, or licorice) It is effective for pain accompanying acute muscle spasms. Due to its effectiveness as a sedative, pain reliever, and anti-spasmotic, Shakuyaku-kanzo-to is prescribed to relieve calf cramps, menstrual, and non-specific abdominal pain and the pain of urinary stone. TS, or Danggui-Shaoyao-San in Chinese herbology, is a mixture of Alisma orientale Rhizoma (Takusha), Angelica acutiloba Radix (Toki), Atractylodes lancea Rhizoma (Sojutsu), Cnidium officinale Rhizoma (Senkyu), Paeonia lactiflora Radix (Shakuyoku), and Poria cocos Hoelen (Bukuryo). It has been reported that TS increases NGF, has an antioxidant action, and has a prophylactic effect against free-radical-mediated neurological disease associated with aging (8).

In the study, SK and TS were given in cyclic therapy, in which the herbs are administered alternately within the menstrual cycle to 17 patients with dysmenorrheal, including recurrent endometriosis and adenomyosis and had received treatment with gonadotropin-releasing hormone agonists or danazol. All the patients obtained complete relief within 3 months when treated with the SK/TS cyclic therapy. Nine of 12 patients treated with the SK/TS cyclic therapy ovulated as determined by biphasic changes in basal body temperature patterns. One of the treated patients, who had a history of 10 repetitive spontaneous abortions, carried the 11th pregnancy to term and gave birth to a normal newborn *(9)*.

These early studies show some promise that TCM herb combinations can be studied using Western scientific methodology. Obviously more data is needed to make strong conclusions, but these ancient formulations may provide viable alternatives to treat difficult chronic pain conditions.

6. SAFETY

In the United States, traditional Chinese herbal products are currently sold as dietary supplements, as defined by The Dietary Supplement Health and Education Act (DSHEA). As a result, although claims about the structure and function of the herbs are allowable under DSHEA regulations, disease claims are not. Like other over-the-counter supplements and botanical preparations, there is no governing body in the United States that regulates content or quality of these herbs *(10)*.

Nevertheless, TCM medicinal products (TCMPs) are increasingly popular. Their current popularity makes the assessment of their safety an urgent necessity. Constituents of TCMPs can be toxic, and numerous examples of liver, kidney, or other organ damage are on record. All TCMPs contain a range of pharmacologically active constituents, which can in certain cases be toxic; this issue of herbal toxicity can be even more complicated by the combination of TCMPs with prescribed drugs. There have been some early attempts at looking at herb-drug interactions (see Table 6). Perhaps an even greater problem is the finding that some TCMPs are contaminated (e.g., with heavy metals) or adulterated (e.g., with prescription drugs) *(11)*. One report from Taiwan suggests that 24% of all samples were contaminated with at least one conventional pharmacological compound. Phenylbutazone, phenytoin, glibenclamide and corticosteroids are some of the adulterants associated with serious adverse events *(12)*.

Concern about the safety of Chinese herbs was brought to national attention with the discovery of aristolochic acid extracted from species of Aristolochia found in some herbal preparations. The condition Chinese herbs nephropathy (CHN) was coined after the report of a rapidly progressive interstitial nephropathy after the introduction of Chinese herbs in a slimming regimen taken by young Belgian women. It is characterized by early, severe anaemia, mild tubular proteinuria, and initially normal arterial blood pressure in half of the patients. Renal histology shows unusually extensive, virtually hypocellular cortical interstitial fibrosis associated with tubular atrophy and global sclerosis of glomeruli decreasing from the outer to the inner cortex. Urothelial malignancy of the upper urinary tract develops subsequently in almost half of the patients. Suspicion that the disease was due to the recent introduction of Chinese herbs in the slimming regimen was reinforced by identification in the slimming pills of the nephrotoxic and carcinogenic aristolochic acid (AA) extracted from species of Aristolochia. Given the positive identification of AA as the cause, this condition is better called aristolochic acid nephropathy (AAN). AAN is not restricted to the Belgian cases. Similar cases have been observed throughout the world. This has led to the withdrawal in several countries of herbs known to have AA as a constituent *(13)*.

Therefore, several health institutions, including the United States Food and Drug Administration, have published safety information related to the presence of AA in botanical products and dietary supplements in order to prevent more cases of intoxication. These plants include *Aritolochia* species (spp.), *Asarum* spp., *Bragantia* spp., *Stephania* spp., *Menispernum* spp., *Akebia* spp., and *Cocculus* spp. Meanwhile, in traditional Chinese medicine, some herbs share the same Chinese names, which may lead to significant confusion. For instance, AA-containing *Aristolochia Fangji* (Guang fang ji) is often mistakenly used because both the nontoxic herb *Stephania tetrandra ST* (Han fang ji) and *Aristolochia Fangji* (Guang fang ji) are usually called Fangji. The herbal regulatory agencies in China and other countries have developed a number of rapid and sensitive method to detect AA in these Chinese medicinal plants such as high-performance liquid chromatography (HPLC) and thin-layer chromatography and cyclic voltammetry (CV) *(14)*.

There have also been reports of severe hepatitis after taking Chinese herbal remedies for minor complaints. Two products appear to be implicated frequently: Jin bu huan was taken by 11 patients, and Dictamnus dasycarpus was taken by 6 patients, including both fatal cases. It is difficult to provide conclusive evidence of what caused hepatitis, as these products are mixtures that may contain adulterants. These cases highlight not only the potential dangers of these products to consumers but also the need for greater control of their manufacture and use *(15)*.

In response to these safety issues, a network of herb growers and health-care practitioners that use herbs in the United States have formed the Medicinal Herb Network to support sustainable production and appropriate use of high-quality medicinal herbs by bringing together experienced and knowledgeable growers, herbalist health-care practitioners, and other professionals to improve the production, processing, marketing, and use of medicinal herbs and research and develop standards of quality *(16)*.

7. INTEGRATION INTO A PAIN CLINIC

The integration of Chinese herbal medicine into modern medical practices must take into account the interrelated issues of quality, safety, and efficacy. In a number of countries, herbal medicines are unregulated, which has led to product quality differences. The lack of pharmacological and clinical data on the majority of herbal medicinal products is a major impediment to the integration of herbal medicines into conventional medical practices. For valid integration, pharmacological and especially, clinical studies, must be conducted on those plants lacking such data. Adverse events, including drug–herb interaction must also be monitored to promote a safe integration of efficacious herbal medicine into conventional medical practices *(17)*.

TCM herbal specialists in the United States are predominantly also trained in acupuncture but not exclusively. By a quirk of the licensing mechanism in the United States, practitioners that do not also provide acupuncture services are not regulated by any governing body such as the state medical board, because herbs fall under the DSHEA and thus are considered "safe" as would be a dietary or nutritional supplement. In contrast, non-physician acupuncturists who perform TCM herbal therapy are regulated by the state medical boards and thus are more accountable for the quality of their practice and will have to demonstrate evidence of continuing education credits in acupuncture and herbal medicine to maintain their license. In addition, the National Certification Committee for Acupuncture and Oriental Medicine (NCCAOM) has set higher standards for acupuncturists to sit for the certification test in Chinese Herbology. This is the primary non-physician acupuncture organization of the United

States. They oversee the traditional acupuncture training programs, which consist of 3–4-year accredited schools that vary widely in the scope of their instruction, with many including course-work in herbs, bodywork, tai-chi, meditation, and Eastern philosophy. The website is www.nccaom.com.

Before working with or hiring a TCM herbalist, one should ensure that the following standards have been met:

- Successful completion of written and oral examinations (completion to be verified by the NCCAOM examination board), the Clean Needle Technique course, and state oral and/or practical examination if required by relevant local medical board rules and practices. Valid, active state acupuncture license
- Since 2004, certification in Chinese herbology requires a minimum of 2,050 hours in an Accreditation Commission for Acupuncture and Oriental Medicine (ACAOM) approved acupuncture school (must include 410 clinical hours in acupuncture and herbs).
- Evidence of at least five consecutive years of clinical experience since licensure [with an average of at least 500 patient visits per year].
- Three letters of recommendation from peer practitioners.

8. RESOURCES

8.1. Web-Based Articles

http://www.healingchronicpain.org/content/introduction/comp_herbal.asp
http://rheumatology.oxfordjournals.org/cgi/content/full/40/7/779
http://www.ancientway.com/catalog/product_info.php?products_id=2566&
    osCsid=6f604fa7af13dee78978a60cebc10f49
http://www.chineseherbsdirect.com/product_info.php?manufacturers_id=&
    products_id=47
http://beyondwellbeing.com/headaches/xue-stag.shtml
http://content.nhiondemand.com/moh/media/TCMHC1.asp?objID=100903&
    ctype=tcmhc
http://www.acupuncture.com/conditions/backpain1.htm
http://www.acupuncture.com/herbs/bloodstagn.htm
http://www.healthy.net/scr/Article.asp?Id=1953
http://www.giovanni-maciocia.com/articles/pain.html
http://www.highbeam.com/library/docFree.asp?DOCID=1G1:85131521
http://www.arthritis.org/research/Bulletin/Vol52No12/Boswellia_Serrata.asp
http://qualitycounts.com/fpcurcumin.html
http://tcm.health-info.org/Common%20Diseases/low.back.pain.htm#_Blood_
    Stagnation_–_Low_Back_Pain.

8.2. Books

Chinese Herbal Patent Formulas, A Practical Guide. Jake Fratkin; Shya Publications, Boulder, CO 1997.

The Energetics of Western Herbs, Vol.1 and Vol.2. Peter Holms; Artemis Press, Boulder, CO 1989.

Formulas and Strategies. Dan Bensky and Randel Barolet; Eastland Press Seattle, WA 1990.

Outline Guide to Chinese Herbal Patent Medicines in Pill Form. Naeser M., Boston Chinese Medicine, Boston, MA 1990.

8.3. Recommended Herbal Companies

Crane Herb Company distributes a variety of prepared formulas and can supply the practitioner with catalogs and printed information. Crane Herb Company, 745 Falmouth Road, Mashpee, MA 02649. Tel: 508-539-1700, Fax: 508-539-2369 info@craneherb.com or http://www.craneherb.com.

Golden Flower: P.O Box 781, Placitas, NM 87043. (800) 729-8509, (505) 821-8857. Fax: (505) 821-3285.

Health Concerns: 8001 Capwell Drive, Oakland, CA 94621. Orders: 1-800-233-9355, Fax: 1-510-639-9140. http://www.healthconcerns.com.

Three Treasures: http://www.giovanni-maciocia.com/herbal/default.html.

Secara: http://www.secara.com/site/Home.html 1 (888) 732-2721.

Blue Poppy Enterprises, Inc.: http://www.bluepoppy.com or 800-487-9296.

Seven Forest herbal formulas: ITM, 2017 SE Hawthorne Blvd., Portland, Oregon 97214 Phone: (503) 233-4907 Fax: (503) 233-1017. http://www.itmonline.org/

Mayway: 1338 Mandela Parkway; Oakland, CA 94607. 1-800-262-9929. www.mayway.com.

9. CONCLUSIONS

In spite of the lack of rigorous research for many botanicals and Chinese herbal preparations, it is highly likely that many patients will continue to seek out these therapies especially as there is greater public awareness about the health hazards of many conventional pharmacological options *(18)*. Chinese herbal formulas are particularly difficult to study, given the issues inherent in standardizing the dose of combinations of dried herbs. Notwithstanding the immense value of identifying the pharmacological activity of a TCM herb in order to create a chemical suitable for pharmaceutical development, another approach to safe and efficacious herbal products is to develop a standardized herbal extract *(19)*. There is a growing trend in the pharmaceutical industry for traditional companies to ally themselves with Chinese herbal companies with the goal of investigating many of what are considered the active ingredients in the common formulas in the hopes of discovering novel medications for a variety of medical conditions *(20)*. The problem with this trend is that is that such studies do not give us adequate information about the benefit of the native formula, especially when prescribed to patients using TCM differential diagnoses. Another major hurdle to overcome if Chinese herbal medicine is going to integrate successfully into Western medical clinics is the fear of widespread heavy metal and other contaminants in herbal preparations, potential toxicities of the native herb, and unknown herb–drug interactions (see Table 6). Physicians who decide to avoid herbal medicine altogether over these concerns may miss the fact that their patients are still using them, and this needs to be assessed. Patients may not be forthcoming about the use of herbal medicine— even if it causes severe adverse effects—because they fear censure. Clinicians must ask patients about their use of herbs in a non-judgmental way to encourage full disclosure. The patient should be treated as a partner in watching out for adverse reactions or interactions, and should be told about the lack of information on interactions and the need for open communication about the use of herbal remedies. Formulation, brand, dose, and reason for use of herbs should be documented on the patient's charts and updated regularly.

Table 6
**Clinical Reports of Herb–Drug Interactions (modified with permission from Fugh-Berman A.
Herb–drug interactions. Lancet 2000;355:134–38.)**

Herb and drug(s)	Results of interaction	Comments
Betel nut *(Areca catechu)*		
Flupenthixol and procyclidine	Rigidity, bradykinesia, jaw tremor	Betal contains arecoline, a cholinergic alkaloid
Fluphenazine	Tremor, stiffness, akithesia	
Prednisone and salbutamol	Inadequate control of asthma	Arecoline challenge caused dose-related bronchoconstriction in six asthma patients
Danshen *(Salvia miltiorrhiza)*		
Warfarin	Increased INR, prolonged PT/PTT	In rats, danshen decreases elimination of warfarin. Danshen is in at least one brand of cigarettes
Dong quai *(Angelica sinensis)*		
Warfarin	Increased INR and widespread bruising	Dong quai contains coumarins
Eleuthero or Siberian ginseng *(Eleutherococcus senticocus)*		
Digoxin	Raised digoxin concentrations	Herb probably interfered with digoxin assay (patient had unchanged ECG despite digoxin concentration of 5·2 nmol/L)
Ginkgo *(Ginkgo biloba)*		
Aspirin	Spontaneous hyphema	Ginkgolides are potent inhibitors of PAF.
Paracetamol and ergotamine/ caffeine	Bilateral subdural haematoma	May not be interaction but due to ginkgo alone. Subarachnoid haemorrhage and subdural haematoma have been reported with the use of ginkgo alone
Warfarin	Intracerebral haemorrhage	
Thiazide diuretic	Hypertension	This effect may be an unusual adverse reaction to the drug or herb; ginkgo alone has not been associated with hypertension
Ginseng *(Panax spp)*		
Warfarin	Decreased INR	In rats, concomitantly administered ginseng had no significant effect on the pharmacokinetics or pharmacodynamics of warfarin

Phenelzine	Headache and tremor, mania	Patient with mania also ingested bee pollen, and had previously had unipolar depression
Alcohol	Increased alcohol clearance	In mice, ginseng increases the activity of alcohol dehydrogenase and aldehyde dehydrogenase
Karela or bitter melon (Momordica charantia)		
Chlorpropamide	Less glycosuria	Karela decreases glucose concentrations in blood
Liquorice (*Glycyrrhiza glabra*)		
Prednisolone	Glycyrrhizin decreases plasma clearance, increases AUC, increases plasma concentrations prednisolone	11-dehydrogenase converts endogenous cortisol to cortisone; orally administered glycyrrhizin is metabolised mainly to glycyrrhetinic acid
Hydrocortisone	Glycyrrhetinic acid potentiates of cutaneous vasoconstrictor response	Glycyrrhetinic acid is a more potent inhibitor of 5-, 5-reductase and 11 -dehydrogenase than is glycyrrhizin
Oral contraceptives	Hypertension, edema, hypokalaemia	Oral contraceptive use may increase sensitivity to glycyrrhizin acid; women are reportedly more sensitive than men to adverse effects of liquorice.
Saiboku-to (Asian herbal mixture)		
Prednisolone	Increased prednisolone AUC	Contains all the same herbs as sho-saiko-to, and *Poria cocos*, *Magnolia officinalis*, and *Perillae frutescen*
Sho-saiko-to or xiao chai hu tang (Asian herb mixture)		
Prednisolone	Decreased AUC for prednisolone	Contains liquorice (*Glycyrrhiza glabra*), *Bupleurum falcatum*, *Pinellia ternata*, *Scutellaria baicalensis*, *Zizyphus vulgaris*, *Panax ginseng*, and *Zingiber officinale*

ACE = angiotensin-converting enzyme; INR = international normalised ratio; PT = prothrombin time; PTT = partial hromboplastin time; ECG = electrocardiogram; PAF = platelet-activating factor; AUC = area under the concentration/time curve.

Hopefully, as physicians begin to work more closely with experienced acupuncturists who have had adequate training in Chinese herbal medicine, they will develop a greater comfort level with the benefits of this approach. Important in this integrative process is to familiarize oneself with reputable herbal companies (see list above) that have high quality control measures in place to prevent contamination. If the theories presented in this chapter eventually prove to be correct, the potential benefits of Chinese herbs to chronic pain sufferers is manifold, opening a window to healing and disease modification rather than just symptom management. However, to reach this ideal, much more research and clinical experience is needed in the West, and integrative health practitioners can be leaders in providing this experience.

REFERENCES

1. Kao ST, Chang CH, Chen YS, et al. Effects of Ding-Chuan-Tang on bronchoconstriction and airway leucocyte infiltration in sensitized guinea pigs. Immunopharmacol Immunotoxicol 2004;26(1):113–124.
2. Zhu Y-P, Woerdenbag HJ, Traditional Chinese herbal medicine. Pharm World Sci 1995; 17(4): 103–112
3. A very good article on the differential diagnosis of pain according to Traditional Chinese Medicine is written by Giovanni Maciocia at http://www.giovanni-maciocia.com/articles/pain.html.
4. Ahmed S, Anuntiyo J, Malemud CJ, et al. Biological basis for the use of botanicals in osteoarthritis and rheumatoid arthritis: a review. Evid Based Complement Alternat Med 2005;2(3): 301–308.
5. Canter PH, Lee HS, Ernst E. A systematic review of randomised clinical trials of *Tripterygium wilfordii* for rheumatoid arthritis. Phytomedicine 2006;13(5):371–377.
6. Cao Y, Shi Y, Zheng Y, et al. Blood-nourishing and hard-softening capsule costs less in the management of osteoarthritic knee pain: a randomized controlled trial. eCAM 2005;2(3) 363–368.
7. Teekachunhatean S, Kunanusorn P, Rojanasthien N, et al. Chinese herbal recipe versus diclofenac in symptomatic treatment of osteoarthritis of the knee: a randomized controlled trial BMC Complement. Altern Med 2004;4:19.
8. Hatip-Al-Khatib I, Egashira N, Mishima K, et al. Determination of the effectiveness of components of the herbal medicine Toki-Shakuyaku-San and fractions of angelica acutiloba in improving the scopolamine-induced impairment of rat's spatial cognition in eight-armed radial maze test. J Pharmacol Sci 2004;96:33–41.
9. Tanaka T. A novel anti-dysmenorrhea therapy with cyclic administration of two Japanese herbal medicines. Clin Exp Obstet Gynecol 2003;30(2–3):95—98.
10. Chang J. Scientific evaluation of traditional Chinese medicine under DSHEA: a conundrum. Dietary Supplement Health and Education Act. J Altern Complement Med 1999;5(2):181–189.
11. Ernst E. Risk of herbal medicinal products. Pharmacoepidemiol Drug Saf 2004;13(11):767–771.
12. Ernst E. Adulteration of Chinese herbal medicines with synthetic drugs: a systematic review. J Intern Med 2002;252(2):107–113.
13. Cosyns JP. Aristolochic acid and 'Chinese herbs nephropathy': a review of the evidence to date. Drug Saf 2003;26(1):33–48.
14. Sun Z, Liu L, Zheng X, et al. An easy and rapid method to determine aristolochic acids I and II with high sensitivity. Anal Bioanal Chem 2004;378:388–390.
15. McRae CA, Agarwal K, Mutimer D, et al. Hepatitis associated with Chinese herbs. Eur J Gastroenterol Hepatol 2002;14(5):559–562.
16. Hassel CA, Hafner CJ, Soberg R, et al. Using Chinese medicine to understand medicinal herb quality: an alternative to biomedical approaches? Agric Hum Values 2002;19:337–347.
17. Fong HH. Integration of herbal medicine into modern medical practices: issues and prospects. Integr Cancer Ther 2002;1(3):287–293.
18. Goldkind L, Simon LS. Patients, their doctors, nonsteroidal anti-inflammatory drugs and the perception of risk. Arthritis Res Ther 2006;8(2):105.

19. Chang J. Scientific evaluation of traditional Chinese medicine under DSHEA: a conundrum. Dietary Supplement Health and Education Act. J Altern Complement Med 1999;5(2): 181–189.
20. Tatsumi S, Mabuchi T, Abe T, Xu L, Minami T, Ito S. Analgesic effect of extracts of Chinese medicinal herbs Moutan cortex and Coicis semen on neuropathic pain in mice. Neurosci Lett 2004;370(2–3):130–134.

IV   INTEGRATIVE MODELS

22 Integrative Pain Medicine Models
Women's Health Programs

Allison Bailey and Meryl Stein

Summary

Recognition of the important biological differences between men and women when it comes to pain processing is key to providing optimum care to women with both subacute and chronic musculoskeletal and pain conditions. Pregnancy, labor, and delivery, hormonal fluctuations of the menstrual cycle and the decrease in gonadal hormones that accompany menopause may all affect the musculoskeletal and neurological systems in varied and complex ways that may result in painful conditions. The precise mechanisms by which these changes occur remain under investigation. Nevertheless, pain programs in Women's Health should be designed to address the needs of women with a variety of health issues including, but not limited to, pregnancy and postpartum-related musculoskeletal problems, pelvic pain and pelvic floor muscle dysfunction, fibromyalgia and myofascial pain, osteoporosis and its complications, and general musculoskeletal health and fitness. In addition, Women's Health programs should recognize the effects of the sex hormones on pain processing and attempt to address underlying issues of hormone imbalance. An integrative model of care that combines high-quality complementary and alternative medicine (CAM) services with those of conventional medicine when appropriate may be the optimal setting in which to treat women with such pain disorders.

Key Words: women's health, sex hormones, pelvic floor muscle dysfunction, pelvic pain, urinary incontinence, fibromyalgia, myofascial pain, osteoporosis, back pain, pregnancy, postpartum, sacroiliac joint dysfunction

From: *Contemporary Pain Medicine: Integrative Pain Medicine: The Science and Practice of Complementary and Alternative Medicine in Pain Management*
Edited by: J. F. Audette and A. Bailey © Humana Press, Totowa, NJ

1. INTRODUCTION

Recognition of the important biological differences between men and women when it comes to pain processing is key to providing optimum care to women with both sub-acute and chronic musculoskeletal and pain conditions. Besides the now well-recognized differences in pain modulation between the sexes, women's bodies also tend to undergo greater changes over the course of a lifetime than do men's. Pregnancy, labor and delivery, hormonal fluctuations of the menstrual cycle, and the decrease in gonadal hormones that accompany menopause may all affect the musculoskeletal and neurological systems in varied and complex ways that may result in painful conditions. The precise mechanisms by which these changes occur remain under investigation. Nevertheless, pain programs in Women's Health should be designed to address the needs of women with a variety of health issues including, but not limited to, pregnancy and postpartum-related musculoskeletal problems, pelvic pain and pelvic floor muscle dysfunction, fibromyalgia and myofascial pain, osteoporosis and its complications, and general musculoskeletal health and fitness. In addition, Women's Health programs should recognize the effects of the sex hormones on pain processing and attempt to address underlying issues of hormone imbalance.

Integrative pain medicine is frequently helpful in managing such disorders and many women may prefer a range of therapeutic options that include appropriate pharmacological and procedural treatments offered within an allopathic medical framework, but also allow choices of less invasive therapies that may be associated with lower risk for adverse events when incorporated into the total plan of care. The National Center for Health Statistics found, in their 2002 National Health Interview Survey, that women are more likely than men to use CAM therapies (1). This may be due to the higher incidence in women of many chronic conditions, which allopathic medicine is typically poor in treating, or alternatively due to psychosocial factors affecting women's preferences for providers with greater emphasis on patient-doctor communication and collaboration. This chapter will start with an introduction to some of the hormonal issues specific to women and pain processing. Various painful conditions that should be addressed within the framework of a comprehensive women's health program in pain management will then be discussed with an emphasis on how these conditions may be optimally treated within an integrative pain medicine model of care.

2. SEX DIFFERENCES IN PAIN

2.1. Introduction

Pain is well known to be a complex experience, influenced by many variables. Interest in the influence of sex on the experience of pain is increasingly emerging within the field of pain medicine. The fact that there are sex differences when it comes to pain is now a well-recognized phenomenon and is no longer debated by pain medicine experts. However, what these differences are and why they exist remains controversial (2,3). This is likely because of the multiple interacting factors involved. Traditionally, these sex differences have mainly been attributed to psychological, behavioral, and sociocultural variables, in particular a perceived greater willingness on the part of women to report painful symptoms. Although these factors are likely to be important in mediating sex differences in pain, evidence is mounting for a strong role of biological factors in shaping the differing pain experiences of men and women.

The role that biological factors play in these differences has too long gone under emphasized. There are likely many reasons for this including the fact that psychosocial and behavioral factors tend to be more easily observable and, therefore, more easily studied in human populations. Secondly, the current state of the evidence for the biological reasons underlying these differences remains somewhat in its infancy and, therefore, difficult to interpret. As tends to be the case in medicine, when the biological reasons that explain a condition are poorly understood greater emphasis is often placed upon the influence of psychological factors. However, as our understanding of the biological explanations for these differences grows, a shift in emphasis is likely to occur with increasing attention given to the importance of biological differences, in particular, hormonal factors, in modulating pain responses.

2.2. Sex Differences in Experimental Pain

Despite the widespread popular belief that women are better able to endure pain due to the fact that they give birth, laboratory studies of experimentally induced painful stimuli have repeatedly demonstrated that women, in fact, have lower pain thresholds and lower pain tolerances than men (2,4). The magnitude and consistency of these findings, however, have been shown to vary based on the type of stimulus that was used. In a meta-analysis of studies examining sex differences in experimental pain responses, moderate to large effect sizes were found for the various stimuli with pressure pain being the most consistent and showing the largest effect sizes and thermal pain being the least consistent in demonstrating sex differences in pain responses (5). Although the exact mechanism underlying these findings remains under investigation, evidence is mounting for the influence of biological factors, and, in particular, hormonal variables to explain these differences.

These sex differences in pain responses also extend to more sophisticated measures. For example, women show greater temporal summation of thermal pain, which indicates the process of wind up or amplification of peripheral nociceptive input at the level of the dorsal horn of the spinal cord (6). Women also have been shown to have greater pupillary dilation in response to painful pressure (7), and it has been observed that different brain regions are activated in women than in men in response to painful stimuli (8). These findings suggest that underlying physiological mechanisms play a role in sex differences in pain responses and that purely psychosociocultural factors appear to be an incomplete explanation for these differences.

2.3. Sex Differences in Clinical Pain Conditions

In order, of course, better to understand the clinical relevance of these findings, we must consider sex differences in endogenous pain experience. Women are known to be affected by many chronic pain conditions and painful conditions of the musculoskeletal system in overwhelmingly greater numbers than are men (3). These conditions that occur with higher incidences in women include migrainous and non-migrainous headache, fibromyalgia, tempomandibular joint disorder (9), irritable bowel syndrome, chronic pelvic pain, interstitial cystitis, carpal tunnel syndrome, patellofemoral pain syndrome, DeQuervain's tenosynovitis, and rheumatoid arthritis. Women are also at greater risk of joint pain due to arthritis (10) and of developing disability specifically due to pain than are men (11). However, when chronic pain is looked at in general, grouping all conditions together (such as in chronic pain clinic settings, for example), there does not appear to be a clear female predominance in either the prevalence or severity of chronic pain overall *(12)*. Despite this, women have been reported to experience more recurrent pain and widespread pain, or pain at multiple body regions, than men *(2)*. This may indicate that there is more of a qualitative rather than quantitative difference between the sexes when it comes to pain. One possible explanation for this phenomenon could be decreased neuromodulation of pain on the part of women, which could potentially be mediated hormonally.

2.4. Hormones and Pain in Animal Studies

More and more, evidence is accumulating that the sex hormones, estrogen, progesterone, and testosterone, are in fact involved in pain processing *(13–16)*. Thus far, much of the research examining the effect of the sex hormones on pain remains in the realm of animal studies. How these studies apply to humans obviously remains unclear. Nevertheless, they are helpful to examine from a basic science perspective in order to understand the effects of specific hormones on pain responses. For example, studies in rats have suggested a potential pronociceptive effect of estrogen. When exposed to injection of the inflammatory compound formalin, female rats show greater rates of hindpaw licking (pain behavior) than their male counterparts. When administered estradiol, however, these same male rats increase their rate of hindpaw licking to that of females *(13)*. Testosterone, on the other hand, has been shown to have a potentially protective effect on pain responses in rats. In one study, formalin injections were given to both intact and gonadectomized male rats once a week for 3 weeks. With each injection, the intact rats showed decreasing pain behavior demonstrating adaptation over time to the painful stimulus, while the gonadectomized rats continued to show baseline levels of pain behavior, never adapting to the stimulus. In addition, the gonadectomized rats showed increased levels of c-fos expression in the central nervous system (CNS), while these changes in c-fos expression did not occur in the intact rats. This seems to indicate that the intact male rats were protected from neuroplastic change that occurred in the setting of lower testosterone levels in the gonadectomized rats. However, it should also be noted that, in addition to lower testosterone levels, the gonadectomized male rats had higher estradiol levels than the intact rats *(17)*.

A role for progesterone in pain modulation has also been suggested by studies in rats. Injection of Complete Freud's Adjuvant, an inflammatory agent, was given to four groups of rats: (1) those with normal estrus cycles, (2) those that were lactating, (3) ovarectomized (OVX) rats given progesterone supplementation, and (4) ovarectomized (OVX) rats given normal saline. Lactating rats have comparatively high progesterone levels and their estrogen to progesterone balance is said to mimic the luteal phase of the human menstrual cycle. Paw withdrawal latency to painful stimulation of the inflamed paw was then measured in each group. This showed that the lactating rats and those OVX rats that received progesterone supplementation had significantly longer paw withdrawal latencies than the normally cycling rats or those that received normal saline. Additionally, these findings were associated with less C-fos expression in the dorsal horn of the lactating rats and further study revealed significantly less pain behavior in the lactating rats when administered an NMDA receptor agonist *(16)*. Therefore, progesterone appeared to be protective in terms of pain responses in the lactating rats and this action seemed to be mediated through lower NMDA receptor activation.

2.5. Menstrual Cycle Variations in Pain Sensitivity

It is, of course, vital to examine the effects of the sex hormones on pain response in humans. In terms of human studies, there are two main lines of evidence examining the effects of the sex hormones on pain modulation; studies that have looked at menstrual cycle variations in pain sensitivity and those that have looked at exogenous hormone use and pain sensitivity. Multiple studies have been done examining changes in pain sensitivity across the menstrual cycle. Among the methodological problems with these studies is the manner in which cycle phase was determined. In the majority of studies this was done by self-report of the subject of the first day of the last menstrual period. This not only has the inherent problem of recall bias, but also fails to account for inter-subject variation in the day of ovulation, which makes it difficult to determine phase precisely by this method. Surprisingly few of these studies attempted to measure hormone levels in order to determine phase. Because of this lack of objective data, the menstrual phases in most of these studies were statically described as either estrogen dominant (the follicular phase) or progesterone dominant (the luteal phase). In fact, great fluctuations in hormone levels occur over the course of both these phases. For example, the mid-luteal phase, which is characterized by relatively high levels of progesterone, is hormonally quite different from the late-luteal (or premenstrual) phase when both estrogen and progesterone levels are rapidly falling and is the time period known to be associated with various psychological and physiological symptoms, such as PMS (late luteal phase dysphoric disorder) and migraine headache. Few of these studies, unfortunately, attempted to distinguish this premenstrual phase from the rest of the luteal phase. Due to this methodological diversity, interpretation of the findings from such studies is somewhat problematic.

Recently, however, Riley and colleagues performed a meta-analysis, attempting to clarify the available data. This revealed significant differences in pain sensitivity across the menstrual cycle with the findings varying based on the type of experimental pain stimulus that was applied *(15)*. For the majority of stimuli used, there was less pain sensitivity during the follicular phase or estrogen dominant phase of the cycle. However, for electrical stimulation the pattern reversed itself, showing less pain sensitivity in the luteal or progesterone dominant phase, with small to moderate effect sizes seen for all. These results, of course, raise the question of what type of experimental pain stimulus is most important or clinically relevant. The answer to this clearly remains debatable. However, pressure as an experimental pain stimulus is particularly intriguing, since tenderness to pressure palpation is frequently used in clinical practice and, in fact, is the main diagnostic tool used in fibromyalgia syndrome (FMS), a clinical pain condition with strong sex differences.

On closer review, only two of the studies in the above meta-analysis looked at response to pressure palpation as a pain stimulus. One of these studies compared pain responses in the mid-follicular phase of the cycle to the premenstrual (late luteal) phase *(18)* and the other compared the periovulatory (late follicular phase) to the menstrual and premenstrual phases *(19)*. Therefore, neither of these pressure pain studies examined responses in the mid-luteal phase of the cycle when progesterone levels are high. This raises considerable doubt about the authors' conclusions that pressure pain sensitivity is higher during the luteal, or progesterone dominant, phase of the cycle *(15)*.

Another study, not included in this meta-analysis, examined sensitivity to pressure pain across the menstrual cycle in a slightly different way. Tender point count by palpation was measured at 13 spots bilaterally in 36 women with normal menstrual cycles and 30 oral contraceptive users with correlation made to menstrual cycle phase as determined by self-report. The number of tender points to palpation was significantly greater during the follicular (estrogen dominant) phase of the cycle than during the luteal (progesterone dominant) phase of the cycle in the women with normal menstrual cycles. No significant variations in tender point count were noted in users of oral contraceptives *(14)*. This illustrates a potentially protective role for the sex hormone progesterone in terms of pain responses. Although the mechanism to explain these types of transient changes in tissue sensitivity currently remains unclear, one could hypothesize that hormonal fluctuations could be promoting the process of peripheral sensitization through complex interactions with the immune system.

2.6. Exogenous Hormone Use and Pain Sensitivity

The other set of human studies looking at the effects of sex hormones on pain sensitivity are those involving exogenous hormone use. One study of experimental pain responses in postmenopausal women on and off hormone replacement therapy (HRT) and men found that heat pain threshold and tolerance was significantly lower in women on HRT as compared to both women not on HRT and men. When the women in this study were grouped together regardless of HRT status, their pain thresholds and tolerances were significantly lower than the men's *(20)*. This illustrates the importance of hormonal status as a variable in research on pain responses. All of the clinical studies in this arena are cross-sectional in design making it impossible, therefore, to draw cause and effect conclusions. However, clinical studies have shown an increased frequency of tempomandibular joint disorder, increased severity of orofacial pain symptoms, and increased low back pain (LBP) and impairment due to LBP in HRT users as compared to non-users *(21–23)*.

The studies involving oral contraceptive (OC) use and pain are more varied in terms of conclusions with some showing no difference in pain sensitivity between users and non-users, some showing less pain sensitivity in OC users, and still others showing increased pain sensitivity in OC users versus non-users *(21,24–26)*. There are several likely reasons for this phenomenon, including the cross-sectional design of such studies, relatively short follow up times, and wide variability in the specific hormonal formulations used. Although the studies of short-term use of exogenous hormones in premenopausal women remain inconclusive at this time, another important question to be clarified in future research is what the effects of long-term oral contraceptive use on the pain modulatory system are.

2.7. Summary

Although many questions remain to be answered regarding the effects of the gonadal hormones on pain conditions, it does seem clear that there are important differences between the sexes for many clinical pain disorders that may be at least partially explained by hormonal mechanisms. Therefore, assessment of hormonal factors may play an important role in both evaluating and researching pain conditions in women. Many pain conditions are associated with menstrual cycle related fluctuations in pain complaints, and attention to menstrual cycle phase and irregularities should be part of the assessment of women with pain disorders. In addition, exogenous hormone use, at least in the case of HRT formulations previously in widespread use, appears to increase the risk of certain pain disorders. Women with chronic pain disorders should be discouraged when possible from use of such hormonal preparations. Currently, due to the results of the Women's Health Initiative Study, hormone replacement therapy in lower doses and alternate formulations is being examined *(27–30)* However, because of stereo-specificity of hormones *(31)*, use of bio-identical hormonal compounds may be important *(32–35)* In addition, the rate of change of hormone levels may be a vital factor, and rapid changes such as those that occur after hysterectomy or with abrupt initiation or cessation of HRT may have the most profound impact on pain processing systems. Also, the balance between interacting hormones may be more critical than one specific hormone in terms of pain responses *(31)*.

Finally, there may be many confounding factors playing a role in hormonal effects on pain. For example, percent body fat is likely important in postmenopausal women, as significant aromatization of androgens to estrogens occurs in fat tissue. There are also many dietary and environmental hormonal factors that are either difficult or impossible to account for, such as the presence of hormones in meat and dairy products and the presence of xenoestrogens in the environment *(36)*. As a general rule, women with pain problems should be advised to decrease consumption of both meat and dairy products and to eat, as much as possible, organic pesticide-free fruits and vegetables.

3. PREGNANCY AND POSTPARTUM-RELATED PAIN

3.1. Introduction

Painful conditions of the musculoskeletal and neurological systems and back and pelvic pain, in particular, occur commonly both during and after pregnancy. Retrospective and prospective studies estimate that somewhere between 50–60% of pregnant women experience new onset back pain during pregnancy with at least one third of these experiencing disabling symptoms *(37,38)*. However, despite the high frequency of such problems, recognition of them as treatable conditions remains low, and medical care of the pregnant woman, except in extreme life and health-threatening situations, tends to focus on the health of the fetus to an extreme degree, likely in part because of the litigious environment in which medicine is currently practiced. In addition, the postpartum time period has been recognized as one in which women experience multiple health problems, including fatigue, incontinence, back pain, headache and depression, however, these issues are frequently neglected by healthcare professionals *(39)*. In general, the traditional response to such complaints by pregnant and postpartum women has been that pain is a normal and expected part of these time periods and that these issues will spontaneously resolve without treatment.

Women who experience musculoskeletal pain during pregnancy are frequently told to rest and await resolution of their symptoms after delivery. This gives the impression that the only treatment available for pain during pregnancy is rest. However, rest is an unacceptable treatment for back and other pain conditions occurring during pregnancy for several reasons. Rest is no longer considered an appropriate treatment for low back pain (LBP), in general; and, in fact, greater than three days of bed rest for acute LBP has been shown to be detrimental to recovery *(40,41)*. If that is the case, then certainly several months of rest could impede the recovery process by contributing to significant deconditioning and functional limitations. Secondly, many women are not able to rest during pregnancy, as they may be working full time, caring for other children, and are simply unable to put their lives on hold for nine months. It is, therefore, essential that healthcare providers find ways of helping them in order to limit their pain and preserve their functional integrity. In addition, there are several safe, though not rigorously studied, treatments available for back and pelvic pain of pregnancy. The scarcity and poor methodological quality of available research on this topic, however, should not limit the treatments that are offered to individual patients when deemed of low risk to both mother and fetus.

Multiple studies suggest that pain frequently persists during the postpartum period, which can interfere with childcare responsibilities and inhibit return to normal function, and may in certain cases become chronic in nature. The possible reasons for this will be reviewed at the conclusion of this section. In a retrospective cross-sectional study, a history of low back pain during pregnancy was shown to be a strong risk factor for low back pain in later life; 10–15% of women in this study with chronic low back pain reported the onset of their symptoms during pregnancy *(42)*. Recently, a prospective study examining factors associated with postpartum back pain identified a 21% prevalence of persistent pain at 2 years postpartum. Severe, early onset pain and inability to reduce weight to its normal prepartum level were strongly correlated with poor regression of symptoms postpartum *(43)*. These patients should be identified early on as being at high risk of developing chronic back pain symptoms and available treatments should be offered to them aggressively.

3.2. Brief Review of the Literature

Unfortunately, despite how common this condition is, very little well done research has examined treatments for LBP in pregnancy. In fact, the Cochrane Pregnancy and Childbirth group identified only 3 studies of sufficient methodological quality for inclusion in their review as of October 2001 *(44)*. This included a randomized trial of water gymnastics performed weekly as compared to a no treatment control group. The study reported a statistically significant decrease in visual analog scores (VAS) one week after birth *(45)*.

Another study compared acupuncture as a treatment for back pain of pregnancy to group physical therapy (PT). A total of 48 women were randomized to receive either ten 30–minute individual sessions of acupuncture over one month's time or ten group PT sessions, each lasting 50 minutes, over 6 to 8 weeks. The PT group had a 40% drop-out rate. The acupuncture group showed significantly greater reductions in VAS than the PT group. In addition, 27/28 acupuncture subjects rated their treatment as good or excellent, while only 14/18 PT participants did likewise. One important explanation for this phenomenon is the lack of individualization of treatment in PT group, which can have important psychological and physical consequences *(46)*.

Finally, a 2-week crossover design study of 92 pregnant women examined the efficacy of a specialized maternity pillow, the Ozzlo pillow, with a standard pillow for preventing poor sleep due to nighttime back pain. The Ozzlo pillow is a specially designed hollowed out, nest shaped pillow used for supporting the lower abdomen. Sixty-three women reported moderate or better sleep with the Ozzlo pillow compared with only 39 women who reported sleep improvement with the standard pillow *(47)*. Unfortunately, this specific pillow does not currently appear to be on the market in the United States or Europe.

One likely reason for the paucity of studies showing effective treatments for back pain of pregnancy is the generally poor understanding of the etiology of the problem. Proposed theories include mechanical stress due to increased weight gain and postural factors, venous congestion due to pressure from the gravid uterus, ligamentous laxity leading to sacroiliac joint and pubic symphysis pain, discogenic pain, spondylolithesis, and hip joint pathology. Myofascial pain is another cause of back and pelvic pain that likely goes greatly under-recognized in pregnant patients as it does in the general non-pregnant population. Problems arise, both in clinical care and research, when the majority of subjects with LBP are grouped into one diagnostic category without recognition that a proper differential diagnostic approach should apply. This problem is true of studies examining LBP in non-pregnant subjects and may apply even more so to pregnant women with back pain, who are generally told that their pain is due to mechanical factors. These patients are frequently diagnosed, therefore, with mechanical LBP of pregnancy similar to the patient with so-called non-specific mechanical LBP. This term, however, is often applied when a more specific diagnosis is not established, which may be based mainly on the limitations of the diagnostician rather than any other factor.

The evidence for generic mechanical factors contributing to LBP of pregnancy is limited and more specific diagnoses should be sought whenever possible. For example, no association has been found between the amount of weight gained or the weight of the baby and the incidence of LBP in pregnancy, although there does appear to be a relationship between pre- and post-pregnancy maternal weight and BMI and LBP and pelvic pain during pregnancy *(48,49)*. In addition, the incidence of back pain pregnancy increases during the first trimester, long before such mechanical factors should have much effect. Therefore, it is vital in each pregnant patient to establish as specific a diagnosis as possible. This allows for specificity in treatment and may result in improved outcomes for patients. However, this does require an understanding of the most likely historical factors associated with various diagnoses presenting as back or pelvic pain in pregnancy, familiarity with examination of the musculoskeletal system, and a high comfort-level with diagnosing and treating pregnant women with musculoskeletal problems.

3.3. Lumbar Disc Disease

Lumbar disc herniation is one cause of back (and lower extremity) pain that remains part of the differential diagnosis but is not extremely common during pregnancy. Lumbar disc herniation occurs in only about 1 of 10,000 cases of back pain in pregnancy *(50)*. Prior to the advent of Magnetic Resonance Imaging (MRI), it had been suggested that pregnancy may predispose women to disc disease of the lumbar spine. However, studies employing MRI technology have not shown any greater disc pathology in pregnant versus non-pregnant and parous versus nulliparous women *(51)*. However, when disc herniation is suspected during pregnancy, based on history and physical exam findings, MRI can supposedly be performed safely, although the long-term effects on the fetus are unknown *(52,53)*. For this reason, in cases of suspected disc herniation without neurological deficit, management may begin conservatively without imaging while symptoms are monitored closely. Physical therapy for education in body mechanics and postural training and stretching exercises for the lower extremities with progression to strengthening of core musculature in positions of comfort may be initiated. Acupuncture may be an additional form of non-pharmacological pain control that is deemed safe during pregnancy *(54)*. Epidural steroid injection (ESI) for severe intractable pain due to lumbar radiculopathy has been performed safely in pregnancy, and laminectomy for radiculopathy associated with progressive neurological changes has also been performed safely. When there has been a known disc herniation during pregnancy, delivery is typically by scheduled Cesarean section to avoid progression of the herniation due to labor. This, however, has not been studied, and based on clinical experience appears overly conservative.

3.4. Pregnancy and Spondylolithesis

Spondylolithesis, which is the forward slip of one vertebra on the other, can occur for various reasons, including degeneration of the facet joints and surrounding ligamentous structures (degenerative spondylolithesis). This type occurs most commonly at the L4–5 level and is four times as common in women as it is in men. The reason for this increased incidence in women is unknown, but the role of pregnancy has been implicated. In order to investigate this relationship further, Sanderson and Fraser reviewed the database of all female patients (n = 949) presenting with LBP to one spinal surgeon's practice from 1990–1995. Each woman completed a questionnaire on how many children they had borne, and each underwent plain films of the lumbar spine that were examined for evidence of spondylolithesis. Those with isthmic (congenital) spondylolithesis and a history of lumbar spine surgery were excluded. These patients were compared to a control group of 120 male patients in same age range presenting to same surgeon with complaints of LBP. Ninety-six of the women were nulliparous and 853 had borne one or more children. The incidence of degenerative spondylolithesis was 28% in the parous women, 16.7% in the nulliparous, and 7.5% in the men. There was a trend towards increased incidence in the parous women with increasing number of pregnancies, but these numbers did not reach statistical significance *(55)*. The authors proposed that the increased incidence in the parous versus nulliparous women may be due to longstanding changes in joint and ligamentous laxity induced by pregnancy and that the hormonal changes of pregnancy may affect collagen in a more permanent way. They also propose that the increased incidence may be due to deconditioning of and long-term changes in abdominal muscle strength due to a history of pregnancy. One of the senior surgeons stated his clinical observation that during anterior surgery on the lumbar spine in multiparous women the rectus abdominis muscle often is widely separated with associated wasting of the abdominal musculature. However, clearly the increased incidence in women observed in this study cannot be entirely attributed to pregnancy, since the nulliparous women showed a significantly increased incidence as compared to men. One must consider, therefore, the possible influence of estrogen and progesterone on ligamentous and joint laxity as contributing factors. In addition, other studies have shown no increase in degree of slippage or symptoms during pregnancy in those women with a prior history of known spondylolithesis *(56)*.

3.5. Hip Disorders in Pregnancy

Pain emanating from the hip joint occurs relatively infrequently during pregnancy, but is critical to identify, as its causes may result in serious consequences if left undiagnosed *(57)*. Although hip joint pain typically radiates to the groin, anteromedial thigh, and lateral trochanteric region, it can also frequently cause buttock pain or pain in the sacroiliac joint (SIJ) area. Therefore, hip ROM and provocative hip joint tests should be performed on any pregnant patient complaining of lower back or pelvic pain. Transient osteoporosis of pregnancy and osteonecrosis of the femoral head are rare diagnoses typically presenting in the third trimester with painful weightbearing and an antalgic gait. MRI is the study of choice to rule out these uncommon, yet serious, diagnoses when suspicion arises *(58)*. Treatment for transient osteoporosis is with protected weightbearing to avoid femoral neck fracture *(57)*. The use of bisphosphonates and/or calcitonin has been shown to shorten the duration of symptoms, but their use in pregnancy is controversial *(59–61)*. In cases of avascular necrosis, restricted weight-bearing is the treatment of choice with aspiration being considered in the postpartum period if necessary *(62)*.

3.6. Sacroiliac Joint Dysfunction

Pelvic ligamentous laxity is commonly implicated as contributing significantly to LBP and pelvic girdle pain (PGP) of pregnancy. The pelvis is a bony ring joined to the sacrum posteriorly through the two sacroiliac (SI) joints and joined together anteriorly through the fibrocartilaginous pubic symphysis. The SI joints are synovial joints surrounded by a capsule. They are fairly flat joints with a slight C or L shape making them optimal for horizontal load transfer from the lower extremities. This shape, however, leaves them vulnerable to vertical shear loads such as occur with a fall onto a single limb or impact from a motor vehicle accident (MVA). They are surrounded by many strong ligaments that are important in the stability of the joint, and the surrounding musculature is important in providing compression and added stability. Therefore, anything that contributes to loosening of the ligamentous structures or weakening of the surrounding muscles can lead to increased SI joint instability.

During pregnancy, hormonal changes lead to increased ligamentous laxity. This is frequently attributed to the hormone relaxin, which increases during the first trimester peaking at about the 12th week of pregnancy. Subsequently, relaxin levels decline until the 17th week and stabilize at approximately 50% of the peak value *(38)*. In vitro and animal studies have shown that relaxin decreases the synthesis and secretion of interstitial collagen with these changes being much more dramatic in the setting of elevated estrogen levels. Relaxin's role in human pregnancies has been somewhat less clear with some studies showing no relationship to the degree of ligamentous laxity and serum relaxin levels *(63)*. However, this same study did reveal increased laxity in the elbows, knees and MCP joints of pregnant women that persisted into the postpartum state suggesting a role for other hormonal influences such as elevated estrogen and progesterone.

Although increased ligamentous laxity is often cited as a reason for increased SI joint pain in pregnancy and postpartum, an association between the degree of laxity and presence or severity of SI joint pain is difficult to establish due to the lack of specificity of diagnostic tests for SI joint dysfunction *(64,65)*. However, in the pregnant and postpartum population, specifically the posterior pelvic pain provocation (PPPP) test and the active straight leg raise (ASLR) tests have been documented as reliable, sensitive and specific diagnostic tests to diagnoses SI joint pain *(66,67)*. However, more recently Doppler imaging has been established as a reliable objective method of measuring the degree of laxity in the SI joints. Using Doppler imaging in 163 pregnant women, 73 with moderate to severe posterior pelvic pain and 90 with no or mild pain, there was no association between the degree of SI joint laxity and the presence and severity of SI joint pain *(68)*. However, there was a clear association between asymmetric SI joint laxity (a significant side to side difference in degree of laxity) and SI joint pain. There was also a significant association between asymmetric laxity and visual analog score (VAS) and score on the Quebec Back Pain Index (QBPI). In a subsequent study, asymmetric laxity also predicted pain that persisted into the postpartum period *(69)*. Although the reasons for this asymmetrical laxity being so predictive of pain remain unclear, it could be that they are more likely to result in structural or postural asymmetries such as a pelvic obliquity that then perpetuates myofascial strain patterns, leading to increased pain.

Multiple muscle groups, including those of the abdominal region, lumbar spine, gluteal area, lower extremities and pelvic floor, play prominent roles in stabilizing the SI joint. This is important to recognize as anything that leads to increased SI joint instability could lead to imbalance in these muscle groups and subsequent myofascial pain. In addition, anything that results in weakness or strain patterns in these muscle groups, such as deconditioning or postural changes due to pregnancy, can cause or perpetuate SI joint dysfunction. Particularly important groups of muscles contributing to SI joint stability that are affected for obvious reasons during pregnancy are the pelvic floor muscles beneath, the transversus abdominis (TA) in the front and sides and the multifidus group of extensors posteriorly. There is often a great deal of attention focused on the TA and multifidus in terms of lumbar and pelvic stabilization exercises, but unless the patient is treated within the framework of experienced women's healthcare providers, assessment and training of the pelvic floor muscles may be forgotten or ignored.

Treatment of sacroiliac joint pain during pregnancy and in the postpartum period should focus on maintaining strength and motor control in these pelvic stabilizing muscles. One randomized controlled trial of 81 subjects with postpartum SI joint pain showed significantly better outcomes for both pain as measured by VAS and physical functioning in those subjects given specific pelvic stabilizing exercises as opposed to those in a traditional physical therapy control group *(70)*. In addition, these differences were maintained at both one and two years postpartum *(70)*. A subsequent study examined standard physical therapy to standard physical therapy plus acupuncture to stabilizing exercises for the treatment of pregnant women with pelvic girdle pain. The acupuncture group had less morning and night pain than the standard group and less night pain than the stabilizing exercise group after one week of treatment *(71)*. Further follow-up data was not provided.

Associated myofascial pain should be addressed concomitantly with joint malalignment or dysfunction. Gentle osteopathic manipulation techniques can be performed safely during pregnancy to correct structural asymmetries. In addition, treatment by dry needling or structural acupuncture can release myofascial trigger points in key muscles that may be maintaining strain patterns. The piriformis muscle is commonly involved in cases of SI joint dysfunction and can result in posterior thigh pain that may mimic true "sciatica." This is likely a common cause of lower extremity pain in pregnant patients with SI joint dysfunction and should be addressed accordingly. Depending on the patient and the degree of disability, use of an SI joint stability belt may be necessary for the duration of the pregnancy. Weaning from the belt and training of the pelvic stabilizers should begin shortly into the postpartum period. For the less debilitated patient, working with an experienced women's health yoga therapist may be appropriate. Many yoga poses can focus on stretching of the appropriate musculature and strengthening of the pelvic stabilizers in a safe and gentle way both during and after pregnancy.

3.7. Pubic Symphysis Pain

At times pregnancy-related ligamentous laxity may give rise to pain at the pubic symphysis rather than in the lower back, buttock or SI joint regions. Symphyseal pain may be due to inflammation, osteitis pubis, or rarely separation of the joint. Inflammation may respond to ice and a short period of limited weightbearing. Osteitis pubis is characterized by sclerosis and bony changes around the pubic symphysis that can lead to chronic pubic pain. This pain commonly refers to the groin or medial thigh but may also refer to the pelvis or lower abdomen. This disorder may be associated with chronic adductor tightness that should be addressed as part of a comprehensive treatment program. Again, dry needling for associated myofascial trigger points and gentle osteopathic manipulation to restore structural integrity may be necessary. Acupuncture may be a helpful method of non-pharmacological pain control. For severe or persistent postpartum symptoms, steroid and lidocaine injection may be considered. True separation (>1cm) of the pubic symphysis is rare and when occurs is usually the result of birth trauma. Treatment typically consists of bedrest and progressive weightbearing as tolerated with need for surgical intervention being rare *(57)*.

3.8. Peripartum Neuropathies

Peripheral nerve injuries occur frequently in the peripartum period. During pregnancy these tend to be compressive in nature due to increased fluid retention and subsequent increased perineural pressure. Lower extremity neuropathy occurring after labor and delivery are a well-recognized phenomenon that has gone by multiple names with multiple mechanisms having been proposed. Names given this condition include maternal birth palsy, obstetrical neurapraxia, traumatic neuritis of the peurerium, maternal obstetrical paralysis, and idiopathic neuritis. The condition, therefore, remains somewhat poorly understood. That being the case this can be a difficult problem for women to encounter during the postpartum period that is a stressful time when they are faced with new childcare responsibilities. Frequently this may give rise to a great deal of psychosocial distress that may be interpreted by healthcare providers as the cause rather than result of their sometimes strange symptoms. As the majority of these neuropathies will resolve gradually over time without other intervention, the majority of patients require reassurance and support by a provider with an understanding of the problem.

The incidence of postpartum lower extremity neuropathy cited in the literature has varied widely from 0.0008–0.5% depending on methodological differences between studies with most being retrospective in nature *(72–74)*. One prospective study of 6,048 women with lower extremity neuropathy symptoms postpartum found an incidence of 0.92%. After controlling for many confounding variables the disorder was significantly associated with nulliparity and prolonged second stage of labor. Women with nerve injury were also more likely to spend greater time in lithotomy position than women without injury. However, this was difficult to control for as the majority of women were positioned this way. In addition, as 70% of the women in this study underwent epidural analgesia, it was impossible to establish any potential contribution of epidural use to nerve injury *(75)*.

This study also attempted to localize the site of the neurological lesion based on physical examination by a physiatrist, rather than on electromyography (EMG) and nerve conduction studies (NCS). The most common nerve involvement was the lateral femoral cutaneous nerve followed by the femoral nerve, nerve root injury and then the peroneal nerve and lumbosacral plexus *(75)*. Injury to the lateral femoral cutaneous nerve, also called meralgia paresthetica, occurs commonly during pregnancy as well as in the postpartum time period. One study of patients with this disorder found an incidence of 4.3 per 10,000 with recent or current pregnancy being the most significantly associated factor *(76)*. Treatment for this condition mainly consists of reassurance, as most cases tend to resolve postpartum. However, education regarding postpartum weight loss and exercise should also be provided. An exercise program should consist of hip flexor stretching and strengthening of core musculature. A comprehensive structural assessment may reveal potentially contributing asymmetries that could be addressed through osteopathic or chiropractic manipulation. When pain persists postpartum or is intolerable, additional treatment options include low dose tricyclic antidepressants (TCAs) or other anti-neuropathic pain agents, nerve block procedures, transcutaneous electrical nerve stimulation (TENs), and acupuncture.

Postpartum footdrop is a disorder with a wide differential diagnosis, including L4/5 radiculopathy, lumbosacral plexopathy, sciatic neuropathy, and peroneal nerve palsy. In a case series of seven patients with postpartum footdrop who underwent detailed neurological exam and EMG/NCS testing, the neuroanatomical lesion in all cases was localized to the lumbosacral trunk of the lumbosacral plexus *(77)*. The lumbosacral trunk (also called the cord) is formed primarily by the L5 root with some contribution from the L4 root, and travels in close contact with the ala of the sacrum adjacent to the SI joint (see Figure 1). The trunk is cushioned by the psoas muscle through much of its course except at the terminal portion near the pelvic brim where it can be compressed by the fetal head as it descends through the pelvis. This study illustrates the potential usefulness of EMG/NCS in lesion localization. In addition, EMG/NCS may also be helpful for prognosis in those patients who appear to be having an unusually prolonged recovery course. In the Wong et al. study the median duration of nerve injury symptoms was 2 months (range 1 week to 18 months). No difference was seen in symptom duration for the various nerve injury distributions or for those patients experiencing sensory versus motor symptoms *(75)*. This time range likely reflects differences between neurapraxia (myelin sheath injury, segmental demyelination, recovery within days to weeks) versus axontomesis (axonal injury, recovery over months, may be incomplete) type of nerve injuries.

3.9. Other Postpartum Concerns

As mentioned earlier, although pregnant women are often told that pain problems will resolve postpartum, evidence exists that the postpartum time period is one in which women encounter a spectrum of persistent or new health problems that may go unaddressed by the healthcare community. The reasons for this are most likely multifactorial with deconditioning and untreated structural lesions in the setting of increased demands of nursing and childcare making the musculoskeletal system vulnerable to injury. In addition, the postpartum hormonal milieu may be a factor. Many inflammatory (rheumatoid arthritis) and autoimmune (multiple sclerosis) disorders that improve during pregnancy are known to worsen postpartum for unclear reasons. Finally, any pain problem that is allowed to persist without treatment increases the risk of giving rise to peripheral and central sensitization. One question that often arises for patients in the setting of persistent postpartum back pain is the role that epidural analgesia may play in their symptoms. Retrospective studies had suggested a possible link between epidural use and postpartum back pain. However, a well-done prospective study that

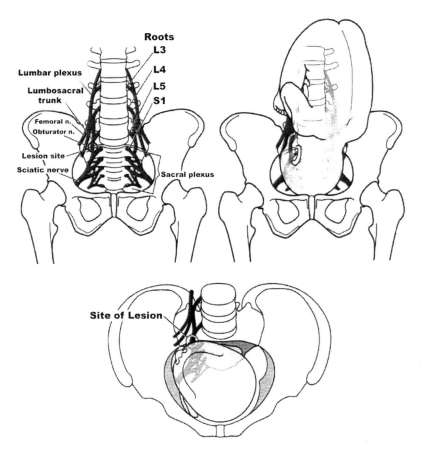

Fig. 1. Descent of fetal head compressing lumbosacral trunk at pelvic brim. (reprinted from Katirji B, Wilbourn AJ, Scarberry SL, et al. Intrapartum Maternal Lumbosacral Plexopathy. Muscle and Nerve 2002;26:340–347 with permission from Wiley Periodicals, Inc.)

followed 1,042 women up to 2 months postpartum found no significant difference in back pain rates based on epidural use. The most significant associated factors in this study were back pain during pregnancy and greater postpartum weight *(78)*. This suggests a role for deconditioning in the persistence of pain during the postpartum period and also emphasizes the importance of treating back pain that occurs during pregnancy.

The postpartum time period is one of relative deconditioning. One study of 63 women showed significant decreases in aerobic fitness and strength as compared to pre-pregnancy performance with improvement by the 27th postpartum week but not to baseline levels. The women were not followed beyond this time period *(79)*. Therefore, it remains unclear what percentage of women return to their prepartum level of physical fitness. The numbers may be low due to increased scheduling demands due to childcare responsibilities. In addition, persistent or new muscuoskeletal problems and structural asymmetries may make it difficult to resume normal exercise routines. For example, up to 66% of women in the third trimester of pregnancy are estimated to develop a rectus diastasis due to stretching and thinning of the linea alba. This condition may persist into the postpartum period in anywhere from 30–60% of women. Performing traditional abdominal muscle exercises, such as abdominal crunches, may actually worsen this condition. Although it is unknown the exact effect that these changes have on abdominal muscle strength, one study revealed significant decreases in abdominal muscle function during pregnancy that was persistent at 8 weeks postpartum and paralleled the structural changes in the abdominal musculature that also remained unresolved *(80)*. Deconditioning, soft tissue tightness, decreased core strength, and overweight status are all risk factors for back pain in general and these may also contribute to persistent pain in postpartum women. Therefore, treatment of unresolved musculoskeletal issues and counseling regarding proper return to fitness after pregnancy is important for general health and well-being, but may also be helpful in avoiding more long-term pain problems.

3.10. Exercise and Pregnancy

Historically, conventional wisdom dictated pregnant women should refrain from exercise, or at least reduce its intensity. Today, however, most authorities encourage exercise for pregnant women as part of a general health maintenance program. For non-pregnant individuals, both the Centers of Disease Control and Prevention and the American College of Sports Medicine recommend at least 30 minutes of cumulative moderate exercise on most if not all days of the week *(81)*. In the absence of either medical or obstetric complications, these recommendations extend to pregnant women.

Exercise conveys the same general health benefits to pregnant women as it does to the general population. It improves endurance and other cardiovascular parameters. For many, it improves their mood and reduces stress. Additionally, some studies suggest exercise may reduce the risk of gestational diabetes, especially in morbidly obese women. The American Diabetes Association has endorsed exercise as "a helpful adjunctive therapy" for gestational diabetes when diet alone fails *(82,83)*.

In non-pregnant individuals, moderate exercise can be defined as a percentage of maximal heart rate. However, pregnancy blunts the heart rate's response to exercise. Thus, the Borg Scale of Perceived Exertion can define moderate exercise. Pregnant women should aim for a rating of 12–14 ("somewhat hard"), meaning they should be able to comfortably converse *(84)*.

While exercise is safe in pregnancy, pregnant women should abide by certain precautions. They should wear loose fitting clothing and exercise in well-ventilated areas to avoid persistently elevated body temperatures. They should also ensure that they remain euglycemic. Since exercise increases both maternal and fetal glucose demand, pregnant women should be careful to avoid hypoglycemia while exercising *(84)*. After the first trimester, the women should modify their routine to adjust to pregnancy's cardiovascular changes. They should avoid lying supine for long time periods as well as prolonged motionless standing because these positions impede venous return resulting in reduced cardiac output and orthostatic hypotension *(85)*.

Before prescribing an exercise program for pregnant women, however, the physician must perform a thorough history and physical exam (See Tables 1 and 2 for absolute and relative contraindications to exercise and Table 3 for warning signs to terminate exercise while pregnant). Additionally, pregnant women should avoid activities that could potentially endanger themselves or their fetus. Contact sports, such as ice hockey, soccer and basketball should be avoided. Additionally, any sport with a significant fall risk, such as gymnastics, skiing, or horseback riding should be avoided. Scuba diving should also be avoided due to the significant risk that the fetus could develop compression sickness because fetal circulation cannot filter bubble formation *(86)*.

Table 1

Absolute Contraindications to Aerobic Exercise During Pregnancy (reprinted with permission from the American College of Obstetricians and Gynecologists. Exercise During Pregnancy and the Postpartum Period [Committee Opinion No. 267], Washington, DC © ACOG 2002)

Hemodynamically significant heart disease
Restrictive lung disease
Incompetent cervix/ cerclage
Multiple gestation at risk for preterm labor
Persistent second or third trimester bleeding
Placenta previa after 26 weeks of gestation
Premature labor during the current pregnancy
Ruptured membranes
Pre-eclampsia/pregnancy induced hypertension

Exercise at altitudes up to 6,000 feet also appears to be safe. However, any woman exercising at high altitudes should understand the signs and symptoms of altitude sickness, and if she develops these findings she should descend and seek medical help immediately *(87)*.

Aquatic exercise may be ideal for many pregnant women, especially for previously inactive women. Exercise in temperate water reduces or eliminates many of exercise's stressors on the body. Buoyancy unloads the joints and the water reduces heat storage and sweat loss. Aquatic exercise also has less dramatic effects on increases in maternal heart rate *(84)*.

Although exercise is considered safe in pregnancy, pregnant women who were previously inactive or who have a complicated pregnancy should seek medical advice before beginning an exercise program. According to the 2003 Canadian clinical practice guidelines for exercise in pregnancy, previously inactive women should begin with 15 minutes of continuous exercise three times per week with the goal of 30 minutes four times per week. More frequent exercise has been associated with an increased risk of

Table 2

Relative Contraindications to Aerobic Exercise During Pregnancy (reprinted with permission from the American College of Obstetricians and Gynecologists. Exercise During Pregnancy and the Postpartum Period [Committee Opinion No. 267], Washington, DC © ACOG 2002)

Severe anemia
Unevaluated maternal cardiac arrhythmia
Chronic bronchitis
Poorly controlled type 1 diabetes
Extreme morbid obesity
Extremely underweight (BMI <12)
Previous extremely sedentary lifestyle
Intrauterine growth retardation during pregnancy
Poorly controlled hypertension
Orthopedic limitations
Poorly controlled seizure disorder
Poorly controlled hypothyroidism
Heavy smoker

Table 3
Warning Signs to Terminate Exercise While Pregnant (reprinted with permission from the American College of Obstetricians and Gynecologists. Exercise During Pregnancy and the Postpartum Period [Committee Opinion No. 267], Washington, DC © ACOG 2002)

Vaginal Bleeding
Dyspnea prior to exertion
Dizziness
Headache
Chest pain
Muscle weakness
Calf Pain
Preterm labor
Decreased fetal movement
Amniotic fluid leakage

a low birth weight infant. Notably, however, low-birth-weight infants of women who exercised during pregnancy do not necessarily have the usual complications of low birth weight *(84)*.

Exercise is also safe during the postpartum period. For the first 4–6 weeks, many of the physiologic changes of pregnancy persist. Women may return to a comfortable exercise program as soon as their bodies allow. Women, who exercised prior to pregnancy but not during pregnancy, will be deconditioned when they resume their former routine. Their return to exercise should be gradual. In addition, examination for persistent rectus diastasis, SI joint dysfunction, or other related musculoskeletal problems may be helpful to avoid complications related to return to exercise in the postpartum population.

3.11. Summary

In conclusion, integrated pain programs in women's health should be capable of offering a variety of treatment options to the pregnant or postpartum woman with musculoskeletal pain. Pharmacological options for treating pain in pregnancy exist but are relatively limited. In addition, pregnant and nursing women, in particular, may wish to avoid medications and seek other methods of treatment such as physical or occupational therapy or CAM modalities. An integrated, interdisciplinary women's health program consisting of providers knowledgeable in pregnancy and postpartum-related conditions is often the ideal setting in which women can get help for such problems, as well as obtain guidance regarding exercise during pregnancy and return to fitness postpartum.

4. PELVIC PAIN AND PELVIC FLOOR MUSCLE DYSFUNCTION

4.1. Introduction

Pelvic pain and pelvic floor muscle dysfunction are common problems among women of childbearing age and these issues may persist without appropriate treatment. In addition, many women during the postmenopausal years may suffer from urinary incontinence or painful symptoms in the pelvic region due to the extensive hormonal changes occurring during that time period. Women with pelvic pain and disorders of the pelvic floor may benefit from treatment in an interdisciplinary setting where they are offered conservative therapeutic options that may replace or act in an adjunctive manner to surgical interventions and/or pharmacological modalities when outcomes are sub-optimal or risks are unacceptable. The complex and sensitive nature of pelvic problems demands compassionate and knowledgeable women's health providers who are comfortable with the multi-specialty collaboration that is often required in their management. Pain management specialists in women's health should build reliable referral sources within the fields of gynecology, urology, gastroenterology, endocrinology, and psychology/psychiatry, as well as within the disciplines of physical and occupational therapy and with alternative health providers who are experienced in dealing with women's health issues.

4.2. Chronic Pelvic Pain

Chronic pelvic pain is defined as pain in lower abdomen, groin, upper thighs, vulva, or posterior pelvis of greater than six months in duration. It is estimated that over 10 million women are affected and 15% of women between ages 15 and 50 years of age are thought to suffer from this condition. Chronic pelvic pain accounts for 10% of all gynecologic office visits and is the main reason underlying 20% of laparoscopies (88). In addition, 10–15% of hysterectomies are performed as a treatment for chronic pelvic pain (89). After laparoscopic evaluation for chronic pelvic pain, 61% of women will remain undiagnosed (90). Depending on the healthcare provider they see, these women may be led to believe that their pain is entirely psychological in nature and may not be referred on for further diagnosis and management of their pain problem. Such women are clearly at high-risk of developing a chronic pain syndrome with the associated morbidity of impaired function, altered work and family roles, extensive deconditioning, sleep disturbance, and depression and anxiety. Patients with chronic pain syndromes typically develop pain that is beyond that expected due to the underlying pathology and is unresponsive to usual treatments. Although such findings may be due to the process of sensitization of the nervous system, these patients are frequently labeled as having purely psychological sources of their pain. Compassionate interdisciplinary and multi-specialty care is almost universally needed to help such patients.

The differential diagnosis of chronic pelvic pain is extensive and includes gynecologic, urologic, gastrointestinal, neurological, and musculoskeletal etiologies. Many of these diagnoses, such as pain of myofascial origin, are poorly recognized by traditional providers caring for women with pelvic pain problems. Again, this may lead to the determination that the patient's pain is purely psychogenic. However, more often than not psychological symptoms and signs of depression and anxiety are a result of unremitting pain and loss of function rather than the sole cause of such symptoms. When physical symptoms are not fully accounted for by a medical condition this more often represents stress reactivity rather than a true somatization disorder. In addition, chronic pelvic pain is often likely to be multifactorial. Through the process of visceral to somatic conversion (see Chapter 2), disorders of the internal organs can lead to myofascial trigger points (91). Unless the patient is treated comprehensively addressing both the visceral and the somatic pathology, recovery will be incomplete at best.

Characteristic qualities of visceral pain are its lack of association with visceral injury, its referral to other locations, its diffuse and poorly localized nature, and its accompanying motor and autonomic reflexes. The diffuse and poorly localized nature of visceral pain is due to the relative paucity of visceral afferent pathways as compared to those from somatic tissue *(92)*. Once visceral pain becomes referred to somatic structures, it tends to become sharper and more localized. Frequently, hyperalgesia will develop in the muscle layers within the referral zone, but may even extend to the skin and subcutaneous tissues in severe cases *(93)*. Muscle hyperalgesia within the zones of referred pain has been shown to develop in patients with various visceral pathologies including renal and biliary colic and primary dysmenorrhea *(93)*. This is likely due to the mechanisms of central and peripheral sensitization, as well as reflex arcs resulting in sustained musculature contraction. In addition, the process of viscero-visceral hyperalgesia can result in pain in one internal organ due to a painful process in another organ whose segmental afferent innervation is at least partially overlapping such as that of the female reproductive organs and the urinary tract that share T10-L1 as common segments *(94)*.

In addition, myofascial dysfunction due to trigger points may give rise to visceral dysfunction in organs sharing segmental innervation *(95)*. Thus, trigger points in the pelvic floor and hip girdle muscles may lead to painful bladder or uterine symptoms. In this manner, injuries to the musculoskeletal system can provoke symptoms in visceral organs and may lead to chronic pelvic pain of myofascial origin with associated visceral dysfunction. For example, residual SI joint dysfunction from prior traumatic injury or pregnancy (see above section) may lead to trigger points in the piriformis and other pelvic stabilizing muscles including the pelvic floor. Then, through the process of somatic to visceral convergence this could cause urinary frequency and urgency symptoms. In such instances, treatment of the myofascial pain results in symptoms resolution. Therefore, the majority of patients with chronic pelvic pain complaints would benefit from a full evaluation of the musculoskeletal system including a structural and myofascial examination.

Among the integrative therapies that may benefit the patient with pelvic pain and/or pelvic muscle dysfunction are biofeedback, electrical stimulation, manual myofascial release, pelvic floor muscle exercises, trigger point injections, osteopathic manipulation, yoga, and acupuncture. In addition, dietary and lifestyle modifications may be of benefit and a substantial amount of treatment time should be devoted to counseling the patient regarding these issues. Although many of these treatments may not be covered by health insurance companies, some of these, such as biofeedback, electrical stimulation, and manual therapy may be provided by physical and occupational therapists as part of the overall treatment plan. Referring providers should be sure that the treating therapists are experienced in these modalities and optimal results are most likely obtained with a collaborative team approach.

Patients with chronic pelvic pain, dypareunia, and vulvodynia may benefit from such integrative therapies. Biofeedback is a commonly used treatment for disorders of the pelvic floor and may help to decrease painful symptoms by helping patients to regain a sense of pelvic floor muscle relaxation. Feedback can be provided to the patient with either internal measurements of pelvic floor muscle tone via perineometers or surface electromyography. Perineometers that measure pelvic floor muscle activity internally are inserted into the vagina and sense intravaginal pressure changes. Information regarding normal values is limited to one study of 142 asymptomatic women that found an average resting intravaginal pressure of 5 mm HG with increases to an average of 15 mm Hg with voluntary pelvic floor muscle contraction *(96)*. Surface EMG electrodes also appear to provide good estimations of pelvic floor muscle tone when placed superficially on the pelvic floor 1 cm anterior to the anus *(97)*. Research regarding this technique is limited and generally of poor quality. However, one study found significantly reduced pain scores and analgesic use in a small group of patients with chronic rectal pain and tenderness of the levator ani muscle after a course of biofeedback *(98)*. EMG biofeedback has also been studied in women diagnosed with vulvodynia demonstrating decreased pain levels and resumption of sexual activity in a significant percentage of subjects *(99–101)*.

Electrical stimulation and manual therapy may also be helpful treatments for painful disorders of the pelvis. In a retrospective review of 66 women with pelvic pain and levator ani muscle spasm treated with transvaginal electrical stimulation, 68% had improvement of symptoms at the conclusion of the study with the majority of patients undergoing three or less sessions *(102)*. Thiel was the first to develop specific techniques of rectal massage for coccygodynia and levator ani muscle pain. He reported cures in 70% of 324 of his patients treated with this technique combined with treatment of anal infection when necessary *(103)*. A separate study evaluated Thiel's massage technique combined with relaxation exercises and rectal diathermy and found 59% of subjects reported marked or complete resolution of pelvic floor pain *(104)*. Other studies have focused on manual therapy for interstitial cystitis that is often associated with levator ani muscle tenderness or spasm *(105,106)*. Although thought to be a neuroinflammatory disorder of the bladder, treatment of associated myofascial dysfunction appears to be helpful in a subset of patients *(107)*.

In clinical practice, any one pelvic floor treatment technique is rarely applied in isolation for painful symptoms. A typical evaluation and treatment regimen for the patient with symptoms of pelvic pain, dypareunia, and/or vulvodynia would involve gynecological evaluation followed by referral to the pain specialist for examination of the musculoskeletal and neurological systems. This examination should focus on uncovering signs of peripheral and central sensitization, ensuring normal neurological function to rule out underlying central or peripheral nervous system disorder, and identifying musculoskeletal risk factors for pelvic pain such as sacroiliac joint malalignment and myofascial pain in the pelvic floor, hip rotators and lumbar spine. Depending on the clinical findings, referral is then made to various allied health or alternative providers usually in combination with appropriate medication management for more severely affected patients. For example, patients with evidence of extensive structural issues and associated myofascial findings but minimal signs of sensitization, frequently benefit from a program that includes localized trigger point injections and exercises to stretch the hip rotators and pelvic floor muscles followed by progressive strengthening of the pelvic stabilizers. This exercise program could be taught by a physical therapist specializing in women's health. In addition, yoga therapists with an interest in women's health issues can help patients to develop a similar exercise program with the added benefits of awareness, relaxation and stress reduction. For patients with limited voluntary pelvic floor muscle control, biofeedback or electrical stimulation may also be prescribed. In those patients with significant sensitization, direct and invasive treatments are limited, especially during the initial phases of treatment. These patients are often started on oral agents such as low-dose tricyclic antidepressants or anticonvulsants to decrease sensitivity and increase tolerance of other therapies. For those patients wishing to avoid medications, acupuncture is a less direct needling technique than trigger point injections that can help to decrease sensitization in certain patients. Another benefit to acupuncture is the concomitant treatment of visceral and somatic dysfunction, as well as the potential to improve hormone imbalance issues that may be present.

4.3. Urinary Incontinence

In addition to chronic pelvic pain, many patients with pelvic floor muscle disorders suffer from urinary incontinence. It is estimated that approximately 13 million Americans are affected by this condition that can be extremely functionally limiting *(108)*. Despite the widespread nature of the problem, a very small percentage of women with this condition seek medical care *(109)*. Urinary incontinence is not limited to elderly or multiparous women. In one study, nearly one-third of nulliparous female athletes reported loss of urine during participation in their sport *(110)*. A multidisciplinary treatment approach focusing on rehabilitation of the pelvic floor muscles may be helpful to women with mild to moderate urinary incontinence. In general, surgery is considered more beneficial to those women with severe incontinence or organ prolapse, but need not entirely exclude non-surgical approaches *(111)*.

Pelvic floor muscle rehabilitation has also been studied in the treatment of urinary incontinence. Many of these studies offered combined treatment regimens, including biofeedback, pharmacotherapy, manual treatments, exercises, and electrical stimulation, making it difficult to separate out the effects of any one modality. One study comparing pelvic floor muscle training with a home biofeedback unit versus pelvic floor exercise alone for female stress urinary incontinence found significantly greater improvement in the biofeedback group at 12 weeks *(112)*. However, at one year follow up the two groups were found to be equal in terms of their symptoms, which were significantly improved compared to their baseline *(113)*. In a study comparing pelvic floor muscle training with pelvic floor muscle exercises, biofeedback and electrical stimulation begun 2 months postpartum versus no treatment, the incidence of stress urinary incontinence was significantly reduced in the treatment group at 10 months postpartum *(114)*. Pelvic floor electrical stimulation has also been successfully used in the treatment of stress urinary incontinence *(115)*. Frequencies of 20–50 Hz with pulse durations of 1–5 ms have been reported to be the most effective for urethral closure *(116)*.

4.4. Summary

In conclusion, pelvic pain and urinary incontinence are significant problems that affect substantial numbers of women. However, many women go without diagnosis and treatment for these issues. Surgical approaches to pelvic pain are often of incomplete or temporary benefit. Although the surgical treatment of stress urinary incontinence is reported to be successful, this may be of unacceptable risk for many patients. Pharmacological treatments are frequently of partial benefit and may also be associated with side effects. Many women may prefer conservative treatment options. More complex patients are unlikely to benefit without an interdisciplinary, multimodal approach to their issues. Integrative pain programs in women's health should provide women with various conservative treatment options and are ideally led by a pain specialist who can determine on an individual basis, which patients are most likely to benefit from certain integrative treatment regimens. In this way, combined treatments can be applied on a patient-by-patient basis with improved outcomes for sometimes complicated and longstanding problems as the goal.

5. FIBROMYALGIA

5.1. Introduction

Fibromyalgia is a widespread central nervous system–mediated chronic pain disorder. The diagnosis of fibromyalgia (FM) is primarily a clinical one, but should be considered a diagnosis of exclusion occurring in the absence of other systemic illness that may explain the patient's symptoms, for example other rheumatoglic disorders. The prevalence of FM in the United States has been estimated at 3.4% of women and 0.5% of men, for a total of 3.7 million Americans *(117,118)*. The reasons for the preponderance of women who suffer from this disorder remain unclear but one hypothesis is differences in pain processing between men and women due to sex hormone differences as discussed in the first section of this chapter. However, good qualities studies on the influence of sex hormones in fibromyalgia are lacking at this time.

The diagnosis of FM is based on at least a 3-month history of widespread pain that is bilateral and includes the upper and lower body and spine, as well as the presence of excessive tenderness when 4 kg of pressure is applied to 11 of 18 muscle tendon sites *(119)*. Recognizing associated symptoms—such as non-restorative sleep, daytime fatigue, dysmennorhea, irritable bowel/bladder syndrome, restless leg syndrome, dysautonomia, endocrine dysfunction, cognitive dysfunction, dizziness, cold intolerance, headaches, and mood disorders—is integral to successful functional improvement and treatment. Osteoarthritis and other musculoskeletal problems can concur with FM and if suspected, may require further evaluation and treatment or specialty referral.

Like other chronic pain syndromes, FM is often defined by subjective symptoms and lacks specific and unique pathophysiologic characteristics. Thus, the nature and existence of illnesses such as FM are often questioned. The comorbidity of mood disorders leads to concern about whether this is a stress-related or somatization disorder; however, evidence of abnormal pain processing via brain imaging and higher concentrations of cerebrospinal fluid substance P when compared to healthy controls supports a pathophysiologic process in FM syndrome, as seen in other chronic pain syndromes. Nevertheless, research continues to demonstrate that the clinical expression of FM and related disorders depends greatly on psychosocial factors. Because of these psychosocial factors, treatment can be very challenging.

5.2. Treatment and Management

Upon diagnosis of FM, a stepwise program is recommended based on current evidence *(120)*. Recent research has delineated clusters of FM patients in order to help identify the most efficacious treatment plan for each patient (Table 4) *(121)*. It is important to validate the patient's symptoms and emphasize the nondestructive nature of FM. Patients may be hoping for a "magic pill" or "quick fix"; therefore, education regarding the goal of FM treatment as improved functioning, and not the complete elimination of all symptoms, is vital to avoid unrealistic expectations. It is important to clearly explain all aspects of treatments and stress the significance of the patient's active role in any treatment.

Level I Treatment (Patient Education and Lifestyle Changes)

Patient education and lifestyle modification may adequately treat patients who fall into clusters 1 and 3. A healthy lifestyle, including the avoidance of caffeine, eating a healthy diet, regular exercise, stress reduction, and proper sleep hygiene, may help to

Table 4
Subgroups of Fibromyalgia Patients

Cluster 1: "Typical FM Patient in Primary Care"
- Low tenderness
- Moderate depression/anxiety
- Moderate catastrophizing
- Moderate control over pain

Cluster 2: "FM Patient in Tertiary Care"
- High tenderness
- High depression/anxiety
- High catastrophizing
- Low control for pain

Cluster 3: "FM Patient With Neurobiologic Presentation"
- High tenderness
- Low depression/anxiety
- Low catastrophizing
- High control over pain

control many symptoms. Much of this education can take place in the physician's office. Exercise is a mandatory component, with the caveat that the patient begins slowly and advances as tolerated. Patients should be counseled regarding gentle exercise rather than vigorous, jarring body movements. Swimming, walking, and low-impact aerobics are generally well-tolerated *(122,123)*. Another option would be one-on-one instruction in alternative forms of exercise such as gentle yoga or Tai Chi to help patients understand their individualized needs and limitations. Once patients are sufficiently aware of such they may choose to practice on their own at home or in a class setting suing the knowledge they gained from one-on-one instruction to guide them.

Level II Treatment (Monitored Pharmacologic Treatment With Skilled Care)

Healthcare providers may consider initiating medications and referrals to monitored or supervised therapies for cluster 2 patients or patients who do not respond to level 1 treatment *(120)*.

5.3. Drug Therapies

In FM, medications are typically geared toward symptom management and generally require a combination of agents *(124)*. Pharmacotherapy has been most successful with central nervous system agents, including medications in the classes of antidepressants, muscle relaxants, and anticonvulsants. These medications have effects on various neurochemicals (e.g., serotonin, norepinephrine, substance P), which in turn affect activity in the brain and spinal cord, including modulation of pain sensation and tolerance. To date, the US Food and Drug Administration has not approved any of the medications reviewed here for treatment of FM, although this is likely to change in the future with new developments in randomized, controlled trials. Medications with moderate to strong efficacy for the treatment and management of FM syndrome are summarized in Table 5.

Tricyclic antidepressants, especially amitriptyline, have shown the strongest efficacy in FM management, including improving quality of sleep and sense of well-being and relieving fatigue and pain *(125)*. Other antidepressant medications, such as the selective serotonin reuptake inhibitor (SSRI), fluoxetine, have shown moderate efficacy

Table 5
Medications for Fibromyalgia Syndrome

Tricyclic antidepressants
Amitriptyline 25–50 mg at bedtime
Nortriptyline 30 mg at bedtime
Cyclobenzaprine 10–30 mg at bedtime
Analgesics
Tramadol with or without acetaminophen 200–300 mg/d
SSRIs
Fluoxetine 20–80 mg with or without tricyclic at bedtime
Sertraline 50 mg
SNRIs**
Venlafaxine 75 mg/d
Milnacipran <200 mg/d
Duloxetine 60 mg bid
Anti-convulsants*
Pregabalin 450 mg/d

*Selective serotonin reuptake inhibitor
**Serotonin norepinephrine reuptake inhibitor

in managing FM symptoms. Adding a second antidepressant or medication is often necessary *(126–128)*. Selective norepinephrine reuptake inhibitors (SNRIs) have the added benefit of raising both serotonin and norepinephrine levels. Several of these agents have demonstrated efficacy with FM patients *(129,130)*. Analgesic medications including tramadol, taken with or without acetaminophen, have demonstrated efficacy in reducing pain in 3 randomized, controlled trials of FM patients *(131–133)*. Cyclobenzaprine has been found to be as effective as amitriptyline *(134–136)*. NSAIDs may be useful for pain relief when combined with TCAs, although there is no evidence that these drugs are effective when used alone *(137)*.

FM patients may be taking many other medications, dietary supplements, or herbal remedies with the potential for adverse interactions and are often more sensitive to side effects. Patients should be asked about any over-the-counter or nonprescription medications they are taking. Some antidepressants lower the seizure threshold and, when combined with other agents, such as tramadol, could lower this threshold further. SSRIs may cause drug interactions because of their inhibition of the cytochrome P-450 system. Since the cardiovascular effects of tricyclic antidepressants include postural hypotension, FM patients with dysautonomia, hypotension, heart disease, including cardiac conduction abnormalities or arrhythmias should avoid the use of these drugs. An ECG is indicated to rule out prolonged QT interval or other rhythm abnormalities in any patient for whom there is concern of beginning a tricyclic antidepressant. They should also be used with caution in patients with hepatic dysfunction, since antidepressant medications are eliminated through the liver.

5.4. Skilled Therapy

Physical therapy is shown to be highly beneficial for patients with FM *(123,138,139)*. Because patients will likely experience an increase in pain, soreness, and discomfort as they embark on a physical therapy treatment and an exercise routine, they should be educated about the difference in "protective" acute pain and "nonprotective" chronic pain. It is also important to teach patients how to self-manage flare-ups using a variety of modalities, including ice, heat, self-massage, and self–trigger point release. Strength training and aerobic exercise have confirmed efficacy *(123,138–140)*, while stretching and flexibility exercises have shown weak to no efficacy *(141)*. Pool exercise and indoor walking are often well-tolerated *(142–144)*.

5.5. Psychological and Mind–Body Therapies

FM patients are at high risk for developing secondary mood disorders such as depression and anxiety. It is important to recognize and treat psychological problems in the early stages, as mood symptoms will interfere with successful treatment. Psychological treatment can strengthen self-efficacy and help the patient develop tools for dealing with stress to reduce the impact of FM on all aspects of the patient's life *(145)*. Cognitive behavioral therapy (CBT), conducted by a psychologist with expertise in behavioral medicine and aimed at cognitive restructuring and improving functional status, has been shown to be highly beneficial. Research has shown that CBT can provide significant abatement in pain and fatigue and improvement in social and occupational functioning *(146–149)*. Mind–body techniques, such as meditation, relaxation, and self-hypnosis, have also demonstrated benefit for FM patients *(150)*.

5.6. Other Nondrug Therapies

These treatment components can be utilized and recommended to patients at any point in the presentation of symptoms. Education and support groups are among the therapies with moderate to strong efficacy, and they can assist with coping and validation of symptoms. Acupuncture, biofeedback, hypnotherapy, and balneotherapy have also demonstrated efficacy in management of FM symptoms *(151–154)*. Massage and connective tissue manipulation have been shown to reduce severity of pain and amount of analgesics used *(155,156)*. There is mild evidence for the efficacy of chiropractic treatment, electrotherapy, and trigger point injections *(157,158)*. Patients who are employed report less pain and fatigue and better overall functioning *(159,160)*. An occupational therapist may be involved to assist patients in making environmental modifications for continuing or returning to work.

Level III Treatment (Multidisciplinary Program)

Patients for whom levels 1 and 2 treatment have failed and the majority of patients in cluster 2 should be referred to a multidisciplinary treatment program *(161–163)*. The team of providers in such centers have familiarity with the treatment of a variety of chronic pain conditions such as fibromyalgia; they include physicians, psychologists, psychiatrists, nurses, physical therapists, occupational therapists, vocational counselors, social workers, and other specialized healthcare providers. Such programs emphasize structured rehabilitation and typically include education, progressive exercise, individual or group cognitive behavioral therapy, and medical management of pain, fatigue, mood, and other symptoms in a coordinated fashion.

5.7. Summary

Fibromyalgia is a chronic condition characterized by widespread pain with multiple tender points, fatigue, sleep disturbances, mood disorders, and clinically significant functional impairments. Patients with FM pose a challenge to healthcare practitioners because the condition affects multiple aspects of physical as well as psychological functioning. Upon diagnosis, a stepwise program of evidence-based treatments is recommended. Empirically supported treatments include a combination of healthy lifestyle modifications, medication, physical therapy, and psychological treatment for the optimal outcome. The healthcare provider plays a vital role in educating the patient about FM. It is important to validate the patient's experience while emphasizing the nondestructive nature of FM. Healthcare providers should be very clear with patients that the ultimate goal is an improvement in quality of life and level of functioning, not the total elimination of pain. However, they can reassure patients that there is evidence showing that these goals are realistic and achievable based on the collaboration and active participation of the primary healthcare provider, allied FM specialists, and the patient.

6. OTHER MUSCULOSKELETAL ISSUES IN WOMEN

6.1. Osteoporosis

6.1.1. INTRODUCTION

Osteoporosis is the most common metabolic bone disease in the United States. In most cases, primary osteoporosis develops over a lifetime. Failure to accumulate adequate bone mass during the first three decades of life, failure to maintain adequate bone mass during the middle decades, and then accelerated bone loss at menopause all contribute to the disease. Genetic, hormonal, environmental, and nutritional factors cause the rate of bone degradation (resorption) to exceed that of bone formation, resulting in reduced bone mineral density. The reduced bone mineral density is primarily in the trabecular bone mass but the bone's mineral content remains unchanged.

Decreased bone mineral density is a major risk factor for fracture. It is estimated that over 1.3 million osteoporotic fractures occur each year in the United States. Approximately one-half of these fractures are vertebral fractures, one-quarter are hip fractures, and one-quarter are Colles' fractures *(164)*. Pelvic and hip fractures are associated with increased mortality, although the premorbid conditions associated with the fracture account for most of the deaths *(165)*. Hip fracture rates are approximately 10-fold higher in the nursing home residents *(166)*. Ability to transfer independently, which is a marker of ambulatory status, is an independent predictor of fracture in these women *(167)*.

Osteoporosis has many risk factors, including tobacco use, sedentary lifestyle, low body weight, and female gender. Female gender predisposes to osteoporosis due to lower baseline mean peak bone mass and accelerated bone loss after menopause *(168)* After age 50, a hip or vertebral fracture is three times more likely for a woman than for a man (16 to 18 percent versus 5 to 6 percent) and a Colles fracture is six times more likely for a woman (16 percent versus 2.5 percent) *(169)*.

Bone loss begins in early menopause, most significantly due to estrogen deficiency. After menopause, the ovary secretes little or no estrogen. Estrogen deficiency changes the balance between osteoblastic cells (involved in bone building) and osteoclastic cells (involved in bone destruction) because osteoblastic cell function requires estrogen. Estrogen receptors have been identified osteoblastic cells, and in vitro studies have demonstrated the hormone's direct effect on the proliferation and differentiation of these cells *(170)*. Relative estrogen deficiency also occurs in women with anorexia nervosa. These women tend to have low bone density, and has been found to be more than two standard deviations below normal in 50% *(171)*. The bone loss is caused by low production of both estrogen and insulin-like growth factor-1 *(172)*.

Exogenous administration of estrogen in postmenopausal women results in decreased bone resorption, increased plasma 1,25 vitamin D levels, increased gastrointestinal calcium absorption, and increased renal tubular calcium reabsorption. Ultimately, estrogen decreases the rate of bone resorption *(173)*. Long-term estrogen therapy in postmenopausal women reduces the incidence of fractures of the vertebrae, distal forearm, and hip by approximately 50% *(174)*. The excess bone loss in women can be prevented by estrogen therapy *(175)*. However, estrogen is no longer a first-line therapy for prevention of bone loss, due to its other potential cardiovascular and breast cancer risks. Progestins, selective estrogen receptor modulators (SERMs), and bisphosphonates have replaced estrogens treatment.

Some studies estimate that as much as 75 percent of bone lost in the years after menopause can be attributed to estrogen deficiency rather than age *(176)*. Women lose approximately 50% of their trabecular bone and 35% of cortical bone during their lifetime. Although the lifetime effects of dietary, environmental, and age-associated factors contribute to bone loss, estrogen deficiency alone causes an estimated that 25% of the trabecular bone loss and 15% of cortical bone loss *(177)*. Menopause-related bone loss lasts for about 10 years. After this time, the rate of bone loss is diminished to near the rate with aging *(178)*. Age-related bone loss compounds osteoporosis in post-menopausal women. Beginning in the fourth or fifth decades, cortical and trabecular bone masses decrease in both men and women *(179)*. This age-related bone loss continues into the 9th and 10th decades in women, and may be partially due to decreased calcium absorption and is a factor which is attenuated by calcium supplementation.

Race also likely influences osteoporosis. In a longitudinal study of approximately 2300 premenopausal and early perimenopausal women, lumbar spine bone density measurements (adjusted for other factors known to affect bone density) in women under 70 kg was similar for African-American, Japanese, and Chinese women, but lower in Caucasians *(132)*. In these same studies, Asian women were also found to have a lower bone density-specific fracture risk than Caucasian women. Asian women appear to have a lower risk of fracture than Caucasian women *(180)*. This can perhaps also be attributed to increased soy in their diet.

6.1.2. TREATMENT

Prevention and treatment of osteoporosis consist of both non-drug and drug therapies. In the past, estrogen therapies were used to prevent and treat postmenopausal osteoporosis. Additionally, estrogen reduced menopausal symptoms and was believed to reduce cardiovascular disease. However, when data from the Women's Health Initiative (WHI) revealed that estrogen-progestin therapy does not reduce the risk of coronary heart disease, and increases the risk of breast cancer, stroke, and venous thromboembolic events, other therapies were sought *(181)*. As a result of these findings, other antiresorptive agents are now the drugs of choice, and are prescribed more frequently for the prevention and treatment of osteoporosis in postmenopausal women *(182)*.

There are three major components to the non-drug therapy of osteoporosis: diet, exercise, and smoking cessation. In addition, affected patients should avoid, if possible, drugs that increase bone loss, such as glucocorticoids.

An optimal diet for treatment (or prevention) of osteoporosis includes an adequate calorie, calcium, and vitamin D intake. In general, premenopausal women require greater than 1000 mg/day in premenopausal women and postmenopausal women require greater than 1500 mg/day (if they are not taking estrogen) (183). Postmenopausal women (and older men) should take supplemental calcium, in divided doses, at mealtime, such that their total calcium intake, inclusive of food calcium, approximates 1,500 mg/day. Women should also ingest a total of 800 IU of vitamin D daily. Higher doses are required if they have malabsorption or rapid metabolism of vitamin D due to anticonvulsant drug therapy.

In addition to supplemental calcium and Vitamin D, phytoestrogens have garnered attention as alternative treatments for osteoporosis. A phytoestrogen is a compound with estrogen-like effects on the central nervous system, induces estrus, and stimulates growth of the genital tract of female animals. More than 300 plants have been identified to have sufficient estrogenic activity to induce estrus in animals.

Phytoestrogens can be divided into three classes: isoflavones, coumestans, and lignans. All have chemical structures similar to natural and synthetic estrogens and estrogen antagonists. Isoflavones and coumestans are the most common phytoestrogens. Soybeans and soy foods are the most significant sources of isoflavones. Chickpeas and other legumes, as well as clover and bluegrass, are also sources of isoflavones. Coumestans are found in plants, with only a few isomers having estrogenic activity, such as those found in alfalfa, clover, and other fodder crops. Legumes and seeds, such as split peas, pinto bean seeds, lima bean seeds, and soybean sprouts, contain small amounts of coumestrol. Lignans are found primarily in flax seeds, pumpkin seeds, rye, broccoli, soybeans, and some berries. Flax seed oil is often refined and therefore depleted of the lignans. Thus, if using flax seed oil, find a product that is unfiltered and unrefined.

Animal studies have shown that soy isoflavones may prevent estrogen-related bone loss, but few data are available in humans, especially in the Asian populations. One double-blind placebo controlled randomized trial showed soy isoflavones have a mild, but significant, independent effect on the maintenance of hip BMC in postmenopausal women with low initial bone mass (184). The study enrolled 233 Chinese women, age 48–62, and randomly assigned them to one of three groups: daily doses of placebo (1 g starch; n = 67), mid-dose (0.5 g starch, 0.5 g soy extracts, and $\sim$40 mg isoflavones; n = 68), and high dose (1.0 g soy extracts and $\sim$80 mg isoflavones; n = 68). All were given 12.5 mmol (500 mg) calcium and 125 IU vitamin D_3 . Bone mineral density (BMD) and bone mineral content (BMC) of the whole body, spine, and hip were measured using dual energy x-ray absorptiometry at baseline and 1 year post-treatment. Multiple statistical analyses showed that women in the high dose group had mild, but statistically significantly, higher favorable change rate in BMC at the total hip and trochanter ($p < 0.05$) compared with the placebo and mid-dose groups. Further stratified analyses revealed that the positive effects of soy isoflavone supplementation were observed only among women with lower initial baseline BMC (median or less).

The effective dosage of total isoflavones to significantly reduce bone turnover is estimated at 90–100 mg/d (30–40 g soy protein), based on the limited available data. This amounts to 2–4 daily servings of soy food. Soy milk alternatives include soy beverages, yogurt, cheeses, sour cream, and frozen desserts. Soy flour, derived from ground soybeans, can be purchased as full fat, low fat, and defatted. In cooking, soy flour can be substituted for one-third of the all-purpose flour in most recipes, except in making yeast bread (Only substitute approximately 15% of the flour). There are many commercially prepared soy food products available, including textured soy protein items, such as patties, hot dogs, sausage links, and nuggets. In general, the products that are manufactured from textured soy protein, such as links, franks, and nuggets, have lower isoflavone content than minimally processed soy foods *(185)*.

Exercise is an excellent nonpharmacologic therapy for osteoporosis. Bone responds to mechanical stress by increasing its mass and strength, either by the direct impact from the weight-bearing activity or by the action of attached muscle. The incidence of hip fracture has been found to be 20–40% lower in individuals who report being physically active than in those who report being sedentary *(186)*. Inactive elderly women and men (i.e., rare stair climbing, gardening, or other weight-bearing activities) were more than twice as likely to sustain a hip fracture as those who were physically active, even after adjusting for differences in body mass index, smoking, alcohol intake, and dependence in daily activities *(187)*. A prospective study of more than 30,000 Danish men and women found that the incidence of hip fracture in active people who became sedentary was twice as high as in those who remained physically active *(188)*. The Nurses' Health Study of more than 61,000 postmenopausal women suggested that the relative risk of hip fracture was reduced by 6% for every 3 MET.h.WK^{-1} of physical activity, which is roughly equivalent to 1 h of walking per week *(189)*. Women reporting walking at least 4 h.WK^{-1} had a 41% lower risk of hip fracture compared with sedentary peers who walked less than 1 h.WK^{-1}, suggesting that even low-intensity weight-bearing activity, such as walking, may be beneficial in lowering fracture risk, even though minimal changes in BMD would be expected.

To be beneficial, exercise does not have to be done by the young. Older postmenopausal women and even the frail elderly can tolerate and potentially show improvements in muscle strength and BMD in response to strength training and resistive exercise programs. As an example, in a prospective cohort study of over 61,000 postmenopausal women, women who walked four hours or more per week had a 41 percent lower risk of hip fracture than those who walked one hour per week (RR 0.6; 95 percent CI 0.4 to 0.9) *(190)*. Exercise also appears to minimize the bone loss in anorexic women *(191)*, and bone density improves with recovery and resumption of normal menses *(192)*.

Women with osteoporosis (or those seeking to prevent it) should exercise (prudently) for at least 30 minutes three times per week *(193)*. Recommendations include weight-bearing exercise in the form of walking, mild- to moderate-impact aerobics, and resistance exercises as tolerated. Any weight-bearing exercise regimen, including walking, is can improve bone mineral density. The benefits of exercise were illustrated by the following two studies and one meta-analysis:

- A two-year trial investigated the effects of exercise and calcium supplementation on peak bone mass in 127 young women (aged 20 to 35 years). The women were randomly assigned to either an aerobics and weight training program or to a stretching program, and all received supplemental calcium (up to 1,500 mg/day, including dietary intake).

The aerobic/resistance training group demonstrated significant increases in bone mineral density in the spine (2.5%), femoral neck (2.4%), trochanter (2.3%), and calcaneus (6.4%), but the stretching group demonstrated no statistically significant improvement *(194)*.

- A one-year randomized controlled study of 40 postmenopausal women (aged 50 to 70 years) evaluated the effect of high-intensity strength training exercises upon bone mineral density. Femoral neck and lumbar spine density in the strength-trained women increased by 0.9% and 1.0%, respectively. In contrast, bone mineral density decreased by 2.5% and 1.8%, respectively, in the control group *(195)*.

The exercise regimen does not have to be intense; there is no convincing evidence that high-intensity exercise such as running is more beneficial than lower intensity exercise such as walking. Because continuation of the regimen is important (the benefits of exercise are quickly lost after the woman stops exercising) *(196)*, the patient should select a weight-bearing exercise regimen she enjoys to ensure long-term compliance. Balance training should be included in exercise programs for older individuals at risk of falling. Tai chi is an alternative form of exercise that can provide benefit for bone health and balance (see Chapter 12).

However, although weight-bearing exercise appears maintain or increase bone density at the lumbar spine and hip in postmenopausal women, no evidence suggests that it directly decreases fractures *(197)*. Indirectly, however it has been shown to reduce the risk of fall and fracture with muscle strengthening and improved balance. Reducing fall risk is crucial, but many factors contribute to falling, including diminished postural control, poor vision, reduced muscle strength, reduced lower limb range of motion, and cognitive impairment, as well as such extrinsic factors as psychotropic medications and tripping hazards.

Ultimately, exercise reduces falls only if it is directed to individuals who fall because they have poor muscle strength, balance, or range of motion. Reviews and meta-analyses of randomized trials suggest that exercise trials that included balance, leg strength, flexibility, and/or endurance training effectively reduced risk of falling in older adults. Regular exercise increases muscle mass and strength, improves balance and coordination, and has been shown to reduce the risk of falls by about 25% in frail elderly persons *(198)*. Weight-bearing aerobic activities should be done four days per week; resistance training (especially back extension and abdominal strengthening) two or three days per week; flexibility training five to seven days per week. Tai-chi and yoga are particularly helpful for balance training. However, a proper exercise regimen must be established with a health care professional prior to beginning.

While exercising, the intensity should be 40–70% VO_2 reserve for aerobic activities; progressive resistance training (PRT) (Borg RPE at 13 to 15)should include one or two sets of 8 to 10 repetitions. Pain status should dictate the exercise plan; patients limited by pain should consult a physician before initiating an exercise program. Patients with osteoporosis should avoid explosive movements and high-impact loading (e.g., jumping, jogging) and dynamic abdominal exercise with excessive trunk flexion and twisting (e.g., sit-ups, golf swing, bending while picking up objects) *(196)*.

Although exercise is widely believed to be important in the prevention and treatment of osteoporosis, several studies have found little or no effect of exercise interventions on the incidence of falls. A Cochrane database review concluded that exercise alone does not reduce fall risk in elderly women and men *(197)*. One possible reason for these negative results is that these studies frequently study very frail nursing home residents, who likely had multiple risk factors for falling which are unlikely to be improved by exercise (e.g., poor vision). Further, if the exercise intensity is too low (common in studies of the frail elderly), only minimal gains in muscle strength that might help reduce falling risk are achieved. Lastly, it must be recognized that the opportunity for falling probably increases as people become more physically active, particularly in community-dwelling elderly *(198)*.

In addition to exercise, other interventions that reduce the fall risk are crucial in managing osteoporosis. Patients should be counseled to remove loose rugs and cords, to ensure adequate lighting in their residence, and to avoid walking on ice or in unfamiliar areas outside. Although there are some conflicting data, hip protectors may be a valuable addition to a fall prevention program in nursing homes.

6.1.3. SUMMARY

Osteoporosis is a common problem among women, especially those of postmenopausal status. Women's health providers should have an understanding of the recommendations regarding prevention and treatment of this disease. Ultimately, prevention using an integrative approach is the best medicine when it comes to osteoporosis, as treatment can prove difficult and consequences, such as hip fractures, may be devastating.

7. KNEE PAIN IN WOMEN

7.1. Introduction

Some of the most common chronic painful conditions of the knee occur more commonly in women than in men. These conditions include knee osteoarthritis (OA) in older women *(199,200)*, patellofemoral pain syndrome (PFPS), and sports-related knee injuries such as tears of the anterior cruciate ligament (ACL) *(201,202)*. Women also do more poorly than men in long-term follow-up studies after menisectomy surgery *(203,204)* and may also have a greater risk than men of developing symptoms of complex regional pain syndrome (CRPS) following menisectomy *(205,206)*, although there is little published on this topic. The reasons behind these sex differences in knee pain remain incompletely understood and are likely to be multifactorial. Proposed theories include anatomical, neuromuscular, biomechanical, hormonal and environmental factors. This section will briefly outline some of the unique features of knee pain in women and how these conditions may be optimally treated within an integrative women's health pain management program.

7.2. Etiology

Given the higher rates of multiple knee problems in women, hormonal differences between the sexes have been implicated as a possible causative factor. The sex hormones may exert effects on various aspects of knee problems that may include differences in pain sensitivity as discussed earlier in this chapter, neuromuscular factors such as reaction time and coordination of muscle contraction, and biomechanical factors like ligamentous laxity. The role of ligamentous laxity needs to be further clarified but has been implicated in PFPS *(207)*, non-contact ACL tears *(208)*, and progression of knee OA *(209)*. In general, women tend to have more laxity of their ligaments than do men and this difference may be due to hormonal factors. Estrogen and relaxin have been implicated in ligamentous laxity of pregnancy and relaxin receptors have been identified on the human ACL *(210)*. In addition, significantly increased anterior-posterior (AP) laxity of the knee joints has been identified in women during pregnancy that appears to persist through at least 6 weeks postpartum *(63)*. This may be due to hormonal influences of pregnancy such as elevated estrogen and relaxin levels. However, it is unclear if ligaments ever fully regain their pre-pregnancy strength. In addition, the influence of ligamentous laxity may be more dramatic around the pelvic joints as discussed in the above section on pregnancy and postpartum-related problems. This could result in structural asymmetries such as pelvic obliquities that also affect knee alignment and mechanics. Such asymmetries may be particularly important in knee conditions that are associated with structural risk factors such as genum valgum, foot pronation and increased quadriceps angle (Q angle). The term "Miserable Malalignment syndrome" is used to describe a constellation of structural factors consisting of increased Q angle, femoral neck anteversion, genu valgum, external tibial torsion, and compensatory foot pronation that in combination greatly increase the risk of musculoskeletal injuries in women (Figure 2).

7.3. Patellofemoral Pain Syndrome

Patellofemoral pain syndrome (PFPS) is a term describing non-arthritic anterior knee pain emanating from the patellofemoral joint. This is one of the most common painful conditions affecting the knee and accounts for 25% of all knee injuries treated in sports medicine clinics *(211)*. This common and painful knee disorder has been found to occur significantly more frequently in women as compared to men *(212)*. The reasons for this remain unclear and are likely multifactorial as described above. The diagnosis is made clinically based on history and physical examination findings, although no one finding is pathognomonic. Patients often complain of a diffuse, vague ache of insidious onset most commonly felt in the anterior knee but sometimes with radiation to the popliteal fossa. The pain is commonly worse after prolonged sitting (theater sign), stair climbing, and deep knee bending. They may experience clicking in the knee and the sense of instability, but no true mechanical symptoms. The physical exam should focus on a structural evaluation, assessment of muscle strength and flexibility, careful examination of the patella itself, and active testing of patellar tracking *(213)*.

Once diagnosed, the treatment of PFPS should be considered threefold: (1) control symptoms, (2) correct biomechanical problems, and (3) address muscle imbalance issues. For symptom control, relative rest from pain-provoking activities and use of ice or heat is frequently recommended. Based on recent systematic reviews, there is limited evidence for the use of non-steroidal anti-inflammatories (NSAIDs) for short-term pain reduction and no clear usefulness of ultrasound in the treatment of PFPS *(214,215)*. Acupuncture has also been shown to be an effective treatment for symptom control in PFPS and may be preferable to patients who wish to avoid the adverse effects and potential morbidity of NSAID use *(216)*. The correction of biomechanical issues in PFPS has traditionally been through the use of McConnell taping or other orthoses that support the patella. In patients with over pronation, medial arch support foot orthoses may be helpful. However, structural issues along the entire kinetic chain may be corrected through various osteopathic manipulation techniques (see Chapter 15). Muscle imbalance should be addressed with an exercise program that not only focuses on stretching and strengthening of the lower extremities when specific deficits are noted but also on increasing core stability in order to promote improved posture and

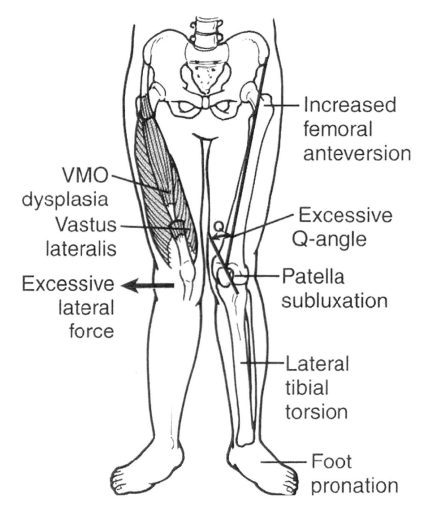

Fig. 2. Miserable malalignment syndrome: Illustration of the forces on the knee that can lead to patellofemoral tracking disorders (reprinted with permission from Magee, D. 2002 Orthopedic Physical Assessment, 4th edition. Saunders: Philadelphia, PA).

body mechanics. Yoga and/or pilates may help to achieve these goals in patients who may not require physical therapy. When myofascial trigger points exist in association with PFPS, these should be addressed through needling techniques in order to increase the effectiveness of prescribed exercises.

7.4. Knee Osteoarthritis

Osteoarthritis (OA) is the most prevalent musculoskeletal condition that causes joint pain and the knee is the most commonly affected joint *(217)*. In the United States, OA is the second leading cause of workplace disability *(218)*. The condition has both a greater prevalence in older women as compared to men and symptoms and disability due to knee OA are also worse in women *(200)*. The etiology and pathogenesis of OA remains incompletely understood but is thought to be due to a combination of biomechanical, biochemical, and genetic factors. Risk factors for the development of knee OA include increasing age, female gender, obesity, joint trauma, and knee malalignment. The contribution of factors such as physical activity and muscle weakness, in particular in the quadriceps muscles remains somewhat controversial. There currently remains no curative treatment for the disorder, and the only definitive surgical treatment is joint replacement surgery. Therefore, significant attention must be given to managing pain and preventing and treating functional deficits that result.

Because of its significant impact, many integrative treatments have been studied for knee osteoarthritis. The American College of Rheumatology (ACR) has stated in their consensus guidelines regarding the treatment of knee osteoarthritis that all pharmacologic agents should be considered additions to nonpharmacologic measures *(219)*. The American Geriatrics Society panel on the management of chronic pain in older persons agrees that drug treatment of pain is most effective when combined with nonpharmacological strategies *(220)*. Among the ACR guidelines for nonphar-macologic management are patient education and self-management programs, weight loss, if overweight, aerobic exercise programs, physical therapy for range of motion (ROM), stretching, and strengthening exercises, assistive devices, and patellar taping, orthotics (lateral wedge insoles, valgus brace, neoprene knee sleeve), and occupational therapy for joint protection and energy conservation strategies and assistive devices for activities of daily living (ADLs) *(219)*. Various CAM therapies are frequently used by patients with knee OA, several of which have shown efficacy. These include acupuncture, electromagnetic fields, glucosamine/chondroitin, and various other nutritional supplements, Tai Chi, and yoga. More details on these specific therapies in the treatment of knee OA can be found in the corresponding chapters in this book. In the setting of an integrative pain program patients benefit from a combination of medication, non-medication and CAM treatments. This multimodal type of treatment is commonly necessary in the treatment of chronic pain conditions such as knee OA.

7.5. ACL Injuries

Of additional concern regarding knee pain in women is the issue of female athletes and their increased risk of non-contact ACL tears. The female athlete has a 4- to 6-times greater risk of ACL injury as compared to male athletes competing at similar levels in the same sports *(202)*. These injuries can result in loss of entire seasons or sports careers *(221)*. In addition, ACL injury appears to have long-term consequences including increased risk of degenerative joint disease of the knee, a major cause of disability in older women *(222)*. As a result, increasing research interest has been given to the possible underlying etiological factors involved in injury to the ACL in female athletes and to various neuromuscular training strategies aimed at prevention *(223)*.

In terms of ACL injury in general, risk factors can be divided into several general categories including environmental, anatomical, hormonal, and neuromuscular. Several studies have examined various environmental factors, including playing surface, footwear and knee braces, but their contribution to ACL injury remains unclear. The Hunt Valley group, however, concluded that there may be some evidence that harder surfaces and longer cleats increase the risk of ACL injury by increasing the shoe-surface traction. More interesting, however, in regard to female ACL injuries are the anatomical, hormonal and neuromuscular differences between men and women that may contribute to the increased risk in female athletes *(223)*.

Among the anatomical risk factors identified as potential contributors to injury to the ACL are increased Q angle, knee valgus alignment, foot pronation, and the size of the femoral notch. Women are known to have increased Q angles as compared to men due to increased width of the pelvis amongst other anatomical factors. One study has shown that the Q angle of athletes sustaining knee injuries were significantly larger that those in uninjured athletes *(224)*. However, it is not clear if it is the Q angle per se that contributed directly to knee injury but the effects of an increased Q angle on other aspects of lower extremity static and dynamic alignment, in particular increased knee valgus angulation. This may be particularly important during landing from jumps as a valgus knee position is thought to be contribute to positions of risk for ACL injury *(225)*. In addition, increased Q angle appears to explain anywhere from 32% to 46% of the difference in varus-valgus positions in men versus women *(226)*. Other static postural faults that possibly contribute are excessive navicular drop, knee recurvatum, and excessive subtalar joint pronation *(227)*. Numerous studies have been conducted on femoral notch geometry and ACL injury without clear associations being found at this time, with possible increased injury associated with smaller femoral notches, which is generally true in females versus males *(221)*.

Hormonal differences between men and women also appear to contribute to the increased risk of ACL tears in female athletes. Animal studies had identified estrogen receptors on the ACLs of animals but results were conflicting regarding the effects of estradiol on ACL tissue in these models *(223)*. However, more recently studies have examined the effects of estrogen and progesterone on human ACL. In vitro studies revealed decreased fibroblast proliferation and type I procollagen synthesis in human ACL cell cultures with increasing doses of 17β-estradiol that plateaued at supraphysiologic levels. Increasing concentrations of progesterone, however, attenuated the inhibitory effects of estradiol on both fibroblast and collagen synthesis. In addition, control of estradiol levels resulted in increasing synthesis of type I procollagen and fibroblast proliferation with increasing levels of progesterone *(228,229)*. Clinical studies have therefore attempted to investigate the relationship between menstrual cycle phases/hormone levels and knee laxity as well as the relationship between knee laxity and risk of ACL tears. Problems with menstrual cycle related studies as mentioned earlier in this chapter are lack of clearly defined phases and failure of many studies to confirm phases with hormone measurements resulting in conflicting results. Still, significantly more noncontact ACL injuries appear to occur during the periovulatory phase of the menstrual cycle when estrogen levels are high, as compared to the luteal phase of the cycle, which is considered progesterone dominant *(230,231)*. These results appear consistent with the basic science research. In addition, no study has demonstrated increased risk of ACL injury during the luteal phase of the cycle, suggesting a possibly protective role for progesterone in preventing injury *(223)*.

Neuromuscular risk factors that have been suggested to contribute to ACL injury in women include altered movement patterns, altered muscle activation patterns, and inadequate muscle stiffness *(223)*. This has resulted in a large number of research articles examining a variety of training strategies to help prevent ACL injury in female athletes. Hewett et al. conducted a meta-analysis to attempt to make sense of these studies. This group found 6 studies that fulfilled their criteria with the overall results showing a decreased number of ACL injuries in the training group versus the control group. In analyzing the studies separately, it appeared that regimens emphasizing plyometrics combined with biomechanical analysis and technique training were important components of the studies that demonstrated decreased risk of ACL injury. Balance training alone did not appear to be effective *(202)*. However, single leg core stability training did appear beneficial in decreasing the rate of ACL injury in elite female handball players over two seasons *(232)*.

7.6. Conclusions

Women are at increased risk of developing knee pain throughout the lifecycle most likely due to a combination of interacting factors, including differences in sex hormones, ligamentous laxity, anatomical, biomechanical, and neuromuscular differences. Great attention should be given to prevention of knee injury in the young female athlete as considerable short-term and long-term consequences can result. Women may not respond as favorably as men to surgical treatments of knee problems and when possible conservative measures should be employed aggressively prior to surgical consideration. Among the integrative treatments that may benefit women with knee pain are acupuncture, trigger point injections, alternative forms of exercise such as Yoga and Tai Chi, osteopathic manipulative techniques, nutritional supplementation, weight loss if necessary, and neuromuscular athletic training programs for the athlete. Women presenting with knee pain would benefit from evaluation and treatment by a musculoskeletal pain specialist with an interest and knowledge of the important differences between men and women when it comes to knee problems.

8. UPPER EXTREMITY PAIN IN WOMEN

Women are at increased risk as compared to men of developing musculoskeletal pain of the upper extremities. The reasons for this are, again, multifactorial. An understanding of the myriad of upper extremity conditions that women may be affected by, the underlying reasons for this, and the recommended treatments is essential to the women's musculoskeletal health and pain medicine provider.

After age 10–12 years there are significant differences in physical performance between males and females. Females reach physiological and skeletal maturity and peak height velocity earlier than males. Women also have more body fat and less lean body mass than males, a difference that can be attributed to increased estrogens in the female and increased androgens in the male *(233)*. Females have less upper body strength, which even with training remains 30% to 50% less than that of males. Lower extremity strength is much closer in parity *(234)*. Despite these differences women show the same physiological training changes as males and experience significant increases in strength, power, and muscular endurance *(235)*.

Physiologic gender differences predispose women to upper extremity musculoskeletal disorders. Women have shorter upper extremities, an increased valgus-carrying angle, decreased upper extremity strength, and increased ligamentous laxity compared with males *(234)*. The shoulder, which is the body's most mobile joint, is particularly vulnerable. In younger females, increased joint laxity and decreased strength can cause shoulder problems. The vicious cycle of physiological joint instability, rotator cuff weakness, pain, posterior capsule tightness, and further imbalance results in persistent pain and dysfunction in overhead activities. Care should be taken to address scapular dysfunction. A specific diagnosis of the cause of the pain should be made. Restoration of normal range of motion and strength with proper sport biomechanics should be the goal.

Shoulder instability is a problem for young women. However, as she ages, a woman because susceptible to adhesive capsulitis, otherwise known as ''frozen shoulder.''

Frozen shoulder is defined by progressive pain and global loss of motion in the shoulder. Underlying rotator cuff tendinitis or bicipital tendinitis predispose a person to this disorder, but it is also associated with stroke, myocardial infarction, cervical radiculopathy, diabetes and pulmonary disease. Treatment is directed toward pain relief and functional restoration, often with a combination of exercises, local heat, ultrasonography, and NSAIDs or mild analgesic medications. Complete rehabilitation of a frozen shoulder often requires 1 to 2 years. Suprascapular nerve blockade, short courses of systemic steroids, and joint distention with intra-articular steroids have been shown to provide short-term benefit in some studies. Manipulative therapy or intra-articular steroid injections combined with physical therapy may provide improvement over longer periods. Surgical procedures and capsular distention with saline injection have reportedly proved useful in individual cases.

Acupuncture is frequently used to treat shoulder pain, despite sparse scientific evidence of its efficacy. A recent Cochrane database review evaluated nine trials of varying methodological quality. In all the trials, the intervention was poorly described and most used a different placebo. Two trials assessed short-term success (post intervention) of acupuncture for rotator cuff disease and could be combined in meta-analysis. There was no significant difference in short-term improvement associated with acupuncture when compared to placebo, but the studies' small sample size may produce a false negative. However, the results of a small pilot study demonstrated some benefit of both traditional and ear acupuncture plus mobilization over mobilization alone. Ultimately, the authors of the Cochrane review declared the sparse evidence inconclusive *(236)*.

Although the shoulder is the most lax joint, a woman's increased joint laxity predisposes her to injury in all of her joints. At the elbow, the female athlete can suffer from osteochondritis dissecans of the elbow with possible loose body formation and elbow dislocations. Osteochondritis dissecans, in particular, should be considered as a diagnosis in axially loading sports such as gymnastics, diving, cheerleading, and tumbling. Elbow dislocations most frequently occur in sports requiring aerial maneuvers. These conditions require surgical evaluation.

Although the bony elbow injuries require surgical evaluation, musculotendinous disorders at the elbow can often be treated by alternative means. Older women, althletic or not, frequently suffer from lateral epicondylitis ("tennis elbow"), which results from repetitive wrist extension. Appropriately aggressive stretching and strengthening of the arm and forearm musculature is frequently used to treat this condition. When exercise alone fails to relieve the pain, many people consider cortisone injections to the lateral epicondyle. A good alternative is trigger point injections to the associated upper extremity musculature.

Wrist, hand, and finger pain are also common in women. Women are often affected by painful osteoarthritis of the fingers and hands for reasons that remain unclear. Yoga, which is an ancient Indian practice, may be a useful treatment of musculoskeletal pain due to osteoarthritis. One study examined yoga as a complementary therapy for OA of the fingers *(237)*. Seventeen patients were randomly assigned either a yoga-based 10-week program or no additional treatment beyond the drugs received by both groups. The intervention subjects received eight 60-minute group sessions focusing on stretching and strengthening exercises emphasizing upper body extension and alignment. The yoga group showed significantly greater decreases in pain and tenderness and improved range of motion; no differences were found in grip strength or joint circumference.

Finger discomfort, particularly numbness, may also be caused by carpal tunnel syndrome (CTS). With advanced CTS, patients may notice decreased grip strength. In general, CTS is the most common peripheral nerve entrapment syndrome. It typically occurs in people older than 30 and is three times more common in women than in men. In most cases, the cause is unknown. However, people who use their hands and wrists repetitively are predisposed to it. Such activities include typing, driving, using vibratory tools and sports such as racketball and handball. Several systemic diseases also predispose to CTS, namely diabetes, pregnancy, menopause rheumatoid arthritis, hypothyroidism, acromegaly, gout, renal failure, and obesity.

Treatment of CTS generally depends upon disease severity. Activity modification is a crucial first step, particularly avoiding repetitive wrist and hand motions, implementing ergonomic work-stations, and reduced use of vibratory tools. Wrist splints, oral NSAIDs and local corticosteroid injections can also be helpful in the early stages. In some cases, however, CTS is a progressive disease and many patients ultimately require surgery. CAM treatments that have shown benefit in the treatment of carpal tunnel syndrome include yoga and acupuncture *(238,239)*.

Stenosing tenosynovitis, or "trigger finger," is a condition involving the flexor tendon of the thumb or individual finger causing catching or "locking" of the digit in flexion. Triggering is usually localized to the region of the first annular (A1) pulley of the flexor tendon sheath. Patients often report pain located at the proximal interphalangeal (PIP) joint of the finger or the interphalangeal (IP) joint of the thumb. Trigger finger is the most common entrapment tendonitis in the hand and wrist. Trigger Finger is found more commonly in women, with a frequency two to six times that observed in men. It usually presents in the fifth and sixth decades of life *(240)*. The thumb is most frequently involved, followed by the fourth and middle fingers.

Conventional initial treatment aims to reduce the inflammation around the tendon. Activity modification, nonsteroidal anti-inflammatory drugs (NSAIDs), splinting, and local steroid injection into the tendon sheath are initial treatment options. Activity modification includes minimizing activities that involve repetitive and prolonged gripping and grasping. A hand-based splint that prevents motion of the MP and PIP/IP joints may be worn at night to prevent excessive flexing and locking during sleep. Caution should be used with the amount of time spent in the splint to avoid permanent stiffness. Patel et al found that 66% of patients with their MP joint splinted at $10°$ to $15°$ of flexion for 6 weeks had relief of symptoms *(241)*. Cortisone injection may also be of benefit. An intial injection relieves symptoms in 84% of trigger fingers and in 92% of trigger thumbs, whereas a second injection increased relief to 91% and 97% of patients, respectively *(242)*. Cortisone injection can be repeated at 3-week intervals for a total of three injections, if necessary *(243)*. Care should be taken to avoid direct tendon injection as this may result in rupture. If three injections fail to provide adequate relief, surgery may be required. Surgical treatment involves percutaneous or open release of the A1 pulley.

After trigger finger, De Quervain tenosynovitis is the second most common stenosing tenosynovitis of the upper extremity. It involves the first dorsal compartment of the wrist, which includes the abductor pollicis longus (APL) and extensor pollicis brevis (EPB). In De Quervain tenosynovitis, the tendons of the APL and EPB become thickened from acute or repetitive trauma and interfere with the normal gliding mechanism through the sheath. Continued thumb motion, along with radial and ulnar deviation of the wrist, perpetuates the inflammation and swelling. Patients complain of pain and tenderness localized to the dorsoradial aspect of the wrist that is exacerbated with thumb and wrist motion. De Quervain tenosynovitis occurs most commonly in women between 30 and 50 years of age *(244)*. Mothers of infants aged 6 to 12 months and day care workers are frequently affected due to repetitive lifting of infants.

Similar to trigger finger, initial treatment aims to decrease the inflammation surrounding the tendons. Activity modification, NSAIDs, splinting, and local steroid injection into the tendon sheath are common treatment options. A pooled quantitative literature evaluation, however, found no benefit for rest or NSAID use. Injection of the tendon sheath of the first distal compartment reduces tendon thickening and inflammation and provides the most effective form of treatment. The first injection has been found to relieve symptoms in roughly 66% to 70% of patients, and a second injection permanently relieves symptoms in another 10% of patients. Use of injections along with splinting has been less effective, providing relief in 57% to 62% of patients *(245)*. Patients who fail injection therapy should be referred for surgical release of the first dorsal compartment.

As women, especially those involved in various athletic activities and repetitive tasks, are at high risk of developing upper extremity pain or injury, healthcare providers in women's health settings should have a high degree of comfort with diagnosing and treating these disorders.

9. CONCLUSIONS

As outlined in this chapter, women are at increased risk as compared to men of developing various musculoskeletal and pain disorders. There are likely to be multiple reasons for this but hormonal differences between the sexes may be important mediating factors and hormone imbalance issues should be sought in women presenting with pain problems. A simple way to accomplish this task is to have female patients fill out a menstrual history and to enquire about various hormone-related symptoms on the initial patient questionnaire. Those responding positively may be asked in more detail about their hormonal status. This is also a good way to uncover bothersome symptoms that a patient may not report of their own accord such as urinary incontinence or pelvic pain. Such symptoms may respond positively to various integrative treatment strategies.

Perhaps most importantly, a women's health program should make every effort to maintain a philosophy of care that emphasizes long-term health benefits and overall wellness. This is particularly important in women's health, as women are prone towards chronic and recurrent pain conditions. Although self-management and maintenance should be encouraged, on-going support for lifestyle changes may be necessary and can be provided by different members of the treatment team depending on individual patient preferences. In this type of supportive setting, women may be able to positively manage and cope with chronic painful conditions that frequently lack curative solutions.

REFERENCES

1. Barnes P, Powell-Griner E, McFann K, et al. Complementary and alternative medicine use among adults: United States, 2002. CDC Advance Data. 2004;343:1250–1270.
2. Berkley KJ. Sex differences in pain. Behavioral and Brain Sciences. 1997;20(3):371ff.
3. Fillingim RB. Sex-related influences on pain: A review of mechanisms and clinical implications. Rehabil Psychol 2003;48(3):165–174.
4. Fillingim RB, Maixner W. Gender differences in the responses to noxious stimuli. Pain Forum 1995;4(4):209–221.

5. Riley JL, Robinson ME, Wise EA, et al. Sex differences in the perception of noxious experimental stimuli: a meta-analysis. Pain 1998;74(2–3):181–187.

6. Fillingim RB, Maixner W, Kincaid S, et al. Sex differences in temporal summation but not sensory-discriminative processing of thermal pain. Pain 1998;75(1):121–127.

7. Ellermeier W, Westphal W. Gender differences in pain ratings and pupil reactions to painful pressure stimuli. Pain 1995;61(3):435–439.

8. Paulson PE, Minoshima S, Morrow TJ, et al. Gender differences in pain perception and patterns of cerebral activation during noxious heat stimulation in humans. Pain 1998;76(1–2):223–229.

9. Riley JL, Gilbert GH, Heft MW. Orofacial pain symptom prevalence: selective sex differences in the elderly? Pain 1998;76(1–2):97–104.

10. Buckwalter JA, Lappin DR. The disproportionate impact of chronic arthralgia and arthritis among women. Clin Orthopaed Relat Res 2000(372):159–168.

11. Rethelyi JM, Berghammer R, Kopp MS. Comorbidity of pain-associated disability and depressive symptoms in connection with sociodemographic variables: results from a cross-sectional epidemiological survey in Hungary. Pain 2001;93(2):115–121.

12. Robinson ME, Wise EA, Riley JL, et al. Sex differences in clinical pain: a multisample study. J Clin Psychol Med Setting 1998;5(4):413–424.

13. Aloisi AM, Ceccarelli I. Role of gonadal hormones in formalin-induced pain responses of male rats: modulation by estradiol and naloxone administration. Neuroscience 2000;95(2):559–566.

14. Hapidou EG, Rollman GB. Menstrual cycle modulation of tender points. Pain 1998;77(2):151–161.

15. Riley JL, Robinson ME, Wise EA, et al. A meta-analytic review of pain perception across the menstrual cycle. Pain 1999;81(3):225–235.

16. Ren K, Wei F, Dubner R, et al. Progesterone attenuates persistent inflammatory hyperalgesia in female rats: involvement of spinal NMDA receptor mechanisms. Br Res 2000;865(2):272–277.

17. Ceccarelli I, Scaramuzzino A, Massafra C, et al. The behavioral and neuronal effects induced by repetitive nociceptive stimulation are affected by gonadal hormones in male rats. Pain 2003;104 (1–2):35–47.

18. Kuczmierczyk AR, Adams HE. Autonomic Arousal and pain sensitivity in women with premenstrual-syndrome at different phases of the menstrual-cycle. J Psychosom Res 1986;30(4):421–428.

19. Amodei N, Nelsongray RO. Reactions of dysmenorrheic and nondysmenorrheic women to experimentally induced pain throughout the menstrual-cycle. J Behav Med 1989;12(4):373–385.

20. Fillingim RB, Edwards RR. The association of hormone replacement therapy with experimental pain responses in postmenopausal women. Pain 2001;92(1–2):229–234.

21. LeResche L, Saunders K, VonKorff MR, et al. Use of exogenous hormones and risk of temporo-mandibular disorder pain. Pain 1997;69(1–2):153–160.

22. Wise EA, Riley JL, Robinson ME. Clinical pain perception and hormone replacement therapy in postmenopausal women experiencing orofacial pain. Clin J Pain 2000;16(2):121–126.

23. Musgrave DS, Vogt MT, Nevitt MC, et al. Back problems among postmenopausal women taking estrogen replacement therapy—the study of osteoporotic fractures. Spine 15 2001;26(14):1606–1612.

24. Brynhildsen J, Lennartsson H, Klemetz M, et al. Oral contraceptive use among female elite athletes and age-matched controls and its relation to low back pain. Acta Obstet Gynecol Scand 1997;76(9):873–878.

25. Thompson HS, Hyatt JP, DeSouza MJ, et al. The effects of oral contraceptives on delayed onset muscle soreness following exercise. Contraception 1997;56(2):59–65.

26. Bouchard C, Brisson J, Fortier M, et al. Use of oral contraceptive pills and vulvar vestibulitis: A case-control study. Am J Epidemiol 2002;156(3):254–261.

27. Anderson GL, Limacher M, Assaf AR, et al. Effects of conjugated, equine estrogen in postmenopausal women with hysterectomy—The women's health initiative randomized controlled trial. JAMA-J Am Med Assoc 2004;291(14):1701–1712.

28. Cushman M, Kuller LH, Prentice R, et al. Estrogen plus progestin and risk of venous thrombosis. JAMA-J Am Med Assoc 2004;292(13):1573–1580.

29. Manson JE, Hsia J, Johnson KC, et al. Estrogen plus progestin and the risk of coronary heart disease. N Engl J Med 2003;349(6):523–534.

30. Chlebowski RT, Hendrix SL, Langer RD, et al. Influence of estrogen plus progestin on breast, cancer and mammography in healthy postmenopausal women—The women's health initiative randomized trial. JAMA-J Am Med Assoc 2003;289(24):3243–3253.

31. Smith SS. Female sex steroid-hormones—from receptors to networks to performance—actions on the sensorimotor system. Prog Neurobiol 1994;44(1):55–86.

32. Clarkson TB, Cline JM, Williams JK, et al. Gonadal hormone substitutes: effects on the cardiovascular system. Osteoporosis Int 1997;7:43–51.

33. Delignieres B, Vincens M. Differential-effects of exogenous estradiol and progesterone on mood in post-menopausal women—individual dose effect relationship. Maturitas 1982;4(1):67–72.

34. Miyagawa K, Rosch J, Stanczyk F, et al. Medroxyprogesterone interferes with ovarian steroid protection against coronary vasospasm. Nat Med 1997;3(3):324–327.

35. Wagner JD, Martino MA, Jayo MJ, et al. The effects of hormone replacement therapy on carbohydrate metabolism and cardiovascular risk factors in surgically postmenopausal cynomolgus monkeys. Metabol Clin Exp 1996;45(10):1254–1262.

36. Aloisi AM, Della Seta D, Rendo C, et al. Exposure to the estrogenic pollutant bisphenol A affects pain behavior induced by subcutaneous formalin injection in male and female rats. Brain Res 2002;937(1–2):1–7.

37. Ostgaard HC, Andersson GBJ, Karlsson K. Prevalence of back pain in pregnancy. Spine 1991;16(5):549–552.

38. Kristiansson P, Svardsudd K, vonSchoultz B. Back pain during pregnancy—a prospective study. Spine 1996;21(6):702–708.

39. Glazener CMA. Postpartum problems. Br J Hosp Med 1997;58(7):313–316.

40. Hagen KB, Jamtvedt G, Hilde G, et al. The updated cochrane review of bed rest for low back pain and sciatica. Spine 2005;30(5):542–546.

41. Arnau JM, Vallano A, Lopez A, et al. A critical review of guidelines for low back pain treatment. Eur Spine J 2006;15(5):543–553.

42. Svensson HO, Andersson GBJ, Hagstad A, et al. The relationship of low-back-pain to pregnancy and gynecologic factors. Spine 1990;15(5):371–375.

43. To WWK, Wong MWN. Factors associated with back pain symptoms in pregnancy and the persistence of pain 2 years after pregnancy. Acta Obstet Gynecol Scand 2003;82(12):1086–1091.

44. Young G, Jewell D. Interventions for preventing and treating pelvic and back pain in pregnancy. Cochrane Database Syst Rev 2002;Issue 1(Art. No.: CD001139.):DOI:10.1002/14651858.CD14001139.

45. Kihlstrand M, Stenman B, Nilsson S, et al. Water-gymnastics reduced the intensity of back/low back pain in pregnant women. Acta Obstet Gynecol Scand 1999;78(3):180–185.

46. Wedenberg K, Moen B, Norling A. A prospective randomized study comparing acupuncture with physiotherapy for low-back and pelvic pain in pregnancy. Acta Obstet Gynecol Scand 2000;79(5):331–335.

47. Thomas IL, Nicklin J, Pollock H, et al. Evaluation of a maternity cushion (ozzlo pillow) for backache and insomnia in late pregnancy. Aust NZ J Obstet Gynaecol 1989;29(2):133–138.

48. Mogren IM, Pohjanen AI. Low back pain and pelvic pain during pregnancy—prevalence and risk factors. Spine 2005;30(8):983–991.

49. Fast A, Shapiro D, Ducommun EJ, et al. Low-back-pain in pregnancy. Spine 1987;12(4):368–371.

50. Laban MM, Perrin JCS, Latimer FR. Pregnancy and the herniated lumbar-disk. Arch Phys Med Rehabil 1983;64(7):319–321.

51. Weinreb JC, Wolbarsht LB, Cohen JM, et al. Prevalence of lumbosacral intervertebral-disk abnormalities on Mr images in pregnant and asymptomatic nonpregnant women. Radiology 1989;170(1):125–128.

52. Evans JA, Savitz DA, Kanal E, et al. Infertility and pregnancy outcome among magnetic-resonance-imaging workers. J Occup Environ Med 1993;35(12):1191–1195.

53. McCarthy SM, Filly RA, Stark DD, et al. Magnetic-resonance imaging of fetal anomalies in utero—early experience. Am J Roentgenol 1985;145(4):677–682.

54. Schmitt H, Zhao JQ, Brocai DRC, et al. Acupuncture treatment of low back pain. Schmerz 2001;15(1):33–+.

55. Sanderson PL, Fraser RD. The influence of pregnancy on the development of degenerative spondylolisthesis. J Bone Joint Surg-Br Vol 1996;78B(6):951–954.

56. Saraste H. Spondylolysis and Pregnancy—a Risk Analysis. Acta Obstet Gynecol Scand 1986;65(7):727–729.

57. Heckman JD, Sassard R. Musculoskeletal Considerations in Pregnancy. J Bone Joint Surg Am Vol 1994;76A(11):1720–1730.

58. Takatori Y, Kokubo T, Ninomiya S, et al. Transient osteoporosis of the hip—magnetic-resonance-imaging. Clin Orthop Relat Res 1991(271):190–194.

59. Arayssi TK, Tawbi HA, Usta IM, et al. Calcitonin in the treatment of transient osteoporosis of the hip. Sem Arthritis Rheum 2003;32(6):388–397.

60. La Montagna G, Malesci D, Tirri R, et al. Successful neridronate therapy in transient osteoporosis of the hip. Clin Rheumatol 2005;24(1):67–69.

61. French AE, Kaplan N, Lishner M, et al. Taking bisphosphonates during pregnancy. Can Fam Phys 2003;49:1281–1282.

62. Vandenveyver I, Vanderheyden J, Krauss E, et al. Aseptic necrosis of the femoral-head associated with pregnancy—a case-report. Eur J Obstet Gynecol Reprod Biol 1990;36(1–2):167–173.

63. Schauberger CW, Rooney BL, Goldsmith L, et al. Peripheral joint laxity increases in pregnancy but does not correlate with serum relaxin levels. Am J Obstet Gynecol 1996;174(2):667–671.

64. Slipman CW, Sterenfeld EB, Chou LH, et al. The predictive value of provocative sacroiliac joint stress maneuvers in the diagnosis of sacroiliac joint syndrome. Arch Phys Med Rehabil 1998;79(3):288–292.

65. Dreyfuss P, Michaelsen M, Pauza K, et al. The value of medical history and physical examination in diagnosing sacroiliac joint pain. Spine 1996;21(22):2594–2602.

66. Ostgaard HC, Zetherstrom G, Rooshansson E, et al. Reduction of back and posterior pelvic pain in pregnancy. Spine 1994;19(8):894–900.

67. Mens JMA, Vleeming A, Snijders CJ, et al. Reliability and validity of the active straight leg raise test in posterior pelvic pain since pregnancy. Spine 2001;26(10):1167–1171.

68. Damen L, Buyruk HM, Guler-Uysal F, et al. Pelvic pain during pregnancy is associated with asymmetric laxity of the sacroiliac joints. Acta Obstet Gynecol Scand 2001;80(11):1019–1024.

69. Damen L, Buyruk HM, Guler-Uysal F, et al. The prognostic value of asymmetric laxity of the sacroiliac joints in pregnancy-related pelvic pain. Spine 2002;27(24):2820–2824.

70. Stuge B, Veierod MB, Laerum E, et al. The efficacy of a treatment program focusing on specific stabilizing exercises for pelvic girdle pain after pregnancy—a two-year follow-up of a randomized clinical trial. Spine 2004;29(10):E197–E203.

71. Elden H, Ladfors L, Olsen MF, et al. Effects of acupuncture and stabilising exercises as adjunct to standard treatment in pregnant women with pelvic girdle pain: randomised single blind controlled trial. Br Med J 2005;330(7494):761–764A.

72. Ong BY, Cohen MM, Esmail A, et al. Paresthesias and motor dysfunction after labor and delivery. Anesth Analg 1987;66(1):18–22.

73. Vargo MM, Robinson LR, Nicholas JJ, et al. Postpartum femoral neuropathy—relic of an earlier era. Arch Phys Med Rehabil 1990;71(8):591–596.

74. Holdcroft A, Gibberd FB, Hargrove RL, et al. Neurological complications associated with pregnancy. Br J Anaesth 1995;75(5):522–526.

75. Wong CA, Scavone BM, Dugan S, et al. Incidence of postpartum lumbosacral spine and lower extremity nerve injuries. Obstet Gynecol 2003;101(2):279–288.

76. van Slobbe AM, Bohnen AM, Bernsen RMD, et al. Incidence rates and determinants in meralgia paresthetica in general practice. J Neurol 2004;251(3):294–297.

77. Katirji B, Wilbourn AJ, Scarberry SL, et al. Intrapartum maternal lumbosacral plexopathy. Muscle Nerve 2002;26(3):340–347.

78. Breen TW, Ransil BJ, Groves PA, et al. Factors associated with back pain after childbirth. Anesthesiology 1994;81(1):29–34.

79. Treuth MS, Butte NF, Puyau M. Pregnancy-related changes in physical activity, fitness, and strength. Med Sci Sport Exerc 2005;37(5):832–837.

80. Gilleard WL, Brown JMM. Structure and function of the abdominal muscles in primigravid subjects during pregnancy and the immediate postbirth period. Phys Ther 1996;76(7):750–762.

81. American College of Sport Medicine. 2000. ACSM's Guidelines for Exercise Testing and Prescription. Sixth edition. Philadelphia: Lippincott, Williams and Wilkins.

82. JovanovicPeterson L, Peterson CM. Exercise and the nutritional management of diabetes during pregnancy. Obstet Gynecol Clin N Am 1996;23(1):75–&.

83. Bung P, Artal R. Gestational diabetes and exercise: a survey. Semin Perinatol 1996;20(4):328–333.

84. Borg-Stein J, Dugan SA, Gruber J. Musculoskeletal aspects of pregnancy. Am J Phys Med Rehabil 2005;84(3):180–192.

85. Clark SL, Cotton DB, Pivarnik JM, et al. Position change and central hemodynamic profile during normal 3rd-trimester pregnancy and post-partum. Am J Obstet Gynecol 1991;164(3):883–887.

86. Camporesi EM. Diving and pregnancy. Semin Perinatol 1996;20(4):292–302.

87. Artal R, Fortunato V, Welton A, et al. A Comparison of cardiopulmonary adaptations to exercise in pregnancy at sea-level and altitude. Am J Obstet Gynecol 1995;172(4):1170–1180.

88. Reiter RC. A profile of women with chronic pelvic pain. Clin Obstet Gynecol 1990;33(1):130–136.

89. Keshavarz H, Hillis S, Kieke BA. Hysterectomy surveillance, United States, 1994–1998. Am J Epidemiol 2001;153(11):S140–S140.

90. Scialli AR, Barbieri RL, Glasser MH, et al. Chronic pelvic pain: an integrated approach. Med Educ Collab Assoc Prof Gynecol Obstet 2000:3–9.

91. Gerwin RD. Myofascial and visceral pain syndromes: Visceral-somatic pain representations. J Musculoskeletal Pain 2002;10(1–2):165–175.

92. Cervero F. Visceral pain—central sensitisation. Gut 2000;47:56–57.

93. Giamberardino MA, Affaitati G, Lerza R, et al. Neurophysiological basis of visceral pain. J Musculoskeletal Pain 2002;10(1–2):151–163.

94. Giamberardino MA, De Laurentis S, Affaitati G, et al. Modulation of pain and hyperalgesia from the urinary tract by algogenic conditions of the reproductive organs in women. Neurosci Lett 18 2001;304(1–2):61–64.

95. FitzGerald MP, Kotarinos R. Rehabilitation of the short pelvic floor. I: background and patient evaluation. Int Urogynecol J Pelvic Floor Dysfunct 2003;14(4):261–268.

96. Levitt EE, Konovsky M, Freese MP, et al. Intra-vaginal pressure assessed by the kegel perineometer. Arch Sex Behav 1979;8(5):425–430.

97. Workman DE, Cassisi JE, Dougherty MC. Validation of surface Emg as a measure of intravaginal and intraabdominal activity—implications for biofeedback-assisted kegel exercises. Psychophysiology 1993;30(1):120–125.

98. Heah SM, Ho YH, Tan M, et al. Biofeedback is effective treatment for levator ani syndrome. Dis Colon Rectum 1997;40(2):187–189.

99. McKay E, Kaufman RH, Doctor U, et al. Treating vulvar vestibulitis with electromyographic biofeedback of pelvic floor musculature. J Reprod Med 2001;46(4):337–342.

100. Glazer HI, Rodke G, Swencionis C, et al. Treatment of vulvar vestibulitis syndrome with electromyographic biofeedback of pelvic floor musculature. J Reprod Med 1995;40(4):283–290.

101. Glazer HI, Romanzi L, Polaneczky M. Pelvic floor muscle surface electromyography—reliability and clinical predictive validity. J Reprod Med 1999;44(9):779–782.

102. Fitzwater JB, Kuehl TJ, Schrier JJ. Electrical stimulation in the treatment of pelvic pain due to levator ani spasm. J Reprod Med 2003;48(8):573–577.

103. Thiel GH. Coccygodynia: cause and treatment. Dis Colon Rectum 1963;11:422–436.

104. Sinaki M, Merritt JL, Stillwell GK. Tension myalgia of pelvic floor. Mayo Clin Proc 1977;52(11):717–722.

105. Lilius HG, Valtonen EJ. Levator Ani spasm syndrome—clinical analysis of 31 cases. Ann Chirurgiae Gynaecol 1973;62(2):93–97.

106. Weiss JM. Pelvic floor myofascial trigger points: manual therapy for interstitial cystitis and the urgency-frequency syndrome. J Urol 2001;166(6):2226–2231.

107. Lukban JC, Parkin JV, Holzberg AS, et al. Interstitial cystitis and pelvic floor dysfunction: a comprehensive review. Pain Med 2001;2(1):60–71.

108. Urinary Incontinence Guideline Panel. 1992. Urinary incontinence in adults: clinical practice guideline. Agency for Health Care Policy and Research, Public Health and Human Services. No. 92–0038.

109. Harrison GL, Memel DS. Urinary-incontinence in women—its prevalence and its management in a health promotion clinic. Br J Gen Pract 1994;44(381):149–152.

110. Nygaard IE, Thompson FL, Svengalis SL, et al. Urinary-incontinence in elite nulliparous athletes. Obstet Gynecol 1994;84(2):183–187.

111. Visco AG, Figuers C. Nonsurgical management of pelvic floor dysfunction. Obstet Gynecol Clin N Am 1998;25(4):849–+.

112. Aukee P, Immonen P, Penttinen J, et al. Increase in pelvic floor muscle activity after 12 weeks' training: a randomized prospective pilot study. Urology 2002;60(6):1020–1023.

113. Aukee P, Immonen P, Laaksonen DE, et al. The effect of home biofeedback training on stress incontinence. Acta Obstet Gynecol Scand 2004;83(10):973–977.

114. Meyer S, Hohlfeld P, Achtari C, et al. Pelvic floor education after vaginal delivery. Obstet Gynecol 2001;97(5):673–677.

115. Yamanishi T, Yasuda K, Sakakibara R, et al. Pelvic floor electrical stimulation in the treatment of stress incontinence: an investigational study and a placebo controlled double-blind trial. J Urol 1997;158(6):2127–2131.

116. Suhel P. Adjustable non-implantable electrical stimulators for correction of urinary-incontinence. Urol Int 1976;31(1–2):115–123.

117. Wolfe F, Cathey MA. Prevalence of primary and secondary fibrositis. J Rheumatol 1983;10(6): 965–968.

118. Wolfe F, Cathey MA. The epidemiology of tender points—a prospective-study of 1520 patients. J Rheumatol 1985;12(6):1164–1168.

119. Wolfe F. 1990 American-college-of-rheumatology criteria for fibromyalgia—reply. Arthritis Rheum 1990;33(12):1863–1864.

120. Goldenberg DL, Burckhardt C, Crofford L. Management of fibromyalgia syndrome. JAMA-J Am Med Assoc 2004;292(19):2388–2395.

121. Giesecke T, Williams DA, Harris RE, et al. Subgrouping of fibromyalgia patients on the basis of pressure–pain thresholds and psychological factors. Arthritis Rheum 2003;48(10):2916–2922.

122. Martin L, Nutting A, MacIntosh BR, et al. An exercise program in the treatment of fibromyalgia. J Rheumatol 1996;23(6):1050–1053.

123. Gowans SE, deHueck A, Voss S, et al. A randomized, controlled trial of exercise and education for individuals with fibromyalgia. Arthritis Care Res 1999;12(2):120–128.

124. Rao S, Bennett R. Pharmacological therapies in fibromyalgia. Best Pract Res Clin Rheumatol 2003;17:611–627.

125. Arnold LM, Keck PE. Antidepressant treatment of fibromyalgia: a meta-analysis and review. Psychosomatics 2000;41:104–113.

126. Goldenberg D, Mayskiy M, Mossey C, et al. A randomized, double-blind crossover trial of fluoxetine and amitriptyline in the treatment of fibromyalgia. Arthritis Rheum 1996;39(11):1852–1859.

127. Cantini F, Bellandi F, Niccolo L, et al. Fluoxetine combined with cyclobenzaprine in the treatment of fibromyalgia. Minerva Med 1994;85:97–100.

128. Celiker R, Cagavi Z. Comparison of amitriptyline and sertraline in the treatment of fibromyalgia syndrome. Arthritis Rheum 2000;43(9):S332–S332.

129. Vitton O, Gendreau M, Gendreau J, et al. A double-blind placebo-controlled trial of milnacipran in the treatment of fibromyalgia. Hum Psychopharmacol Clin Exp 2004;19:S27–S35.

130. Arnold LM, Lu YL, Crofford LJ, et al. A double-blind, multicenter trial comparing duloxetine with placebo in the treatment of fibromyalgia patients with or without major depressive disorder. Arthritis Rheum 2004;50(9):2974–2984.

131. Biasi G, Manca S, Manganelli S, et al. Tramadol in the fibromyalgia syndrome: a controlled clinical trial versus placebo. Int J Clin Pharmacol Res 1998;18(1):13–19.

132. Russell IJ, Kamin M, Bennett RM, et al. Efficacy of tramadol in treatment of pain in fibromyalgia. JCR-J Clin Rheumatol 2000;6(5):250–257.

133. Bennett RA, Kamin M, Karim R, et al. Tramadol and acetaminophen combination tablets in the treatment of fibromyalgia pain: a double-blind, randomized, placlebo-controlled study. Am J Med 2003;114(7):537–545.

134. Carette S, Bell MJ, Reynolds WJ, et al. Comparison of amitriptyline, cyclobenzaprine, and placebo in the treatment of fibromyalgia—a randomized, double-blind clinical-trial. Arthritis Rheum 1994;37(1):32–40.

135. Bennett RM, Gatter RA, Campbell SM, et al. A comparison of cyclobenzaprine and placebo in the management of fibrositis—a double-blind controlled-study. Arthritis Rheum 1988;31(12): 1535–1542.

136. Tofferi JK, Jackson JL, O'Malley PG. Treatment of fibromyalgia with cyclobenzaprine: a meta-analysis. Arthritis Rheum-Arthritis Care Res 2004;51(1):9–13.

137. Goldenberg DL, Felson DT, Dinerman H. A randomized, controlled trial of amitriptyline and naproxen in the treatment of patients with fibromyalgia. Arthritis Rheum 1986;29(11):1371–1377.

138. McCain GA, Bell DA, Mai FM, et al. A controlled-study of the effects of a supervised cardio-vascular fitness training-program on the manifestations of primary fibromyalgia. Arthritis Rheum 1988;31(9):1135–1141.

139. Smith M, Gokula RRM, Weismantel A. Does physical therapy improve symptoms of fibromyalgia? J Fam Pract 2003;52(9):717–719.

140. Schachter CL, Busch AJ, Peloso PM, et al. Effects of short versus long bouts of aerobic exercise in sedentary women with. Fibromyalgia: a randomized controlled trial. Phys Ther 2003;83(4):340–358.

141. Jones KD, Burckhardt CS, Clark SR, et al. A randomized controlled trial of muscle strengthening versus flexibility training in fibromyalgia. J Rheumatol 2002;29(5):1041–1048.

142. Jentoft ES, Kvalvik AG, Mengshoel M. Effects of pool-based and land-based aerobic exercise on women with fibromyalgia/chronic widespread muscle pain. Arthritis Rheum-Arthritis Care Res 2001;45(1):42–47.

143. Mannerkorpi K, Nyberg B, Ahlmen M, et al. Pool exercise combined with an education program for patients with fibromyalgia syndrome. A prospective, randomized study. J Rheumatol 2000;27(10):2473–2481.

144. Mannerkorpi K, Ahlmen M, Ekdahl C. Six- and 24-month follow-up of pool exercise therapy and education for patients with fibromyalgia. Scand J Rheumatol 2002;31(5):306–310.

145. Creamer P, Singh BB, Hochberg MC, et al. Sustained improvement produced by nonpharmacologic intervention in fibromyalgia: results of a pilot study. Arthritis Care Res 2000;13(4):198–204.

146. Nielson WR, Walker C, McCain GA. Cognitive behavioral treatment of fibromyalgia syndrome—preliminary findings. J Rheumatol 1992;19(1):98–103.

147. White KP, Nielson WR. Cognitive-behavioral treatment of fibromyalgia syndrome—a follow-up assessment. J Rheumatol 1995;22(4):717–721.

148. Hadhazy VA, Ezzo J, Creamer P, et al. Mind-body therapies for the treatment of fibromyalgia. A systematic review. J Rheumatol 2000;27(12):2911–2918.

149. Singh BB, Berman BM, Hadhazy VA, et al. A pilot study of cognitive behavioral therapy in fibromyalgia. Altern Ther Health Med 1998;4(2):67–70.

150. Kaplan KH, Goldenberg DL, Galvinnadeau M. The impact of a meditation-based stress reduction program on fibromyalgia. Gen Hosp Psychiatry 1993;15(5):284–289.

151. Berman BM, Ezzo J, Hadhazy V, et al. Is acupuncture effective in the treatment of fibromyalgia? J Fam Pract 1999;48(3):213–218.

152. Deluze C, Bosia L, Zirbs A, et al. Electroacupuncture in fibromyalgia—results of a controlled trial. Br Med J 1992;305(6864):1249–1252.

153. Harris RE, Tian XM, Cupps TR, et al. The treatment of fibromyalgia with acupuncture: effects of needle placement, needle stimulation, and dose. Arthritis Rheum 2003;48(9):S692–S692.

154. Buskila D, Abu-Shakra M, Neumann L, et al. Balneotherapy for fibromyalgia at the Dead Sea. Rheumatol Int 2001;20(3):105–108.

155. Brattberg G. Connective tissue massage in the treatment of fibromyalgia. Eur J Pain 1999;3(3): 235–244.

156. Gambert RG, Shores JH, Russo DP, et al. Osteopathic manipulative treatment in conjunction with medication relieves pain associated with fibromyalgia syndrome. J Am Osteopath Assoc 2002;102: 321–325.

157. Blunt KL, Rajwani MH, Guerriero RC. The effectiveness of chiropractic management of fibromyalgia patients: a pilot study. J Manipulative Physiol Ther 1997;20(6):389–399.

158. Almeida TF, Roizenblatt S, Benedito-Silva AA, et al. The effect of combined therapy (ultrasound and interferential current) on pain and sleep in fibromyalgia. Pain 2003;104(3):665–672.

159. Wolfe F, Anderson J, Harkness D, et al. Work and disability status of persons with fibromyalgia. J Rheumatol 1997;24(6):1171–1178.

160. Waylonis GW, Ronan PG, Gordon C. A profile of fibromyalgia in occupational environments. Am J Phys Med Rehabil 1994;73(2):112–115.

161. Mengshoel AM, Forseth KO, Haugen M, et al. Multidisciplinary approach to fibromyalgia—a pilot-study. Clin Rheumatol 1995;14(2):165–170.

162. Bennett RM. Multidisciplinary group programs to treat fibromyalgia patients. Rheum Dis Clin N Am 1996;22(2):351–&.

163. Bailey A, Starr L, Alderson M, et al. A comparative evaluation of a fibromyalgia rehabilitation program. Arthritis Care Res. 1999;12(5):336–340.

164. Conference CD. Consensus development conference: diagnosis, prophylaxis, and treatment of osteoporosis. Am J Med. 1993;94(6):646–650.

165. Browner WS, Pressman AR, Nevitt MC, et al. Mortality following fractures in older women—the study of osteoporotic fractures. Arch Int Med 1996;156(14):1521–1525.

166. Ensrud KE, Palermo L, Black DM, et al. Hip and calcaneal bone loss increase with advancing age—longitudinal results from the study of osteoporotic fractures. J Bone Min Res 1995;10(11):1778–1787.

167. Chandler JM, Zimmerman SI, Girman CJ, et al. Low bone mineral density and risk of fracture in white female nursing home residents. JAMA-J Am Med Assoc 23 2000;284(8):972–977.

168. Riggs BL, Melton LJ. Involutional osteoporosis. N Eng J Med 1986;314(26):1676–1686.

169. Melton LJ, Chrischilles EA, Cooper C, et al. How many women have osteoporosis. J Bone Min Res 1992;7(9):1005–1010.

170. Benvenuti S, Tanini A, Frediani U, et al. Effects of ipriflavone and its metabolites on a clonal osteoblastic cell-line. J Bone Min Res 1991;6(9):987–996.

171. Rigotti NA, Nussbaum SR, Herzog DB, et al. Osteoporosis in Women with anorexia–nervosa. N Eng J Med 1984;311(25):1601–1606.

172. Counts DR, Gwirtsman H, Carlsson LMS, et al. The effect of anorexia–nervosa and refeeding on growth hormone-binding protein, the insulin-like growth-factors (Igfs), and the Igf-binding proteins. J Clin Endocrinol Metabol 1992;75(3):762–767.

173. Ettinger B, Genant HK, Cann CE. Long-term estrogen replacement therapy prevents bone loss and fractures. Ann Int Med 1985;102(3):319–324.

174. Prince RL, Smith M, Dick IM, et al. Prevention of postmenopausal osteoporosis—a comparative-study of exercise, calcium supplementation, and hormone-replacement therapy. N Eng J Med 1991;325(17):1189–1195.

175. Nordin BEC, Need AG, Bridges A, et al. Relative contributions of years since menopause, age, and weight to vertebral density in postmenopausal women. J Clin Endocrinol Metabol 1992;74(1):20–23.

176. Oursler MJ, Landers JP, Riggs BL, et al. Estrogen effects on osteoblasts and osteoclasts. Ann Med 1993;25(4):361–371.

177. Riggs BL, Melton LJ. Clinical review 8—clinical heterogeneity of involutional osteoporosis—implications for preventive therapy. J Clin Endocrinol Metabol 1990;70(5):1229–1232.

178. Emaus N, Berntsen GKR, Joakimsen R, et al. Longitudinal changes in forearm bone mineral density in women and men aged 45–84 years: The tromso study, a population-based study. Am J Epidemiol 2006;163(5):441–449.

179. Chapuy MC, Arlot ME, Duboeuf F, et al. Vitamin-D(3) and calcium to prevent hip-fractures in elderly women. N Eng J Med 1992;327(23):1637–1642.

180. Rossouw JE, Anderson GL, Prentice RL, et al. Risks and benefits of estrogen plus progestin in healthy postmenopausal women—principal results from the women's health initiative randomized controlled trial. JAMA-J Am Med Assoc 2002;288(3):321–333.

181. Stafford RS, Drieling RL, Hersh AL. National trends in osteoporosis visits and osteoporosis treatment, 1988–2003. Arch Int Med 2004;164(14):1525–1530.

182. NIH Consensus Development Panel on Optimal Calcium Intake. Optimal calcium intake. JAMA-J Am Med Assoc 272(24):1942–1948.

183. Chen YM, Ho SC, Lam SSH, et al. Soy isoflavones have a favorable effect on bone loss in Chinese postmenopausal women with lower bone mass: a double-blind, randomized, controlled trial. J Clin Endocrinol Metabol 2003;88(10):4740–4747.

184. Harkness L, Fiedler K, Sehgal AR, et al. Decreased bone resorption after soy isoflavone supplementation in postmenopausal women (60–78 years of age). J Bone Min Res 2004;19:S313–S313.

185. Marks R, Allegrante JP, MacKenzie CR, et al. Hip fractures among the elderly: causes, consequences and control. Ageing Res Rev 2003;2(1):57–93.

186. Coupland C, Wood D, Cooper C. Physical inactivity is an independent risk factor for hip fracture in the elderly. J Epidemiol Commun Health 1993;47(6):441–443.

187. Hoidrup S, Sorensen TIA, Stroger U, et al. Leisure-time physical activity levels and changes in relation to risk of hip fracture in men and women. Am J Epidemiol 2001;154(1):60–68.

188. Feskanich D, Willett W, Colditz G. Walking and leisure-time activity and risk of hip fracture in postmenopausal women. JAMA-J Am Med Assoc 2002;288(18):2300–2306.

189. Klibanski A, Biller BMK, Schoenfeld DA, et al. The effects of estrogen administration on trabecular bone loss in young-women with anorexia–nervosa. J Clin Endocrinol Metabol 1995;80(3):898–904.

190. Gregg EW, Cauley JA, Seeley DG, et al. Physical activity and osteoporotic fracture risk in older women. Ann Int Med 1998;129(2):81–88.

191. Friedlander AL, Genant HK, Sadowsky S, et al. A 2-year program of aerobics and weight training enhances bone-mineral density of young-women. J Bone Min Res 1995;10(4):574–585.

192. Nelson ME, Fiatarone MA, Morganti CM, et al. Effects of high-intensity strength training on multiple risk-factors for osteoporotic fractures—a randomized controlled trial. JAMA-J Am Med Assoc 1994;272(24):1909–1914.

193. Dalsky GP, Stocke KS, Ehsani AA, et al. Weight-bearing exercise training and lumbar bone-mineral content in postmenopausal women. Ann Int Med 1988;108(6):824–828.

194. Bonaiuti D, Shea B, Iovine R, et al. Exercise for preventing and treating osteoporosis in postmenopausal women. 2002;3:CD000333. Cochrane Database Syst Rev 2002;3:CD000333.

195. Taaffe DR, Duret C, Wheeler S, et al. Once-weekly resistance exercise improves muscle strength and neuromuscular performance in older adults. J Am Geriatr Soc 1999;47(10):1208–1214.

196. McDermott AY, Mernitz H. Exercise and older patients: prescribing guidelines. Am Fam Phys 2006;74(3):437–444.

197. Gillespie LD, Gillespie WJ, Robertson MC, et al. Interventions for preventing falls in elderly people. Cochrane Database Syst Rev 2001;CD000340.

198. Stevens JA, Powell KE, Smith SM, et al. Physical activity, functional limitations, and the risk of fall related fractures in community-dwelling elderly. Ann Epidemiol 1997;7(1):54–61.

199. Tsai CL, Liu TK. Osteoarthritis in women—its relationship to estrogen and current trends. Life Sci 1992;50(23):1737–1744.

200. Oliveria SA, Felson DT, Reed JI, et al. Incidence of symptomatic hand, hip, and knee osteoarthritis among patients in a health maintenance organization. Arthritis Rheum 1995;38(8): 1134–1141.

201. Tumia N, Maffulli N. Patellofemoral pain in female athletes. Sport Med Arthrosc Rev 2002;10(1): 69–75.

202. Hewett TE, Ford KR, Myer GD. Anterior cruciate ligament injuries in female athletes—part 2, a meta-analysis of neuromuscular interventions aimed at injury prevention. Am J Sport Med 2006;34(3):490–498.

203. Roos EM, Ostenberg A, Roos H, et al. Long-term outcome of meniscectomy: symptoms, function, and performance tests in patients with or without radiographic osteoarthritis compared to matched controls. Osteoarthritis Cartilage 2001;9(4):316–324.

204. Englund M, Lohmander LS. Risk factors for symptomatic knee osteoarthritis fifteen to twenty-two years after meniscectomy. Arthritis Rheum 2004;50(9):2811–2819.

205. Kim HJ, Kozin F, Johnson RP, et al. Reflex sympathetic dystrophy syndrome of the knee following meniscectomy—report of 3 cases. Arthritis Rheum 1979;22(2):177–181.

206. Martin VM. Reflex sympathetic dystrophy syndrome of the knee after meniscectomy. Arthritis Rheum–Arthritis Care Res 1980;23(6):780.

207. Krivickas LS. Anatomical factors associated with overuse sports injuries. Sport Med 1997;24(2): 132–146.

208. Uhorchak JM, Scoville CR, Williams GN, et al. Risk factors associated with noncontact injury of the anterior cruciate ligament—a prospective four-year evaluation of 859 West Point cadets. Am J Sport Med 2003;31(6):831–842.

209. Sharma L, Hayes KW, Felson DT, et al. Does laxity alter the relationship between strength and physical function in knee osteoarthritis? Arthritis Rheum 1999;42(1):25–32.

210. Dragoo JL, Lee RS, Benhaim P, et al. Relaxin receptors in the human female anterior cruciate ligament. Am J Sport Med 2003;31(4):577–584.

211. Baquie P, Brukner P. Injuries presenting to an Australian sports medicine centre: A 12-month study. Clin J Sport Med 1997;7(1):28–31.

212. Taunton JE, Ryan MB, Clement DB, et al. A retrospective case-control injuries analysis of 2002 running. Br J Sport Med 2002;36(2):95–101.

213. Fredericson M, Yoon KS. Physical examination and patellofemoral pain syndrome. Am J Phys Med Rehabil 2006;85(3):234–243.

214. Heintjes E, Berger MY, Bierma-Zeinstra SMA, et al. Pharmacotherapy for patellofemoral pain syndrome. Cochrane Database Syst Rev 2004;1(3):CD003470.

215. Brosseau L, Casimiro L, Robinson V, et al. Therapeutic ultrasound for treating patellofemoral pain syndrome. Cochrane Database Syst Rev 2005;1.

216. Bizzini M, Childs JD, Piva SR. Systematic review of the quality of randomized controlled trials for patellofemoral pain syndrome. J Orthop Sport Phys Ther 2003;33(1):4–20.

217. Lane NE, Thompson JM. Management of osteoarthritis in the primary-care setting: an evidence-based approach to treatment. Am J Med 1997;103:25–30.

218. Lawrence RC, Helmick CG, Arnett FC, et al. Estimates of the prevalence of arthritis and selected musculoskeletal disorders in the United States. Arthritis Rheum 1998;41(5): 778–799.

219. Guidelines TACoRSoO. Recommendations for the medical management of osteoarthritis of the hip and knee: 2000 Update. Arthritis Rheum 2000;43:1905–1915.

220. American Geriatrics Society Panel on Chronic Pain in Older Persons. The management of chronic pain in older persons. J Am Geriatric Soc 1998;46:635–651.

221. Dugan SA. Sports-related knee injuries in female athletes—what gives? Am J Phys Med Rehabil 2005;84(2):122–130.

222. Ferretti A, Conteduca F, Decarli A, et al. Osteoarthritis of the knee after Acl reconstruction. Int Orthop 1991;15(4):367–371.

223. Griffin LY, Albohm MJ, Arendt EA, et al. Understanding and preventing noncontact anterior cruciate ligament injuries—a review of the Hunt Valley II Meeting, January 2005. Am J Sport Med 2006;34(9):1512–1532.

224. Shambaugh JP, Klein A, Herbert JH. Structural measures as predictors of injury in basketball players. Med Sci Sport Exerc 1991;23(5):522–527.

225. Ireland ML. Anterior cruciate ligament injury in female athletes: epidemiology. J Athletic Training 1999;34(2):150–154.

226. Buchanan PA, Vardaxis VG. Sex-related and age-related differences in knee strength of basketball players ages 11–17 years. J Athletic Training. 2003;38(3):231–237.

227. Loudon JK, Jenkins W, Loudon KL. The relationship between static posture and ACL injury in female athletes. J Orthop Sport Phys Ther 1996;24(2):91–97.

228. Yu WD, Liu SH, Hatch JD, et al. Effect of estrogen on cellular metabolism of the human anterior cruciate ligament. Clin Orthop Relat Res 1999(366):229–238.

229. Yu WD, Panossian V, Hatch JD, et al. Combined effects of estrogen and progesterone on the anterior cruciate ligament. Clin Orthop Relat Res 2001(383):268–281.

230. Beynnon BD, Johnson RJ, Braun S, et al. The relationship between menstrual cycle phase and anterior cruciate ligament injury—a case–control study of recreational alpine skiers. Am J Sport Med 2006;34(5):757–764.

231. Wojtys EM, Huston LJ, Boynton MD, et al. The effect of the menstrual cycle on anterior cruciate ligament injuries in women as determined by hormone levels. Am J Sport Med 2002;30(2):182–188.

232. Myklebust G, Engebretsen L, Braekken IH, et al. Prevention of anterior cruciate ligament injuries in female team handball players: A prospective intervention study over three seasons. Clin J Sport Med 2003;13(2):71–78.

233. Wilmore JH. The application of science to sport: physiological profiles of male and female athletes. Can J Appl Sport Sci 1979;4:103–115.

234. Ireland ML, Ott SM. Special concerns of the female athlete. Clin Sport Med 2004;23(2):281–+.

235. Baechle TR. Women in resistance training. Clin Sport Med 1984;3(4):791–808.

236. Green S, Buchbinder R, Hetrick S. Acupuncture for shoulder pain. Cochrane Database Syst Rev 2005(2):CD005319.

237. Garfinkel MS, Schumacher HR, Husain A, et al. Evaluation of a yoga based regimen for treatment of osteoarthritis of the hands. J Rheumatol 1994;21(12):2341–2343.

238. Garfinkel MS, Singhal A, Katz WA, et al. Yoga-based intervention for carpal tunnel syndrome—a randomized trial. JAMA-J Am Med Assoc 1998;280(18):1601–1603.

239. Naeser MA, Hahn KAK, Lieberman BE, et al. Carpal tunnel syndrome pain treated with low-level laser and microamperes transcutaneous electric nerve stimulation: a controlled study. Arch Phys Med Rehabil 2002;83(7):978–988.

240. Kale S. Trigger finger. Available at: http://www.emedicine.com/orthoped/topic570.htm, 2006.

241. Patel MR, Bassini L. Trigger fingers and thumb—when to splint, inject, or operate. J Hand Surg Am Vol 1992;17A(1):110–113.

242. Marks MR, Gunther SF. Efficacy of cortisone injection in treatment of trigger fingers and thumbs. J Hand Surg Am Vol 1989;14A(4):722–727.

243. Fauno P, Andersen HJ, Simonsen O. A Long-term follow-up of the effect of repeated corticosteroid injections for stenosing Tenovaginitis. J Hand Surg Br Eur Vol 1989;14B(2):242–243.

244. Meals R. De Quervain tenosynovitis. Available at: http://www.emedicine.com/orthoped/byname/de-quervain-tenosynovitis.htm.

245. Richie CA, Briner WW. Corticosteroid injection for treatment of de Quervain's teosynovitis: a pooled quantitative literature evaluation. J Am Board Fam Pract 2003;16(2):102–106.

23 Integrative Medicine

*History, Overview, and Applications
to Pain Management*

Joseph Mosquera

CONTENTS

"Someday it will just be called good medicine."
*Dr. Andrew Weil in 1996 speaking about Integrative medicine to his first fellowship
class of The Program in Integrative medicine, University of Arizona Medical School.*

Summary

Presently the expansive growth of Integrative medicine has been fueled in part by a public discontent
with conventional medicine and increasing consumer demand for medical advice on the subjects of
lifestyle, nutrition, exercise, and natural therapies. Patients want more emphasis on health, healing and
prevention of chronic illness rather than just diagnosis and treatment. Numerous peer-reviewed, published
studies in the literature reflect the increasing popularity and use of integrative therapies in the populations
of the United States and developed countries. The appearance of many Integrative and Complementary
and Alternative Medicine (CAM) departments in major medical centers and schools (such as Harvard,
Memorial Sloan-Kettering Cancer Center, Stanford, Duke, University of Maryland, Scripps, MD Anderson
and many others), speaks to the wide acceptance and increasing public demand for these services. The
increasing prominence of Integrative Medicine has led to the establishment and growth of the Consortium
of Academic Health Centers for Integrative medicine (CAHCIM), which now includes over 30 medical
schools. Appreciation of the self-healing nature of the human body and the interactions between the mind
and the body are two fundamental principles of integrative medicine. The defining principles of Integrative

From: *Contemporary Pain Medicine: Integrative Pain Medicine: The Science and Practice
of Complementary and Alternative Medicine in Pain Management*
Edited by: J. F. Audette and A. Bailey © Humana Press, Totowa, NJ

Medicine are provided, training resources discussed and then examples of an integrative approach to the treatment of pain conditions are given.

Key Words: complementary and alternative medicine, integrative medicine, botanicals, hypnosis, evidence-based medicine

1. INTRODUCTION

Doctor Andrew Weil's use of natural remedies and recognition of self-healing concepts date back to the early seventies, when following his formal education at Harvard Medical School this inquiring scientist-physician traveled throughout various countries of South America where he lived with and studied the indigenous healing cultures of Colombia, Mexico, Peru, and Bolivia. His passion for botany as an undergraduate at Harvard University provided the basis for his interest in the plant-based medicine of these countries. His investigative immersion in these cultures further helped him develop his theories on the importance of obtaining the proper connections and balance with health, healing, and the natural world in which we live. Dr. Weil's valuable studies and visionary ideas in medicine have since produced ten notable books. These tomes examine the philosophies, strengths, and weaknesses that underlie the practice of a number of medical systems, both conventional and alternative. The outcome of Dr. Weil's investigations led him by the early 1990s to recognize the need for physicians to become better acquainted with complementary and alternative therapies and integrate these concepts with conventional medicine to better promote the optimal health of their patients. This evolution of ideas has fostered the development of what has become known as *Integrative Medicine*, a medical system based not upon disease and treatment but upon health and healing, which is inquiry-driven, evidence-based, and open to new therapeutic paradigms.

Safe and effective evidence based therapies provide the foundation for this new medicine, which focuses on a closer physician-to-patient relationship that takes into account the whole person (mind, body, and spirit), including all aspects of their daily lives. Today, Dr. Weil continues his pioneering efforts into the 21st century, advancing the transformation of healthcare through his creation and directorship of The Program in Integrative Medicine at the University of Arizona Medical School (PIMUA) in 1996. The fundamental principles of his fellowship in Integrative medicine are rigorous scientific research and the recognition of the importance of clinical care that integrates biomedicine, the complexity of human beings, and the healing power of nature into the care and treatment of patients.

Presently the expansive growth of Integrative medicine has been fueled in part by a public discontent with conventional medicine and increasing consumer demand for medical advice on the subjects of lifestyle, nutrition, exercise, and natural therapies with emphasis on health, healing and prevention of chronic illness rather than just diagnosis and treatment. Numerous peer-reviewed, published studies in the literature reflect the increasing popularity and use of integrative therapies in the populations of the US and developed countries *(1)*. The appearance of many Integrative and Complementary and Alternative Medicine (CAM) departments in major medical centers and schools (such as Harvard, Memorial Sloan-Kettering Cancer Center, Stanford, Duke, University of Maryland, Scripps, MD Anderson and many others), speaks to the wide acceptance and increasing public demand for these services.

One of the most visible examples of acceptance and increasing prominence of Integrative medicine has been the establishment and growth of the Consortium of

Academic Health Centers for Integrative medicine (CAHCIM). CAHCIM was originally organized by Dr. Weil at PIMUA to study the abounding diversity of therapeutic
systems and incorporate these within a modern bio-medical paradigm to create new
models of evidence-based clinical care. CAHCIM offers institutional membership to
qualifying North American Colleges of Medicine, which is contingent upon evidence
of commitment and broad-based institutional support for such an initiative. Presently,
30 highly regarded academic medical centers are members of CAHCIM, including The
University of Arizona, Harvard, Georgetown, Duke, and Columbia universities. In the
June 2004 issue of *Academic Medicine*, a core competency in Integrative Medicine for
medical school curricula was proposed by members of the working group of CAHCIM,
which describes the challenges and delineates the values, knowledge, attitudes, and
skills that they believe are fundamental to the field of Integrative medicine. Leading
Fellowship and Residency training programs in Integrative Medicine have utilized this
curricula as a fundamental guideline, including Doctor Woodson Merrell's Continuum
Center for Health and Healing at the Beth Israel Medical Center and Albert Einstein
College of Medicine in New York, David Eisenberg's Division for Research and
Education in Complementary and Integrative Medicine at Harvard, Fredi Kronenberg's
program at Columbia Presbyterian Hospital (Richard and Hinda Rosenthal Center
for Complementary and Alternative Medicine), and the Duke Integrative Medicine
Program with Tracy Gaudet.

In the following discussion we will journey from the origins and development of
Integrative Medicine at the University of Arizona and examine the important distinctions between CAM, allopathic or conventional medicine, and how true integration of
therapies can someday become known as Dr. Weil stated, "just good medicine."

2. DEFINITIONS

Although there are many characterizations of Integrative medicine, the definition
developed at the University of Arizona, which established the first program for
physician fellowship training in this field, is preferred and widely accepted:

Complementary and alternative medicine (CAM) is a group of diverse medical and
healthcare systems, practices, and products that are not presently considered to be
part of conventional medicine. While scientific evidence exists regarding some CAM
therapies, for most there are key questions that have yet to be answered through well-
designed scientific studies; questions such as whether these therapies are safe and
whether they work for the diseases or medical conditions for which they are used.

Integrative Medicine is a healing-oriented medicine that takes into account the whole
person (body, mind, and spirit), including all aspects of lifestyle. It emphasizes the
therapeutic relationship and makes use of all appropriate therapies, both conventional
and alternative.

The defining principles of integrative medicine are:

1. Patient and practitioner are partners in the healing process.
2. All factors that influence health, wellness, and disease are taken into consideration,
   including mind, spirit, and community, as well as the body.
3. Appropriate use of both conventional and alternative methods facilitates the body's
   innate healing response.
4. Effective interventions that are natural and less invasive should be used whenever
   possible.

5. Integrative Medicine neither rejects conventional medicine nor accepts alternative therapies uncritically.
6. Good medicine is based on good science and therefore, Integrative Medicine is inquiry-driven and open to new paradigms.
7. Alongside the concept of treatment, the broader concepts of health promotion and the prevention of illness are paramount.
8. Practitioners of Integrative Medicine should exemplify its principles and commit themselves to self-exploration and self-development.

Appreciation of the self-healing nature of the human body and the interactions between the mind and the body are two fundamental principles of integrative medicine. Conventional medicine, which during the last century has relied primarily on the success of potent medicines (antibiotics, anti-hypertensive, anti-inflammatory, anti-cancer agents) and surgeries, is beginning to recognize again the importance of the mind in physical illness and health. Robert Ader's milestone experiments in the 1970s *(2,3)* demonstrated the strong influence that a mental stimulus can exert on the immune system. His work demonstrated how specific psychological conditioning could destroy a mouse's immune function as effectively as a potent chemotherapeutic agent. In addition to Ader's work on the mind-body connection with conditioned responses, recent study findings further support the role of mind in wellness and disease. From the work of Candice Pert, Ph.D. on chemical communicators *(4)*, Margaret Kemeny, Ph.D. on emotions and the immune system *(5)*, to David Felten, M.D., Ph.D., and his work with the brain and the immune system *(6)*, the connection and therapeutic possibilities of mind-body therapies are gaining scientific support.

Presently there is no desire among trained integrative physicians to transform this field into a separate entity or subspecialty. The goal is that these principles of medical care will truly be integrated into "good medicine" and will be taught and practiced by all physicians. Integrative Medicine (IM) evolved from a desire to expand the practice of medicine beyond the rigid and reductionistic boundaries of modern Western medicine. Despite impressive technological advances, biomedicine has generated great dissatisfaction and neglected the humanistic features of clinical medicine. In addition, important facets of a patient's lifestyle, such as nutrition, mental health, physical activity, and spirituality are not routinely addressed. These are all essential aspects of optimal holistic care, which IM seeks to restore and promote.

3. CREATING A NEW MODEL OF HEALTH CARE AND MEDICAL EDUCATION

When David Eisenberg, a respected internist and researcher at Harvard, astounded the medical community in 1993 with a survey in the *New England Journal of Medicine* demonstrating that more than one-third of the US population had used at least one form of complementary and alternative medicine, recognition of patient dissatisfaction with the conventional medical system reached a watershed moment *(7)*. The success and phenomenal advances of conventional bio-medicine had to be tempered by the strong message of frustrated discontent with the standard, technology-based models of care issued by the results of this survey. More than a decade after Eisenberg's study, the failure to connect with consumers who desired to be treated altruistically, as a whole person, engaged in a healing and empowered relationship with their doctors, often has lead disappointed patients to seek unproven therapies. The goal of integrative medicine is to construct a bridge, which would combine the best of conventional medicine with evidence-based CAM, founded on the philosophy of humanistic, patient-centered care with an emphasis on wellness, prevention, and healing of the whole person (mind, body, spirit) in the hope of creating an improved model of healthcare. Understanding this need, Andrew Weil in 1994 brought together a panel of national leaders in CAM, represented by Jeanne Achtenberg, Ph.D.; Philip Greenman, D.O.; Stuart Hamaroff, M.D.; Joseph Helms, M.D.; Fredi Kronenberg, Ph.D.; Michael Murray, N.D.; Candace Per, Ph.D.; Kenneth Pelletier, Ph.D., M.D.; Martin Rossman, M.D.; and Beverly Rubik, Ph.D. This expert panel convened for two days of dialogue and recommendations to create the initial curriculum for PIMUA. PIMUA accepted its first four clinical fellows who matriculated in 1996. Each was board-certified in a specialty and chosen from a competitive pool of applicants. The Residential Fellowship is a two-year training period that consists of three didactic and four process sections as seen in Table 1. The three didactic sections include philosophical foundations, lifestyle practices, and therapeutic systems with modalities. Clinical integration, personal development and reflection, research education, and leadership make up the four process sections.

There is growing evidence to support the development of an IM curriculum both in medical school and for postgraduate training, to ensure that physicians are aware of the scientific literature in CAM. This is especially seen in the volume of publications listed at The National Center for Complementary and Alternative Medicine (NCCAM) website where journals from *JAMA*, *British Medical Journal*, and *Annals of Internal Medicine* to *Pediatrics and Clinics in Family Practice* have published numerous basic science and clinical studies in CAM and IM. PIMUA was awarded the National Institutes of Health NCCAM Pediatric Center Grant in 1998, which supported the training of pediatricians in research and clinical aspects of integrative medicine, and there is now a NCCAM program grant supporting a 3-year faculty development and research fellowship program in Complementary and Integrative Medical Therapies at Harvard Medical School. Medical schools are beginning to provide elective courses and conferences on IM, which are very popular with students. The Harvard Continuing Medical Education (CME) has provided courses for physicians on Mind Body Medicine and Spirituality for the last fifteen years and during the last 6 years in Acupuncture. These courses are directed and taught by leading experts and researchers such as Herb Benson, M.D. in Mind–Body Medicine, and Joseph Audette, M.D., in Acupuncture.

The PIMUA Associate Fellowship program has evolved since its inception in 1996 and beginning in 2001 has provided a non-residential advanced training program in Clinical Integrative Medicine for physicians who could not commit the necessary two years in Tucson away from their practices and communities. As a result, physicians from throughout the world, including Canada, Japan, Ecuador, and Saudi Arabia, have joined US physicians to bring their unique cultural and diverse experiences in health care to the fellowship program.

This two-year program consists of an innovative and highly regarded distance-learning format with state-of-the-art web based support. Doctors from around the world in different time zones can engage in threaded dialogues and clinical cases after reviewing a particular learning module such as botanical medicine or nutrition. Online patient conferences and scenarios are also presented and evaluated, concluding with a suggested treatment plan of integrative therapies. This exceptional experience, requiring an average of 12 hours per week, allows for a one-of-a-kind contact and exchange of views on a global scale. In addition, the associate fellowship brings every

Table 1

Curriculum in Integrative Medicine of the Program in Integrative Medicine, University of Arizona College of Medicine, 2002

Components of PIM residential training program	Description
Didactic sections	
Philosophical foundation	Shifts the orientation from a disease-oriented model Practitioners are asked to confront their own worldviews and to face the uncertainties of not knowing
Healing-oriented medicine	To understand the nature of the body's healing system; case studies of spontaneous healing; the placebo response as a therapeutically; lifestyle medicine; healing versus curing; and strategies for protecting, enhancing, and activating the healing system
Philosophy of science	To understand the history, philosophy, and limitations of the modern scientific method and enterprise
Medicine and culture	To provide historical and anthropological perspectives on health belief models and healing systems of other cultures
Art of medicine	To explore the doctor as a facilitator of healing; effective communication and the art of suggestion; relationship-centered care; the role of intuition; techniques for motivating behavioral changes; and matching therapeutic approaches
Lifestyle practices	How we live our lives clearly affects our health and disease; Lifestyle practices and prevention are central to this approach
Spirituality and medicine	To explore and experience the role of spirituality in oneself, the patient, and the healing relationship
Mind-body medicine	To explore the breadth and mechanics of mind–body interactions, appreciate a broad range of applied interventions, and learn how to use a variety of mind–body interactions in clinical care
Nutritional medicine	To understand the central role of nutrition in healing: to provide a scientific basis for the integration of nutrition in medicine, in order to practice preventative and therapeutic nutrition

Physical activity	To learn benefits of physical activity, how to prescribe exercise and enhance self-practice
Therapeutic systems & modalities	Explores the distinction between alternative and integrative medicine; the history of CAM; the history, underlying philosophies, scientific basis, and practical applications of various systems of medicine; and the scientific evidence as it pertains to these systems
Botanical medicine	To understand the philosophy, science, safety, efficacy, and use of botanicals in integrative medicine
Manual medicine	To understand the philosophy and scope of manual medicine
Chinese medicine	To develop a general understanding of the principles, safety, and efficacy of traditional Chinese medicine (TCM) and related therapeutic approaches
Homeopathy	To understand the philosophy and scope of homeopathic medicine
Energy medicine	To provide an introduction to the theories, research, and techniques of energy medicine and show how the concept of energy is a fundamental component of integrative medicine
Allopathic medicine	To understand the history, philosophy, scientific basis, and practice of allopathic medicine, including preventing illness through medical screening, patient education, and lifestyle modification
Process sections	
Personal development & reflection	To develop in physicians processes of self-exploration and personal growth, to transform themselves from doctors to healers
Clinical integration	To integrate various medical systems, therapies, and modalities into comprehensive treatment plans for individual patients
Research education	To develop skills in evaluating medical literature, developing research designs, and contributing to scholarly publications
Leadership	To obtain a comprehensive overview and gain practical skills in leading and managing their roles in the academic, political, administrative, advocacy, and personal commitment aspects of integrative medicine

participant together for three residential weeks in Tucson, spread over a two-year period. During the residential weeks, the associate fellows meet and work together with faculty and participate in expanded hands-on skills training and interactive educational seminars. This experience gives the participants the opportunity to develop an overall sense of community and mission to transform our healthcare system. A summary of some online learning modules in the two-year Associate Fellowship in IM can be found in Table 2.

All fellowship graduates are expected, after the program completion, to develop competency in the areas of botanical medicine, nutrition, mind-body medicine, spirituality and medicine, the doctor-patient relationship, and physician wellness. Familiarity with and knowledge of homeopathy, osteopathy, hypnosis/visual imagery and traditional Chinese medicine/acupuncture is required for screening appropriate patients for referral or in some cases, advanced certified training in these areas is obtained guided by a physician's specific interests. For example, following the author's two-year associate fellowship, he trained and obtained certification in Ericksonian hypnotherapy (NYSEPH-New York Society of Ericksonian Psychology and Hypnotherapy certification course) and Acupuncture (Harvard Continuing Medical Education Course, Structural Acupuncture for Physicians), allowing a higher level of expertise and ability to directly treat complex patient cases.

Having the choice of evidence-based treatment options in both allopathic and CAM models gives the physician the ability to provide the patient with a powerful integrative plan. Graduates of the program are provided with a body of resources that include referral contacts, a growing PIMUA research database, conferences, career opportunities, and continued access to all PIMUA community members online. An active alumni association is also available where graduates can participate in Continued Medical Education (CME) learning modules and further their leadership roles in IM. As IM moves forward, the field will need to advance clear treatment guidelines, set credentialing standards, and develop criteria for subspecialty qualification in areas of CAM to ensure that patients will be provided with proven and critically reviewed integrative choices for their care. The Consortium of Academic Health Centers for Integrative Medicine will hopefully lead the way in making recommendations and influencing national policy in this area in the future. As mentioned at the beginning of this chapter, there are several other leading integrative medicine programs where education, research, and clinical applications are also central to their mission. The Center for Continuum Health (Beth Israel Program) in New York City is Directed by Roberta Lee, M.D., a graduate of PIM, and has seen and treated thousands of patients combining CAM and conventional therapies. The Duke Integrative center is directed by Tracy Gaudet, M.D., and expert and author on women's health and also a graduate of PIM. Both centers have training programs and clinics based upon the core curriculum and protocols developed at PIM. Harvard Medical School, with its Mind Body Institute, Osher Institute for Asian Healing, and Structural Acupuncture Course has brought leadership in research and applications of these CAM fields to IM. David Eisenberg's groundbreaking research in the public's use of CAM, Herb Benson's pioneering work in the "relaxation response," and Ted Kapchuk's demystification and applications of Traditional Chinese Medicine have all served to greatly advance IM in the United States.

Table 2

Curriculum in integrative medicine of the Program in Integrative Medicine, University of Arizona College of Medicine, 2002

Components of PIM Associate Fellowship program	Description
Didactic sections	
Medicine and culture	Increase awareness of the dynamics and differences between cultures, and develop ways to accommodate cultural practices and overcome barriers to communication
Art of medicine	An introduction to the integrative care process with focus on the obstacles likely to be confronted and possible solutions such as motivational interviewing techniques and assessing readiness for change
Spirituality and medicine	Exploration of one's own spiritual/philosophical framework by learning about rituals, ceremony and spiritual practice
Mind–body medicine	Research and study of guided imagery, hypnosis, expressive arts, biofeedback, meditation, breath work, mindfulness-techniques, and appropriate referral options; also the role that social support and stress reduction plays with concepts such as self-efficacy, meaning and life purpose
Botanical medicine	History and philosophy, preparations, research, herb-drug interactions, the study of adaptogens and tonics. The study of herbs and medicinal mushrooms, and their applications to women's health, the immune system, the gastrointestinal system, the cardiovascular system, the nervous system, and the respiratory system
Manual medicine	History and applications of various forms of massage, chiropractic, and osteopathy-training, research, regulation, and referral options
Chinese medicine	Foundations, concepts, diagnosis, modalities, techniques, and styles, with introduction to herbs, credentialing and licensing

(Continued)

Table 2
(Continued)

Components of PIM Associate Fellowship program	Description
Diet and nutrition	Self assessment, dietary patterns and research, study of fats, proteins, carbohydrates, fad diets, alcohol, minerals, vitamins, phytochemicals, fluids, and review of food labels and nutrition
Energy medicine	Healing touch, reiki, the philosophy of Barbara Brennan and Rosalyn Bruyere , and evidence-research
Physical medicine	The science, barriers, and recommendations for incorporating physical activity into treatment plans: Fellows see a sample FITT (Frequency, Intensity, Time, and Types of Activity) prescription for a virtual patient and also provide physical activity recommendations to each other
Physician self-assessment	Throughout the program fellows review and journal their own dietary, spiritual, and exercise habits with others in the program
Legal issues and integrative medicine	Become acquainted with regulatory bodies, legal definitions and explore potential problems and solutions to malpractice liability

4. AN INTEGRATIVE MEDICINE OFFICE VISIT

One of the obvious and most important distinctions between a conventional physician and a doctor who practices with an integrative approach is the difference in a medical office visit. A conventional physician is usually focused on making a diagnosis via a quick history of present illness and physical exam to develop an expedient treatment plan, with little or no importance given to the psychosocial portion of the interview, often ending the visit with the prescription of medications and a bewildered patient. An integrative physician recognizes the patient as a whole person, instead of a medical condition, and utilizes his or her motivational interviewing skills to facilitate helping the patient participate in his own healing process. Important areas that are typically covered include the following:

—Upbringing and background (including parents and siblings)
—The nature of relationships (spouse, children, friends, support system, etc.)
—Psychosocial stressors and how they are managed
—Diet and nutritional status
—Physical activities, exercise preferences, and frequency
—The role of spirituality in a person's life
—Relaxation practices

Integrative clinics and exam rooms provide an inviting and warm atmosphere in which the patient is encouraged to feel comfortable and to trust in their surroundings. The initial interview is usually 45 minutes to one hour in length with the goal of better understanding the personal preferences and personality of the patient. A visit in an IM clinic will often begin with a detailed, holistic-oriented interview, where a person's lifestyle habits, support system, and spirituality are considered along with the standard medical history. The prior use of CAM and allopathic modalities should also be carefully noted. Following this initial interview, a complete physical exam and review of systems generally follows conventional practice guidelines.

Ideally, this information can then be reviewed, evaluated, and discussed by a team of healing-oriented practitioners, which could include the integrative physicians, a nutritionist, a psychologist trained in mind-body techniques, a naturopathic physician or botanical expert, a nurse trained in energy medicine, an acupuncturist trained in traditional Chinese medicine, a chiropractor, and an exercise expert. Often one individual can provide expertise in a number of these areas to help make the team size more practical. Afterward the integrative physician chooses an individualized therapeutic strategy based upon proven and peer-reviewed scientific principles that also reflect the realistic preferences of the patient.

Often an IM clinic can manage a wide range of medical conditions from chronic disease to physical and emotional trauma, frequently pain will be the chief complaint. The symptom of pain arises from a variety of physiological pathways, which may be associated with a range physical and emotional dysfunction all of which can cause inappropriate inflammatory responses at the musculoskeletal or visceral levels. These responses are largely regulated by a series of complex biochemical, neurological, hormonal, and immune mechanisms that can be modulated with various therapies. Analgesic and anti-inflammatory medications are often the sole remedy offered by allopathic care, but an integrative approach to pain treatment can provide the patient with multiple non-pharmacological options that frequently are successful in modifying the pain response. In the following paragraphs a review of these integrative options for pain are discussed with a closer view of how nutrition and a mind-body approach utilizing Ericksonian-based hypnotherapy can be effective modalities in the management of pain.

4.1. Evidence-based Care in Integrative Medicine

In providing evidence-based care, the practitioner is trained to use a "sliding scale method" where stronger scientific evidence is demanded of therapies that pose a greater potential for harm. Advancing the scientific basis of CAM is a cornerstone for successful integration. One of the issues that researchers face is that the use of conventional research models in CAM constrain and limit the full richness of the normal application of the modality to such a degree that the results of studies in these areas become difficult to interpret. Indeed, not until the last decade has the safety, efficacy, and mechanism of action of individual CAM therapies been properly studied and clarified with peer-reviewed literature. These reviews include consensus conferences, randomized controlled trials, systematic reviews, and meta-analysis. Trials have now been conducted in such diverse areas of medicine from chiropractic care for infantile colic to homeopathy for warts, to mind/body techniques for pain and insomnia (8). Importantly, there is also growing literature on herb toxicity and drug-herb interactions; for example, the finding of adverse reactions between St John's wort and the prescription drug such as Indinavir (a protease inhibitor used for HIV) (9). In addition, there is increased use of the most sophisticated medical technology in the basic research of the mechanism of action of CAM interventions, including microdialysis techniques (see Chapter 5), functional magnetic resonance imaging (fMRI), and the use of positron emission tomography (PET) (see Chapter 4).

Integrative health care must still accept the challenge of providing the type of credible healthcare outcomes research that physicians are accustomed to when utilizing conventional or allopathic medicine. Integrative Medicine is not just the combination or merger of two medicines (CAM added to conventional), but instead represents a context, within which an effective and supportive physician-patient relationship is established where the wellness and bio-psycho-social-spiritual dimensions of the entire person are emphasized. This philosophical approach, together with multiple conventional and CAM treatments, requires study of the whole person as a complex living system, unlike the reductionistic, bio-medical model, which isolates and studies components of the individual, one at a time. A complex, whole-system theory approach must be the mainstay of the emerging perspective of healthcare outcomes research in IM, where the whole equals more than the sum of its parts (10).

The Integrative Clinic at PIMUA in Tucson serves as a model center where some of these theories are put into real-world application. More than three thousand patients have been evaluated and treated, where each integrative healing plan has been individualized and designed by a multidisciplinary team. Pain is a major symptom in nearly half the cases, often as part of a rheumatologic or immune etiology consistent with a recent study by the CDC (11,12).

5. INTEGRATIVE APPROACHES TO PAIN MANAGEMENT

Our Western model of pain management has mostly relied upon analgesic medications, physical therapy, and localized injections. Our typical analgesic armamentarium includes acetaminophen, aspirin, and non-steroidal anti-inflammatory drugs (NSAIDs), and opiate derivatives for severe pain. Increasingly, antidepressants and seizure medications are also used for neuropathic and other types of chronic pain. Physical therapy is often employed to recover from painful injuries and to lessen joint and musculoskeletal pain. Localized injections often consist of local anesthetic such as lidocaine and/or steroid preparations. Some of these medications are responsible for significant morbidity and mortality. NSAIDs alone are responsible for an average sixty thousand hospitalizations for gastrointestinal (GI) bleeds annually *(13)*.

An Integrative approach to pain management might include these allopathic therapies, but will also study and include the potential role of lifestyle practices. This would include assessment and modification of patient's diet and nutritional practices, their stressors and relaxation practices, the frequency and type of physical activity and exercise, and the role of spirituality in their lives. After obtaining this information a therapeutic system or modality can be offered, specifically designed for the individual patient. Some of the options offered to the patient could incorporate allopathic care combined with botanical, nutritional, manual, chinese, or mind-body therapies. homeopathy, energy medicine, and journaling. Healing and patient participation in pain management are essential concepts to an integrative approach. In the following pages a brief overview of pain remedies are discussed with a closer look at nutrition and the mind-body approach utilizing hypnotherapy and visual imagery.

6. BOTANICAL MEDICINE

Herbal medicine dates back to pre-historic time as the first source of medicine available to mankind and is an integral part of every healing tradition in the world. Egyptian, Greco-Roman, Chinese, and Aruyvedic uses of plants to promote, maintain, or restore health are well documented. Since the mid-19th century, scientific breakthroughs provided methods to identify and extract active constituents of medicinal plants, which led to the replacement of natural remedies with powerful, synthesized, and purified drugs. In the United States today, twenty-five percent of prescription drugs are still extracted from plants or their chemical synthetic copies, and more than one-half of all prescribed drugs use plant chemical constituents as building blocks for synthetic drugs. Despite the wonderful advances in modern medicine in the treatment of infectious disease, the production of vaccines, and in the medicinal cures of illness, 80% of the world's population still relies on herbal remedies as their primary source of health care.

The use of botanicals in modern medicine has undergone explosive growth in the United States largely as a result of increasing consumer demand and the introduction in 1994 of the Dietary Supplement Health and Education Act (DSHEA). This bill deregulated the herbal and supplement industry, allowing misleading health claims and second-rate manufacturing practices to be free of FDA scrutiny. As a result, a strong need for standardization, safety, and appropriate uses of herbal medicines and supplements arose in the US. German, Canadian, and European models have provided an excellent foundation for the future of Botanical Medicine regulation and research here in the United States. Federal regulation of the safety, quality, and effectiveness of herbs and supplements is important to develop consumer trust. Resources such as references and monographs (German E Commission) *(14)* describing active constituents, herb and drug contraindications and interactions, safety, dosage, indications, and mechanism of action are becoming increasingly available to healthcare practitioners and patients *(15)*.

In the discussion below, we will discuss turmeric, ginger, flax, and bromelain as four well studied examples of how herbs and supplements can be included in an integrative pain management plan (see Chapter 2 for more detail on this subject) *(16)*.

6.1. Turmeric or Curcumin

Turmeric or curcumin (*Curcuma longa*) is a perennial herb with yellow to orange colored rhizomes, which gives mustard its color. It has been traditionally used in Chinese medicine for arthritic, neuralgic, and traumatic pain. Today it is one of the most studied herbs, both for its anti-inflammatory effects (curcumin is a dual inhibitor of arachidonic acid metabolism) in pain management as well as its antioxidant properties by reducing lipid oxidation. The active constituents are curcuminoids (phenolic compounds); essential oils (3–5%), containing sesquiterpene ketones (65% including ar-turmerone), zingiberene (25%), phellandrene, sabinene, cineole, and borneol; and yellow pigments (3–6%) known as diarylheptanoids, including curcumin and methoxylated curcumins. Curcumin inhibits both the 5- and 12-lipoxygenase and the COX-2 pathways in vitro (see Chapter 7). Curcumin has also been found to deplete substance P from nerve terminals, in a mechanism similar to capsaicin (substance found in hot peppers). Curcumin inhibits platelet aggregation by interfering with the synthesis of thromboxanes while increasing prostacyclin and therefore requires the monitoring of patients taking anticoagulants or antiplatelet agents. Normal dosing with standardized 95% curcuminoids vary with standardized turmeric extract: one 450 mg capsule three times daily, whole-plant turmeric: up to 2 g/day, and curcumin 400–600 mg three times a day (for therapeutic effect). Turmeric should not be taken in therapeutic doses during pregnancy (uterine contractions), and in patients with gallstones or bile duct obstruction *(16)*.

*6.2. Ginger (**Zingiber officinale***)*

Ginger (*Zingiber officinale*) is also a perennial plant whose knotty and thick tuberous rhizomes are the sources of the dried, powdered spice containing the gingeroles and shogoal as the active constituents. Traditional uses include morning sickness, colic, nausea and dyspepsia. Gingeroles and shogoal are formed during the drying process along with volatile oils, including sesquiterpenes, monoterpenes, alkanes, aldehydes, and sulfide derivatives; all create a pungent taste. The shogoals appear to be the pharmacologically active constituents most responsible for the anti-inflammatory effect of ginger. Ginger acts as a potent inhibitor of arachidonic acid, epinephrine, and adenosine diphospahate (ADP). The positive effects of ginger in arthritis may be due to the inhibition of cylooygenase and 5-lipoxygenase *(15)*. In vitro ginger also inhibits platelet aggregation *(17)* (requiring monitoring of patients taking anti-coagulants). Therapeutic doses in most studies are in the one gram range of dried ginger while the FDA considers doses up to five grams safe for consumption as food. Although, in theory, ginger might enhance the effect of other blood-thinning medications by inhibiting platelet aggregation, one study of healthy volunteers receiving 2 g had no effect on bleeding times *(18)*. I often recommend ginger alone or in combination with turmeric in patients suffering from chronic musculoskeletal pain states such as osteoarthritis or fibromyalgia. Getting the patient to ingest ginger as a functional food instead of pill form is often more desirable and, in my view, increases compliance and participation in dietary and lifestyle modification.

6.3. Flax

Linum usitatissimum has a history of use dating back 5000 years with multiple applications from cloth in the stone age, wrappings of Egyptian mummies, linen garments, and linseed oil, to the more recent uses of the flax seed for constipation and gastrointestinal health. Flax seeds contain alphalinoleic acid (ALA), which in the body is broken down into eicosapentaenoic acid (EPA) and docosahexaenoic acid (DHA), creating favorable prostaglandin effects (see Chapter 7). The omega-3 essential fatty acids (EFAs) are believed to encourage the formation of prostaglandins that may help reduce inflammation and pain in a number of conditions. Flax also contains lignans, especially secoisolariciresinol diglucoside (SDG), which are broken down in the colon and have been shown to have protective effects against breast and colon cancer *(19–21)*. These substances also serve vital physiologic functions in the formation of cell membranes and the health of nerves, the retina, and brain cells. Flax also lowers cholesterol and harmful low-density lipoproteins (LDL). Omega-3 EFAs have clear scientific support in risk reduction for cardiovascular disease as seen in the French study known as the Lyon Heart study, where a threefold increase in Omega-3 dietary intake resulted in dramatic reductions in cardiac morbidity and mortality (>70%) *(22)*. The balance or ratio of dietary intake of Omega-6 to Omega-3 in our country is about 20 to 1, which favors inflammation and heart disease while a 4 to 1 ratio appears to be protective against both. This underscores the importance of an integrative plan, which should include dietary modification to create favorable EFA ratios. Flax consumption is considered quite safe with no known side effects although it is contraindicated in bowel obstruction and may reduce the absorption of other drugs due to its high fiber content. Standardization is to 58% of alpha-linoleic acid with one to two teaspoons a day as oil or 2.5 teaspoons of seed (ground) taken two to three times daily *(23,24)*.

6.4. Bromelain

Ananus comosus was introduced as a therapeutic compound and supplement in 1957 *(25)*. It is the general name for a family of sulfhydryl proteolytic enzymes obtained from the stem of the pineapple plant that exert a wide range of clinical effects. Physiological effects include modulation of the kinin system, the coagulation cascade, the cytokine system, and prostaglandin synthesis, all of which can lead to the reduction of pain and inflammation. Bromelain reduces the generation of bradykinin at the site of inflammation by depleting available plasma bradykinin and limiting the formation of fibrin by reduction of clotting cascade intermediates. Similar to NSAIDs, bromelain has been shown to inhibit prostaglandin PGE_2 and selectively decrease thromboxane production, creating a favorable prostacyclin (PGI_2) balance *(26)*. These actions can lead to significant reductions in pain and edema while enhancing circulation to the site of injury. Bromelain aloe may enhance the absorption and utilization of some antibiotics, chemotherapeutic agents, and glucosamine; a supplement frequently used for osteoarthritis. Drugs or herbs known to increase bleeding may be potentiated by the presence of Bromelain in the higher dosage ranges *(27)*. Although better quality trials and research is needed, Bromelain offers a safe and effective choice to complement pain management. Oral standardized dosage in adults by the German expert panel (Commission E) has recommended 80–320 mg (200–800 FIP units) taken two to three times daily *(14)*. With information about its safety being limited, it is not recommended in children (younger than 18 years) and during pregnancy or breastfeeding. In theory,

Bromelain may increase the risk of bleeding so caution is advised in people who have bleeding disorders or are taking drugs that increase risk of bleeding *(26,27)*.

7. FOOD AS MEDICINE

In his book, *Eating Well for Optimal Health*, Dr. Weil describes why choosing how and what we eat can be a powerful strategy for managing disease and restoring health. Drawing upon Hippocrates' advice in the fifth century B.C. —"Let medicine be thy food and food be thy medicine—Dr. Weil provides valuable insights on how food ingredients and culinary preparations in Asia play a major role in the healing matrix of its cultures. The therapeutic uses of turmuric and ginger in Chinese and Indian cuisine over centuries are examples of healing through food as medicine. In Western culture we are recently discovering the benefits of food in the context of pleasure, social interaction, culture, and as an important strategy to handle disease and promote health. The study of nutrition, food, and diet therapy can provide the modern physician with an effective integrative modality in clinical settings (see Chapter 7).

7.1. Food Elimination

Nutritional interventions in clinical practice can be difficult to implement and pose significant time challenges. Barriers include lack of nutritional training, scarcity of time, and uncertainty about how best to get a nutrition message across effectively. Challenges may involve the unique makeup of each patient, from eating and behavioral patterns to their individual biology. The key to success is for the healthcare provider to establish clear goals, both general and specific, in collaboration with the patient to reach agreed-upon clinical outcomes. Examples of general goals could include, wanting a patient to *care* more about his eating patterns, make better food choices, or recognize the link between eating and health. Specific clinical goals could include improvement of LDL cholesterol levels or decreasing symptoms of Irritable Bowel Syndrome or pain. Once the goals are agreed upon, then an intervention can begin by changing some aspect of food or dietary supplement in a patient's nutrition. This generally involves adding a new food or supplement to the diet, eating more of a food or supplement already in the diet, eating less of a food or supplement already in the diet, or eliminating a food or supplement altogether.

Elimination of a food often requires the proposal of a substitute. An example of a substitute would be to suggest a specific form of exercise or relaxation technique to replace the food as a response to relieve stress. Categories of intervention then can involve general messages about diet to more individualized brief and comprehensive recommendations. Examples of general messages are written materials, magazines, posters or videos in the office or waiting area, as well as brief verbal messages to individual patients. Brief and general recommendations would include the initiation of calcium and vitamin D supplementation for osteopenia, a multivitamin without iron for geriatric patients, or substituting poly-unsaturated for saturated fats when there is a family history of heart disease or rheumatoid arthritis. Examples of more individualized, brief recommendation could include increasing fiber and fluid intake for constipation, avoiding dairy products in otitis media, and increased folic acid and B_{12} supplementation for elevated serum Homocysteine. Examples of a comprehensive and individualized recommendation are managing transient hypoglycemic symptoms by manipulating frequency and timing of meals, reducing cholesterol levels by increasing soluble fiber and decreasing saturated fat, and managing hypertension using the principles of the DASH diet. DASH stands for Dietary Approaches to Stop Hypertension and evolved from a large multicenter study funded by NIH and NHLBI first presented in April of 1997 *(28)*. This study demonstrated the beneficial effects of this 2000-calorie combination diet on blood pressure and involves eating a diet rich in fruits, vegetables, low-fat dairy foods, low in saturated and total fat, low in cholesterol, while high in fiber, potassium, calcium, magnesium, and modestly high in protein.

7.2. Anti-Inflammatory Diets

Many patients present to their healthcare provider with complaints of chronic pain that have an underlying inflammatory etiology as is seen with autoimmune diseases, osteoarthritis, and other chronic musculoskeletal conditions. There is an increasing recognition of the relationship of diet to the development of a pro-inflammatory state and the role it plays in the perpetuation of pain and ill health *(29,30)*. Inflammation, especially when chronic, is, in part, determined by the circulatory balance of specific prostaglandin levels. These prostaglandins are synthesized from fatty acids, making these precursors an integral part in understanding how to influence the inflammatory process with diet. In particular, there are two classes of fatty acids, omega-3 and omega-6, that can affect the inflammatory cascade and can provide an important window for therapeutic intervention with the dietary habits of patients. Both classes of fat are metabolized competitively by oxygenase enzymes via the arachidonic acid pathway to form eicosanoids that include prostaglandins, thromboxanes, leukotrienes, and protacyclins. Omega-3 polyunsaturated fatty acids, abundant in cold-water fish such as salmon and mackerel and also found in flaxseed and walnuts, provide eicosapentanoic acid (EPA), docosahexanoic Acid (DHA), and alpha-linoleic acid (ALA), which can reduce the synthesis of inflammatory prostaglandins (see Chapter 7). In contrast, omega-6 fatty acids tend to increase the synthesis of these inflammatory prostaglandins. Cellular membranes' lipid composition and inflammatory balance is therefore influenced by the ratio of omega-3 and 6 fatty acids in our diets.

Avoidance of fats rich in omega-6 fatty acids such as those derived from safflower oil, sunflower oil, corn oil, vegetable shortening, margarine, and processed foods with partially dehydrogenated oils can favor the synthesis of anti-inflammatory eicosanoids. Dietary inclusion of oils contained in olives, walnuts, flax/hemp, salmon, sardines, and herring will create a favorable ratio to produce more of the anti-inflammatory metabolic pathways and regulators.

The traditional Mediterranean diet seen in countries like Spain, Italy, and Greece offers food choices that naturally support many of these anti-inflammatory principles mentioned. In addition, there is evidence that this diet can lower the incidence of cardiovascular disease, cancer, and obesity *(30–33)*.

When observed in the cultural context of these countries, with their strong family and social bonds, noticeable pleasure in eating, varied cuisine, and daily physical activity, the traditional Mediterranean diet offers important health advantages. Unfortunately Western-style dietary habits with fast food, processed food, and high saturated fat content are rapidly becoming a part of these traditional cultures. Walter Willet, Ph.D., chairman of the department of nutrition at the Harvard School of Public Health and co-investigator of the Harvard Nurses Study, supports the advantages of this diet. The benefits of following such a diet include the following as mentioned by Dr. Weil in his book, *Eating Well for Optimal Health (34)*:

- Great variety of tastes that appeal to people of many different cultures
- Emphasis on whole-grain products as opposed to refined carbohydrates in the Western diet, hence a reduced glycemic load
- Mostly monounsaturated fat and plenty of omega-3 fatty acids from fish, nuts, seeds, and vegetables
- Little meat and poultry compared to the Western diet and more fish and legumes
- Inclusion of some cheese and yogurt
- Wide variety of fruits and vegetables, including low-glycemic index fruits and vegetables, providing fiber and protective phytochemicals
- Emphasis on fresh foods
- Little processed food
- Use of familiar ingredients and good adaptability to locally available ingredients
- Relative ease of preparation

Drawbacks are few but include—

- May not provide enough iron for growing children and pregnant women, unless iron-rich foods are emphasized
- May not provide enough calcium unless calcium-rich foods are emphasized or supplemental calcium is added

Therefore a traditional Mediterranean diet can and should be an important strategy to consider when creating an integrative treatment plan for chronic inflammation and pain.

8. MIND–BODY THERAPIES FOR PAIN: HYPNOSIS

"Each Individual is unique."
"Trust your unconscious. It knows more than you do."
"Psychotherapy should be interesting, appealing and charming."
Milton Erickson, M.D.

Hypnosis involves the development of a trusting relationship between a clinician and a patient where the subject undergoes a shift from external reality to an internal reality or trance, where highly focused, responsive attentiveness is directed at one's internal experience for a period of time. Specific physiological changes occur in a patient's breathing, muscle tone, and nervous system (see Chapter 10). Critical thinking relaxes, permitting active unconscious learning in response to suggestions. This altered trance state of mind, which is not usually accessible through conscious thought, provides the patient with moments when there is an enhanced openness to change and a deep level of learning is possible in response to appropriate suggestions from the clinician.

There are many misconceptions and fears about hypnosis, stemming from the belief that it requires mysterious or special powers of mind control, as well as claims of magical cures. The Bible refers to hypnotic-like methods with the laying on of hands, while in 1773, Franz Mesmer, a Viennese physician claimed that he could control magnetic rays that flowed from his fingers, calling the phenomenon *animal magnetism*. Stage charlatans often exploited people with claims of the occult and black magic. What was being overlooked in all these instances was how the heightened state of suggestibility (trance) was a powerful tool in effecting responses and cures. Other popular fallacies are that hypnosis involves a loss of consciousness, increased gullibility, surrendering of one's will, hypnotic weakening of the mind, and fear of not awakening from trance. The truth is that nothing can be suggested against one's will, and therapeutic hypnosis is a cooperative and learning experience that involves focused attention and mutual trust. There is also a wide spectrum of susceptibility to hypnosis among patients.

8.1. Therapeutic Methods

Most hypnotic practitioners would agree that hypnosis is a unique kind of therapeutic interaction that opens the door to changed behavior and novel experiences that are not possible in a regular waking state. They would, however, differ significantly regarding the specific nature of the hypnotic relationship. Generally, there are three approaches to this relationship: the authoritarian approach, the standardized approach, and the cooperative approach utilized by Milton Erickson. The authoritarian approach focuses on the hypnotist as a powerful individual with special abilities who induces the subject to enter a passive state in which he or she is susceptible to suggestions. An individual's knowledge, beliefs, and capabilities are not taken into account with this approach, thus limiting the possibilities for therapeutic change. The authoritarian approach is exploited by stage hypnotists and by historical figures such as Mesmer, Bernheim, Charcot, and Freud. In the 1890s Freud's jealousy of his colleague Breuer, a general practitioner and one of the best hypnotists of his time, and his frustration with his own poor results made him give up hypnosis and seek other therapeutic methods. Although his decision set back hypnosis many years, the result was Freud's development of free association and dream interpretation. A standardized approach is the dominant method used by experimental psychologists where the subject becomes the unit of study and traits of susceptibility are determined with standardized induction practices. Although this can be a valid way of assessing an individual's hypnotic susceptibility, it is a therapist's role to find an induction method most appropriate for a given person. Just as a person's ability to perform the Foxtrot, Waltz, or Tango may vary, his susceptibility to induction into a trance requires a therapist to adapt or modify their technique.

8.2. Eriksonian Approach to Hypnotherapy

The cooperative approach to hypnotherapy pioneered and used by Milton Erickson is considered the most useful and effective approach in clinical practice. It is based upon the principles of a cooperative relationship between therapist and patient where an intimate intrapersonal experience develops within a safe therapeutic context. Communication is extremely flexible and adaptive to the patient's individual patterns, and a prior detailed medical and psychosocial history given by the patient is contextualized. The intent is to create opportunities for transformational change by trusting that the normally inaccessible or unconscious material that comes up while in the trance state has therapeutic value. The Ericksonian therapist begins a session by creating a context of safety and trust, with the goal of de-mystifying the trance state. The therapist places the patient into a light trance and then proceeds from contextualization to induction, utilization, and reorientation. Induction involves orienting a patient into a trance by skillful use of words and cadence, which can pace and lead the patient's mind into an altered state. Utilization represents the core work where experimental communication takes place while the patient is in trance. This is where skillful methods of adaptive communication using language patterns, metaphors, time distortion, imbedded commands, hypnotic suggestions, confusion techniques, regressive methods, and story-telling with specific themes are utilized. In Reorientation the patient is brought back to their waking state as suggestions are given to the conscious mind.

The principles of hypnosis found in Ericksonian cooperative hypnotherapy can be very useful in the management of pain. The use of hypnosis in dentistry and surgery to lessen pain or eliminate the need for anesthesia is well documented (see Chapter 10). Obtaining a detailed sensory description of the pain can provide important guidance in outlining a hypnotic strategy for a patient. This description as described in D. Corydon Hammond's book would include (1) thermal sensations (e.g., degree of heat vs. cold); (2) kinesthetic sensations and pressure aspects of pain (e.g., dull, sharp, binding, itching, heavy, twisting, drilling, penetrating, stabbing, pounding); and (3) imagery of the pain (size, shape, color, texture, sound). For example, if the patient describes his pain as a flaming red sphere, then one could use the setting sun metaphor during hypnosis; the suggestion is given that as the sun (pain) changes color and sinks into the ocean, disappearing into a tranquil and quiet stillness, so too will the patient experience a more relaxed feeling and diminution of their flaming pain. The following paragraphs will introduce selected and documented hypnotic techniques for pain with models of verbalization from the "Handbook of Hypnotic Suggestions and Metaphors" edited by Hammond *(35)*.

8.3. Techniques of Hypnotic Pain Management

While clinicians will differ in the application, there are four basic methods of achieving hypnotic pain control. The following is a synopsis of these approaches outlined by Joseph Barber *(36)*.

Analgesia or anesthesia can be created in the hypnotized individual by simply suggesting that the perception of pain is changing, diminishing, or that the area is becoming numb, so that the pain gradually disappears. It may be easier for a patient to notice growing *comfort* rather than diminishing pain; thus, a specific feeling of comfort such as that associated with anesthesia can be suggested specifically. For example, *"You may remember the feeling of anesthesia from the past, and begin already imagining that such numbing comfort is beginning, just barely, to become more and more apparent."* Alternatively, the patient can be given a specific focus to notice diminishing pain. For instance, it may be helpful to ask the patient before treatment to rate his or her pain on a scale from 0 to 10; 0 representing no pain at all, and 10 representing the most pain imaginable. Following induction, the hypnotized patient is told, *"Earlier, you were able to rate your pain, using numbers. I'd like you to look up, in the corner of your mind, right now, and notice what number you see, and notice that number beginning to change."* Further suggestions can be given for associating the number with the perception of pain and for perceiving progressively diminishing magnitude of numbers.

Substitution of a painful sensation by a different, less painful sensation can frequently enable a patient to tolerate some persistent feelings in the area but to not suffer from it. A sensation of stabbing pain may be substituted with a sensation of vibration, for example: *"The stabbing needles might become, in a surprising way, somehow more dull, not quite so very hot, so that, at some point in the future, maybe in two minutes, maybe in two hours, you can notice the peculiar buzzing or vibrating feeling of the blunt, warm needles."* For some patients, substitution is easier when the substituted feeling is not thoroughly pleasant; a burning neuralgic pain may become an irritated itch, for instance, or a tickle; a patient who needs, for some reason, to continue to be aware of the stimulus of pain, for instance, may be better with this technique.

Displacement of the locus of pain to another area of the body, or sometimes, to an area outside the body, can again provide an opportunity for the patient to continue experiencing the sensations, but in a less vulnerable, less painful area. The choice of the area is usually based on its lesser psychological vulnerability, and suggestions can leave the choice to the patient. For example: *As you continue to pay careful attention to the discomfort in your abdomen, let me know when you first begin to notice the very slight movement of that feeling...that's right..., now, just notice, as the movement continues, in perhaps a circular way, to increase...is it moving clockwise, or counter-clockwise?... That's fine, now just continue to be curious as you notice how the feeling can continue to move, in an ever-increasing spiral, moving round and round your abdomen, and notice which leg it begins to move into...."* and so on, as the feeling is suggested to move into a limb, perhaps even to the center into a single toe or finger, or to move outside the body altogether.

Dissociation of awareness can be created when the patient does not need to be very functional (e.g., during a medical or dental procedure) or when some condition renders the patient virtually immobile (e.g., during the last stages of terminal illness). The patient can be taught simply to begin to psychologically experience herself as in another time, place, or state, as in a vivid daydream. For instance, one can suggest that the patient experiences himself as floating, and that, *"Your mind, your awareness, can just float easily outside your body, and move over by the window, so you can watch the world outside..."*. One could instead suggest that the patient floats outside the room, and travel to any place he would enjoy. Much of this visual imagery technique is seen in the award-winning foreign movie, "The Sea Inside."

The active unconscious learning which takes place during trance in cooperative hypnotherapy and its beneficial clinical effects are well documented in the literature and research. In many ways Ericksonian methods are very much Integrative in their approach and philosophy. There is strong emphasis placed upon the doctor-patient relationship while constantly being adaptive and providing individualized therapy. Other well-studied integrative therapies can also be successful in pain management. These include Acupuncture, Osteopathy, and exercise therapy with QiGong or Tai Chi (see chapters on acupuncture, osteopathy, Tai Chi). Selection of these modalities should be guided by a physician who takes into account patient preferences, the available scientific research, and the suitability of a particular technique, given the patient's individual medical and psychosocial issues. Remember that integrative medicine is a healing-oriented medicine that takes into account the whole person (body, mind, and spirit), including all aspects of lifestyle while emphasizing the therapeutic relationship and making use of all appropriate therapies, both conventional and alternative. Applying these principles for pain management provides the doctor and patient with a strategy that can maximize benefit and minimize risk.

9. RESOURCES

9.1. Integrative Medicine Training

University of Arizona's Program in Integrative Medicine
http://integrativemedicine.arizona.edu/

University of Michigan Integrative Medicine Fellowship
http://www.med.umich.edu/umim/education/fellowship.htm

Univ of Maryland Integrative Medicine Bravewell Collaborative for Integrative Medicine, Bravewell Fellowship in Integrative Medicine
http://www.compmed.umm.edu/EducationFellow.html

Faculty Development and Fellowship Program in Complementary and Integrative Medical Therapies at Harvard Medical School
http://www.osher.hms.harvard.edu/e_fellowships.asp

9.2. Other Integrative Medicine Training Resources

American Medical Student Association
http://www.amsa.org/ICAM/trainingopps.cfm#opps

UCLA Center for East-West Medicine
http://www.cewm.med.ucla.edu/education/fellow.html

9.3. Articles

Integrative medicine and systemic outcomes research—issues in the emergence of a new model for primary care. Iris Bell, M.D, M.D. (H), P.hD.; Opher Caspi, M.D; Gary R. Shwartz, Ph.D.; Kathryn L. Grant, PharmD; Tracy Gaudet, M.D.; David Rychener, Ph.D., Victoria Maizes, M.D., Andrew Weil, M.D., Archives of Internal Medicine/Volume 162 Jan 28 2002 pages 133–139.

Core competencies in integrative medicine for a medical school curricula: a proposal. Benjamin Kligler, M.D.; Victoria Maizes, M.D.; Steven Schacter, M.D.; Constance M. Park, M.D., Ph.D., Tracy Gaudet, M.D., Rita Benn, Ph.D., Roberta Lee, M.D., and Rachel Naomi Remen, M.D. Academic Medicine, Vol. 79, no. 6/ June 2004.

Viewpoint: what is the best and most ethical model for the relationship between mainstream and alternative medicine: Opposition, integration, or pluralism? Ted Kaptchuk, O.M.D., and Franklin G. Miller, Ph.D., Academic Medicine, Vol. 80, No. 3/March 2005.

The tower of Babel: Communication and medicine—An essay on medical education and complementary-alternative medicine. Opher Caspi, M.D., Iris Bell, M.D., Ph.D.; David Rychener, Ph.D.; Tracy Gaudet, M.D.; Andrew Weil, M.D., Archives of Internal Medicine/Vol. 160, Nov. 27, 2000 3193-3195.

9.4. Books

Yapko, Michael D., *Trancework—An Introduction to the Practice of Clinical Hypnosis,* second edition. 1990 Bruner/Mazel.

Gilligan Stephen G., *Therapeutic Trances—The Cooperation Principle in Ericksonian Hypnotherapy*. Bruner/Mazel 1987.

Rosen Sidney, *My Voice Will Go With You—The Teaching Tales of Milton Erickson.* Norton Publications 1982.

Weil, Andrew, *Health and Healing*. Houghton Miflin Company 1998.

Weil, Andrew, *Eating Well for Optimal Health*. Quill-Harper Collins 2001.

10. CONCLUSIONS

The expansive growth of Integrative medicine has been fueled in part by a public discontent with conventional medicine and increasing consumer demand for medical advice on the subjects of lifestyle, nutrition, exercise, and natural therapies with emphasis on health, healing and prevention of chronic illness rather than just diagnosis and treatment. As resources for training physicians in Integrative Medicine and other CAM modalities continue to grow, the onus will be on the medical community to bring the best of conventional and unconventional therapies into the mainstream of healthcare.

Pain in particular is an arena where many of the standard therapies are ineffective for chronic conditions. Often patients are offered a multitude of medications and procedures that create a vicious cycle of pain and adverse side effects rather than wellness. The problem has two sides, as many patients who come to pain clinics are seeking (and often demanding) quick fixes without the motivation or interest to devote any time or effort into a change in lifestyle and behavior that could often have a more profound effect on pain than what the clinician can provide. The model of Integrative Medicine offers a pathway that can empower both the clinicians and patients by providing real clinical options that promote healing, lifestyle changes, and ultimately the potential for disease modification.

REFERENCES

1. Benjamin Kligler, Roberta Lee. 2004 Principles for Practice of Integrative Medicine. McGraw Hill.
2. Ader R. Behaviorally conditioned immunosuppression. Psychosom Med 1974;36(2):183–184.
3. Ader R, Cohen N. Behaviorally conditioned immunosuppression. Psychosom Med 1975;37(4): 333–340.
4. Pert C. Paradigms from neuroscience: when shift happens. Mol Interv 2003;3(7):361–366.
5. Dickerson SS, Kemeny ME. Acute stressors and cortisol responses: a theoretical integration and synthesis of laboratory research. Psychol Bull 2004;130(3):355–391.
6. Berk LS, Felten DL, Tan SA, et al. Modulation of neuroimmune parameters during the eustress of humor-associated mirthful laughter. Altern Ther Health Med 2001;7(2):62–72 (74–76).
7. Eisenberg DM, Kessler RC, Foster C, et al. Unconventional medicine in the United States, prevalence, costs, and patterns of use. N Eng J Med 1993;328:246–252.
8. NIH Technology Assessment Statement. Integration of Behavioral and Relaxation Approaches into the treatment of Chronic Pain and Insomnia, 1995. Bethesda, NIH pub # PB96113964.
9. Piscitelli SC, Burstein AH, Chaitt D, et al. Indinavir concentrations and St John's wort. Lancet 2000;355(9203):547–548 (Erratum in: Lancet 2001;357(9263):1210).
10. Bell IR, Caspi O, Schwartz GE, et al. Integrative medicine and systemic outcomes research: issues in the emergence of a new model for primary health care. Arch Intern Med 2002;162(2):133–140.
11. Barnes P, Powell-Griner E, McFann K, et al. CDC Advance Data Report #343. Complementary and Alternative Medicine Use Among Adults: United States, 2002. May 27, 2004 (http://nccam.nih.gov/news/camstats.htm)
12. Kaufman DW, Kelly JP, Rosenberg L, et al. Recent patterns of medication use in the ambulatory adult population of the United States: the slone survey. JAMA 2002;287:337–344.
13. Tarone RE, Blot WJ, McLaughlin JK. Nonselective nonaspirin nonsteroidal anti-inflammatory drugs and gastrointestinal bleeding: relative and absolute risk estimates from recent epidemiologic studies. Am J Ther 2004;11(1):17–25.
14. Blumenthal M, Busse W. GoldbergA, et al., Eds. 1998. The Complete German E commission Monographs. Austin, TX: The American Botanical Council, Boston, Integrative Medical Communications.
15. Mills S, Bone K. 2000. Principles and Practice of Phytotherapy Modern Herbal Medicine. Edinburgh:Churchill Livingstone.

16. McGuffin M, Hobbs C, Upton R, et al., Eds. 1997. 1997. The American Herbal Products Association Botanical Safety Handbook. Boca Raton, FL: CRC press.
17. Lumb AB. Effect of dried ginger on human platelet function. Thromb Haemost 1994;71(1): 100–111.
18. Kruth P, Brosi E, Fux R, Morike K, Gleiter CH. Ginger-associated overanticoagulation by phenprocoumon. Ann Pharmacother 2004;38(2):257–260.
19. Jenab M, Thompson LU. The influence of flaxseed and lignans on colon carcinogenesis and beta-glucoronidase activity. Carcinogenesis 1996;17(6):1343–1348.
20. Wallace JM. Nutritional and botanical modulation of the inflammatory cascade—eicosanoids, cyclooxygenases, and lipoxygenases—as an adjunct in cancer therapy. Integr Cancer Ther 2002;1(1):7–37.
21. Serrano M, Thompson LU. Flaxseed supplementation and early markers of colon carcinogenesis. Cancer Lett 1992;63:159–165.
22. de Lorgeril M, Salen P, Martin JL, Monjaud I, Delaye J, Mamelle N. Mediterranean diet, traditional risk factors, and the rate of cardiovascular complications after myocardial infarction: Final report of the Lyon Diet Heart Study, Circulation 1999;99:779–785.
23. Serrano M, Thompson LU, The effect of flaxseed supplementation on the initiation and promotional stages of mammary tumorigenesis. Nutr Cancer 1992;17:153–159.
24. Knight DC, Eden JA. A review of the clinical effects of phytoestrogens. Obstet Gynecol 1996;87(5):897–890.
25. Seligman B. Bromelain: an anti-inflammatory agent. Angiology 1962;13:508–510.
26. Cirelli MG. Five years of clinical experience with bromelains in therapy of edema and inflammation in post-operative tissue reaction, skin infection, and trauma Clin Med 1967;74(6):55–59.
27. Heck AM, DeWitt BA, Lukes AL. Potential interactions between alternative therapies and warfarin. Am J Health Syst Pharm 2000;57(13):1221–1227.
28. Moore TJ, Vollmer WM, Appel LJ, Sacks FM, Svetkey LP, Vogt TM, Conlin PR, Simons-Morton DG, Carter-Edwards L, Harsha DW. Effect of dietary patterns on ambulatory blood pressure: results from the Dietary Approaches to Stop Hypertension (DASH) Trial. DASH Collaborative Research Group. Hypertension 1999;34(3):472–477.
29. Summary of the second report of the National Cholesterol Education Program (NCEP) Expert Panel on Detection, Evaluation, and Treatment of High Blood Cholesterol in Adults (Adult Treatment Panel II). JAMA 1993;269(23):3015–3023.
30. Mantzioris E, James MJ, Gibson RA, et al. Dietary substitution with an alpha-linolenic acid-rich vegetable oil increases eicosapentaenoic acid concentrations in tissues. Am J Clin Nutr 1994;59(6):1304–1309.
31. (a) AHA Scientific Statement: AHA Dietary Guidelines: Revision 2000, #71–0193 Circulation 2000;102:2284–2299; (b) Stroke 2000;31:2751–2766.
32. de Lorgeril M, Salen P. The Mediterranean-style diet for the prevention of cardiovascular diseases. Public Health Nutr 2006;9(1A):118–123.
33. AHA Science Advisory: Lyon Diet Heart Study: Benefits of a Mediterranean-Style, National Cholesterol Education Program/American Heart Association Step I Dietary Pattern on Cardiovascular Disease, #71–0202 Circulation 2001;103:1823–1825.
34. Weil A. 2000. Eating Well for Optimum Health: The Essential Guide to Food, Diet, and Nutrition. New York: Knopf.
35. Hammond DC. 1990. Handbook of Hypnotic Suggestions and Metaphors. New York: Norton Publications.
36. Barber J, Benenke CJ. 1996. Hypnosis and Suggestion in the Treatment of Pain: A Clinical Guide. New York: Norton Professional Books.

INDEX

MIX
Papier aus verantwortungsvollen Quellen
Paper from responsible sources
FSC® C105338

FSC
www.fsc.org

Printed by Books on Demand, Germany